Medical-Surgical Nursing Recall

Tamara H. Bickston, RN, BSN, CCTC

Clinical Transplant Nurse Coordinator
University of Virginia
Charlottesville

Recall Series Editor

LORNE H. BLACKBOURNE, MD

Fellow, Trauma/Critical Care
Department of Surgery
University of Miami
Jackson Memorial Hospital
Miami

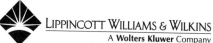
LIPPINCOTT WILLIAMS & WILKINS
A **Wolters Kluwer** Company
Philadelphia · Baltimore · New York · London
Buenos Aires · Hong Kong · Sydney · Tokyo

Staff

Executive Publisher
Judith A. Schilling McCann, RN, MSN

Senior Acquisitions Editor
Elizabeth Nieginski

Editorial Director
David Moreau

Clinical Director
Joan M. Robinson, RN, MSN

Senior Art Director
Arlene Putterman

Editorial Project Manager
Tracy S. Diehl

Clinical Project Manager
Beverly Ann Tscheschlog, RN, BS

Editors
Kevin Haworth, Brenna H. Mayer,
Carol Munson, Rob Traister

Copyeditors
Kimberly Bilotta (supervisor),
Scotti Cohn, Tom DeZego,
Heather Ditch, Dona Hightower,
Judith Orioli, Carolyn Petersen,
Irene Pontarelli, Lisa Stockslager,
Dorothy P. Terry, Pamela Wingrod

Designers
Will Boehm (book design),
Corporate Imagination (project
manager)

Digital Composition Services
Diane Paluba (manager),
Joyce Rossi Biletz, Donna Morris

Manufacturing
Patricia Dorshaw (director),
Beth Janae Orr

Editorial Assistants
Megan L. Aldinger,
Tara L. Carter-Bell,
Arlene Claffee, Linda Ruhf

Indexer
Karen C. Comerford

Library of Congress
Cataloging-in-Publication Data

Bickston, Tamara H., 1969-
    Medical surgical nursing recall / Tamara H. Bickston.
        p. ; cm.
Includes index.
    1. Nursing—Examinations, questions, etc.
    2. Surgical nursing—Examinations, questions, etc.
    [DNLM: 1. Perioperative Nursing—Examination
Questions. 2. Emergency Nursing—Examination
Questions. WY 18.2 B583m 2004] I. Title.
    RT55.B53 2004
    610.73'076—dc22
ISBN 0-7817-4465-2 (alk. paper)   2003019411

Contents

To Steve,
for the immeasurable joy and inspiration
he brings to my life each day

Associate editors, contributors, and consultants

Associate editors

Bonnie F. Angel, RN, MSN, EdD
Clinical Assistant Professor
University of North Carolina at Chapel
    Hill School of Nursing

Robert G. Sawyer, MD
Associate Professor of Surgery, Critical
    Care and Abdominal Transplantation
University of Virginia Health System
Charlottesville

Contributors

Michelle Beard, RN, MSN, ACNP, OCN
Acute Care Nurse Practitioner
University of Virginia Health System
Charlottesville

Laura Beech, RN, BSN, CCRN
Clinician 3, Surgical–Trauma ICU
University of Virginia Health System
Charlottesville

Nan A. Carroll, RN, BSN, CCTC
Liver Transplant Nurse Coordinator
University of Virginia Health System
Charlottesville

Regina M. DeGennaro, RN, MSN, AOCN
Advanced Practice Nurse 1
University of Virginia Health System,
    Cancer Center
Charlottesville

Mary M. Deivert, RN, MSN, ACNP-CS,
CCRN
Trauma Care Coordinator
University of Virginia Health System
Charlottesville

Beth Dierdorf RN, MSN, CS
Advanced Practice Nurse
Digestive Health Center of Excellence
University of Virginia Health System
Charlottesville

Ann Donovan, RN, MSN, CWOCN
Director of Nursing
Bethlen Home
Ligonier, Pa.

Lisa W. Forsyth, RN, MSN
Clinician 4, Nursing Education
    Coordinator
University of Virginia Health System
Charlottesville

Jane S. Kaufman, RN, MS, ANP, CS
Clinical Assistant Professor & Nurse
    Practitioner
University of North Carolina School of
    Nursing & Pulmonary Division
    University of North Carolina
    Hospitals
Chapel Hill

Kelly McAdams, RN, MSN, CCRN
Clinical Nurse Specialist
Palmetto Health Richland
Columbia, S.C.

Laurie Rush McCotter, BS, RD, CDE
Clinical Dietitian
University of Virginia Health System
Charlottesville

Kimberley Ann Popovsky, RN, BSN
Research Coordinator
University of Virginia Health System
Charlottesville

Cindy L. Russell, RN, CCRN, TNCC, ONC
Clinician III
University of Virginia Health System
Charlottesville

Winsor Davis Simmons, RN, BSN, CCTC
Transplant Coordinator
University of Virginia Health System
Charlottesville

Anita K. Sites, RN, BSN
Clinical Transplant Coordinator,
    Kidney & Pancreas
University of Virginia Health System
Charlottesville

Carolyn Teeple-Pauly, RN, BSN, OCN
Cancer Nurse Coordinator
University of Virginia Health System
Charlottesville

**Florence Elizabeth Turrentine,
RN, PhD**
Assistant Professor of Research
University of Virginia Health System
Charlottesville

Brigid Wonderly, RN, MSN
Clinical Research Coordinator
University of Virginia Health System
Charlottesville

Consultants

Susan D. Bell, RN, MS, CNRN, OCN
Neurosurgery Nurse Practitioner
Ohio State University Medical Center
Columbus

Deborah M. Berry, RN, BSN, MS
Clinical Education Specialist
Franklin Square Hospital Center
Baltimore

Dorothy Borton, RN, BSN, CIC
Infection Control Practitioner
Albert Einstein Healthcare Network
Philadelphia

Cheryl L. Brady, RN, MSN
Adjunct Faculty
Youngstown (Ohio) State University

Michelle M. Byrne, RN, MS, PhD, CNOR
Clinical Faculty
North Georgia College & State
    University
Dahlonega

**Marsha L. Conroy, RN, BA, MSN,
APN, CNS**
Instructor of Nursing
Cuyahoga Community College
Cleveland
Adjunct Faculty
Kent (Ohio) State University

Dolores Cotton, RN, BSN, MS
Practical Nursing Coordinator
Meridian Technology Center
Stillwater, Ohio

Mary Ann Dudley, RN, MSN
Nursing Faculty
Laramie County Community College
Cheyenne, Wyo.

Shelba Durston, RN, MSN, CCRN
Adjunct Faculty
San Joaquin Delta College
Stockton, Calif.
Staff Nurse
San Joaquin General Hospital
French Camp, Calif.

Carrin Dvorak, RN, MSN
Assistant Professor of Nursing
Cuyahoga Community College
Cleveland

Ken W. Edmisson, ND, EdD, RNC, FNP
Associate Professor
Middle Tennessee State University
Murfreesboro

Carmel A. Esposito, RN, MSN, EdD
Consultant
Follansbee, W.Va.

Athena A. Foreman, RN, MSN
Nursing Coordinator
Stanly Community College
Albemarle, N.C.

Margaret M. Gingrich, RN, MSN
Associate Professor
Harrisburg (Pa.) Area Community
College

Allen Hanberg, RN, MSN
Associate Professor
Weber State University
ICU Registered Nurse
St. Mark's Hospital
Ogden, Utah

Julia Anne Isen, RN, MS, FNP-C
Nurse Practitioner—Internal Medicine
Veterans Administration
Assistant Professor
University of California San Francisco

Denise C. Johnson, MSN
Assistant Professor
Borough of Manhattan Community
College
New York

Eleftheria T. Karapas, RN, MS
Clinical Consultant
Lemont, Ill.

Kay Luft, RN, MN, CCRN
Assistant Professor
Saint Luke's College
Kansas City, Mo.

Dawna Martich, RN, MSN
Clinical Trainer
American Healthways
Pittsburgh

Catherine Shields, RN, BSN
Instructor of Practical Nursing
Career and Technical Institute
Lakehurst, N.J.

Catherine M. Snelson, RN, MSN
Faculty
Kent (Ohio) State University College
of Nursing

Helen M. Taggart, RN, DSN, CS
Associate Professor
Armstrong Atlantic State University
Savannah, Ga.

Tamara Thell, RN, BSN, PHN
Nurse Educator
Anoka-Hennepin Technical College
Anoka, Minn.

Geraldine M. Wagner, RN, M.Ed, BA,
BSN
Consultant
Wagner's Medical/Educational
Consulting Services
Lompoc, Calif.

Sharon Wing, RN, MSN
Assistant Professor
Cleveland State University

Michele Woodbeck, RN, MS
Associate Professor, Nursing
Hudson Valley Community College
Troy, N.Y.

Demetra C. Zalman, RN, MSN, CCRN
Staff Nurse, Level III
Hospital of the University of
Pennsylvania
Philadelphia

Preface

Medical-Surgical Nursing Recall is a powerful new learning tool designed for nursing students. It provides a succinct review of anatomy and physiology, physical assessment skills, pathophysiology, pharmacology, critical nursing skills, and hundreds of specific nursing interventions — all contained in an innovative and fast-paced question-and-answer format.

This book provides rapid access to a wealth of information, including comprehensive coverage of fundamental nursing principles using a body systems-oriented approach. In addition to 10 body system chapters, *Medical-Surgical Nursing Recall* features chapters on fluids and electrolytes, nutrition, pain management, diagnostic procedures, the surgical experience, common medical-surgical emergencies, and oncology.

Each body system chapter in *Medical-Surgical Nursing Recall* begins with an overview of the anatomy and physiology of specific body systems and continues with a review of the major disease processes associated with that system. A pharmacologic overview is included as well, and lists modes of action, examples of generic and brand names, and common adverse reactions. In addition, the book reviews critical nursing skills relevant to the body system, including a step-wise approach to the proper techniques used to perform particular skills safely and effectively.

Special features of the book include straight-forward illustrations that enhance the student's comprehension of medical-surgical nursing, including anatomy and physiology, disease processes, medical and surgical procedures, and essential nursing skills. Visual learning aids highlight critical information throughout *Medical-Surgical Nursing Recall*:

⚡ designates important clinical alerts

✎ indicates frequently tested content.

The unique question-and-answer format makes testing yourself easy and enjoyable, and promotes active learning. As you read questions in the left-hand column, simply use the enclosed bookmark to cover the right-hand column until you've formulated your answer.

Another key feature of the book is the NCLEX practice test located in the appendix, where students can fine-tune their critical thinking skills by reviewing the 200 multiple-choice NCLEX-style questions with rationales for correct and incorrect answers.

Medical-Surgical Nursing Recall is designed to be an invaluable aid to help nursing students assess and build the knowledge necessary to excel in academic courses, clinical rotations, and licensing examinations as well as provide quality patient care in their professional practice.

Tamara H. Bickston, RN, BSN, CCTC

Acknowledgments

I am deeply grateful for the outstanding support and guidance the editorial and production staffs at Lippincott Williams & Wilkins provided me during the creation of this book. Their professionalism and dedication to excellence in publishing were evident with every interaction. In particular, I want to thank Elizabeth Nieginski for her faith in this project as well as her perseverance in helping it to become a reality. I would also like to thank my clinical editor, Beverly Tscheschlog, for being a constant source of encouragement and support through what developed into very rigorous — and at times daunting — editorial schedules.

In addition, the editorial talents of Tracy Diehl, Joan Robinson, and David Moreau are deserving of special recognition for the guidance they provided me.

I am especially appreciative of the commitment and diligence demonstrated by the associate editors, Drs. Robert Sawyer and Bonnie Angel. Their clinical and teaching expertise were indispensable resources for me, and their contributions helped make this book the invaluable review tool that it is.

Special recognition is also due to the many talented contributing authors and reviewers for the immense amount of work they put into ensuring the content of *Medical-Surgical Nursing Recall* was comprehensive, current, and accurate. Thanks to each of you for the many hours of work you committed to this project.

A final word of appreciation is extended to my family and friends who helped sustain me through it all. Without your love and support, this book would never have been possible.

1

Concepts of nursing practice

The nursing process

What's the nursing process?

The framework providing a cyclical checklist for nurses giving individualized care to patients: assessment, diagnosis, planning, implementation, and evaluation

How does the nursing process differ from the medical process?

The nursing process focuses on a patient's response to illness, whereas the medical process emphasizes the disease process itself.

What are the characteristics of the nursing process?

1. *Systematic:* ordered sequence of interdependent activities
2. *Dynamic:* each activity is fluid and overlaps with the next
3. *Interpersonal:* patient-centered
4. *Goal-directed:* nurses and patients work together toward achieving specific goals
5. *Universally applicable:* enables nursing to be practiced in any setting with any patient population

✎ What are the five components of the nursing process?

Assessment, diagnosis, planning, implementation, and evaluation

What's the nurse's role during the assessment phase?

To collect objective and subjective data through a nursing history, physical, interview, or chart review

✎ What's the nurse's role during the diagnosis phase?

To analyze the data and identify actual or potential health problems as well as identify patient coping skills

What's the nurse's role during the planning phase?

To set goals and priorities as well as devise interventions to accomplish them

What's the nurse's role during the implementation phase?	To set the plan into action
✎ **What's the nurse's role during the evaluation phase?**	To analyze the effectiveness of the previous steps and to measure the extent to which the patient's goals were met (individualized care plans can aid in the evaluation of nursing care)
What's a nursing diagnosis and how does it differ from a medical diagnosis?	A nursing diagnosis identifies and labels human responses to actual and potential health problems, whereas a medical diagnosis identifies a disease process based on clinical signs and symptoms.

Nursing practice

What's a nurse practice act?	A legal standard developed by legislative action and implemented by state-granted authority
✎ **What's the purpose of a nurse practice act?**	1. To determine minimum standards for nursing education 2. To set requirements for licensure or registration 3. To determine when a license may be suspended or revoked
What's credentialing?	The method of defining and upholding competent practice; it includes licensure, registration, certification, and accreditation
What's licensure?	The process by which a government agency grants a legal permit to practice a profession and to use a particular title
What's certification?	Verification that someone has voluntarily met minimum competence standards in specialty areas

Legal issues

✎ **What's a living will?**	An individual's signed request to be allowed to die when life can be supported only by mechanical or heroic measures
✎ **What's a durable power of attorney?**	An individual who has legal responsibility for making health care decisions regarding the provision or withdrawal of life-saving treatments

🔖 What's meant by the term "informed consent"?

A patient's agreement to undergo a course of treatment or a procedure after disclosure of complete information (risks, benefits, alternative therapies)

When is informed consent required?

At the time of admission (for routine care), before each diagnostic or therapeutic procedure, and before patient participation in experimental studies

When is informed consent not required?

In an emergency when there's an immediate threat to life or health or when the patient can't provide consent and the legally authorized person can't be reached

Whose obligation is it to obtain informed consent?

The physician's; the nurse's responsibilities are primarily witnessing and ensuring patient comprehension

🔖 What are the components of informed consent?

1. Voluntary or no coercion
2. Competence
3. Comprehension
4. Full disclosure of risks, benefits, and alternatives

What patients are unable to provide consent?

Minors, unconscious or injured patients who can't give appropriate consent, and mentally ill persons deemed legally incompetent

In what order are family members considered "next of kin" for giving consent?

Patient's spouse, adult children, parents, adult siblings, and legal guardian

🔖 What's a Do-Not-Resuscitate (DNR) order?

One that states no effort is to be made to resuscitate a patient in the event of cardiopulmonary arrest

What are Good Samaritan laws?

Laws designed to protect health care professionals at the scene of an emergency against malpractice claims unless it can be proven there was a significant departure from the normal standard of care

What are statutory laws?

Laws enacted by any legislative body, such as nurse practice acts and Good Samaritan acts

What's a criminal law?

A law that concerns actions against public safety and welfare, such as active euthanasia, possession of controlled substances, and homicide

What's a civil law?

A law concerning relationships between private individuals that protects the rights of individual persons in society

What's a tort law?

A law that defines and enforces private individuals' duties and rights that aren't based on contractual agreements, such as negligence and malpractice; can be intentional or unintentional

What's negligence?

Conduct that falls below the standard of care; it involves omitting something that a reasonable person would do (omission) or doing something that a reasonable person wouldn't do (commission)

What's malpractice?

A type of professional negligence; may include professional misconduct or unreasonable lack of professional skill

What are common malpractice occurrences in nursing?

Medication errors are the most common. Patient falls, mistaken identity, incorrect sponge counts, and failure to note or appropriately respond to patient complaints are also common.

What's an incident report?

An agency record of an accident or any uncommon occurrence that results in (or has the potential to result in) harm to a patient, employee, or visitor

What information should be included in an incident report?

1. Patient name and medical record number
2. Date, time, and location of the incident
3. Facts and circumstances surrounding the incident
4. Witnesses to the incident
5. Equipment and medications involved

What's liability?

The state of being legally responsible for one's obligations and actions, and for making financial restitution for wrongful acts

What's *respondeat superior*?

A type of legal relationship in which the employer assumes responsibility for the conduct of the employee

A hospital is responsible for a nurse's conduct, but the nurse may also be individually liable.

What's a grievance?

Any disagreement arising out of terms of employment

What are the legal obligations of nursing students?

Students are legally responsible for the same professional standard of skill and competence as a registered nurse. They are liable for their own actions and for their own acts of negligence.

Ethical issues

What's the difference between ethics and morals?

Ethics are formal sets of rules or values that are stated publicly, whereas morals refer to personal values or principles.

What's a code of ethics?

A guide for establishing, maintaining, and improving professional standards of practice

What's nonmaleficence?

The obligation to do no harm

What's beneficence?

The act of doing good

2

Fluids, electrolytes, and acid-base balance

Basic concepts of fluids and electrolytes

✎ What's homeo-stasis?

A dynamic state of equilibrium between body compartments achieved through complex coordination of physiologic processes resistant to change

What percentage of the body is composed of water?

Water comprises approximately 60% of the body in adults. Gender (slightly less for females, slightly more for males), age, and body surface area affect total body water (TBW).

What important functions does water serve?

It's the universal solvent that dissolves many different solutes. It aids in the transportation of nutrients to cells and in the removal of waste products produced by cellular metabolism. It assists with body temperature regulation.

What are the two main body compartments that store fluid?

Intracellular (70% TBW) and extracellular (30% TBW) spaces, which are separated by semipermeable membranes; the extracellular fluids (ECF) consist of intravascular (plasma) and extravascular (interstitial or "between cells") fluids, cerebrospinal fluid, and other fluids contained in various body spaces (intraocular, pleural, and joint spaces) as well as GI secretions

What's an electrolyte?

A substance whose molecules split (or dissociate) into electrically charged particles (ions) when placed in water

✎ What are the five major electrolytes?

Sodium (Na), potassium (K), calcium (Ca), phosphorus (P), and magnesium (Mg)

What are the functions of electrolytes?

1. Regulate water distribution (sodium and potassium)
2. Transmit nerve impulses (sodium and potassium)
3. Regulate acid-base balance
4. Aid in blood clotting
5. Generate adenosine triphosphate (ATP) (phosphorus)

What's an ion?

Particles with an electrical charge

◼ *Electrical charge is important because it influences the location of the electrolyte.*

What's a cation?

A positively charged ion, such as sodium (Na⁺) and potassium (K⁺)

What's an anion?

A negatively charged ion such as chloride (Cl⁻)

Movement of fluids and electrolytes

How does fluid move between the intracellular and extracellular spaces?

Via active transport and passive transport mechanisms, such as diffusion, facilitated diffusion, and osmosis

What's active transport?

A process that requires external energy to move molecules or solutes in and out of cells against a concentration gradient; molecules are moved from areas of low concentration to areas of high concentration

What's diffusion?

A process that doesn't require external energy to move molecules or solutes in and out of cells; molecules or solutes move from an area of a higher concentration to an area of a lower concentration

What's facilitated diffusion?

A form of diffusion that requires a carrier molecule to facilitate or accelerate the movement of molecules from an area of high concentration to an area of low concentration; for instance, insulin serves as the carrier molecule for glucose transport into the cell

What's osmosis?

A special form of diffusion in which water moves through a semipermeable membrane from an area of low solute concentration (is more dilute or has more water) to an area of high solute concentration (is more concentrated or has less water)

What's osmotic pressure?

The force created by water movement

What's tonicity?

The tension that osmotic pressure exerts on cell size due to water movement across the cell membrane

What's osmolality?

A measurement of osmotic pressure (used interchangeably with osmolarity, although the units of measure differ)

▧ *The osmolality of surrounding fluids influences cell size.*

✎ **What's an isotonic solution?**

One that has the same osmolality (contains the same amount of water) relative to the cell interior; causes no change in cell size

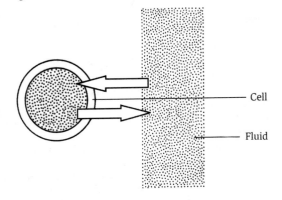

Cell

Fluid

✎ **What's a hypotonic solution?**

One that contains more water relative to the cell and causes a cell to swell; also called a *hypoosmolar solution*

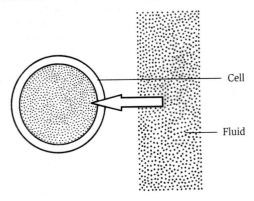

Cell

Fluid

What's a hypertonic solution?

One that contains less water relative to the cell and causes a cell to shrink; also called a *hyperosmolar solution*

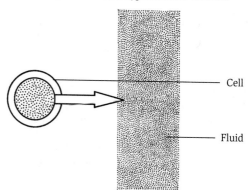

Cell

Fluid

What pressures affect fluid movement in capillaries?

Hydrostatic and oncotic pressures

What's hydrostatic pressure?

The force exerted by a fluid pressing against a wall (blood against capillary walls); it pushes fluid out of the vasculature at the capillary level and into the interstitial space

Hydrostatic pressure then works with oncotic pressure to maintain balance.

What's the relationship between hydrostatic pressure and osmotic pressure?

They are opposing forces that determine the direction and amount of fluid that crosses capillary walls. Fluids will exit a capillary if the net hydrostatic pressure exceeds the net osmotic pressure, and fluids will enter the capillary if the net osmotic pressure is greater than the net hydrostatic pressure.

What's oncotic pressure?

The force exerted by colloids in solution; also called *colloidal osmotic pressure,* it opposes the outward flow of fluid from the interstitial space, causing fluid to remain in the vasculature

The majority of oncotic pressure is due to albumin in the plasma.

What's net filtration?

The end result of fluid movement after the cellular compartments have exerted their forces; also described as Starling's hypothesis

What equation represents Starling's hypothesis?

Net filtration = Forces favoring filtration − Forces opposing filtration

Regulation of fluids and electrolytes

How is water intake controlled?

Through activation of the osmoreceptor system (located in the thirst center of the hypothalamus), due either to a decrease in plasma volume or an increase in plasma osmolality

✎ What factors affect water output?

1. *Pituitary gland:* secretion of antidiuretic hormone when osmoreceptor system detects decreased plasma volume (or increased plasma osmolality)
2. *Adrenal cortex:* secretion of glucocorticoids and mineralocorticoids
3. *Kidneys:* selective reabsorption of glomerular filtrate
4. *Gastrointestinal:* elimination of water in feces
5. *Insensible water loss:* obligatory water loss primarily from the lungs and skin

What's antidiuretic hormone (ADH)?

A hormone secreted by the posterior pituitary gland that causes water reabsorption by the distal tubules and the kidneys' collecting ducts

⧉ *When ADH is secreted, water is reabsorbed and the ECF volume increases.*

What factors affect the secretion of ADH?

Detection of decreased circulating volume (increased plasma osmolality) by osmoreceptors in the hypothalamus, and detection of blood volume or pressure changes by stretch receptors in the heart

What other factors cause the release of ADH and, therefore, water retention?

Dehydration, fever, severe pain, nausea, medications, and stress

What medical condition is associated with ADH secretion despite normal circulating volume and normal plasma osmolality?

Syndrome of inappropriate antidiuretic hormone

What medical condition is associated with absent ADH production?

Diabetes insipidus

What's aldosterone?

A mineralocorticoid secreted by the adrenal cortex that, under complex control of the renin-angiotensin system, causes the distal tubules of the kidneys to reabsorb sodium (water is retained along with sodium)

What factors stimulate aldosterone secretion?

Decreased plasma volume, decreased serum sodium, and increased serum potassium

❧ What's the renin-angiotensin system?

The mechanism that increases serum sodium, resulting in increased blood volume or pressure; decreased blood volume causes the kidneys to secrete renin

Renin activates angiotensinogen to angiotensin I, which is converted in the lungs to angiotensin II. Angiotensin II stimulates secretion of aldosterone, which increases sodium reabsorption.

What's atrial natriuretic factor (ANF)?

A hormone released from the atrial muscles of the heart in response to increased blood pressure (or blood volume); ANF blocks the secretion of renin, aldosterone, and ADH so that blood vessels dilate; enhanced water and sodium excretion, and reduced blood volume and pressure occur

❧ What's the function of sodium?

Regulation of water balance, cell size, acid-based balance, and transmission of nerve impulses (action potential requires sodium)

❧ What factors affect sodium regulation?

Water balance, blood pressure regulation, and both neural and hormonal factors (aldosterone secretion from the kidneys and adrenal glands; ADH secretion from the pituitary gland)

❧ What's the function of potassium?

Transmission of nerve impulses (resting polarization and repolarization depend on potassium), maintenance of cardiac rhythm, and use of glucose by cells

What factors are involved with potassium regulation?

Aldosterone and the hydrogen ion concentration (pH) of the extracellular fluid

▨ *Sodium and potassium levels are inversely related.*

How does the extracellular pH level affect potassium movement?

An acidotic (pH < 7.35) state causes potassium to move out of the cells and be excreted, while an alkalotic state (pH > 7.45) causes potassium to move into the intracellular compartment.

What other factors affect potassium levels?

1. Diuretics (potassium wasting)
2. Other drugs, such as insulin and epinephrine
3. Excessive vomiting, diarrhea, and GI suctioning

◆ What's the function of calcium?

Contraction of skeletal and heart muscle, coagulation of blood, and regulation of cell permeability

The balance of what electrolyte is reciprocally related to calcium balance?

Phosphate; when calcium levels increase, phosphate levels decrease

What's the function of phosphorus?

ATP production provides intracellular energy for active transport across cell membranes, acid-base balance maintenance, oxygen delivery, and bone strength.

◆ What factors regulate serum calcium and phosphate levels?

Vitamin D, parathyroid hormone, and calcitonin

What's the function of magnesium?

Assists in the transport of sodium and potassium across the cell wall as well as transmission of central nervous system signals, which affects neuromuscular activity

What factors affect serum magnesium levels?

Magnesium competes with calcium for absorption in the GI tract and renal tubules, so an increase in one level will cause a decrease in the other.

Assessment and management of fluid and electrolyte disturbances

◆ What are some clinical manifestations of dehydration or water deficit?

Dry mucous membranes, fatigue, thirst, poor skin turgor, decreased urine output (oliguria) with increased serum osmolality (increased blood urea nitrogen [BUN] and hematocrit), decreased weight, tachycardia, a weak and thready pulse, and hypotension

◆ How is dehydration treated?

Replacement of fluid and treatment of the underlying cause of fluid loss such as diarrhea

◆ What are some clinical manifestations of fluid overload or water excess?

Pitting edema (fluid in the interstitial space), pulmonary edema (shortness of breath, dyspnea, cough, and crackles), jugular vein distention, bounding pulse, and hypertension

◆ How is fluid overload treated?

Administration of diuretics, implementation of fluid and sodium restrictions, and dialysis in severe cases

What are some clinical manifestations of hypernatremia (increased sodium)?

Thirst, dry and sticky mucous membranes, lethargy, agitation, restlessness, decreased reflexes, muscular rigidity, tachycardia, oliguria or anuria, hypotension, tremors, seizures, and coma

How is hypernatremia treated?

Increased fluid intake (preferably free water) and decreased sodium intake

✎ What are some clinical manifestations of hyponatremia (decreased sodium)?

Muscle cramps, weakness, fatigue, headache, depression, confusion, coma, and seizures as well as decreased BUN and hematocrit

How is hyponatremia treated?

Implementation of fluid restriction, administration of diuretics, I.V. sodium, and dialysis if renal failure is present

What are some clinical manifestations of hyperkalemia (increased potassium)?

Paresthesia, muscle weakness, cramps, dizziness, confusion, nausea, diarrhea, electrocardiogram (ECG) changes (peaked T waves, depressed S-T segments) as well as possible cardiac arrest

In what disease process is hyperkalemia commonly seen?

End-stage renal disease

✎ How is hyperkalemia treated?

Decreased dietary intake (including salt substitutes), decreased fluid intake, and administration of potassium-binding medications, such as polystyrene sulfonate resin (Kayexalate) or sorbitol
In severe, symptomatic cases, administering 50% glucose, insulin, bicarbonate, calcium and, possibly, dialysis may be necessary.

✎ What are some clinical manifestations of hypokalemia (decreased potassium)?

Muscle weakness or cramps, paresthesia, nausea, vomiting, anorexia, fatigue, lethargy, depression, confusion, constipation or paralytic ileus, and ECG changes (T-wave inversion, U waves), as well as other cardiac symptoms, such as bradycardia and palpitations

✎ How is hypokalemia treated?

Increased dietary intake of potassium (citrus fruits and bananas), administration of potassium supplements, decreased diuretics, and administration of I.V. potassium in more severe cases

✎ What are some clinical manifestations of hypercalcemia (increased calcium)?

Muscle weakness or atrophy, fatigue, hyporeflexia, anorexia, nausea, vomiting, polyuria, polydipsia, constipation, ECG changes (shortening of QT interval and presence of atrioventricular block), ataxia, mental status changes (lethargy, irritability, stupor, coma), pathologic fractures, and development of renal calculi

In what disease processes is hypercalcemia commonly seen?

Cancer and hyperparathyroidism

How is hypercalcemia treated?

Hydration is the primary intervention. Other treatment methods include decreasing calcium intake, administering loop diuretics (furosemide), calcitonin, corticosteroids, and bisphosphonates (alendronate, etidronate) to stop bone resorption, and initiating dialysis in severe cases.

What are some clinical manifestations of hypocalcemia?

Paresthesia, tetany including positive signs of Trousseau (muscular spasm of hand with upper arm compression as with a blood pressure cuff) and Chvostek (twitching of upper lip in response to tapping facial nerve) hyperreflexia, muscle cramps, bronchospasms, mental status changes (depression, memory loss, hallucinations), seizures, and cardiac insufficiency

How is hypocalcemia treated?

Increased dietary intake (dairy products), administration of calcium supplement, administration of vitamin D supplement (to enhance GI absorption of calcium), and administration of intravenous calcium in more severe cases

What are some clinical manifestations of hypermagnesemia?

Diminished deep tendon reflexes, muscle weakness, facial flushing, lethargy, respiratory depression or paralysis, and ECG changes (T-wave elevation, prolonged PR interval, and widened QRS complex)

How is hypermagnesemia treated?

Restriction of magnesium-containing antacids or other preparations, administration of intravenous calcium (direct antagonist of magnesium), and dialysis in severe cases

What are some clinical manifestations of hypomagnesemia?

Hyperreflexia, tetany (positive Chvostek's or Trousseau's signs), muscle weakness, nystagmus, seizures, mental status changes (irritability, disorientation, depression), tachycardia, and ECG changes (prolonged PR and QT intervals)

Because magnesium and calcium excretion are so closely related, symptoms of hypomagnesemia and hypermagnesemia are similar to those of hypocalcemia and hypercalcemia.

How is Chvostek's sign elicited?

To elicit this sign, tap the patient's facial nerve just in front of the earlobe and below the zygomatic arch or between the zygomatic arch and the corner of the mouth, as shown below.

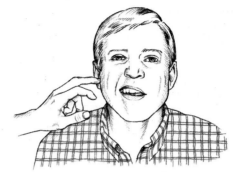

What's a positive response?

A positive response (indicating latent tetany) ranges from simple mouth-corner twitching to twitching of all facial muscles on the side tested. Simple twitching may be normal in some patients. However, a more pronounced response usually confirms Chvostek's sign.

How is Trousseau's sign elicited?

In this test, occlude the brachial artery by inflating a blood pressure cuff on the patient's upper arm to a level between diastolic and systolic blood pressure. Maintain this inflation for 3 minutes while observing the patient for carpal spasm (Trousseau's sign), as shown below.

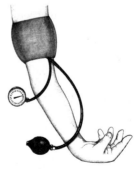

How is hypomagnesemia treated?

Increased dietary intake of magnesium and administration of magnesium supplement; administration of intravenous magnesium in severe cases

What are some clinical manifestations of hyperphosphatemia?

Muscle cramps, tetany, joint pain, and seizures

How is hyperphosphatemia treated?

Administration of aluminum hydroxide binding gels (to limit phosphate absorption and to promote its excretion) and dialysis in severe cases or with renal failure

What are some clinical manifestations of hypophosphatemia?

Muscle weakness, hyporeflexia, paresthesia, fatigue, intention tremor, joint stiffness, bone pain, mental status changes (irritability, apprehensiveness, confusion), and seizures

How is hypophosphatemia treated?

Discontinue any phosphate-binding gels and increase dietary intake of phosphorus. Administration of oral and I.V. phosphate supplements is usually contraindicated in patients with renal failure and hypercalcemia, as it may lead to disseminated calcification.

Why should electrolyte imbalances be corrected slowly?

To prevent overcompensation and resultant complications such as seizures; monitor electrolyte levels frequently during implementation of corrective measures

Basic concepts of acid-base balance

What's an acid?

A molecule that will cause hydrogen to be released into a solution; carbonic acid is the most important acid in determination of pH in the human body

What's a base?

A molecule that combines with hydrogen and removes it from a solution; sodium bicarbonate is the most common base in the body

✎ What's pH and what's a normal pH level for the body?

A term that refers to hydrogen ion concentration; normal extracellular pH is 7.35 to 7.45, a pH < 7.35 is acidic, and a pH > 7.45 is basic

What determines extracellular pH?

The *ratio* (not absolute values) of bicarbonate and carbonic acid, and the degree to which carbonic acid dissociates to form hydrogen and bicarbonate ions

Regulation of acid-base balance

✎ How is acid-base regulated?

By buffering mechanisms (for immediate control), by renal and respiratory mechanisms, and by renal selective conservation of bicarbonate; intracellular and extracellular electrolyte composition also affects pH

What's a buffer and what's a buffer system?	A buffer is a chemical that prevents sudden changes in pH level. A buffer system is composed of a weak acid and the alkali salt of that acid (or a weak base and its acid salt), and will exchange a strong acid for a weak acid (or a strong base for a weak base) in order to maintain a stable pH.
What buffering mechanisms regulate acid-base balance?	Bicarbonate buffers, phosphate buffers, and protein buffers
✎ **How does the respiratory system contribute to acid-base balance?**	By providing a mechanism for the elimination of carbon dioxide (CO_2) into the air. Excessive CO_2 in the blood causes a sudden increase in ventilation (exhalation of CO_2) and a fairly rapid correction of the CO_2 level.
✎ **How does the renal system contribute to acid-base balance?**	By selective conservation (recycling) of bicarbonate and by elimination of excessive hydrogen ions
How is renal bicarbonate conservation achieved?	When CO_2 levels are increased, hydrogen ion secretion exceeds bicarbonate ion filtration, and the urine becomes acidic. Alkaline urine is produced when bicarbonate filtration exceeds hydrogen ion secretion. Urinary pH can vary greatly from 4.5 to 8.0.
What are the mechanisms by which the kidneys can eliminate excessive hydrogen ions (acid)?	1. Secretion of free hydrogen into the renal tubule 2. Combining hydrogen ions with ammonia to produce ammonium 3. Excreting weak acids
What's compensation?	A mechanism that maintains acid-base balance without actually correcting the underlying cause; compensatory mechanisms are utilized in situations in which correction is impossible or can't be achieved immediately, and involves the use of an unaffected body system to maintain normal pH
What's correction?	A means of controlling pH by fixing the underlying cause of an acid-base imbalance; however, it doesn't involve the use of another body system

Acid-base imbalances

✎ **What's acidosis?**	The state of a low pH level (< 7.35) and a high concentration of hydrogen ions

✎ What's alkalosis?   The state of a high pH (> 7.45) and a low concentration of hydrogen ions

How are these imbalances tested?   Arterial blood gas (ABG) analysis, which assesses pH level, CO_2 level, and bicarbonate (HCO_3^-) level

✎ What are the differences between respiratory and metabolic imbalances?   A respiratory imbalance is due to abnormal functioning of the lungs and affects carbonic acid concentrations. A metabolic imbalance is due to abnormal functioning of a body system other than the lungs and affects the bicarbonate concentration.

What are the four acid-base imbalances?   Respiratory acidosis, respiratory alkalosis, metabolic acidosis, and metabolic alkalosis

✎ What's respiratory acidosis? CO_2 retention (elevated partial pressure of carbon dioxide [Pco_2] levels) and carbonic acid excess that occur in the presence of hypoventilation

✎ What's the compensatory mechanism for respiratory acidosis?   Conservation of bicarbonate by the kidneys

✎ What are some of the causes of respiratory acidosis?   Acute causes can include airway obstruction, brain stem trauma (causing decreased respiratory drive), oversedation, neuromuscular diseases, and flail chest related to trauma. Chronic causes may include chronic obstructive pulmonary disease (COPD), such as emphysema, chronic bronchitis, and asthma.

✎ What's CO_2 narcosis?   An acute episode of severe respiratory acidosis that occurs in persons with chronic lung disease with chronically elevated Pco_2 levels (patients with COPD)

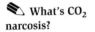 *It's important not to administer normal amounts of oxygen to these patients, because depression of their respiratory drive results.*

✎ What's respiratory alkalosis?   Increased CO_2 excretion (decreased Pco_2 levels) and carbonic acid deficit that occur in the presence of hyperventilation

✎ What's the compensatory mechanism for respiratory alkalosis?   Excretion of bicarbonate by the kidneys

What are some of the causes of respiratory alkalosis?

Anxiety, fever, pain, pulmonary disease, heart failure, salicylate toxicity, and increased blood ammonia levels; can also occur at high altitudes or from mechanical overventilation

What's metabolic acidosis?

HCO_3^- deficit (decreased HCO_3^- levels) that occurs in the presence of acid accumulation (other than carbonic acid) in the blood or decreased bicarbonate in the extracellular fluid

What's the compensatory mechanism for metabolic acidosis?

Excretion of CO_2 by the lungs

What are some of the causes of metabolic acidosis?

Renal failure, shock, starvation, diabetic ketoacidosis, and lactic acidosis

What's metabolic alkalosis?

HCO_3^- excess (elevated HCO_3^- levels) that results from the loss of a strong acid or the gain of a base

What's the compensatory mechanism for metabolic alkalosis?

Retention of CO_2 by the lungs

What are some of the causes of metabolic alkalosis?

Prolonged vomiting, excessive GI suctioning, excessive ingestion of sodium bicarbonate, hyperaldosteronism, and diuretic therapy

What's the milk alkali syndrome?

A condition that results from the consumption of excessive amounts of milk along with alkaline antacids

Assessment and management of acid-base imbalances

What are some clinical manifestations of respiratory acidosis (increased Pco_2)?

Restlessness and nervousness initially; dizziness, confusion, drowsiness, headache, muscle twitching, seizures, and rapid, shallow breathing are later findings

What are typical laboratory findings with respiratory acidosis?

1. Decreased pH (< 7.35)
2. Increased Pco_2 (> 50 mm Hg)
3. Normal HCO_3^-

How is respiratory acidosis treated?	Returning the respiratory drive and ventilation ability to normal, which may involve reversing sedation or placing on mechanical ventilation in severe cases
🔍 **What are some clinical manifestations of respiratory alkalosis?**	Tachypnea may be the first indicator. Later occurrences include dizziness; confusion; paresthesia; tetany, including positive Chvostek's and Trousseau's signs; seizures; and, possibly, coma.
🔍 **What are typical laboratory findings with respiratory alkalosis?**	1. Increased pH (> 7.45) 2. Decreased P_{CO_2} (< 35 mm Hg) 3. Decreased HCO_3^- (< 24 mEq/L)
🔍 **How is respiratory alkalosis treated?**	Instituting measures that increase P_{CO_2} (rebreathing small amounts of expired air) and treating the underlying cause (anxiety, salicylate toxicity, increased blood ammonia)
🔍 **What are some clinical manifestations of metabolic acidosis?**	Headache, weakness, warm and flushed skin, lethargy, confusion, bradycardia, cardiac arrhythmias, stupor and, possibly, coma; deep, rapid respirations (Kussmaul breathing) indicate a respiratory compensation and are commonly seen in diabetic ketoacidosis
🔍 **What are typical laboratory findings with metabolic acidosis?**	1. Decreased pH (< 7.35) 2. Normal CO_2 3. Decreased HCO_3^- (< 24 mEq/L)
How is metabolic acidosis treated?	Treatment of the underlying cause and replacement of fluids and electrolytes
🔍 **What are some clinical manifestations of metabolic alkalosis?**	Confusion, hyperreflexia, muscle hypertonicity, tetany, and seizures
🔍 **What are typical laboratory findings with metabolic alkalosis?**	1. Increased pH (> 7.45) 2. Normal CO_2 3. Increased HCO_3^- (> 29 mEq/L)
🔍 **How is metabolic alkalosis treated?**	Treatment of the underlying cause and replacement of fluids (the alkalosis may worsen with volume depletion and hypokalemia)

3

Nutrition

Physical assessment of nutritional status

✎ What are four important measures of nutritional status?

Weight, intake and output, laboratory values (prealbumin as well as vitamin, mineral, and electrolyte levels), and calorie counts

✎ What are important aspects of a nutritional history to include during a nursing assessment?

Food allergies, food likes and dislikes, difficulties with chewing and swallowing, weight (recent loss or gain), height, exercise habits, stool habits, body image perceptions, and cultural beliefs

How are pounds changed to kilograms?

By dividing the amount of pounds by 2.2

How are kilograms changed to pounds?

By multiplying the amount of kilograms by 2.2

What's ideal body weight (IBW)?

An estimate of optimal weight for optimal health

✎ What's body mass index (BMI)?

A measure of body composition, which measures the level of adiposity to the relationship of weight to height

$$BMI = \text{Weight (in kg) divided by height (in meters)}^2$$

How are underweight, overweight, and obesity defined?

Underweight: Weight 10% < IBW or BMI < 18.5
Overweight: Weight 20% > IBW or BMI > 25
Obesity: Weight 120% > IBW or BMI > 30

What's malnutrition?

A state of either undernutrition or overnutrition

✎ **What clinical outcomes are associated with malnutrition?**

A higher rate of morbidity and mortality, longer hospital stays, a higher rate of hospital admissions and readmissions as well as longer wound healing times postoperatively

What are some causes of inadequate nutritional status?

Poor dietary intake or choices, malabsorption, maldigestion, physical stress, or abnormal nutrient losses caused by wounds, fistulas, or burns

✎ **What are the clinical manifestations of severe malnutrition?**

Lack of periorbital and palmar fat pads, dependent edema, pale skin, poor muscle tone, brittle finger nails, hair loss, swollen mouth and lips, mottled enamel on teeth, missing teeth, and bleeding or spongy gums

Is albumin or prealbumin a better indicator of recent nutritional status?

Prealbumin is a better indicator because fewer variables affect it and it has a longer half-life than albumin. Albumin can be decreased falsely in liver disease, pregnancy, nephrotic syndrome, overhydration, ascites, and hypocalcemia.

Digestion, absorption, and metabolism of nutrients

How many calories per day does a healthy adult need?

25 to 30 cal/kg of body weight

How much protein does a healthy person require daily?

0.8 g/kg of body weight

✎ **What are the six nutrients?**

Protein, carbohydrate, fat, vitamins, minerals, and water

✎ **What are the three macronutrients and what percentage of each should be in a healthy person's diet?**

1. Carbohydrates: 55 to 60%
2. Proteins: 15 to 20%
3. Fats: 20 to 30%

How does the body use proteins?

Growth and maintenance of body tissues, such as skin, connective tissues, and muscles; production of antibodies and enzymes; regulation of fluid balance, electrolyte balance, and nutrient transport

What are the building blocks of proteins?

Amino acids, which are either essential (must be obtained from dietary sources) or nonessential (can be produced by the body)

✎ **What are important dietary sources of proteins?**

Animal products, such as eggs, milk, and meat; legumes, nuts, and seeds also contain large quantities of protein, but are nutritionally incomplete because they lack one or more of the essential amino acids

What disease processes affect protein metabolism?

Those linked to exocrine pancreatic insufficiencies (chronic pancreatitis, cystic fibrosis, pancreatic cancer), as well as liver disease and cirrhosis

What condition results from inadequate protein intake?

Kwashiorkor

What substances make up dietary carbohydrates?

Simple sugars, complex carbohydrates, and fiber (undigested carbohydrates)

What's the main function of carbohydrates?

They're the preferred energy source for the human body, because all are eventually converted to glucose

What metabolic processes are involved with the regulation of glucose?

1. *Glycogenesis:* excess glucose is converted to glycogen (storage form of glucose)
2. *Glycogenolysis:* glycogen is converted to glucose when blood levels decrease
3. *Gluconeogenesis:* fatty acids and amino acids are converted to glucose when glucose reserves have been depleted

✎ **What are important dietary sources of carbohydrates?**

Plant sources (fruits and vegetables) primarily, with the exception of lactose in milk products and small amounts of glycogen in meats

What's the most common deficiency affecting carbohydrate metabolism?

Lactase deficiency, which results in an intolerance to dairy products; this deficiency can be congenital or linked to other diseases, such as Crohn's disease or sprue

How does the body use fats and lipids?

Formation of all cellular membranes (phospholipids), absorption of fat-soluble vitamins, formation of myelin sheaths around nerve fibers (lecithin), production of prostaglandins (linoleic acid), and provision of a concentrated source of energy production (triglycerides)

What substances primarily make up dietary fats?

Triglycerides (fatty acids and glycerol)

What are important dietary sources of fats or lipids?

Saturated fats, which elevate cholesterol levels, are found primarily in meats and dairy foods. Unsaturated fats are found in vegetable oils, seeds, and nuts.

What are essential fatty acids and what purpose do they serve?

They're unsaturated fats that are essential to the diet because the body can't produce them. The two primary categories are omega-3 fatty acids and omega-6 fatty acids, which are important in the production of cholesterol and prostaglandins, in wound healing, and in maintaining the integrity of hair, skin, and nerve fibers.

How is cholesterol used in the body?

It's the structural basis of bile salts and steroid hormones, and it's the major constituent of cell membranes.

What are important dietary sources of cholesterol?

Egg yolks, meats, and milk products

What are lipoproteins?

Lipid-protein complexes that transport fatty acids, triglycerides, and cholesterol; they can be classified as high-density ("good cholesterol"), low-density ("bad cholesterol") and very low-density

What are the byproducts of lipid metabolism that serve as an important fuel source during starvation and uncontrolled diabetes mellitus?

Ketone bodies

What are vitamins?

Vitamins are essential organic compounds that can't be synthesized by the body and are needed for the maintenance of normal metabolic functions. Most act as coenzymes in various catalytic reactions.

How are vitamins classified?

Water-soluble or fat-soluble

What's the primary difference between water-soluble and fat-soluble vitamins?

The body excretes excesses of water-soluble vitamins, whereas it retains fat-soluble vitamins, which may build up to toxic levels.

What are the water-soluble vitamins and their food sources?

1. *Thiamin (B$_1$):* pork, beef, legumes, grains, cereals
2. *Riboflavin (B$_2$):* milk, eggs, organ meats, enriched cereals
3. *Niacin (B$_3$):* meat, poultry, fish, beans, peas, peanuts
4. *Pantothenic acid (B$_5$):* organ meats, salmon, eggs, legumes
5. *Pyridoxine (B$_6$):* meats, cereal grains, yeast, soybeans
6. *Biotin:* liver, kidney, legumes, egg yolk, tomatoes
7. *Cobalamin (B$_{12}$):* meats, liver, shellfish, milk, eggs
8. *Folic acid:* green leafy vegetables, cabbage, asparagus
9. *Ascorbic acid (C):* citrus fruits, tomatoes, potatoes

What are the fat-soluble vitamins and their food sources?

1. *Vitamin A:* organ meats, fish oils, milk, carrots, sweet potatoes
2. *Vitamin D:* cod liver oil, salmon, tuna, milk, cereals
3. *Vitamin E:* vegetable and wheat germ oils, milk, muscle meats, nuts
4. *Vitamin K:* pork, green leafy vegetables, tomatoes, egg yolk

What vitamins are important for wound healing?

Beta-carotene (a derivative of vitamin A), vitamin C, and vitamin E

How is vitamin A deficiency manifested?

Night blindness and dry mucous membranes

How is vitamin D deficiency manifested?

Osteomalacia, bone deformities, and easy fracturing

What are minerals?

Inorganic substances required by the human body; minerals are divided into two groups: macrominerals and trace minerals.

What are examples of macrominerals and in what foods can they be found?

1. *Calcium:* dairy products, dark green leafy vegetables
2. *Phosphorus:* dairy products, meat, poultry, legumes
3. *Magnesium:* whole grains, nuts, legumes, green vegetables
4. *Sodium:* table salt, seafood, meat, various processed foods
5. *Potassium:* bananas, citrus and dried fruits, meats, fish
6. *Chloride:* similar to sodium

In what foods is the trace mineral iron most abundant?

Red meats, legumes, green leafy vegetables, whole grain or enriched breads, and cereals

In what foods is the trace mineral zinc most abundant?

Oysters, milk, cheese, eggs, and liver

Nutrition in patient care

✎ What's a common cause of daily fluctuations in a patient's body weight?

Water weight (edema or dehydration); water comprises 50% to 60% of an adult's total weight

▧ *Weight gains of more than 2 lb (0.9 kg)/day is an indication of water weight gain rather than weight gain related to diet.*

What's an RDA?

The recommended daily allowance (RDA) of a nutrient that preserves normal body functions and meets basic metabolic needs

What's a DRI and how does it differ from an RDA?

Dietary reference intake (DRI) refers to the role of nutrients in long-term health. An RDA considers the relationship between deficiency and disease.

What are the food categories as defined by the Food Guide Pyramid, and how many servings of each should be consumed per day?

1. *Grains (breads, cereals, pasta, and rice):* 6 to 11 servings
2. *Vegetables and fruits:* 3 to 5 servings of vegetables and 2 to 4 servings of fruit
3. *Dairy and meat foods:* 2 to 3 servings of both meat and dairy
4. *Fats and sweets:* should be consumed sparingly

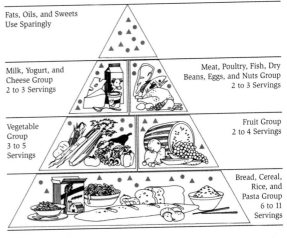

Fats, Oils, and Sweets
Use Sparingly

Milk, Yogurt, and Cheese Group
2 to 3 Servings

Meat, Poultry, Fish, Dry Beans, Eggs, and Nuts Group
2 to 3 Servings

Vegetable Group
3 to 5 Servings

Fruit Group
2 to 4 Servings

Bread, Cereal, Rice, and Pasta Group
6 to 11 Servings

Key:
● Fat (naturally occurring and added)
▲ Sugars (added)

Nutrition in GI disorders

What dietary restrictions are commonly implemented in a patient with cirrhosis or end-stage liver disease?

A 2-g sodium diet and a 1,000- to 2,000-ml fluid restriction to minimize fluid retention; occasionally, a physician can recommend a low-protein diet to assist with the management of encephalopathy (due to ammonia build up from nitrogen breakdown)

What type of diet is used in celiac sprue?

A gluten-free diet; these patients must avoid products made from grains, such as wheat, oats, barley, and rye

What are the dietary guidelines for a patient with gastroparesis?

Small, frequent, low-fat meals to promote gastric emptying

How is the diet advanced for a patient with bowel sounds following gastric surgery?

A progression from clear liquids to a soft diet and, ultimately, to a regular diet

How can the postoperative gastric surgery patient avoid dumping syndrome (diarrhea)?

Avoid concentrated sweets, eat small and frequent meals, and avoid liquids during mealtime

What are the dietary restrictions for ulcer patients?

Because foods don't cause ulcers, there are no specific dietary restrictions, although certain foods may aggravate the symptoms. Therefore, it's recommended that patients with ulcers avoid alcohol, spicy foods, and caffeine (stimulates acid production).

What's the recommended diet for a patient with diverticulosis?

A 25 to 35 g/day high-fiber diet to limit the development of additional diverticula or outpouchings; no specific data exists to support the avoidance of nuts and seeds

What are the recommended dietary restrictions after an episode of acute pancreatitis?

Avoid fried and fatty foods (stimulate bile and pancreatic secretions) as well as alcohol

What types of dietary considerations exist for a patient with inflammatory bowel disease (Crohn's and ulcerative colitis)?

Although no dietary restrictions exist for ulcerative colitis, patients with Crohn's disease may need to avoid high-residue foods (whole grains, nuts, seeds, raw fruits, and vegetables) if they have areas of intestinal stricturing due to inflammation or fibrosis.

✎ What food group should a patient with lactose intolerance avoid?

Dairy products, because these patients are deficient in the enzyme lactase, which is required to digest lactose; adding lactase supplements (LactAid) to the diet may decrease symptoms

Nutrition in cancer

What's cancer cachexia?

A syndrome characterized by significant weight loss, tissue wasting, weakness, and organ dysfunction in a cancer patient

✎ What's radiation enteritis?

A complication of radiation therapy in which the mucosa of the GI tract becomes severely inflamed or damaged, resulting in difficulty swallowing, absorbing, and digesting; total parenteral nutrition or enteral tube feedings may be necessary until the radiation enteritis resolves

✎ What are common nutritional concerns for a cancer patient?

Early satiety, nausea and vomiting, changes in taste (dysgeusia), dry mouth, stomatitis, as well as constipation and diarrhea

✎ What's a neutropenic diet?

A diet that consists of cooked foods and excludes raw fruits and vegetables, dried fruits, fresh squeezed juices, pepper, and yogurt with live, active cultures
It's commonly used when the neutrophil count is less than 1,000/µl as a result of chemotherapy, radiation therapy, or the disease itself, because the patient is at increased risk for infection, including food-borne illnesses; also known as a *low microbial* or *reverse isolation diet.*

Nutrition in renal disorders

✎ What's a renal diet?

A diet that's low in sodium (less than 2 g/day), potassium (less than 1,500 mg/day) and phosphorus (less than 1,200 mg/day); fluids and protein intake (less than 60 g/day) should also be restricted in patients with renal dysfunction

▣ *Many renal patients also have diabetes and will need a diet to aid with glucose management*

◥ What foods have high sodium content?

Processed, cured, or canned foods

◥ What foods have high potassium content?

Citrus fruits, bananas, milk, beans, and many vegetables, such as tomatoes and potatoes

What foods have high phosphorus content?

Foods high in phosphorus are typically high in calcium and include dairy foods, dark soft drinks, and beans

How do nutritional needs differ when a patient starts hemodialysis?

Protein needs increase

How do the nutritional needs of a peritoneal dialysis patient differ from those of a hemodialysis patient?

Because the dialysate in peritoneal dialysis provides a significant number of calories, a patient may receive the equivalent of one extra meal each day through the dialysis solution. In addition, the monitoring of sodium, potassium, magnesium, and fluid is less rigid for peritoneal dialysis patients, and protein restrictions are slightly less (due to protein losses that occur with peritoneal dialysis).

Nutrition in diabetes

◥ What's the major nutrient to manage in a patient with type 1 diabetes?

Carbohydrates; teach total carbohydrate counting to allow flexibility in meal planning and growth for children and adolescents

How does meal planning differ for some patients with type 2 diabetes?

Weight loss should be a goal. Teach carbohydrate counting and appropriate portion sizes of all food groups and encourage a low-fat, moderate-sodium diet due to the increased risk of heart disease in patients with diabetes.

How many carbohydrates should most patients with diabetes consume per day?

45% to 60% of the diabetic diet (typically 160 to 300 g of carbohydrates/day)

◥ Can a patient with diabetes eat sugar?

Yes, if they monitor overall carbohydrate intake; therefore, label reading and carbohydrate counting are crucial

Weight control

✎ What health conditions are associated with obesity?

Diabetes mellitus, hypertension, coronary artery disease, cerebrovascular disease, fatty liver, liver failure, degenerative joint disease, sleep apnea, and some cancers

How is obesity treated?

Diet, exercise, and behavioral modification; employ pharmacologic agents or surgical intervention in some severe cases

One pound of fat is equivalent to how many calories?

3,500 stored calories

What are the two most common eating disorders that cause a patient to be underweight?

Anorexia nervosa and bulimia

What methods can increase body weight?

Provide frequent meals and snacks, decrease activity level, and provide pharmacologic treatment and psychological intervention

How long should an otherwise nutritionally healthy patient have a nothing-by-mouth (NPO) order or have inadequate intake before considering nutritional support (tube feeding or total parenteral nutrition)?

5 to 10 days

Tube feedings

✎ What complications are associated with tube feedings?

Vomiting, diarrhea, constipation, aspiration pneumonia, and refeeding syndrome

What's refeeding syndrome?

A condition that occurs when previously malnourished patients eat high-carbohydrate loads; it involves rapid decreases in serum phosphorus, magnesium, and potassium levels (due to rapid cellular uptake) as well as increased fluid retention

✎ What are possible causes of vomiting with tube feedings?

Feeding too soon after intubation, improper location of the feeding tube, rapid rate of infusion, stenosis or obstruction beyond the distal end of the tube, excessive volume (air and formula), and position of the patient

✎ What are possible causes of diarrhea with tube feedings?

Rapid rate of infusion, high osmolality of formula, high concentration of the formula, low fiber, medication incompatibilities, and infectious causes

What are possible causes of constipation with tube feedings?

Lack of fiber and inadequate fluid intake

What are the advantages of enteral tube feedings with respect to parenteral feedings?

Enteral feedings are generally safer, less expensive, and more physiologic (better used by the GI system) than parenteral feedings

✎ What's the customary manner in which to initiate enteral tube feedings?

Full-strength formula at 10 to 30 ml/hour, increasing by 20 to 30 ml/hour every 6 to 8 hours as tolerated until achieving the target rate

Why are bolus feedings into the small intestine contraindicated?

May produce overdistention and dumping syndrome

What are the advantages of gastric feedings instead of enteral feedings?

Gastric feeding is more physiological, allowing for increased nutrient contact with GI mucosa and increased absorption throughout the entire GI tract. It also allows for bolus feedings 4 to 5 times per day, which the small intestine wouldn't tolerate.

By what methods are gastrostomy feedings administered?

Via gravity drainage bag, push syringe, or feeding pump

What's the optimal patient position for administering gastric tube feedings?

Fowler's position in bed or a sitting position in a chair (a normal position for eating), although a slightly elevated right-side lying position is acceptable if sitting is contraindicated; these positions enhance the gravitational flow of the solution and prevent aspiration of fluid into the lungs

⬚ *Keep the head of the bed elevated 30 degrees during feedings and for at least 1 hour afterwards.*

When should you withhold a tube feeding?	If nausea or vomiting occurs, if discomfort or abdominal distention occurs, or if a gastric residual check obtains a 2-hour volume
When should you withhold an intermittent tube feeding?	If the gastric residual is more than 150 ml, recheck in 3 to 4 hours.
How often should you check a gastric residual for continuous tube feedings?	Every 4 to 6 hours for 24 to 48 hours

TYPES OF FEEDING TUBES

What are the options for placement of feeding tubes?	Stomach (nasogastric or gastrostomy) or small intestine (nasoenteric: nasoduodenal or nasojejunal; jejunostomy)
In what situations are nasogastric (NG) tube feedings appropriate?	When a patient has an intact gag reflex and adequate gastric emptying
What's the primary concern during placement of an NG tube?	Inadvertent pulmonary intubation; must confirm proper placement before using
After what types of surgeries should you *not* manipulate or reposition an NG tube?	After gastric resections or gastric bypass, due to risk of damage the suture line
When are nasoduodenal or nasojejunal tubes more appropriate than nasogastric tubes?	In a critically ill patient who's at higher risk for pulmonary aspiration, in a patient with delayed gastric emptying, or in a patient with pancreatic disease
When are long-term feeding tubes indicated?	When the duration of nutritional support is expected to exceed 2 weeks; long-term feeding tubes can be temporary or permanent
✎ **What are important nursing actions for a patient with a long-term feeding tube?**	1. Inspect the skin daily for irritation or skin breakdown. 2. Clean the skin and external retention device daily with soap and water.

✎ What's a percutaneous endoscopic gastrostomy (PEG) tube? A feeding tube that's placed by endoscopic guidance into the stomach through an opening in the skin, which provides nutrients and fluids directly to the stomach

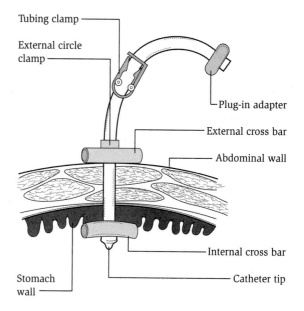

Tubing clamp

External circle clamp

Plug-in adapter

External cross bar

Abdominal wall

Internal cross bar

Stomach wall

Catheter tip

What are the advantages of a PEG tube versus gastric or small intestine feeding tubes?

1. Performed endoscopically with local anesthesia and conscious sedation (decreased risk of aspiration)
2. Less expensive
3. More aesthetically acceptable

What's a PEG/J tube? A dual-access feeding tube in which the G (gastric) lumen can be used for gastric decompression while the J (jejunostomy) lumen is used for enteral feedings; it reduces nausea and vomiting while promoting nutritional support tolerance

What are important considerations for gastrostomy tube size? Use a small-bore (large gauge or small French) tube for feedings and liquid medications only. Use a larger bore tube for administering protein powders or crushed medications.

When is a jejunostomy tube preferred over a gastrostomy tube? When bypassing the stomach is indicated, as in a patient with gastric disease, upper GI obstruction or fistula, absent gag reflex, or significant risk for esophageal reflux and aspiration

✎ What are important nursing considerations for a gastrostomy tube?	1. Don't administer tube feeds immediately after placement due to risk of ileus (typically wait at least 6 hours). 2. Assess the site daily for erythema, skin breakdown, or drainage. 3. Clean the skin and external rotation device daily with soap and water or saline. 4. If the tube has a balloon, check the volume every 7 to 10 days.
✎ What's an appropriate nursing action when a gastrostomy or jejunostomy tube is dislodged?	Contact the physician immediately, because the stoma will close quickly (as few as 20 minutes in the case of a jejunostomy) unless it's replaced.

Parenteral nutrition

What's total parenteral nutrition (TPN)?	Administration of nutritional support through a peripheral or central I.V. catheter ◾ *Use peripheral lines for less concentrated solutions with a lower caloric load. Use central lines for rapid dilution of high protein and glucose solutions.*
What are common indications for TPN therapy?	1. Long-term (more than 10 days) supplemental nutrition secondary to inability to obtain adequate energy, protein, and other requirements through oral or enteral feedings (chemotherapy, radiation therapy, intractable vomiting or hyperemesis gravidarum) 2. Severe gut dysfunction (massive small bowel obstruction, inflammatory bowel diseases, radiation enteritis) 3. Inability to tolerate enteral feedings 4. High catabolic conditions in which the gut can't be used within 1 week (severe burns, major trauma, closed head injury)
✎ **How should TPN therapy be initiated?**	Gradually, for the first 48 to 72 hours to allow the pancreas to adapt to the increased circulating glucose and to prevent refeeding syndrome (electrolyte abnormalities); may require insulin due to increase in circulating glucose
What types of central lines may be utilized for TPN infusion?	Peripherally inserted central catheter, Hickman, Groshong, Port-A-Cath, or temporary central line

❧ What are the potential complications of TPN therapy?

Infection (fungal and bacterial) and sepsis, metabolic disturbances, and problems with the central line catheter (insertion complications, dislodgment, and thrombosis of a great vein) as well as the development of a fatty liver (steatosis) with chronic use

❧ What's the concern with abrupt discontinuation of TPN?

Hypoglycemia; because TPN solutions typically have high glucose concentrations, hyperinsulinemia can result unless therapy is tapered gradually (over 4 to 6 hours while increasing oral intake)

Total parenteral nutrition

❧ What nursing assessments should you perform for a patient receiving TPN?

1. Obtain daily weights.
2. Monitor intake and output every shift.
3. Monitor blood glucose at least daily.
4. Use an infusion pump to ensure accurate infusion rate.
5. Observe for signs of phlebitis.
6. Observe for signs of hyperglycemia, hyperkalemia, hypokalemia, and electrolyte abnormalities.
7. Check the expiration date and assess for signs of contamination of TPN solution before administration.

❧ What are safety considerations for a patient receiving TPN therapy?

1. Don't use the central line for TPN infusion until catheter placement is confirmed by X-ray.
2. Refrigerate solution until 30 minutes prior to administration.
3. Use aseptic technique when connecting the I.V. tubing and filter to the central catheter as well as when changing the occlusive dressing over the insertion site.
4. Never add anything to TPN solution (it must be prepared by pharmacist or trained technician using aseptic technique under hooded laminar air flow).
5. Don't use the TPN lumen of a central catheter for administration of blood products or antibiotics, for drawing blood, or for monitoring central venous pressure.

❧ How often should you rotate the administration site for a patient receiving peripheral TPN?

Every 48 to 72 hours; sooner if symptoms of infiltration or infection develop

✎ **What are important nursing actions involved in the care of TPN tubing?**	1. Change the tubing every 72 hours (lipid tubing every 24 hours). 2. Label the tubing and occlusive dressing with the time and date of each change.

Types of diets

What's a regular diet?	A diet without restrictions, typically adequate in amounts of all nutrients
For what reasons are patients ordered to have nothing by mouth?	1. Preoperative procedure or immediately postoperative procedure 2. Severe nausea and vomiting 3. Inability to chew or swallow 4. Known or suspected intestinal obstruction 5. Severe, acute pancreatitis
✎ **What foods are permitted on a clear liquid diet?**	Broth, pulpless juices, coffee, tea, flavored ices, and clear liquid nutritional supplements such as Resource
✎ **What foods are permitted on a full liquid diet?**	All of those on a clear liquid diet in addition to milk, ice cream, cream soups, Cream of Wheat, and nutritional supplements, such as Boost or Ensure
✎ **What's a soft diet?**	A regular diet that has been modified to eliminate hard-to-digest and hard-to-chew foods (typically eliminates high-fiber and high-fat foods) that may be prescribed for patients with chewing or swallowing difficulties or extreme weakness Exclude raw fruits and vegetables, tough meats, and chewy breads. A soft diet may also be recommended to alleviate mild intestinal or stomach discomfort. For this reason, exclude spicy or heavily seasoned foods as well as fried, greasy foods.
✎ **What's a mechanical soft diet?**	A solid diet in which fruits and vegetables are soft-cooked or puréed, and meats are usually ground and moistened with gravy or sauce to ease chewing and swallowing A mechanical soft diet is typically indicated for persons with dysphagia (swallowing difficulty), or esophageal stricture and those recovering from head, neck, or mouth surgery. However, it isn't intended for patients with severe dysphasia (inability to speak) due to risk for aspiration.

What's a puréed diet?

Foods that are blended to the consistency of mashed potatoes, which is the easiest consistency for a dysphasic patient to swallow

What types of foods are included in a post-Nissen fundoplication diet?

Very soft, moist foods; attempt clear liquids first, followed by a progression to solids, such as scrambled eggs, meats in a casserole or with gravy, and well-cooked vegetables; avoid fresh fruit with skins, nuts, dried fruit, and crunchy peanut butter

What dietary considerations exist for a patient after a Whipple procedure (pancreaticoduodenectomy)?

1. Limit fat intake to 10 to 15 g/meal.
2. Eat smaller, more frequent meals.
3. Monitor glucose and count carbohydrates (high incidence of diabetes).

What's the recommended diet following gastric bypass surgery?

A diet of puréed foods in small proportions for a specified number of weeks with a slow progression to solid food as tolerated; avoid sugar

▪ *The "new" stomach following gastric bypass can hold about 3 tbs of food per meal.*

What's an anti-dumping diet?

A diet low in refined sugar and other simple carbohydrates, which prevents diarrhea following gastric surgery (gastrectomy, vagotomy, pyloroplasty); encourage small, frequent meals with high protein content and fluid consumption between meals rather than during them

What's a low-sodium diet?

A diet restricting sodium to less than 2 g; typically prescribed for patients with hypertension as well as those with renal, hepatic, or cardiac disease

What's a cardiac diet?

A diet low in fat (less than 50 to 65 g/day), sodium (less than 3 to 4 g/day), and cholesterol (less than 200 mg/day)

What's a low-fat diet?

A diet in which fat is restricted to 10 to 20 g/meal; it's intended for postpancreatitis patients or for certain medical tests

What's a consistent carbohydrate diet?

A diabetic diet in which a set number of carbohydrates (usually 45 to 70 g) are provided per meal to better regulate postprandial blood sugars

What's a high-fiber diet?

A diet high in indigestible fiber (whole grains, raw vegetables, nuts, and seeds); recommended for patients with diverticulosis or constipation; may reduce the risk of colon cancer; the American Dietetic Association recommends 25 to 35 g of fiber per day

✎ What's a low-residue diet?

A diet low in indigestible fiber used to decrease stool output; commonly used after an intestinal obstruction due to inflammatory bowel disease; avoid whole grains, raw fruits, raw vegetables, and juices with pulp, nuts, and seeds

✎ When is a low-tyramine diet recommended?

When a patient is taking a monoamine oxidase inhibitor; avoid cheese, smoked fish, non-fresh meats such as liver, vermouth wines, meat extracts, yeast extracts, brewer's yeast, sauerkraut, beer, and ale

✎ When is a low-phenylalanine diet recommended?

For persons with phenylketonuria (PKU), because they're unable to convert excess amounts of phenylalanine (essential amino acid) to tyrosine; accumulation of phenylalanine in the blood can result in progressive brain damage and mental retardation.

Because most foods containing protein also contain phenylalanine, persons with PKU should avoid meats, eggs, fish, milk, legumes, and cheese. Diet sweeteners such as aspartame (Nutrasweet) that contain phenylalanine should also be avoided.

Nursing skills

What's the proper technique for inserting a nasogastric (NG) tube?

1. Explain the procedure to the patient.
2. Assess the nares for obstructions or deformities.
3. Estimate how far to insert the tube by measuring from the tip of the patient's nose to the tip of her earlobe (a), and then from this point to the tip of the sternum (b).

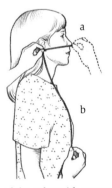

4. Lubricate the tip of the tube with a water-soluble lubricant. Consider an anesthetic lubricant such as viscous lidocaine.

5. Instruct the patient to hyperextend her neck and insert the tube (natural curve toward patient) along the floor of the nostril towards the ear on that side.
6. Instruct the patient to tilt her head forward and drink through a straw or swallow repeatedly as the tube is advanced into the nasopharynx.
7. Assess placement to ensure proper positioning in the stomach after the tube is advanced to the estimated point.
8. Secure the tube by taping it to the bridge of the patient's nose to prevent dislodgment.

What are important safety considerations after placement of a new NG tube?

1. Observe closely for signs of obvious distress and ask the patient to speak or hum to ensure the tube isn't in the trachea (may interfere with speaking abilities).
2. Avoid feeding through the tube until proper placement is confirmed.

◥ *Coughing and choking are more likely to occur when an NG tube has entered the respiratory tract.*

◥ What methods can determine proper positioning of a large-bore NG feeding tube?

1. Making radiographic verification (most reliable; perform after initial placement)
2. Measuring external length of tube and compare before each feeding, or assessing markings on the tube
3. Testing aspirate pH (1.0 to 3.0 for stomach contents, although pH may be neutral to basic in patients receiving a proton-pump inhibitor)
4. Insufflating 5 to 20 ml of air into the tube and auscultating for a gurgling, whooshing, or bubbling sound over the stomach
5. Assessing for presence of bile in aspirate

At what intervals should a nurse assess proper placement of an NG tube?

Before each intermittent feeding and at regular intervals (at least once per shift) when administering continuous feedings

◥ How is an NG tube irrigated?

30 to 60 ml of irrigating solution is slowly injected into the tube, followed by gentle aspiration of the solution.

How is an NG tube flushed?

By instilling 20 to 30 ml of tepid water via a large syringe (30 to 60 ml)

◥ *A smaller syringe increases the risk of rupture of the tube.*

When should you suspect a tube dislodgment?

After episodes of intense coughing, sneezing, and vomiting, or if the tape becomes loose and the distance between the nares and the tip of the tube appears longer

What's the proper technique for removing an NG tube?

1. Explain the process to the patient and provide a tissue for wiping his nose after tube removal.
2. Detach the tube from the suction apparatus.
3. Instill 50 ml of air into the tube (to clear any contents).
4. Detach the tape securing the tube to the nose.
5. Ask the patient to take a deep breath and hold it (this closes the glottis and prevents aspiration).
6. Pinch the tube and quickly withdraw the tube.
7. Encourage the patient to blow his nose and clear the nostrils.
8. Measure and record the amount of gastric drainage.

4

Pain management

Basic concepts of pain management

What's pain?
An unpleasant sensory and emotional experience commonly associated with tissue damage

What's pain threshold?
The least level of pain that an individual can perceive

What's pain tolerance?
The greatest level of pain that an individual can tolerate

What's a nociceptor?
A receptor preferentially sensitive to noxious stimuli (chemical, mechanical, and thermal)

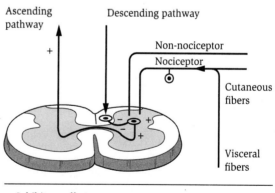

Ascending pathway

Descending pathway

Non-nociceptor

Nociceptor

Cutaneous fibers

Visceral fibers

− Inhibitory effect
+ Excitatory effect

What's a noxious stimulus?
One that's potentially or actually damaging to body tissue

✎ What's analgesia?
Absence of pain in response to stimulation that would normally be painful

✎ What's anesthesia?
Absence of all sensory modalities

✎ What's paresthesia?
An abnormal sensation, either spontaneous or provoked

✎ What's neuralgia?
Pain that occurs in the distribution of a nerve or nerves

✎ What's neuropathy?
A disturbance of function or pathologic change in a nerve

What's radiculopathy?
A disturbance of function or pathologic change in one or more nerve roots

✎ What's radiating pain?
Pain that travels to another body area, such as jaw or shoulder pain with a myocardial infarction (MI)

✎ What's intractable pain?
Pain that persists despite using maximal interventions

✎ What's referred pain?
Pain experienced in an area distant from the site of the stimulus; it occurs when nerve fibers serving the area of the body distant from the site of the stimulus pass in close proximity to the stimulus
An example is myocardial ischemia, which can be experienced as left arm, shoulder, or jaw pain.

What's phantom pain?
Painful sensations in an amputated extremity, as if the part were still attached

How is acute pain defined?
Normal response to injury or painful stimulus; short duration (less than 6 months); has an identifiable, immediate onset and a predictable and limited duration; usually subsides when the stimulus is removed and healing occurs

How is chronic pain defined?
Abnormal processing of sensory input by the nervous system; duration more than 6 months (constant or intermittent); specific cause may not be identified; may exist despite healing and irrespective of physical cause

Biology of pain

✎ What causes pain in tissue injury?

The release of prostaglandins, bradykinins, histamine, serotonin, acetylcholine, and substance P, which depolarize adjacent nociceptors

What are prostaglandins?

Hormone-like chemicals made in response to cell injury that are the chief mediators of inflammation; they're also involved in wound healing, nerve growth, differentiation of immune cells, ovulation, and initiation of labor

What's cyclooxygenase (COX)?

The enzyme necessary for the conversion of arachidonic acid to prostaglandins; the two known forms are COX-1 and COX-2

⚡ *COX-1 protects the stomach lining and intestines. COX-2 produces prostaglandins involved in the inflammatory response.*

How is pain transmitted?

Peripheral nociceptors detect a noxious stimulus and send signals (action potentials) along myelinated A and unmyelinated C nerve fibers to the dorsal horn of spinal cord. The signals then travel to the spinothalamic tract of the spinal cord to the cortex and thalamus of the brain where pain is perceived.

⚡ *Myelinated A nerve fibers are responsible for rapid transmissions and sharp pain. Unmyelinated C nerve fibers are responsible for slow transmissions and burning sensation.*

What's the function of the efferent pathway?

Modulation or inhibition of afferent pain signals

Assessment of pain

How does the body inhibit pain transmission?

By releasing enkephalins and endorphins (endogenous morphines), which block pain impulse transmission in the spinal cord and brain by inhibiting the release of excitatory neurotransmitters

What factors should you include in a pain assessment?

1. *Location:* verbal response or by marking the location of the pain on a drawing of the body
2. *Intensity:* patient's self-reporting using a pain scale
3. *Duration:* onset, length, and pattern of pain (steady, constant, intermittent, periodic)
4. *Frequency:* how often pain occurs over a specific time period
5. *Character:* identifies the quality of pain (sharp, throbbing, stabbing)

What types of scales can you use to assess pain intensity?

1. *Numeric:* graphic scale from 0 (no pain) to 10 (worst pain imaginable)
2. *Faces:* series of descriptive faces ranging from happy to crying (children and adults with language barriers)
3. *Visual analog:* 10-cm line with no pain on the left end and worst pain on the right end; distance of the patient's mark from the zero is measured and reported in cm

How do you select a pain scale?

Based on the patient's age, cognitive ability, and preference

How do you assess pain in an unconscious patient?

Physiologic responses

What factors affect perception of pain?

Patient's experience of pain (different for each person), as well as physical and psychological factors

What effect does anxiety have on pain perception?

Increases pain perception

What physiologic changes commonly occur with acute pain?

Pain causes an increased sympathetic response, which can lead to tachycardia, increased cardiac workload, increased oxygen consumption, hypertension, perspiration, and pallor.

Treatment of pain

What interventions treat pain?

1. *Nonpharmacologic:* distraction, relaxation, guided imagery, therapeutic touch, biofeedback, massage, acupuncture, hypnosis, transcutaneous electrical nerve stimulation (TENS) unit, neuroablation, and surgery
2. *Pharmacologic:* nonopioid analgesics, opioid analgesics, adjuvant analgesics, and anesthetics (local and systemic)

What's distraction and how does it treat pain?

A technique in which attention is directed away from the pain with active or passive cognitive distracters

What's relaxation and how does it treat pain?

It elongates muscle fibers, decreases the neural impulses sent to the brain, and reduces the activity of the brain and body systems. The relaxation response is triggered by techniques that incorporate a repetitive mental focus.

What's biofeedback?

It's used as a supplement to relaxation exercises to assist the patient in learning how to control specific autonomic system responses.

How does biofeedback treat pain?

It uses instruments to provide visual or auditory information concerning autonomic physiologic functions of the body (muscle tension and skin temperature).

What's guided imagery and how does it treat pain?

Using the conscious mind to create mental images; these images evoke physical changes in the body through distraction from pain

What's therapeutic touch and how does it treat pain?

Involves realignment of the body's energy fields, which demonstrate aberrant patterns when body systems are insulted; the clinician directs her own interpersonal energy to flow through her hands to help another

What's massage and how does it treat pain?

Manipulation of soft tissue to increase circulation; it improves muscle tone and promotes relaxation

What's acupuncture and how does it treat pain?

A method of producing analgesia or improving health by inserting needles into specific points on the body thought to enhance the flow of *chi,* or "life energy"

What's hypnosis and how does it treat pain?

A therapy involving conscious relaxation in association with clinician-designed suggestions and exercises that promotes increased energy and more restful sleep as well as decreased pain perception

✎ **What's TENS and how does it treat pain?**	The delivery of an electrical current through electrodes applied to the skin at trigger points, over painful areas, or over a peripheral nerve; TENS decreases pain by stimulating nonpain receptors in the same area as the fibers that transmit the pain
✎ **What are nerve blocks and how do they treat pain?**	Infiltration of a local anesthetic (lidocaine or bupivacaine) around a peripheral nerve to produce anesthesia in an area supplied by the nerve; corticosteroids may also be injected with the anesthetic agent to reduce edema and irritation, which can provide analgesia for several weeks
What's neuroablation and how does it treat pain?	Using chemical (alcohol) or thermal (radiofrequency) agents to destroy neural tissue to control chronic pain and reduce regional sympathetic overactivity
How does surgery treat pain?	Neurosurgical interventions destroy the sensory division of a spinal or peripheral nerve (sympathectomies)

✎ **What are nursing action in designing a pain treatment plan?**

1. Individualize the route of administration and use the least invasive route unless contraindicated.
2. Monitor the patient closely for drug effectiveness and for development of adverse reactions, especially when beginning or changing analgesic regimens.
3. Educate the patient about sensations expected during and following interventions to minimize anxiety.
4. Inform the patient that decreased activity due to pain increases the risk of complications of immobility.

✎ **How can you assess the effectiveness of pain treatment interventions?**

1. Patient rating of intensity (pain scales)
2. Hemodynamic changes (blood pressure, pulse)
3. Behavioral indicators (withdrawing, grimacing)
4. Affective indicators (depression, anxiety)
5. Socioeconomic indicators (level of disability)
6. Sociocultural indicators (family interactions)

Pharmacology related to pain management

Nonopioid analgesics

SALICYLATES (ASPIRIN)

What are common uses of aspirin?	Treat thrombolytic disorders and prophylaxis against MI and stroke
What life-threatening complications are associated with aspirin?	Reye's syndrome

What are contraindications to using aspirin?	Bleeding diathesis (thrombocytopenia, uremia, liver failure), glucase 6 phosphate dehydrogenase deficiency, immenent surgery, pregnancy, and in children under age 12 with suspected influenza or chicken pox
How does aspirin affect bleeding time?	It's doubled for about 1 week after taking 2 aspirin.

■ *Discontinue aspirin 1 week prior to surgery or an invasive procedure*

NONSTEROIDAL ANTI-INFLAMMATORY DRUGS (NSAIDs)

How do NSAIDs work?

Inhibit prostaglandin synthesis by inhibiting the enzyme cyclooxygenase (COX), decrease platelet aggregation, and vasodilate peripheral vessels (antipyretic activity)

What are the common uses of NSAIDs?

1. Relieve mild to moderate pain associated with rheumatoid arthritis, osteoarthritis, dysmenorrhea, gout, and musculoskeletal disorders
2. Decrease inflammation
3. Reduce fever (antipyretic)

What are examples of NSAIDs?

1. *Nonselective COX inhibitors:* ibuprofen (Motrin, Nuprin, Advil) and naproxen (Aleve, Anaprox)
2. *COX-1 and COX-2 inhibitors:* celecoxib (Celebrex), ketorolac (Toradol), diclofenac (Voltaren, Cataflam), piroxicam (Feldene), and indomethacin (Indocin), rofecoxib (Vioxx), valecoxib (Bextra)

✎ What adverse reactions are commonly associated with NSAIDs?

Dyspepsia, nausea, vomiting, rash, bruising, bleeding, and fluid retention

✎ What life-threatening complications are associated with NSAIDs?

GI bleeding, seizures, hepatitis (long-term), pancytopenia, angioedema, nephrotoxicity

✎ What are contraindications to using NSAIDs?

Peptic ulceration, asthma (can induce bronchospasm), impaired renal function, hypersensitivity to NSAIDs, hypersensitivity to sulfonamides (Celebrex).

What drugs, when used in combination with NSAIDs, increase the risk of gastric ulceration?

Glucocorticoids, alcohol, and bisphosphonates (Fosamax, Actonel)

What are clinical manifestations of NSAID toxicity?

Tinnitus, blurred vision, GI distress, nausea, vomiting, lethargy, confusion, headache

What are important nursing actions when administering NSAIDs?

1. Advise the patient to take with food, milk, or water.
2. Instruct the patient to avoid alcohol.
3. Instruct the patient to notify the physician if gastric irritation is persistent or severe.
4. Instruct the patient to report decreased urine output or significant fluid retention.
5. Warn the patient about photosensitivity.

What's a common use of ketorolac, a COX-1 inhibitor?

Because it's the only NSAID approved for I.V. administration, it's the drug of choice for managing moderate postoperative pain (during nothing-by-mouth status) when opioids are inadvisable.

What are the advantages of selective COX-2 inhibitors?

Provide anti-inflammatory and analgesic effects with a decreased risk of GI bleeding and other adverse effects associated with nonselective COX inhibitors

ACETAMINOPHEN (TYLENOL)

How does acetaminophen work?

Decreases prostaglandin synthesis in the central nervous system (CNS) (heat-regulating center of the hypothalamus); however, it lacks anti-inflammatory and antirheumatic activities

What are common uses of acetaminophen?

Treatment of mild to moderate pain and fever reduction

What are the common adverse reactions of acetaminophen?

Nausea, vomiting, abdominal pain, and rash

What are serious reactions associated with acetaminophen?

Anaphylaxis, hepatotoxicity, nephrotoxicity, pancytopenia, hemolytic anemia, and angioedema

What are relative contraindications to using acetaminophen?

Hypersensitivity, impaired renal or hepatic function, or chronic alcohol use

What drug is used in the treatment of acetaminophen overdose?

N-acetylcysteine (Mucomyst)

What are important nursing actions in preventing acetaminophen overdose?	1. Instruct the patient to avoid alcohol. 2. Instruct the patient to limit consumption of acetaminophen to 4 g/day (risk of hepatotoxicity).

Opioid analgesics

How do opioids work?	Bind to the opioid receptors and mimic actions of the endogenous regulatory molecules; opioids reduce pain perception without a loss of consciousness
What's the common use for opioid analgesics?	Management of severe pain arising from deep or visceral structures
✎ **What are common adverse effects of opioid analgesics?**	Dry mouth, nausea, vomiting, pruritus (histamine release), sedation, confusion, miosis, respiratory depression (decreased sensitivity of respiratory centers to carbon dioxide), cough suppression, hypotension from vasodilation, constipation, biliary spasm, and urinary retention (increased smooth muscle tone)
✎ **What life-threatening reactions are associated with opioid analgesics?**	Respiratory depression and hypotension are the most common. Others include bradycardia, anaphylaxis, laryngospasm (fentanyl), bronchoconstriction (fentanyl), circulatory collapse, arrhythmias, cardiac arrest, increased intracranial pressure (ICP) (meperidine), and seizures (meperidine and hydrocodone).
What are relative contraindications to using opioid analgesics?	1. Hypersensitivity to opioids 2. Head injury, increased ICP, or seizure disorder 3. Impaired renal function or prostatic hyperplasia 4. Impaired hepatic function 5. Asthma, emphysema, or chronic lung disease 6. Impaired cardiovascular function or hypotension 7. Inflammatory bowel disease, bowel obstruction, or biliary disease 8. Pregnancy (fetus can become addicted and develop withdrawal symptoms after birth) or breast-feeding
✎ **What drugs should you use with caution in combination with opioid analgesics?**	1. CNS depressants, such as antihistamines, tranquilizers, seizure medications, muscle relaxants, and sleep aids 2. Monoamine oxidase inhibitors, especially in combination with meperidine 3. Tricyclic antidepressants, such as amitriptyline (Elavil) 4. Anticoagulants, such as warfarin (Coumadin) 5. Rifampin 6. Zidovudine (AZT, Retrovir)

✎ **What are important nursing actions when administering opioid analgesics?**

1. Assess pain level on a pain scale.
2. Assess vital signs, especially respiratory rate.
3. Instruct the patient to change positions slowly (orthostatic hypotension).
4. Assist with ambulation and putting up side rails while in bed.
5. Instruct the patient to avoid alcohol and other CNS depressants.
6. Instruct the patient to avoid driving or operating heavy machinery.
7. For long-term use, educate the patient about withdrawal symptoms (nausea, vomiting, cramps, and fever).

▨ *If the respiratory rate is less than 12 breaths/minute, withhold the drug and notify the physician.*

How is codeine commonly used?

Cough suppression and relief of mild to moderate pain

How is hydrocodone (Hycodan) commonly used?

Moderate pain relief and cough suppression

How is methadone (Dolophine) commonly used?

Severe, chronic pain as well as opiate withdrawal and heroin addiction

How is oxycodone (Percocet, Percodan, OxyContin) commonly used?

Treatment of moderate to severe pain

How is morphine (Duramorph, MS Contin) commonly used?

Treatment of severe pain

▨ *Due to first pass metabolism, oral morphine dosing must be larger than parenteral doses.*

How is hydromorphone (Dilaudid) commonly used?

Severe pain in cancer patients (eight times more potent than morphine)

How is fentanyl (Sublimaze, Duragesic) commonly used?

General anesthetic (100 times more potent than morphine) and prolonged analgesia for chronic pain (72 hours for transdermal patches)

What are the advantages of using fentanyl instead of morphine?

Less histamine release than morphine, so patients experience less hypotension and skin rash

How is pentazocine (Talwin) commonly used?

Treatment of moderate to severe pain

How is meperidine (Demerol) commonly used?

Treatment of acute pain (only a few days duration), pain from biliary spasms, and management of medication-induced rigors

Avoid meperidine and pentazocine in patients with cardiovascular risks, because they may increase myocardial oxygen demand.

Avoid meperidine in patients with a history of seizures and renal impairment.

How is propoxyphene (Darvon-N) commonly used?

Treatment of mild to moderate pain

Aside from respiratory depression, what life-threatening condition is associated with propoxyphene?

Hyperthermia (especially in elderly patients)

How is butorphanol (Stadol) commonly used?

Treatment of moderate to severe pain and migraines

How is nalbuphine (Nubain) commonly used?

Treatment of moderate to severe pain, especially in patients with cardiovascular risks

How is tramadol (Ultram) commonly used?

Management of moderate to severe pain

How does tramadol work in relation to other opioids?

It's a central analgesic with weak opioid action that inhibits noradrenaline and serotonin reuptake. The major advantages are that it doesn't cause histamine release and it doesn't affect heart rate.

What are examples of combination analgesics?

1. Oxycodone and acetaminophen (Percocet, Endocet, Roxicet, and Tylox)
2. Oxycodone and aspirin (Percodan)
3. Hydrocodone and acetaminophen (Vicodin, Lortab, Lorcet)
4. Hydrocodone and ibuprofen (Vicoprofen)
5. Hydrocodone and guaifenesin (Vicodin Tuss, Hycotuss)
6. Propoxyphene and acetaminophen (Darvocet N)

What types of drugs are used as adjuvant analgesics?	Antidepressants and anticonvulsants such as gabapentin (Neurontin)
What's patient-controlled analgesia (PCA)?	An infusion pump activated by the patient to deliver a preset dose of an I.V. (or epidural) opioid; a specified timing interval (lock-out period) between doses and a maximal hourly limit (to prevent an overdose) are programmed into the pump; a continuous infusion (basal rate) may also be programmed
What advantages are associated with PCA use?	More consistent plasma drug level, decreased respiratory depression (I.V. route), and improved patient satisfaction (control)
What medications do PCA infusions administer?	Fentanyl (Sublimaze) and morphine ◪ *Instruct patients to activate the pump prior to painful activities, such as ambulation and dressing changes.*
What's an epidural infusion?	Delivery of a continuous infusion of medication into the epidural space (L2) through a catheter
What's the advantage of epidural opioid therapy?	Decrease in systemic adverse effects
✎ **What are important nursing actions for a patient with an epidural infusion catheter?**	1. Monitor neurologic, respiratory, motor, and sensory status. 2. Assess for pruritus, nausea, vomiting, and bladder distention. 3. Instruct the patient to report any leg numbness or weakness. 4. Assess the integrity of epidural catheter system and occlusive dressing.

OPIOID OVERDOSE

✎ **What's the triad of signs of opioid overdose?**	Respiratory depression, pinpoint pupils, and obtundation (decreased mental status)
How does an opioid antagonist work?	Reverses the effects of opiates by preventing drugs and endogenous regulatory molecules from activating receptors

➤ What antagonist treats opioid overdose?	Naloxone (Narcan); because it's shorter-acting than opioids, repeat dosing may be necessary until respiratory and CNS depression are resolved

▶ *Naloxone (Narcan) treats opioid overdose and naltrexone (ReVia) treats opioid addiction.*

OPIOID ADDICTION AND WITHDRAWAL

What's tolerance?	A decreased responsiveness to the pharmacologic effects of a drug, resulting in the need for increased dosage to achieve the same effect
What's physical dependence?	Physical reliance on a drug that results in withdrawal symptoms if the drug is discontinued suddenly or reversed by an antagonist
What's addiction?	A pattern of compulsive drug use characterized by a continued craving for an opioid effect other than pain relief
➤ What drugs treat opioid addiction?	Naltrexone (ReVia) and methadone (heroin addiction)
➤ What are the clinical manifestations of opioid withdrawal?	Nausea, vomiting, diarrhea, anxiety, agitation, insomnia, tachycardia, fever, diaphoresis, piloerection (goose bumps), pupillary dilatation, lacrimation, rhinitis, severe muscle cramps, and abdominal pain

▶ *Withdrawal symptoms peak at 2 days and typically last up to 10 days.*

➤ What's the best method for minimizing withdrawal effects?	Taper the opioid dose gradually over 7 to 10 days.
What supplemental drugs can you use to control opioid withdrawal symptoms?	Clonidine and beta-adrenergic blockers; avoid opioid antagonists such as naloxone, because they will exacerbate withdrawal symptoms

5

Diagnostic and therapeutic procedures

General radiologic studies

Why are contrast agents used in some radiologic studies?

To highlight details of certain pathologic conditions

How are contrast agents classified?

1. *Radiopaque:* impenetrable to X-rays or other forms of radiation
2. *Radiolucent:* permits only partial transmission of X-rays

What are the two most commonly used contrast agents?

Barium (GI tract examinations) and iodine (GI and intravascular procedures); carbon dioxide, gadolinium, and water-soluble agents, such as Gastrografin, are also frequently used

✎ What complications can occur in association with contrast?

Adverse reactions can range from mild conditions, such as nausea and vomiting, to exacerbation of renal dysfunction and, possibly, severe anaphylactic reactions with cardiovascular collapse.

▷ Emergency equipment and supplies should be readily available when contrast agents are used due to the risk of anaphylaxis.

✎ What are possible contraindications for the use of contrast?

History of previous allergic reaction to contrast (three times more likely to have a subsequent reaction, although not necessarily more severe) and history of renal impairment (creatinine greater than 1.4 mg/dl) or diabetes (due to increased risk of renal failure)

▷ Persons with asthma or hay fever are more likely to experience an adverse reaction with iodine contrast.

✎ **What are impor-
tant nursing actions
for a patient undergo-
ing an imaging study
with contrast?**

1. Assess the patient for allergies to iodine-containing foods (shellfish, kale, cabbage, turnips, iodine salt).
2. Maintain nothing-by-mouth status before administering I.V. iodine contrast (must be at least 90 minutes apart).
3. Instruct the patient who is taking metformin (Glucophage) to stop the medication at the time of or just prior to the procedure, due to the risk of kidney dysfunction. Metformin should be withheld for 48 hours following a procedure involving a contrast agent.
4. Instruct the patient to increase fluid intake, if appropriate, after the procedure to facilitate iodine excretion.

◤ *Examinations that don't involve contrast should be scheduled before examinations that do involve contrast.*

◤ *Examinations involving iodine should precede those involving barium.*

X-ray

What's an X-ray?

A noninvasive procedure that projects X-ray beams through soft and bony body tissues to create images on film

**What are examples of
X-rays?**

Chest X-ray, mammogram, upper GI series, KUB (kidneys, ureters, bladder), excretory urography, barium enema study, and cholangiogram

◤ *The greater the structural density means the greater the degree of X-ray absorption. Therefore, dense structures appear white and air-filled areas are black.*

**What risks are
associated with X-ray?**

Exposure to small amounts of radiation

◤ *Pregnant women should avoid radiographic and fluoroscopic studies of the abdomen, pelvis, and lumbar spine whenever possible.*

**How should a patient
be prepared for an
X-ray?**

1. Instruct the patient to remove all metal and jewelry from the area being studied.
2. Place a metal shield over the genital area and abdominal organs to protect reproductive organs.
3. Inform the patient of the need to remain motionless and of the possible need to hold his breath for a brief period.

4. Explain to the patient that a change in position on a table or chair may be necessary, depending on the type of X-ray.
5. Explain to the patient that the test usually takes less than 30 minutes.

Angiography

What's angiography?	An invasive X-ray procedure used to visualize arteries and veins via catheterization using a radiopaque contrast agent
What are common uses of angiography?	Detecting vascular abnormalities, such as aneurysms, malformations, or occlusions as well as hypervascular tumors
✎ What risks are associated with angiography?	Development of embolus, damage to the blood vessel wall and bleeding are the most serious; other risks include infection at the incision site or allergic reaction to the contrast medium
What are possible contraindications for angiography?	Allergy to iodine or contrast agents; pregnancy (known or suspected); renal impairment; and coagulopathy (warfarin therapy, decreased platelets)

⚡ *Anticoagulants should be discontinued several days (preferably 1 week) before angiographic procedures.*

How should a patient be prepared for angiography?

1. Maintain nothing-by-mouth status at least 2 hours before the test.
2. Explain to the patient that the injection site is scrubbed with an antiseptic soap.
3. Explain to the patient that a sedative may be administered, but that he'll remain alert during the procedure.
4. Stress to the patient the importance of remaining as still as possible during the procedure (motion artifacts cause poor images).
5. Clarify with the patient that either the femoral artery (groin) or the brachial artery (upper arm) will be used as the catheter insertion site; contrast dye will be injected into the vessel being studied (some patients may need to have the injection site shaved).
6. Inform the patient that contrast dye injection may cause sensation of hot flashes and palpitations.
7. Explain to the patient that X-rays will be taken of the vessels to assess blood flow.

8. Explain to the patient that the catheter will be withdrawn and pressure will be applied to the puncture site. A pressure dressing, which should remain intact for at least 24 hours, will be applied.
9. Tell the patient that the test usually takes 30 minutes to 3 hours.

✎ What nursing care is required after angiography?

1. Keep the patient flat in bed for 4 to 6 hours without flexion of punctured extremity; normal bed rest until the next day.
2. Monitor vital signs and perform neurovascular checks at frequent intervals (Rule of Four: every 15 minutes for 1 hour; every 30 minutes for 2 hours; every hour for 4 hours and then every 4 hours).
3. Assess puncture site for bleeding, swelling, hematoma, or bruits. Check distal pulses of affected limb.
4. Maintain functional I.V. access.
5. Encourage fluids to facilitate excretion of contrast agent, unless contraindicated.

◤ *Notify the physician if an extremity develops numbness, tingling, decreased or absent pulses, blanching, coolness, or excessive blood loss following an angiographic procedure.*

Ultrasound

What's an ultrasound?

A noninvasive procedure that uses high-frequency sound waves to produce images that can determine the position, size, form, and nature of organs and body structures; it's especially useful to study soft tissues

What are examples of ultrasound?

Obstetric (fetal) ultrasound, echocardiogram, carotid duplex scan, and upper or lower extremity duplex scan

What's a Doppler ultrasound?

A form of ultrasound used to determine the patency of blood vessels and to determine blood flow characteristics (direction, velocity, disturbances)

What potential risks are associated with ultrasound?

No known adverse effects (painless)

How should a patient be prepared for an ultrasound?

1. Explain to the patient that a cool gel will be applied to the body area being studied to enhance sound wave conduction.
2. Explain to the patient that a probe will be moved across the specific body area.

3. Tell the patient that the test usually takes 30 minutes.
4. Explain to the patient that no specific preparation or posttest care is necessary, unless otherwise directed.

Magnetic resonance imaging

What's magnetic resonance imaging (MRI)?

A noninvasive procedure that combines magnetism, radio waves, and a computer to produce three-dimensional images of tissues and structures in the body; most useful for examining the head, central nervous system, and spine; also used for identifying tumors, strokes, degenerative diseases, inflammation, or infection in other organs or soft tissues

What are possible contraindications for an MRI?

1. Known or suspected presence of internal metallic objects (surgical clips, Greenfield filter, metal flakes in eyes from welding, lodged bullets, pacemakers, prosthetic devices, artificial joints)
2. Renal dysfunction or failure
3. Allergy to contrast agent
4. Pregnancy (may increase amniotic fluid temperature)

▶ *A screening X-ray should be performed prior to an MRI if the presence of metallic objects is suspected because they may distort the images.*

What potential risks are associated with MRI?

May increase temperature of amniotic fluid

✎ How should a patient be prepared for an MRI?

1. Maintain nothing-by-mouth status (or clear liquids) before abdominal or pelvic study.
2. Remove all metal objects (jewelry, hairpins, hearing aids, glasses, wigs with metal clips, hair extensions, nonpermanent dentures, keys, credit cards).
3. Explain to the patient that he'll lie on a movable bed that's placed inside a large tube surrounded by a circular magnet.
4. Explain to the patient that he'll hear loud, repetitive clicking noises throughout the procedure.
5. Stress the importance of remaining still during the test.
6. Explain to the patient that an intercom system will be available for constant communication with the staff during the test.
7. Make it clear to the patient that a mild sedative may be provided, if he's claustrophobic.
8. Tell the patient that the test usually takes 30 to 90 minutes.

What's magnetic resonance cholangiopancreatography? (MRCP)

MRI study of the pancreas and bile ducts

What's magnetic resonance angiography?

MRI study of blood vessels used to locate, diagnose, and treat cardiac disorders, stroke, and vascular diseases

Computed tomography scan

What's a computed tomography (CT) scan?

An X-ray procedure that combines many radiologic images with the assistance of a computer to produce cross-sectional images (slices) of internal organs and body structures without superimposing tissues on one another; may require contrast (oral or I.V.) if hollow vicera (intestines) and blood vessels are being studied

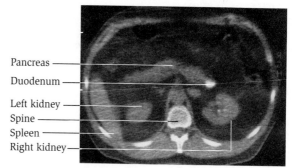

Pancreas
Duodenum
Left kidney
Spine
Spleen
Right kidney

What are the common uses of a CT scan?

Differentiating between normal and abnormal body structures (tumors from normal soft tissue, clotted blood from normal blood), and guiding placement of instruments for procedures

Bone appears white, air appears black, and soft tissues appear as varying shades of gray on CT scans.

What's a spiral (helical) CT?

A form of CT that uses a continuous corkscrew-scanning pattern to create three-dimensional data

What are potential risks of a CT scan?

Minimal radiation exposure

What are the most common adverse reactions to a CT scan?

Allergic reactions and renal impairment related to the contrast agent

✎ What are possible contraindications to a CT scan?	Allergy to iodine and renal dysfunction (especially in patients with diabetes) or failure

How should a patient be prepared for a CT scan?

1. Maintain nothing-by-mouth status (no solid foods on day of test and no clear liquids within 2 hours of the test).
2. Remove all metal objects.
3. Explain to the patient that he'll lie on a sliding table inside a large, donut-shaped machine.
4. Explain to the patient that periodic breath holding may be necessary during the test.
5. Explain to the patient that an intercom will be available for communication between him and staff throughout the test.
6. Tell the patient that the test usually takes 30 to 90 minutes.

✂ *CT equipment may be threatening to a patient because it's large and may be noisy. Appropriate patient preparation is imperative.*

Nuclear medicine

What's nuclear medicine?

A diagnostic modality that uses radioactive isotopes to evaluate the physiology of organ systems

What are examples of nuclear medicine tests?

Positron emission tomography (PET) scan, myocardial perfusions scans (exercise and pharmacologic stress tests, multiple-gated acquisition scan), ventilation-perfusion scan, thyroid scan, bone scan, and bone densitometry (dual energy X-ray absorptiometry scan)

What risks are associated with nuclear medicine?

Minimal radiation exposure (less than with chest X-ray) or reaction to radiopharmaceutical agent

✂ *Pregnancy is a contraindication for nuclear medicine tests; breast-feeding women should discard their breast milk for 3 days after a nuclear medicine study.*

How should a patient be prepared for a nuclear medicine test?

1. Obtain the patient's weight (dose is calculated by weight).
2. Explain to the patient that an isotope will be given orally or I.V. followed by a waiting period of 60 minutes before scanning the specific body part.

3. Instruct the patient to avoid foods high in iodine, such as seafood or table salt, for 3 days prior to the test if iodine will be used (thyroid scan).

Positron-emission tomography scan

What's a positron-emission tomography (PET) scan?

A computerized radiographic technique that utilizes radioactive substances to assess the metabolic activity of various body structures; images of molecular-level physiologic functions, including oxygen utilization, glucose metabolism, blood flow, and tissue perfusion, are produced as a result of the radioactivity emitted

What are common uses of a PET scan?

1. *Oncology:* early tumor detecting, tumor grading, and differentiation of new growth from necrotic tissue
2. *Cardiology:* determining blood flow, myocardial perfusion, and myocardial viability
3. *Neurology:* evaluating epilepsy, stroke, dementia from Alzheimer's or Parkinson's disease, and schizophrenia

What are potential risks of a PET scan?

Minimal radiation exposure; reaction to radiopharmaceutical agent

How should a patient be prepared for a PET scan?

In addition to the general patient preparation for a CT scan, the patient will be given a radioactive substance (usually I.V.). Fasting is required for all noncardiac PET scans.

The integumentary system

Skin biopsy

What's a skin biopsy?

A minimally invasive procedure for removal of a small (3 to 6 mm) skin sample for histopathologic study

What are common uses of a skin biopsy?

Diagnosing infection, malignancy, inflammatory disorders, or other growths of the skin

By what methods can a skin biopsy be obtained?

1. *Shave:* scraping of the outer part of the lesion
2. *Punch:* cutting of top layer of skin using an instrument and twisting motion
3. *Excision:* removal of the entire lesion using the end of a sharp blade

4. *Incision:* removal of the lesion with a scalpel blade when larger specimen is needed; sutures are usually required to close the incision

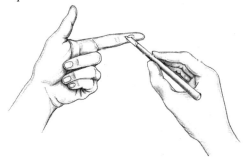

What risks are associated with a skin biopsy?	Infection and bleeding as well as possible scarring (minimal)
How should a patient be prepared for a skin biopsy?	1. Explain to the patient that the area being tested will be cleaned and then numbed by an anesthetic agent before the biopsy. 2. Explain to the patient that a small bandage or stitches may close the area. 3. Explain to the patient that any excessive erythema or drainage at the biopsy site should be reported to the physician.

The musculoskeletal system

Electromyography

What's electromyography (EMG)?	A minimally invasive study of the electrical activity generated in muscle at rest and during contraction; commonly used in conjunction with electroneurography
✎ **What are common uses of EMG?**	Identifying the site and cause of disorders that affect the muscles, peripheral nerves, and spinal cord; myasthenia gravis, muscular dystrophy, Guillain-Barré syndrome, and poliomyositis are conditions for which EMG is useful
What risks are associated with EMG?	Risks are minimal: rare occurrence of infection, mild discomfort related to needle insertion, and possible hematoma formation at the needle site
How should a patient be prepared for an EMG?	1. Explain to the patient that anticoagulants should be avoided for several days before an EMG (risk of hematoma).

2. Stress to the patient that smoking and caffeine should be avoided 2 to 3 hours before an EMG.
3. Explain to the patient the importance of relaxation; movement can cause false results.
4. Advise the patient that electrodes will be placed on the skin and several small needle electrodes will be placed into specific muscles.
5. Explain to the patient that *weak* electrical currents will record electrical activity of nerves and muscles.
6. Advise the patient that contraction of muscles may be necessary to evaluate the response to the weak electrical stimulation.
7. Tell the patient that the test usually takes 60 minutes (for each extremity).
8. Explain to the patient that warm compresses or mild analgesic may relieve mild discomfort associated with the electrical stimulation.

◤ *It's important to obtain baseline enzyme levels that are associated with muscle activity (creatine kinase, lactate dehydrogenase, aspartate aminotransferase) because they may be elevated for several days following an EMG.*

Myelography

What's a myelogram?

An invasive procedure that allows X-ray visualization of the spinal subarachnoid space and nerve roots after the introduction of a contrast agent

What are the common uses of myelography?

Identifying and assessing spinal cord stenosis or compression, herniated disks, and tumors

What are potential risks of myelography?

Infection, allergy to the contrast agent, and exposure to small amounts of radiation

✎ How should a patient be prepared for myelography?

1. Instruct the patient to discontinue metformin (Glucophage) 48 hours before the test and for several days after the test (increases risk of renal failure with contrast).
2. Withhold anticoagulants for several days before the test and obtain prothrombin time (PT) and International Normalized Ratio.
3. Assess pregnancy status of all females of childbearing age.
4. Provide the patient adequate hydration the evening before the test to prevent dehydration, which may cause posttest vomiting.
5. Inform the patient that he'll be placed on nothing-by-mouth status 4 hours before the test.

6. Explain to the patient that he'll be in a side-lying position with his legs curled up on a table. (The table may be tilted during the test, but the patient will be fastened securely.)
7. Advise the patient that the skin will be numbed using a small needle.
8. Explain to the patient that contrast dye may be injected into a lumbar site, which may result in feelings of pressure, nausea, headache, or warmness.
9. Advise the patient that a series of X-rays will be taken in several positions.
10. Stress to the patient that bed rest will be required for several hours after the test.
11. Tell the patient that the test may take up to 90 minutes.

✎ What are important nursing actions after a myelogram?

1. Elevate the head of the bed 45 degrees for a minimum of 8 hours to prevent headache from upward dispersion of contrast agent.
2. Obtain frequent vital signs (at least every 4 hours) for 24 hours.
3. Encourage fluid intake (reduces risk of headache, facilitates contrast excretion, and minimizes metallic taste).
4. Assess for bladder distention and appropriate output.
5. Administer analgesics for discomfort at injection site, as directed by the physician.

Arthrocentesis

What's arthrocentesis?

An invasive procedure involving the puncture of the space around a joint with a needle, which allows aspiration of fluid samples around the joint

What are the common uses of arthrocentesis?

Diagnosing infection, gout, or certain types of arthritis as well as draining accumulated fluid from a joint

What risks are associated with arthrocentesis?

Infection and bleeding at the puncture site

How should a patient be prepared for arthrocentesis?

1. Explain to the patient that the skin over the joint area will be cleaned and possibly numbed with a local anesthetic.
2. Advise the patient that a needle will be inserted into the fluid around the joint and aspirated until the desired amount is obtained.
3. Explain to the patient that slight pressure and a bandage will be applied after the needle is removed.

4. Explain to the patient that an ice pack or mild analgesic may be used to minimize discomfort at the puncture site.
5. Tell the patient that the test usually takes less than 30 minutes.

Bone marrow aspiration or biopsy

What's a bone marrow aspiration or biopsy?

An invasive procedure involving the aspiration of a sample of bone marrow (commonly from the iliac crest)

What are common uses of bone marrow aspiration or biopsy?

Diagnosing hematologic conditions (leukemias, multiple myeloma, lymphoproliferative disorders, severe anemia, thrombocytopenia, toxicity) or infectious diseases (tuberculosis, histoplasmosis)

What risks are associated with bone marrow aspiration or biopsy?

Bleeding is the most common; infection and fracture at the insertion site may also occur

How should a patient be prepared for a bone marrow aspiration or biopsy?

1. Explain to the patient that a local anesthetic will be used at the puncture site and that a mild sedative may be administered.
2. Explain to the patient that a needle will be inserted to collect a marrow sample.
3. Inform the patient that moderate discomfort may be experienced during the procedure.
4. Explain to the patient that a pressure dressing will be applied on the site once the needle is removed and that discomfort may be experienced for several days afterward.
5. Stress to the patient that bed rest will be required for at least 30 minutes after the test is completed.
6. Explain to the patient that analgesics or a sedative may be administered if necessary.
7. Tell the patient that the aspiration site will be observed closely for 24 hours for signs of bleeding.

Dual energy X-ray absorptiometry scan

What's a dual energy X-ray absorptiometry (DEXA) scan?

A minimally invasive procedure that involves a scanner and low-dose radiation beams to measure the density of the spine, hip, and forearm; also called bone densitometry

What are the common uses of a DEXA scan?

Diagnosing osteoporosis or osteopenia and predicting risk of bone fractures related to low bone density; fracture risk is determined by comparing the patient's bone mass to that of 25- to 35-year-old patients, which is measured in standard deviations. Risk of fracture increases 1½ to 2½ times for each standard deviations

What's a T-score?

Number of standard deviations for the patient in relation to normal young adults with mean peak bone mass

What risks are associated with a DEXA scan?

Minimal radiation exposure

How should a patient be prepared for a DEXA scan?

1. Assess whether the patient underwent a barium study, CT scan, or MRI with an I.V. contrast agent within 7 days (residual barium and contrast dye can interfere with the findings).
2. Stress to the patient that he must avoid calcium supplements for at least 24 hours before the study.
3. Explain to the patient that he'll lie on a table and may need to change positions for the scanner to measure different areas.
4. Tell the patient that the test usually takes 20 minutes for the hip and spine.

Bone scan

What's a bone scan?

A minimally invasive procedure that uses a radioisotope (usually technetium) for visualization of the skeleton to indicate areas of increased bone repair activity

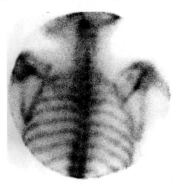

What are common uses of a bone scan?

Locating the presence of increased bone activity associated with metastatic disease, tumor, or infection

What risks are associated with a bone scan?

Minimal exposure to radiation

How should a patient be prepared for a bone scan?

1. Explain to the patient that it's important to void before the study to prevent obscuring of pelvic bones.
2. Advise the patient that a radioisotope will be administered I.V. followed by a 2- to 3-hour wait before the scanning process begins.
3. Explain to the patient that pictures will be taken for detection of concentrated areas of the isotope.
4. Explain to the patient that fluids will be encouraged after the scan to facilitate excretion of the isotope.
5. Tell the patient that the test usually takes less than 60 minutes.

◪ *The radioisotope mimics the physiologic effects of calcium (higher concentrations in areas of increased metabolic activity).*

The neurosensory system

EEG

What's an EEG?

A noninvasive test that measures and records the electrical impulses of the brain

What are the common uses of an EEG?

Diagnosing epilepsy, tumors, subdural hematomas, intracranial hemorrhages, cerebral infarcts, narcolepsy, Alzheimer's disease, and brain death; can also monitor cerebral activity during surgical anesthesia

✎ How should a patient be prepared for an EEG?

1. Explain to the patient that consuming caffeine should be avoided 12 hours before the test and that smoking just before the test should also be avoided.
2. Stress to the patient that his hair and scalp should be clean and that it shouldn't contain styling products.
3. Explain to the patient that electrodes will be attached to the scalp with gel.
4. Explain to the patient that *very weak* electrical stimulation will be used to record brain activity.
5. Stress to the patient the importance of remaining very still in a recumbent position with his eyes closed during the EEG.
6. Explain to the patient that he may be instructed to breathe deeply and quickly (hyperventilate).
7. Explain to the patient that he may be exposed to a rapidly flashing light (photostimulation).
8. Tell the patient that the test usually takes 60 minutes.

What's a sleep-EEG? An EEG performed after the patient has been awake the night before the test; the patient is then encouraged to sleep or rest during the test

Evoked potentials

What's an evoked potentials EEG?
A noninvasive procedure that uses EEG recording techniques and computer data processing to evaluate electrical responses in various regions of the brain in response to specific stimuli; provides information about auditory, sensory, and visual pathways

What are the common uses of an evoked potentials EEG?
Diagnosing multiple sclerosis and various hearing and visual disorders; also aids in assessing and diagnosing optic nerve disorders, tumors, brain stem function, and brain death

How should a patient be prepared for an evoked potentials EEG?
1. Discuss the EEG preparation.
2. Make sure that all jewelry is removed.
3. Explain to the patient that he may be asked to focus on a pattern of visual stimulation with one eye at a time.
4. Explain to the patient that there may be clicking sounds heard through earphones or small electrical stimuli delivered to peripheral nerves, during which the brain's response is recorded.

Lumbar puncture

What's a lumbar puncture?
An invasive procedure involving the collection of a small amount of cerebrospinal fluid (CSF) using a hollow needle inserted between lumbar vertebrae (usually between L3 and L4, or L4 and L5)

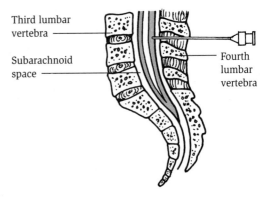

Third lumbar vertebra

Subarachnoid space

Fourth lumbar vertebra

What are common uses of a lumbar puncture?

Obtaining samples for the diagnosis of infections or inflammatory conditions, such as meningitis, encephalitis, multiple sclerosis, hemorrhage, lymphoma, or leukemia; injecting contrast medium or air for diagnostic studies

✎ What risks are associated with a lumbar puncture?

Infection or leakage of CSF

◤ *Lumbar punctures shouldn't be performed on patients with skin infections at or near the puncture site due to the risk of introducing organisms into the CSF.*

✎ How should a patient be prepared for a lumbar puncture?

1. Instruct the patient to empty his bladder before this procedure as a comfort measure.
2. Explain to the patient that he'll be on his side with his knees and head tucked toward his chest (increases space between vertebrae).
3. Explain to the patient that a local anesthetic will be injected with a small needle and a larger needle will then be inserted to drain the fluid.
4. Stress to the patient the importance of remaining as still as possible.
5. Explain to the patient that there may be slight pressure as the needle is inserted.
6. Explain to the patient that the needle will remain in the lumbar area for at least 1 minute before being removed, and a small bandage will then be placed over the site.
7. Tell the patient that the test usually takes 30 minutes and that it's usually performed at the bedside.
8. Inform the patient that he may experience a headache after the test and that lying flat, drinking fluids, and taking a mild analgesic will minimize symptoms.

✎ What are important nursing actions after a lumbar puncture?

1. Instruct the patient to remain flat in bed for at least 4 hours after the test.
2. Encourage fluids to prevent or minimize spinal headache.
3. Assess the puncture site for leakage and hematoma formation.

◤ *A physician should be notified immediately if leakage is noted from a lumbar puncture site.*

The endocrine system

Oral glucose tolerance test

What's an oral glucose tolerance test (OGTT)?

A minimally invasive test performed to assess blood glucose levels at timed intervals and to determine how the body metabolizes carbohydrates

What are common uses of an OGTT?	Diagnosing diabetes mellitus or other disorders that affect carbohydrate metabolism

How should a patient be prepared for an OGTT?

1. Instruct the patient to eat a high-carbohydrate diet and avoid alcohol for 3 days before the test.
2. Maintain nothing-by-mouth status 12 to 16 hours before the test; water is permitted during fasting period.
3. Explain to the patient that a fasting blood glucose and possibly a urine glucose will be checked the morning of the test.
4. Explain to the patient that he'll consume an oral solution of 100 to 300 g of glucose within a 5-minute time frame.
5. Explain to the patient that blood and urine samples will be collected 30, 60, and 120 minutes after he consumes the glucose solution. A 3-hour sample may be drawn to diagnose diabetes in pregnant women, and a 5-hour sample may be drawn to evaluate possible hypoglycemic episodes.

Water deprivation test

What's a water deprivation test?

A test that evaluates one's response to withholding water

What are common uses of water deprivation tests?

Assessing levels of antidiuretic hormone when disorders such as diabetes insipidus are suspected

How should a patient be prepared for a water deprivation test?

1. Withhold water for at least 4 hours (and perhaps up to 18 hours) before the test.
2. Explain to the patient that measuring the volume and osmolality of the urine will test the patient's response to the water deprivation; serum osmolality may also be tested.

Dexamethasone (cortisol) suppression test

What's a dexamethasone suppression test?

A minimally invasive test performed by administering dexamethasone (a synthetic steroid) to determine the effect on cortisol (a naturally occurring steroid hormone) production; in normal conditions, dexamethasone suppresses corticotropin, which then decreases cortisol levels

What are common uses of dexamethasone suppression tests?

Evaluating suspected overproduction of cortisol and diagnosing Cushing's syndrome

What risks are associated with dexamethasone suppression tests?

Minimal risk of bleeding or infection at venipuncture sites

How should a patient be prepared for a dexamethasone suppression test?

1. Advise the patient that medications (especially cortisol, estrogens, birth control pills, tetracycline, phenytoin, and spironolactone) should be discontinued at least 24 hours before the study.
2. Explain to the patient that two baseline blood cortisol levels will be drawn (8 a.m. and 4 p.m.).
3. Explain to the patient that dexamethasone (usually 1 mg) will be administered at 11 p.m. and a blood cortisol level will be drawn at 8 a.m. the next morning.
4. Advise the patient that fasting is required for the 8 a.m. blood draws.

Cortrosyn stimulation test

What's a cortrosyn stimulation test?

A minimally invasive test that measures plasma cortisol levels at specific time intervals after the administration of I.V. cortrosyn (a synthetic form of corticotropin)

What are common uses of cortrosyn stimulation tests?

To screen for adrenocortical insufficiency as occurs with Addison's disease

What risks are associated with cortrosyn stimulation tests?

Minimal risk of allergic reaction to cortrosyn

How should a patient be prepared for a cortrosyn stimulation test?

1. Explain to the patient that a baseline blood cortisol level will be drawn.
2. Explain to the patient that cortrosyn will be administered I.V.
3. Advise the patient that blood cortisol levels will be obtained again at 30- and 60-minute intervals after cortrosyn administration.

The respiratory system

Pulmonary function tests

What are pulmonary function tests (PFTs)?

A group of noninvasive tests used to evaluate pulmonary dysfunction based on perfusion, diffusion, and ventilation assessments; can determine cause of pulmonary dysfunction to be restrictive, obstructive, or both

What are common uses of PFTs?

1. Assessing respiratory status before surgery
2. Screening for pulmonary disease, such as asthma and emphysema
3. Evaluating the effects of a prescribed therapy
4. Measuring progression of pulmonary disease
5. Identifying preoperative patients at risk for development of pulmonary complications postoperatively

How should a patient be prepared for a PFT?

1. Advise the patient to avoid eating a heavy meal or smoking 4 to 8 hours before the test.
2. Advise the patient to wear nonrestrictive clothing.
3. Explain to the patient that he'll wear nose clips during the test.
4. Advise the patient that he'll breathe into a flexible tube (spirometer); he may be asked to change breathing patterns by inhaling and exhaling very quickly or very deeply.
5. Explain to the patient that he may inhale helium, nitrogen, or pure oxygen before or during testing.
6. Tell the patient that the test usually takes 45 minutes.

Adequate patient preparation is essential to alleviate the fear of breathlessness patients with respiratory impairment commonly experience.

Bronchoscopy

What's a bronchoscopy?

An endoscopic procedure that allows visualization of the larynx, trachea, and bronchi

What are common uses of a bronchoscopy?

1. Assessing for a foreign body, tumor, or other obstruction
2. Obtaining tissue biopsy or sputum sample
3. Aiding in diagnosis of cancer, tuberculosis, infection, and causes of bleeding

What risks are associated with a bronchoscopy?	Aspiration, hypoxemia, pneumothorax, bronchospasm, laryngospasm, infection, arrhythmias, and bleeding at biopsy site

How should a patient be prepared for a bronchoscopy?

1. Keep the patient on nothing-by-mouth status for 6 hours before the test (decreases risk of aspiration).
2. Remove the patient's dentures before the test.
3. Explain to the patient that a sedative may be given for relaxation and atropine may be given to decrease secretions.
4. Explain to the patient that a local anesthetic will be sprayed to numb his throat (general anesthesia is necessary if a rigid bronchoscope is used).
5. Advise the patient that a tube will be passed through his mouth and into the trachea for visualization of bronchioles and collection of tissue samples.
6. Caution the patient that some patients experience a false sensation of not being able to breathe as the scope is passed.
7. Tell the patient that the test usually takes 30 to 60 minutes.

What nursing care is required after bronchoscopy?

1. Place the patient in semi-Fowler's position to prevent aspiration of secretions.
2. Monitor vital signs, pulse oximeter, respiratory rate, lung sounds, and skin and nail bed color.
3. Assess for the return of the gag reflex and development of respiratory distress at frequent intervals (due to laryngeal edema).
4. Provide gargles to soothe pharyngitis (after return of gag reflex).
5. Explain to the patient that a small amount of blood in sputum is common if a tissue biopsy was collected.

Notify the physician immediately if the patient develops inspiratory stridor, pallor, or increasing dyspnea

Thoracentesis

What's a thoracentesis?

An invasive procedure involving the insertion of a needle into the pleural space for aspiration of fluid or air

What are common uses of a thoracentesis?

1. Determining cause of effusions (exudates or transudates)
2. Cytologic examination for red and white blood cell counts; protein, glucose, and amylase concentration; and infections (tuberculosis, empyema) or malignant cells

⚡ *Exudates are fluid collections that accumulate as a result of an inflammatory process. Transudates are fluid collections that result from noninflammatory processes.*

✎ What risks are associated with a thoracentesis?

Bleeding, infection, and pneumothorax

✎ How should a patient be prepared for a thoracentesis?

1. Assess vital signs and respiratory status before the procedure.
2. Stress to the patient that remaining still and not coughing during the procedure are important.
3. Explain to the patient that a sedative may be given to help with relaxation.
4. Stress to the patient the necessity of a sitting or leaning forward position (may use a bedside table with head resting on folded arms).
5. Advise the patient that a local anesthetic will be used to numb the insertion site.
6. Explain to the patient that a needle with a syringe will be inserted into the pleural space for fluid or tissue sample withdrawal, and pressure will be applied at the puncture site.
7. Explain to the patient that a small bandage may cover the site after the procedure is completed.
8. Tell the patient that the test usually takes less than 30 minutes.

✎ What nursing care is required after thoracentesis?

1. Position the patient on the unaffected side, with the tested side up for at least 1 hour.
2. Monitor vital signs at frequent intervals (every 15 minutes for 1 hour, every 2 hours for 4 hours, and then as ordered).
3. Assess the puncture site for bleeding.
4. Explain to the patient that a chest X-ray will be ordered to rule out pneumothorax.

⚡ *Notify the physician immediately if hypotension, tachycardia, dyspnea, or hemoptysis occur following a thoracentesis.*

Lung biopsy

What's a lung biopsy?

An invasive procedure involving the collection of lung tissue via bronchoscopy or a percutaneous transthoracic needle; may be performed open (surgically) under general anesthesia if indicated

What are common uses of a lung biopsy?	Diagnosing parenchymal changes, pulmonary diseases, tumors, or rejection of a transplanted lung
What risks are associated with a lung biopsy?	Pneumothorax, bleeding, and infection

How should a patient be prepared for a lung biopsy?

Preparation for lung biopsy:
1. Keep the patient on nothing-by-mouth status for 6 hours before the test (decreases risk of aspiration).
2. Remove the patient's dentures before the test.
3. Explain to the patient that a sedative may be given for relaxation and atropine may be given to decrease secretions.
4. Explain to the patient that a local anesthetic will be sprayed to numb his throat (general anesthesia is necessary if a rigid bronchoscope is used).
5. Advise the patient that a tube will be passed through his mouth and into the trachea for visualization of bronchioles and collection of tissue samples.
6. Caution the patient that some patients experience a false sensation of not being able to breathe as the scope is passed.
7. Tell the patient that the test usually takes 30 to 60 minutes.

Preparation for a percutaneous transthoracic biopsy:
1. Assess vital signs and respiratory status before the procedure.
2. Stress to the patient that remaining still and not coughing during the procedure are important.
3. Explain to the patient that a sedative may be given to help with relaxation.
4. Stress to the patient the necessity of a sitting or leaning forward position (may use a bedside table with head resting on folded arms).
5. Advise the patient that a local anesthetic will be used to numb the insertion site.
6. Explain to the patient that a needle with a syringe will be inserted into the pleural space for fluid or tissue sample withdrawal, and pressure will be applied at the puncture site.
7. Explain to the patient that a small bandage may cover the site after the procedure.
8. Tell the patient that the test usually takes less than 30 minutes.
9. Inform the patient that his skin will be numbed and a needle will be inserted quickly to obtain a piece of lung tissue.

The cardiovascular system

Electrocardiography

What's electrocardiography (ECG)?

A noninvasive test in which the electrical impulses that stimulate the heart to contract are recorded

What are the common uses of ECG?

Determining the source of pathologic rhythms and the location of myocardial ischemia or infarction

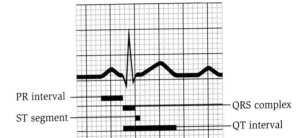

What does a P wave represent?

Atrial depolarization

What does the QRS complex represent?

Ventricular depolarization

What does a T wave represent?

Ventricular repolarization (resting stage between beats)

What might ST-segment elevations and T-wave inversions represent?

Myocardial ischemia or infarction

How should a patient be prepared for ECG?

1. Tell the patient to avoid heavy meals and smoking for at least 30 minutes before the test.
2. Advise the patient to relax as much as possible during the test.
3. Inform the patient that a supine position is best.
4. Explain to the patient that 12 electrodes, also called *leads*, will be placed at various places on the body.
5. Tell the patient that the test is painless and usually takes 10 minutes or less.

Holter monitoring

What's a Holter monitor?

Continuous recording of cardiac functioning through ECG for prolonged periods of time (usually 24 hours); a battery-powered taping device is worn over the shoulder or around the waist; a diary is also used to record the time of any symptoms experienced as well as the activity status

What are common uses of a Holter monitor?

1. Documenting known or suspected rhythm disturbances
2. Evaluating function of pacemakers or implantable defibrillator devices
3. Evaluating effectiveness of drug therapy or treatments

How should a patient be prepared for Holter monitoring?

1. Caution the patient not to use lotions or creams before electrode placement.
2. Explain to the patient that electrodes will be placed on his chest and attached to a small recorder.
3. Stress to the patient that electrodes should be kept dry (no shower or bath) and shouldn't be manipulated.
4. Stress to the patient the importance of avoiding electric blankets, heating pads, hair dryers, and electric shavers during test.
5. Keep a diary of activities for 24 hours; include the time that activities were performed and symptoms experienced.
6. Explain to the patient that electrodes are usually removed the next day; results are evaluated within a few days.

Echocardiogram

What's an echocardiogram?

An ultrasound study used to determine cardiac size, to assess the movements of the chambers and valves, and to evaluate the velocity of blood flow

What are common uses of an echocardiogram?

1. Visualizing cardiac chambers, valves, and blood vessels
2. Evaluating murmurs, valve conditions, and congenital defects
3. Measuring the thickness and size of chambers
4. Assessing fluid around the heart (pericardial effusion)
5. Evaluating the direction and velocity of blood flow through the heart

🔍 **How should a patient be prepared for an echocardiogram?**

1. Explain to the patient that the position for procedure is lying on a table (may also be performed at bedside).
2. Explain to the patient that a cool gel will be applied to his chest.
3. Explain to the patient that a transducer will be moved over his chest area.
4. Advise the patient that he may be asked to change position, hold his breath, or inhale or exhale slowly during test.
5. Tell the patient that the test usually takes 30 to 60 minutes.

What's a transesophageal echocardiography (TEE)?

A form of echocardiography that uses an endoscope to advance the transducer into the esophagus; used in obesity, chronic obstructive pulmonary disease, or when there has been trauma to the chest wall

A patient must be on nothing-by-mouth status for at least 4 hours prior to a TEE.

Cardiac stress test (myocardial perfusion scan)

What's a cardiac stress test?

A nuclear medicine test in which cardiac electrical activity is recorded at rest and during periods of increased oxygen demand; types of stress tests include exercise (treadmill) tests and pharmacologic (dipyridamole, adenosine, dobutamine) tests

What are common uses of cardiac stress tests?

Diagnosing ischemic heart disease, differentiating between ischemia and infarction, detecting myocardial wall defects, and predicting risk of perioperative ischemic events

What risks are associated with cardiac stress tests?

Chest pain, cardiac arrhythmias, and myocardial infarction

🔍 **How should a patient be prepared for an exercise stress test?**

1. Avoid caffeine for at least 12 hours before the test.
2. Explain to the patient that nothing-by-mouth status is necessary and to avoid smoking for at least 2 hours before the test.
3. Tell the patient to wear comfortable clothing and walking shoes for exercise testing.
4. Explain to the patient that the test consists of two phases: a rest scan and a stress scan.
5. Explain to the patient that electrodes will be placed on his chest and arms.

6. Advise the patient that an I.V. will be placed for injection of the radioisotope (thallium or technetium).
7. Advise the patient that a baseline ECG, blood pressure, and pulse will be obtained.
8. Explain to the patient that for an exercise stress test, walking on a treadmill or pedaling on a stationary bike will be gradually increased while his blood pressure, pulse, and the ECG are continuously monitored.
9. Explain to the patient that for a pharmacologic stress test, a medication will be administered that mimics the effects of exercise on the heart.
10. Advise the patient that any symptoms of discomfort, dizziness, or shortness of breath should be reported immediately.
11. Tell the patient that the test may take several hours, but may require 2 days for rest and stress scans (depending on hospital protocol).

◤ *Pharmacologic stress testing is used when the patient can't tolerate, or isn't physically able to, exercise on a treadmill or bike.*

Coronary angiography (cardiac catheterization)

What's coronary angiography?

An invasive study of the coronary vessels that involves insertion of a flexible catheter through the femoral (groin) or brachial (arm) artery into the heart and injecting contrast medium to visualize and evaluate the blood flow through fluoroscopy (X-ray)

What are common uses of coronary angiography?

1. Determining patency of coronary arteries (or confirm suspected heart disease)
2. Diagnosing valvular and chamber defects
3. Measuring cardiac output and hemodynamic pressures within the heart chambers and great vessels

✎ **What risks are associated with coronary angiography?**

Arrhythmias, bleeding, infection, embolism, perforation of an artery, or allergic reaction to contrast medium

How should a patient be prepared for coronary angiography?

1. Maintain nothing-by-mouth status at least 2 hours before the test.
2. Explain to the patient that the injection site is scrubbed with an antiseptic soap.
3. Explain to the patient that a sedative may be administered, but he'll remain alert during the procedure.

4. Stress to the patient the importance of remaining as still as possible during the procedure (motion artifacts cause poor images).
5. Clarify with the patient that either the femoral artery (groin) or the brachial artery (upper arm) will be used as the catheter insertion site; contrast dye will be injected into the vessel being studied (some patients may need to have the injection site shaved).
6. Inform the patient that contrast injection may cause sensation of hot flashes and palpitations.
7. Explain to the patient that X-rays will be taken of the vessels to assess blood flow.
8. Explain to the patient that the catheter will be withdrawn and pressure will be applied to the puncture site. A pressure dressing, which should remain intact for at least 24 hours, will be applied.
9. Tell the patient that the test usually takes 30 minutes to 3 hours.

What are important nursing actions after cardiac catheterization?

1. Keep the patient flat in bed for 4 to 6 hours without flexion of punctured extremity; normal bed rest until the next day.
2. Monitor vital signs and perform neurovascular checks at frequent intervals (Rule of Four: every 15 minutes for 1 hour; every 30 minutes for 2 hours; every hour for 4 hours; and then every 4 hours).
3. Assess puncture site for bleeding, swelling, hematoma, or bruits. Check distal pulses of affected limb.
4. Maintain functional I.V. access.
5. Encourage fluids to facilitate excretion of contrast agent, unless contraindicated.

What's coronary angioplasty?

A form of coronary angiography involving the insertion of a catheter with a balloon through an artery in the groin and into a blocked artery in the heart; the balloon is repeatedly inflated and deflated to open the narrowed portion of the artery, during which time the patient may experience mild chest pressure or discomfort

Notify the physician if an extremity develops numbness, tingling, decreased or absent pulses, blanching, coolness, or excessive blood loss following an angiographic procedure.

The GI system

Upper GI or barium swallow

What's an upper GI or barium swallow?

A form of gastric radiography that allows real-time visualization of the mucosal lining of the esophagus, stomach, duodenum, and upper portion of the jejunum by using a contrast agent (barium or Gastrografin) and fluoroscopy

What are the common uses of an upper GI or barium swallow?

To diagnose ulcers, hiatal hernias, pyloric stenosis, gastritis, and gastric tumors

What risks are associated with an upper GI or barium swallow?

Small radiation exposure, allergy to the contrast, and constipation

How should a patient be prepared for upper GI or barium swallow?

1. Maintain nothing-by-mouth status and stress the importance of avoiding smoking after midnight before the test.
2. Advise the patient to take only necessary medications (other than metformin) with small sips of water.
3. Advise the patient to remove all jewelry before the test.
4. Assess the patient for allergies to the contrast agent.
5. Assess pregnancy status of all women of childbearing age.
6. Explain to the patient that an oral contrast agent will be ingested before the test.
7. Explain to the patient that various positions on the X-ray table will be required.
8. Stress to the patient the importance of remaining still and following breathing instructions during the test.
9. Explain to the patient that stools may be white or pink up to 72 hours after the test.
10. Tell the patient that the test may take up to several hours.

Upper GI series or barium swallows should be performed after barium enemas or gallbladder series to prevent interference with other examinations.

What are important nursing actions after a barium contrast study?

1. Inform the patient that regular diet and activity may be resumed.
2. Encourage extra fluids and a laxative to prevent or minimize constipation from the contrast agent.
3. Document stool color and consistency.

Lower GI or barium enema

What's a lower GI or barium enema?	Radiographic examination of the colon with contrast agent (barium)
What are the common uses of a lower GI or barium enema?	To detect diverticulitis, mass lesions, polyps, colitis, active bleeding, or obstruction
What risks are associated with a lower GI or barium enema?	Small amount of radiation exposure, allergy to contrast, constipation, and electrolyte imbalances (hypokalemia) from enemas

How should a patient be prepared for a lower GI or a barium enema?

1. Keep the patient on a clear liquid diet the day before test (no milk products); maintain nothing-by-mouth status after midnight before the test.
2. Instruct the patient to take only necessary medications (except metformin) with small sips of water before the test.
3. Stool softeners, laxatives, and enemas may be ordered before the examination (a poor bowel prep will result in inadequate visualization and possible repeat testing).
4. Explain to the patient that barium will be administered by a rectal enema while in a side-lying position on an X-ray table.
5. Inform the patient that there may be mild cramping and the urge to defecate during the procedure.
6. Inform the patient that barium may be present in the stool for several days after the procedure.
7. Instruct the patient to drink plenty of liquids following the test to prevent fecal impaction.

What are important nursing actions after a barium enema?

1. Inform the patient that regular diet and activity may be resumed.
2. Encourage extra fluids and a laxative to prevent or minimize constipation from the contrast agent.
3. Document stool color and consistency.

What's a contraindication for a barium enema?

Known or suspected bowel perforation

Cholescintigraphy
(Hydroxyiminodiacetic acid [HIDA] scan)

What's a cholescintig-raphy or HIDA scan?	A nuclear imaging study used to diagnose bile duct ob-struction, diseases of the gallbladder and bile leaks; in-volves I.V. injection of a radioisotope and possibly chole-cystokinin to contract the gallbladder

Cholangiography

What's a cholangio-gram?	Injection of iodinated contrast to allow indirect visualiza-tion of gallbladder and biliary system
What are the common uses of a cholangio-gram?	Detecting intraductal mass lesions and calculi

By what methods can a cholangiogram be performed?

1. *I.V.:* intravenous injection of contrast agent
2. *T tube:* injection of contrast into a drainage tube (T tube) in the common bile duct
3. *Percutaneous transhepatic:* percutaneous injection of contrast into the liver
4. *Operative:* injection of contrast into exposed cystic duct during surgery

How should a pa-tient be prepared for a cholangiogram?

1. Maintain nothing-by-mouth status for several hours before the test.
2. Instruct the patient to take only necessary medications (except metformin).
3. Make sure that all jewelry is removed.
4. Assess pregnancy status of all female patients of child-bearing age.
5. Assess the patient for allergy to iodine.
6. Instruct the patient to remain still and follow breath-ing instructions during test.
7. Inform the patient that he may experience a pressure sensation during contrast agent injection.
8. Tell the patient that the test may take up to 2 hours.

What are impor-tant nursing actions after a cholangiogram?

1. Monitor vital signs at frequent intervals.
2. Assess for reaction to iodine (nausea, vomiting, inter-mittent fever).
3. Monitor for hemorrhage, peritonitis, or pneumothorax after percutaneous transhepatic approach.

Endoscopic studies

What are endoscopic studies?

Visualization of the esophagus (esophagoscopy), stomach (gastroscopy), colon (sigmoidoscopy), rectum (proctoscopy), or biliary system (retrograde cholangiopancreatography) using a hollow tube with a lighted end

✎ What are the major potential complications of endoscopic procedures?

Perforation through the structure being scoped; aspiration; hemorrhage from biopsy sites; reaction to anesthetic agents, medications or sedatives; hypotension; bradycardia; laryngospasm; and respiratory distress

> ⚡ *Anticoagulants and antiplatelet agents including nonsteroidal anti-inflammatory drugs should be discontinued at least 4 to 5 days before endoscopic studies.*

✎ What are common signs of perforation after an endoscopic procedure?

Sudden temperature spike, bleeding, and pain

> ⚡ *Temperature should be checked every 15 to 30 minutes for 1 to 2 hours after endoscopic procedures.*

✎ What are important nursing actions after an endoscopic procedure?

1. Obtain vital signs at least every 30 minutes for 2 hours.
2. Withhold food and liquids for at least 2 hours after an endoscopic examination.
3. Place the patient in a side-lying position with side rails up until sedation has worn off (prevents aspiration).
4. Encourage the use of lozenges to minimize sore throat when swallow reflexes return (upper endoscopies).
5. Observe the patient for complications (bleeding or blood in stool, fever), and notify the physician immediately if any develop.

> ⚡ *Assess for return of gag reflex and ability to swallow before offering food and fluids after endoscopic studies.*

Esophagoduodenostomy/upper endoscopy

What are the common uses of upper endoscopy?

Evaluating problems with the esophagus, stomach, and duodenum; evaluating upper abdominal pain, nausea, vomiting, difficulty swallowing, and anemia; and detecting ulcers and tumors

✎ How should a patient be prepared for upper endoscopy?

1. Explain to the patient that dentures should be removed before the procedure.
2. Advise the patient that his throat will be numbed with a spray.

3. Explain to the patient that I.V. sedation and pain medications will be given before the test.

4. Explain to the patient that a mouthpiece will be inserted to prevent biting of the endoscope and to prevent injury to teeth and other oral structures.

5. Explain to the patient that a left side-lying position is used.

6. Explain to the patient that a finger-thick scope (that doesn't interfere with breathing) will be passed through his mouth and advanced slowly into the stomach and duodenum.

7. Advise the patient that during the test there may be pressure or bloating sensations from air insufflation.

8. Caution the patient that after the test he may experience a mild sore throat or abdominal distention.

9. Inform the patient that a normal diet can be resumed within several hours after the procedure.

Flexible sigmoidoscopy

What's flexible sigmoidoscopy?

Passage of a flexible fiber-optic scope into the anus to examine the rectum and sigmoid colon

What are the common uses of flexible sigmoidoscopy?

Evaluating rectal bleeding, change in bowel habits, and rectal clinical findings, such as pain and persistent diarrhea, as well as screening for colon cancer (every 3 to 5 years for people over age 50) and surveying for polyps

How should a patient be prepared for a flexible sigmoidoscopy?

1. Instruct the patient to consume only clear liquids the evening before the test.

2. Explain to the patient the need for bowel cleaning, involving enemas and laxatives the evening before and the morning of the test (preparation may be waived if diarrhea is present).

3. Explain to the patient that a left side-lying position is used.

4. Advise the patient that a strong urge to defecate and a sensation of bloating or abdominal cramping may be felt during the procedure.

5. Tell the patient that the test usually takes 20 minutes.

6. Stress to the patient the importance of early ambulation after the test.

Colonoscopy

What's colonoscopy?	Passage of a flexible fiber-optic scope through the anus to the ileocecal valve for visualization of the mucosa of the large intestine; colonoscopy is a longer version of a flexible sigmoidoscopy
What are common uses of colonoscopy?	Evaluating polyps and lower GI bleeding as well as screening for colon cancer and differentiating neoplastic disease from polypoid lesions via biopsy

✎ How should a patient be prepared for colonoscopy?

1. Discontinue iron supplements and anticoagulants for 4 to 5 days before the procedure.
2. Place the patient on a clear liquid diet for 48 hours before the procedure; maintain nothing-by-mouth status after midnight before the procedure.
3. Order the patient laxatives for several days before the procedure, and order him an enema the evening before the test. Or, order ingestion of oral saline laxative (Go-LYTELY) taken the evening before the procedure (one 12 oz glass every 10 minutes until only clear liquid is expelled).
4. Explain to the patient that a mild sedative will be administered, but that he'll be awake during the procedure.
5. Advise the patient that a left side-lying position is used.
6. Explain to the patient that deep breaths should be taken as the scope is introduced into the bowel.
7. Advise the patient that he may experience sensations of abdominal cramping and pressure caused by air insufflation during the procedure.

⚡ *Notify the physician immediately if a patient develops fever, malaise, rectal bleeding, abdominal pain, distention, or tenesmus following colonoscopy, as these can be signs of perforation.*

Endoscopic retrograde cholangiopancreatography

What's endoscopic retrograde cholangio-pancreatography (ERCP)?	An endoscopic procedure that involves the use of a long, flexible scope inserted through the mouth to examine the duodenum, papilla of Vater, bile ducts, gallbladder, and pancreatic duct; can be diagnostic or therapeutic (stent placement, sphincterotomy)

What are the common uses of ERCP?

Evaluating gallstones; bile duct obstruction by strictures, calculi, or cancer; and pancreatic disease

✎ How should a patient be prepared for ERCP?

1. Discontinue anticoagulants and antiplatelet agents at least 5 days before the procedure.
2. Assess pregnancy status of females of childbearing age.
3. Maintain nothing-by-mouth status after midnight the day of the procedure.
4. Explain to the patient that his throat will be numbed with an anesthetic spray, and an I.V. will be started.
5. Advise the patient that the position for the test will be left side-lying with his knees flexed on an X-ray table.
6. Explain to the patient that a sedative (and possibly prophylactic antibiotics) will be provided.
7. Explain to the patient that the scope will be passed through his mouth.
8. Advise the patient that a contrast agent will be injected and fluoroscopy will be performed.
9. Inform the patient that the test may last 15 minutes to 1 hour.
10. Advise the patient that there may be temporary bloating or nausea after the procedure.
11. Advise the patient that normal activity may be resumed the next day.

✎ What's the most common complication of ERCP?

Pancreatitis; bowel perforation and infection are other potential risks

✎ What are important nursing actions after ERCP?

1. Monitor vital signs at frequent intervals.
2. Maintain nothing-by-mouth status until return of gag reflex.
3. Observe for complications (infection, urine retention, cholangitis, pancreatitis).
4. Provide ice chips, fluids, lozenges, or gargles for relief of sore throat (after return of gag reflex).

Laparoscopy (peritoneoscopy)

What's laparoscopy?

Use of a laparoscope to view inside the abdomen and pelvis through small incisions (ports)

What are common uses of laparoscopy?

Diagnosing and surgically treating abdominal (laparoscopic cholecystectomy) and pelvic disorders

What risks are associated with laparoscopy?

Displacement of carbon dioxide, bleeding or infection at the puncture site, and thermal burn

✎ How should a patient be prepared for laparoscopy?

1. Discontinue all anticoagulants 4 to 5 days before the procedure.
2. Administer an enema or a suppository to prepare the bowel.
3. Explain to the patient that the position during the procedure will be back-lying .
4. Explain to the patient that an I.V. will be started and anesthesia will be administered.
5. Advise the patient that a urinary catheter will be placed to minimize the risk of bladder perforation.
6. Explain to the patient that several small abdominal incisions will be made to allow insertion of the laparoscope.
7. Explain to the patient that carbon dioxide will be instilled into the abdomen for better visualization.
8. Advise the patient that a few stitches or adhesive strips will be necessary to close the incisions.
9. Inform the patient that he may experience abdominal and shoulder discomfort for 1 to 2 days after the procedure (due to retained carbon dioxide).

What are important nursing actions after laparoscopy?

1. Monitor vital signs at frequent intervals.
2. Evaluate for complications (infection, hemorrhage, or bowel or bladder perforation).
3. Instruct the patient to sit in semi-Fowler's position to minimize abdominal or shoulder discomfort.
4. Observe the incision site for signs of infection or hematoma.

What are the advantages of laparoscopy compared to open surgical procedures?

1. Abbreviated postoperative period
2. Decreased postoperative pain
3. Avoidance of large abdominal incisions (which decreases cardiac and pulmonary postoperative complications)
4. Decreased mortality

Paracentesis

What's paracentesis?

Insertion of a needle into the abdominal cavity to remove fluid for diagnostic or therapeutic purposes

✎ What risks are associated with paracentesis?

Pneumothorax and bowel perforation

How should a patient be prepared for paracentesis?

1. Encourage voiding before the procedure.
2. Explain to the patient that the position for the procedure is lying supine with the head of the bed raised slightly.
3. Explain to the patient that the skin will be cleaned and an anesthetic will be injected before a long needle is inserted into the abdomen.
4. Advise the patient that fluid will be withdrawn slowly.
5. Advise the patient that a small dressing will be applied once the needle is removed.

What are important nursing actions after paracentesis?

1. Monitor vital signs at frequent intervals, especially temperature and respiratory effort.
2. Turn the patient to the *unaffected* side for 1 hour.
3. Assess dressing at frequent intervals.
4. Maintain bed rest until vital signs are stable.

Liver biopsy

What's liver biopsy?

An invasive procedure involving the insertion of needle into the liver through the skin to obtain a sample of liver tissue for microscopic examination

What are the common uses of liver biopsy?

Evaluating chronic hepatitis and portal hypertension, confirming the diagnosis of alcoholic liver disease and space occupying lesions

What risks are associated with liver biopsy?

Hemorrhage from biopsy site, pneumothorax, lacerations of other organs, bowel perforation, and bile peritonitis (painful leakage of bile into peritoneum)

How should a patient be prepared for liver biopsy?

1. Assess prothrombin time, hemoglobin level, and platelet count.
2. Maintain nothing-by-mouth status for at least 2 hours before the biopsy.
3. Explain to the patient that the procedure is usually performed at the bedside under local anesthesia.
4. Advise the patient that the position for the procedure is supine or left lateral with his right arm over his head.
5. Explain to the patient that the physician will instruct him to take a deep breath, blow it out, and then hold it at this point while the needle is inserted (minimizes risk of pneumothorax).
6. Inform the patient that strict bed rest will be required for at least 2 hours after the biopsy.

⬟ In what position should a patient be placed immediately after liver biopsy?

Right side-lying position for at least 2 hours (to splint puncture site)

⬟ What are important nursing actions after liver biopsy?

1. Monitor vital signs at frequent intervals (every 15 minutes for 1 hour; every 30 minutes for 2 hours; and every hour for 4 hours).
2. Maintain bed rest with the patient lying on his right side for a minimum of 2 hours to splint puncture site.
3. Assess the biopsy site for bleeding, hematoma, and bile leakage when obtaining vital signs.
4. Instruct the patient to avoid coughing or straining for at least 2 hours after the biopsy and to avoid heavy lifting and strenuous activities for 1 week.

The genitourinary system

Cystoscopy

What's cystoscopy?

An invasive procedure that allows direct visualization of the urethra, bladder, and the male prostate gland by using a small, lighted scope that's inserted into the urethra

What are common uses of cystoscopy?

1. Evaluating chronic urinary tract infections, hematuria, incontinence, or retention as well as prostatic hyperplasia
2. Obtaining biopsy to diagnose bladder or urethral cancer; removing tumors
3. Crushing and retrieving small stones from the lower urinary tract

⬟ What risks are associated with cystoscopy?

Infection, sepsis (gram-negative shock), perforation of bladder wall, or bleeding from biopsy site

⬟ How should a patient be prepared for cystoscopy?

1. Prepare the patient's bowel (if extensive procedure is anticipated).
2. Give the patient a full liquid breakfast the morning of the procedure to promote urine formation.
3. Explain to the patient that the position for the test is lithotomy with his legs in stirrups.
4. Advise the patient that an I.V. will be started for sedative administration.
5. Inform the patient that external genitalia will be cleaned with antiseptic solution.

6. Explain to the patient that a local anesthetic jelly will be used to numb the urethra before the cystoscope is inserted and passed into the bladder.

7. Explain to the patient that fluids will be infused into the bladder throughout the procedure (distention allows better visualization of bladder wall). The bladder will be drained when it becomes filled with 300 to 500 ml.

8. Advise the patient that there may be an urge to void while the bladder is distended, and there may be a slight pinch if biopsies are obtained.

9. Advise the patient that he may experience a slight burning sensation when voiding and pink-tinged urine for up to 2 days after the procedure.

10. Tell the patient that the test usually takes 30 to 45 minutes.

What are important nursing actions after cystoscopy?

1. Monitor vital signs at frequent intervals.
2. Encourage fluid intake when sedation wears off.
3. Assess voiding patterns (formation of clots may cause difficulty passing urine).
4. Provide catheter care for retention or ureteral catheters.
5. Evaluate for development of edema. If present, provide warm Sitz baths to prevent urinary retention or dribbling.

◤ *Notify the physician immediately if the patient develops fever, chills, hypotension, tachycardia, or back pain following a cystoscopy.*

Excretory urography

What's excretory urography?

An X-ray procedure in which contrast agent is injected I.V. and a series of X-rays are taken at specific time intervals to visualize the kidneys, ureters, and bladder

What are common uses of excretory urography?

Evaluating infections, calculi, or tumors of the bladder or kidneys

✎ **What risks are associated with excretory urography?**

Allergic reaction to contrast agent, minimal exposure to radiation, and renal impairment from contrast agent

How should a patient be prepared for excretory urography?

1. Assess pregnancy status of all women of childbearing age.
2. Assess the patient for iodine allergies.
3. Instruct the patient to maintain nothing-by-mouth status after midnight before the test
4. Explain to the patient that a laxative will be necessary the night before the test and an enema will be given the morning of the test.
5. Advise the patient that the position for the test is supine.
6. Explain to the patient that a baseline X-ray is taken to assess the location of the kidneys and to ensure that the bowel is empty.
7. Advise the patient that the contrast agent will be injected I.V. (commonly via antecubital access).
8. Explain to the patient that he may experience sensations of warmth, facial flushing, and nausea during contrast injection.
9. Inform the patient that at least three more X-rays will be taken at specific time intervals after contrast injection.
10. Explain to the patient that it's necessary to void prior to the last X-ray being performed (to assess bladder emptying).
11. Inform the patient that the test usually takes approximately 1 hour.

What are important nursing actions after excretory urography?

1. Assess for allergic reaction to the contrast agent.
2. Encourage the patient to increase his fluid intake (facilitates contrast excretion).
3. Instruct the patient to resume previous activities and diet.

Retrograde pyelogram

What's retrograde pyelogram?

A series of X-rays taken after a contrast agent has been injected through a urinary catheter into the bladder that outlines the lining of the ureters and renal pelvis

What are common uses of retrograde pyelogram?

Evaluating obstructive tumors or calculi of the ureters as well as congenital defects of the ureters and renal pelvis

What risks are associated with retrograde pyelogram?

Infection, exposure to small amounts of radiation, and allergic reaction to the contrast agent

How should a patient be prepared for retrograde pyelogram?

1. Assess pregnancy status of all women of childbearing age.
2. Assess the patient for allergy to iodine.
3. Maintain nothing-by-mouth status after midnight before the test.
4. Assess the patient's recent renal function (creatinine level).
5. Administer suppositories, laxatives, or enemas the night before and the morning of the test.
6. Explain to the patient that the urethra will be cleaned and numbed with a topical anesthetic before the insertion of a urinary catheter.
7. Explain to the patient that a contrast agent will be injected into the bladder and ureters, and multiple X-rays will be taken.
8. Advise the patient that the catheter will be removed and the contrast agent will be excreted in the urine.
9. Advise the patient that there may be a slight burning sensation and pink-tinged urine when voiding for the first 2 days after the test.

What are important nursing actions after retrograde pyelogram?

1. Monitor vital signs at frequent intervals for 24 hours, if hospitalized.
2. Assess for allergic reactions to iodine.
3. Encourage fluid intake.
4. Record urine output and appearance for 24 hours.
5. Monitor for development of infection as a result of instrumentation.

Renal biopsy

What's renal biopsy?

The percutaneous (through the skin) removal of a renal tissue sample for microscopic examination

What are common uses of renal biopsy?

Evaluate renal functioning and disease

What risks are associated with renal biopsy?

Infection and bleeding

How should a patient be prepared for renal biopsy?

1. Discontinue the patient's anticoagulants 4 to 5 days before the procedure.
2. Explain to the patient that the location of the kidney will be determined by X-ray and marked on the skin with ink.
3. Inform the patient that he'll be in a prone position with a pillow under his abdomen.

4. Advise the patient that a local anesthetic will be injected at the biopsy site.
5. Explain to the patient that a biopsy needle will be inserted into the kidney and then quickly withdrawn.
6. Explain to the patient that direct pressure will be applied to the biopsy site for 20 minutes followed by application of a pressure dressing and sandbag once in a supine position.
7. Inform the patient that bed rest will be maintained for at least 6 hours (typically at least 2 hours flat and 4 hours sitting up).
8. Stress to the patient that all heavy lifting should be avoided for 10 days.

What are important nursing actions after renal biopsy?

1. Monitor vital signs at frequent intervals.
2. Assess biopsy site at frequent intervals.
3. Maintain bed rest for at least 6 hours after the biopsy (at least 2 hours flat bed rest and 4 hours sitting up).

Papanicolaou smear

What's a Papanicolaou (Pap) smear?

A minimally invasive procedure involving the scraping of cells from the surface of the cervix for microscopic examination

What are common uses of a Pap smear?

Diagnosing inflammation, infection, and precancerous or cancerous conditions of the cervix

How should a patient be prepared for a Pap smear?

1. Instruct the patient to avoid vaginal medications, douches, spermicidal creams, tampon usage, and sexual intercourse at least 24 hours before the test.
2. Assess whether the patient is currently menstruating. Pap smears are ideally performed 2 weeks after the first day of the last menstrual period.
3. Promote the use of relaxation techniques for the apprehensive patient.
4. Explain to the patient that clothing from the waist down should be removed.
5. Explain to the patient that the position for the test is lithotomy on an examination table with her feet resting in stirrups.
6. Advise the patient that a warmed, lubricated speculum will be inserted into the vagina to enable visualization of the cervix.
7. Explain to the patient that cells will be gently scraped from the cervix with a small spatula or brush.
8. Advise the patient that a slight cramping sensation may be felt during the procedure and a small amount of bleeding may occur after the test.

Prostate biopsy

What's prostate biopsy?

An invasive procedure that uses a transrectal ultrasound probe with a needle attached to obtain tissue and cell samples from the prostate gland

What are common uses of prostate biopsy?

Evaluating for prostate cancer

What risks are associated with prostate biopsy?

Infection and bleeding

◼ *Sepsis is a potential life-threatening complication of a transrectal biopsy. Any signs of infection should be reported to the physician immediately.*

✎ How should a patient be prepared for prostate biopsy?

1. Explain to the patient that an enema will be given on the morning of the examination.
2. Inform the patient that the position during test will be side-lying, with his knees bent as an ultrasound probe is inserted into the rectum.
3. Advise the patient that a needle biopsy of the prostate is performed, which may cause brief discomfort.
4. Inform the patient that there may be a small amount of blood in the urine or ejaculate for several days after the procedure.

6

Overview of surgery

Surgery

What are the two classifications of surgery?
Elective and urgent or emergency

What different purposes can surgery serve?
Diagnostic or exploratory, resectional, ablative or destructive, palliative, reconstructive or constructive, and curative

What are the four types of surgical methods?
1. Open
2. Laparoscopic or thoracoscopic
3. Endoscopic
4. Electrosurgery or laser

Types of anesthesia

GENERAL ANESTHESIA

What's general anesthesia?
The production of amnesia, analgesia, hypnosis, and relaxation by central nervous system (CNS) depression

How is general anesthesia administered?
Via a breathing mask, endotracheal (ET) tube, laryngeal mask airway, or I.V.

What are common adjuncts to general anesthesia?
1. *Hypnotics:* midazolam (Versed), diazepam (Valium), lorazepam (Ativan), propofol (Diprivan), etomidate
2. *Opioid analgesics:* morphine, meperidine (Demerol), fentanyl (Sublimaze)
3. *Neuromuscular blocking agents:* pancuronium (Pavulon), atracurium (Tracrium), succinylcholine, vecuronium, rocuronium, cisatracurium

✎ What adverse reactions are associated with general anesthesia?

Allergic reactions, respiratory depression, decreased seizure threshold, bradycardia, hypotension, and decreased GI motility

✎ What life-threatening reaction is associated with general anesthesia?

Malignant hyperthermia, a hypermetabolic state triggered by exposure to some anesthetic agents; symptoms include hypercarbia (increased carbon dioxide), tachypnea, tachycardia, arrhythmias, and skeletal muscle rigidity; late manifestations include temperature elevation and cyanosis; a genetic predisposition is suspected

Why are ET tubes used during surgery?

To maintain airway patency in a patient who can't protect the airway due to anesthetic agents; may also be used to administer medications

What complications are associated with ET intubation?

Improper neck extension, improper tube placement (esophagus, right or left mainstem bronchus), trauma to vocal cords, and swollen lips as well as broken teeth and caps

When are ET tubes removed?

When the patient is awake enough to protect his own airway, can follow commands, and has adequate inspiratory effort

✎ What nursing interventions are appropriate when providing care for a patient receiving general anesthesia?

1. Maintain nothing-by-mouth status preoperatively and postoperatively until gag reflex returns.
2. Monitor vital signs frequently postoperatively (especially respiratory status).
3. Monitor the patient's airway and have oxygen and other resuscitative equipment available.
4. Ensure patient safety due to decreased sense of awareness (side rails up while in bed with call bell within reach).
5. Administer opioids cautiously to prevent excessive sedation.
6. Provide lozenges or anesthetic sprays for sore throat relief only after return of gag reflex.

REGIONAL ANESTHESIA

How does regional anesthesia work?

Produces loss of sensation in one body area due to blockage of sensory impulses to the spinal cord and brain while the patient remains conscious

What are examples of regional anesthesia?

Epidural, spinal, nerve block, and local anesthesia

LUMBAR EPIDURAL

What's a lumbar epidural?

Injection of an anesthetic agent into the epidural space (outside the spinal canal), which then infiltrates the tissues producing a loss of sensation in a band around the body at the level of injection

In what situations are lumbar epidurals commonly used?

Surgery involving the lower limbs, during labor, and for postoperative pain management

What adverse reactions are associated with lumbar anesthesia?

Hypotension and headache

SPINAL ANESTHESIA

What's spinal anesthesia?

Injection of an anesthetic agent into the subarachnoid space via a lumbar puncture in order to achieve loss of sensation in a particular body area by interrupting nerve impulses

For what purposes is spinal anesthesia commonly used?

Lower abdominal, pelvic, rectal, or lower extremity surgeries

What adverse reactions are most commonly associated with spinal anesthesia?

Hypotension and severe headache

What are the advantages of epidural anesthesia compared to spinal anesthesia?

1. Decreased incidence of spinal headache
2. Duration; spinal anesthesia is administered once and may last up to 6 hours; epidural catheters can be left in place so that anesthesia can be administered continuously through the postoperative period.

What are important nursing interventions when caring for a patient who has received spinal anesthesia?

1. Make sure the patient lies *flat* for 4 to 6 hours after surgery (prevents spinal headache).
2. Make sure that an unconscious or semiconscious patient remains in a side-lying position (prevents aspiration and occlusion of the pharynx by the tongue).
3. Ensure adequate hydration (minimizes spinal headache and hypotension).

NERVE BLOCK

What's a nerve block?   Injection of an anesthetic agent into a nerve plexus to induce a loss of sensation in a specific area of the body

How are nerve blocks commonly used?   To control intractable pain (frequently in cancer patients) and for minor to moderate surgeries involving the extremities

LOCAL ANESTHESIA

What's local anesthesia?   Blockage of nerve impulse conduction to produce a loss of sensation in a small area of tissue; the anesthetic may be applied topically or injected; the patient remains conscious throughout the procedure

For what situations is local anesthesia commonly used?   Minor surgeries, such as skin or superficial biopsies

What are commonly used local anesthetic agents?   Lidocaine (Xylocaine) and bupivacaine (Marcaine)

✎ What adverse reaction is associated with local anesthesia?   Allergic reaction and toxicity

✎ Why is epinephrine sometimes used in conjunction with local anesthetics?   It enhances the duration of the anesthetic effect

   ▶ *Epinephrine shouldn't be used on ears, nose, fingers, toes, or genitalia due to risk of tissue necrosis.*

Commonly prescribed medications

Why are preoperative medications given?   To reduce anxiety, promote relaxation, reduce oropharyngeal and gastric secretions, and decrease the amount of anesthetic required for induction and maintenance

SEDATIVE OR HYPNOTIC

Why are sedatives and hypnotics administered preoperatively?   To produce sedation in small doses and sleep in larger doses as well as to treat situational anxiety by central nervous system depression

What are examples of sedatives and hypnotics used preoperatively?

1. *Barbiturates:* phenobarbital (Luminal), secobarbital (Seconal)
2. *Benzodiazepines:* midazolam (Versed), diazepam (Valium), flurazepam (Dalmane)
3. *Nonbarbiturates, nonbenzodiazepines:* propofol (Diprivan), etomidate, hydroxyzine (Vistaril)

ANALGESICS

Why are analgesics used preoperatively?

To alleviate postoperative pain and to provide antipyretic as well as anti-inflammatory activity

What are the two main classes of analgesics?

Opioids and nonopioids (including nonsteroidal anti-inflammatory drugs)

ANTICHOLINERGICS

✎ Why are anticholinergics used preoperatively?

To decrease secretions before surgery

What are examples of anticholinergics used preoperatively?

Atropine and scopolamine

HISTAMINE-2 (H$_2$) ANTAGONISTS

✎ Why are H$_2$-antagonists used preoperatively?

To decrease gastric acid secretion, to minimize postoperative nausea and vomiting, and to prevent gastric ulcers resulting from the stress of surgery

What are examples of H$_2$-antagonists used preoperatively?

Omeprazole (Prilosec), esomeprazole (Nexium), nizatidine (Axid), ranitidine (Zantac), famotidine (Pepcid), and pantoprazole (Protonix) given I.V.

ANTIEMETICS

Why are antiemetics used preoperatively?

To decrease postoperative nausea and vomiting

What are examples of antiemetics used preoperatively?

Droperidol (Inapsine), trimethobenzamide (Tigan), ondansetron (Zofran), and promethazine (Phenergan)

Preoperative care

✎ What screening tests are routinely performed in the preoperative phase?

1. Blood tests
2. Chest X-ray (if the patient is symptomatic or has smoking history)
3. Electrocardiogram (if the patient is elderly or has cardiac history)
4. Urinalysis (if the patient is symptomatic)
5. Pregnancy test for women of childbearing age

✎ What blood tests are commonly obtained in the preoperative phase?

1. Type and screen or cross (for possible transfusion)
2. Complete blood count, including platelet count
3. Chemistry panel, especially electrolytes
4. Prothrombin time or partial thromboplastin time

✎ What medical conditions increase a patient's risk for surgery?

1. Cardiac conditions: coronary artery disease, angina, recent myocardial infarction, severe hypertension, and severe heart failure
2. Blood coagulation disorders
3. Upper respiratory infection or chronic obstructive pulmonary disease such as emphysema
4. Renal dysfunction
5. Diabetes mellitus, particularly if poorly controlled
6. Liver disease and alcoholism
7. Uncontrolled neurologic diseases such as epilepsy
8. Morbid obesity
9. Steroid-dependence

What other factors affect a patient's surgical risk?

Age (very young or very old), nutritional status, fluid and electrolyte status, general state of health, medications, and mental health

✎ What information is important to include in preoperative teaching?

1. The possible need for screening tests as well as skin and bowel preparations
2. Action and administration of preoperative medications
3. The need for an I.V. line as well as possible urinary catheter and nasogastric tube
4. Food and fluid restrictions after midnight before surgery
5. Anticipated length of surgery and hospitalization afterward
6. The need for removal of jewelry, makeup, and devices, such as dentures or hearing aids
7. Time and location of where to report on the day of surgery (if outpatient or same-day admission)
8. Postoperative routines and exercises
9. The need for smoking cessation at least 30 days prior to surgery (improves wound healing and decreases pulmonary complications)

10. The need for good diabetic control (diabetics have a higher rate of infections)
11. Action and administration of a patient-controlled analgesia (PCA)

What's the purpose of preoperative skin preparation?

To remove transient microbes and to reduce residual microbial count (inhibits rapid regrowth of microbes postoperatively)

What methods of skin preparation are used preoperatively?

Cleaning with an antimicrobial soap or solution, clipping excessive hair over the surgical site, and applying topical antiseptics, such as povidone-iodine or chlorhexidine (unless contraindicated), to the skin over the surgical site

Skin preparation solutions are also available in an applicator that combines isopropyl alcohol and iodine to form a water-insoluble film that isn't washed away by blood or body fluids; DuraPrep is an example.

What's the purpose of preoperative GI preparation?

Decreases number of bacteria in the GI tract and decreases the amount of solid stool

What are methods of preoperative GI preparation?

1. Clear liquids the evening before surgery; then nothing-by-mouth after midnight
2. Laxatives, enemas, or Go-LYTELY
3. Oral antibiotics (neomycin, erythromycin)

✎ What information is important to include when preparing a patient for postoperative routines?

1. Type and frequency of postoperative assessments
2. Why and how to deep breathe, cough, and use incentive spirometry; demonstrate splinting techniques

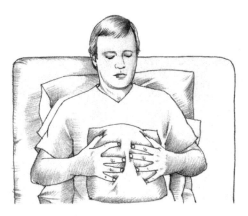

3. Typical dietary and activity restrictions
4. Pain management and use of PCA
5. Location and purpose of drains and dressings
6. Leg exercises and use of sequential compression devices

How should a patient be prepared for daytime surgery?

1. Confirm the date, time, and location of surgery.
2. Discuss food and fluid restrictions (depends on type of surgery).
3. Instruct the patient to leave valuables at home.
4. Advise the patient to wear clothing with large sleeves to accomodate bulky dressings.
5. Discuss the need for someone to drive the patient home.

What nursing activities occur in the immediate preoperative period?

1. Final patient identification
2. Confirmation of the procedure to be performed and of the anatomic site
3. Verification of a signed informed consent form in the chart

What are important nursing actions to ensure proper patient identification preoperatively?

1. Ask the patient to state his full name, the surgeon's name, the operation to be performed, and the site of the operation (right or left).
2. Compare the hospital identification number with the number on the patient's medical band.

Intraoperative care

What are the primary nursing responsibilities intraoperatively?

1. Protect the patient from injury.
2. Monitor the patient's physical response (and psychological response when appropriate).
3. Document intraoperative care.

What preoperative physical data is important for the operating room nurse and surgical team to have available?

1. Baseline vital signs
2. Weight and height (actual)
3. Age
4. Skin condition
5. Skeletal or muscle impairments, or limitations in range of motion (ROM)
6. Sensory (hearing, vision) and neurologic deficits
7. Level of consciousness (LOC)
8. Any source of pain or discomfort
9. Allergies
10. Implants

What are important nursing considerations when positioning a patient intraoperatively?

1. Protect the patient's skin from injury when moving and positioning.
2. Maintain a safe and comfortable position (within the limits of the involved limb's ROM, minimize pressure on pressure points).
3. Ensure exposure and accessibility of surgical site, but avoid unnecessary exposure.
4. Use appropriate safety devices (safety straps).

What are some of the responsibilities of the circulating nurse?

1. Assist in helping the surgical team members put on their gowns.
2. Ensure integrity of sterile field.
3. Open and provide supplies to scrub nurse (using sterile technique).
4. Collect, label, and dispose of specimens.
5. Perform sharps, sponge, and instrument counts with scrub nurse throughout the case.

What are some of the responsibilities of the scrub nurse?

1. Provide surgical instruments to surgeon.
2. Ensure integrity of sterile field.
3. Perform sharps, sponge, and instrument counts with circulating nurse throughout the case.

What documentation factors are important intraoperatively?

Number of needles, instruments, and sponges; dressings; drains; specimens and cultures obtained; medications administered; patient position; use of safety devices and monitors; patient outcome; and personnel in the room

What are important nursing actions when preparing for the postoperative patient?

1. Securing the appropriate equipment (I.V. poles, suction, oxygen equipment)
2. Obtaining report from recovery room nurse

✎ What patient information should the recovery room nurse provide upon patient transfer back to the nursing unit postoperatively?

1. Type of procedure and patient's medical condition
2. Vital signs
3. LOC
4. Number, type, and location of drains, tubes, and dressings
5. Number and location of I.V. accesses as well as type of I.V. solutions infused
6. Input and output volumes, including estimated blood loss
7. Names and times of medications administered, especially analgesics
8. Any perioperative complications (hypotension, nausea, vomiting)
9. Family location and needs

Asepsis and aseptic practices

What's disinfection?

The process of destroying active microorganisms, with the exception of spores

What's sterilization?

The process of destroying all microorganisms, including spores

What methods can sterilize equipment in the operating room?

Autoclaving, using chemical agents or gas, boiling, steaming under pressure, and radiating

What's asepsis?

The prevention of microbial contamination by ensuring only sterile supplies and equipment come in contact with a surface and by ensuring that airborne transmission of microorganisms is reduced

✎ What's medical asepsis (clean technique)?

Practices that confine a specific microorganism to a specific area, limiting the number, growth, and spread of microorganisms

What's surgical asepsis (sterile technique)?

Practices that keep an area (air, operative site) or an object (drape, instrument, gown, glove) free from all microorganisms and spores

▨ *Sterile technique is required for all invasive procedures so that microorganisms are prevented from entering body tissues.*

What's the primary goal of surgical asepsis?

Prevention of contamination of the surgical site by isolating it from the surrounding nonsterile environment

✎ What are the basic principles of surgical asepsis?

1. The operative site is the center of sterile field.
2. Only sterile items may be used within the sterile field.
3. Sterile persons or items become nonsterile when they come in contact with a nonsterile person or item.
4. Staff is considered sterile after performing a surgical scrub and putting on a gown, a mask, and gloves.
5. Gowns are considered sterile only above the waist to the shoulders in the front and 2″ (5 cm) above the elbows to the sleeve cuffs.
6. Gloved hands should be kept away from the face, and elbows should remain at the sides.
7. Only the top of a sterile table is sterile (edges and sides are considered nonsterile). The 1″ (2.5 cm) outer edge of the sterile draped table is considered nonsterile.
8. Sterile items that are dropped below waist level or otherwise out of sight are considered nonsterile.

9. Everyone, especially nonsterile persons, should avoid reaching, coughing, sneezing, or talking over a sterile field.
10. Sterile fields are created as close to the time of use as possible (minimizes chance of environmental contamination from air droplets).

⚑ *Never turn away from a sterile field.*

⚑ *Sterile items should be placed inside the outer edges (1″ [2.5 cm]) of a sterile field.*

 What are examples of actions that compromise sterility?

1. Reaching over a sterile field by a nonsterile person
2. Holding sterile gloved hands below waist or table level
3. Turning your back to a sterile field
4. Talking, coughing, or sneezing over sterile field
5. Spilling liquid (even if it's sterile) on a sterile paper field
6. Touching nonsterile part of sterile gown (shoulders, back, neckline, axillae) with sterile gloved hands
7. Placing sterile item within 1″ outer edge of sterile field
8. Piercing a hole in sterile gloves
9. Extending sterile supplies over the edge of the table

What are appropriate actions if a sterile field becomes nonsterile?

The contaminated field must be discarded and a new sterile field set up

How is the sterility of a package determined?

1. Inspect the integrity of packaging for perforation, puncture, or moisture contamination (may attract microorganisms from the air or draw them in by capillary action).
2. Inspect the expiration dates.
3. Inspect the package for sterilization indicators (tape).

⚑ *Never assume an item is sterile.*

If the sterility of a package is unknown, what's the most appropriate action?

Assume it's nonsterile and discard.

Why is scrubbing necessary for persons working in the sterile field?

Because skin can't be sterilized, it's a potential source of infection. Performing a surgical scrub and putting on a sterile gown, gloves, and a cap minimize the risk of contaminating the operative site.

Why should the hands be held higher than the elbows after surgical hand washing?	To prevent forearm contaminants (most contaminated area) from spreading to the hands (least contaminated area)
Why are masks necessary?	Masks reduce the risk of contamination by areas that can't be scrubbed (mouth, nose).
Why is filtered air used in some operating rooms?	Because air contains dust and droplets that can contaminate the operative site, filtered air (and laminar air flow when necessary) may be used in some operating rooms.

How should individuals who are wearing sterile surgical attire (gown, mask, gloves, cap) move about in the operating room?

1. Move only from one sterile area to another.
2. Maintain a safe distance from one another when changing positions with another sterile person.
3. Pass by each other turning back-to-back or face-to-face.
4. Keep arms and hands within sterile field at all times. Maintain 12″ (30.5 cm) "margin of safety" with nonsterile items or persons.

How should individuals wearing nonsterile attire move about in the operating room?

1. Avoid contact with any sterile areas.
2. Contact only nonsterile items or persons to prevent contamination.
3. Avoid walking between two sterile fields.
4. Always face the sterile field on approach.
5. Maintain a 12″ "margin of safety" with sterile items or persons.
6. Avoid reaching over a sterile field.

What's the "margin of safety"?	The boundary between sterile and nonsterile areas; examples include the 1″ (2.5 cm) outer edge of a sterile wrapper and the 12″ distance between a nonsterile person and a sterile field
What's the purpose of a sterile drape?	Minimizes the passage of microorganisms from nonsterile to sterile areas; the patient (with the exception of the incisional site), furniture, and equipment to be used within the sterile field should be covered with a sterile drape

What rules apply to sterile drapes?

1. Only sterile persons should handle sterile drapes.
2. They should be placed higher than the operating table.
3. They shouldn't be moved or repositioned once established.
4. Only the top surface of the drape is considered sterile.

Postoperative care

✎ What's the pre-ferred position for an unconscious patient in the immediate postoperative phase?

Side-lying position, without a pillow; after reflexes return, the patient can be placed in a back-lying position

⚡ *Side-lying with the face in a slightly downward position prevents the tongue from occluding the pharynx and reduces the risk of aspiration by allowing drainage of mucus or vomitus out of the mouth.*

What are the primary nursing responsibilities postoperatively?

1. Monitor the patient cardiovascular status, fluid balance, and neurologic status.
2. Provide comfort.
3. Ensure safety.
4. Encourage mobility.
5. Prevent postoperative complications (deep vein thrombosis, pneumonia, infection).
6. Monitor for bleeding or hemorrhage.

✎ What factors should be assessed in a postoperative patient?

1. Patency of airway
2. Baseline vital signs, breath sounds, and level of consciousness
3. Patency and placement of any tubes (maintain negative pressure in portable wound drainage systems) and drainage characteristics
4. Dressing integrity
5. Intake and output status
6. Level of pain and any adverse reactions to analgesics, such as oversedation and respiratory depression

✎ How often should deep breathing and coughing be encouraged in the postoperative patient who received general anesthesia?

At least every 2 hours while awake for the first few days

✎ How often should leg exercises be encouraged postoperatively?

At least every 2 hours during waking hours

✎ How frequently should a patient be repositioned postoperatively?

Turn from side to side at least every 2 hours

⚡ *Turning from side to side allows maximum expansion of the uppermost lung and protects skin integrity.*

Why *shouldn't* pillows or rolls be placed under a postoperative patient's knees?

Thrombus formation may result from pressure on the popliteal blood vessels, which impedes the blood circulation to and from the lower extremities.

What are important nursing actions for initial dressing care?

Circle any drainage on dressings (note date and time) and reinforce surgical dressings.

What are important nursing actions when a patient first awakens from general anesthesia?

1. Reorient to person, place, and time.
2. Encourage coughing and deep breathing when the patient can cooperate.
3. Assess vital signs every 15 minutes until stable (or per hospital protocol), every hour for the next 2 hours, and every 4 hours for the next 24 hours.
4. Maintain I.V. therapy as ordered.
5. Assess level of pain and instruct the patient on the use of patient-controlled analgesia.
6. Orient the patient to the call light.
7. Monitor the dressing and surgical site for bleeding or hematomas.

Notify the surgeon immediately if hemorrhage is known or suspected (profuse bleeding, hypotension).

When does the level of pain typically peak in the postoperative period?

12 to 36 hours following surgery

When is a patient allowed to begin ambulating?

Ambulation is generally encouraged the evening of surgery or by the first postoperative day but should be started as soon as possible in accordance with the surgeon's orders.

Why is early ambulation important?

It prevents respiratory, circulatory, urinary, and GI complications as well as muscle weakness.

What are important nursing actions when a patient first ambulates after surgery?

1. Instruct the patient to sit on the edge of the bed, dangle his legs, and take slow, deep breaths before standing (minimizes orthostatic hypotension and may prevent falls).
2. Administer analgesics before ambulating to minimize discomfort.

What position is favored if a patient can't ambulate?

A sitting position because it allows for the greatest lung expansion

Why is maintaining adequate hydration important in the post-operative patient?

1. To prevent dehydration that may occur secondary to preoperative fasting, preoperative medications, and loss of body fluid
2. To keep mucous membranes and respiratory secretions moist, which facilitates the expectoration of mucus

What factors are important when assessing a patient's hydration status?

Skin turgor, blood pressure, intake and output, presence of edema, and drainage from wounds or tubes

How often should a patient's hydration status be assessed?

Every 1 to 4 hours for the first day

When is a patient allowed to resume a diet?

When awake enough to protect the airway and when bowel function returns

What factors inhibit the return of peristalsis postoperatively?

Anesthetics, opioids, intraoperative intestinal manipulation, immobility, and alterations in fluid and food ingestion

When should the return of peristalsis be anticipated in a postoperative patient?

2 to 3 days after major abdominal surgery

What's the typical diet progression postoperatively?

Ice chips to small sips of water to clear liquids to a soft diet to a regular diet, as the patient tolerates

What treatment measures are appropriate for nausea in the postoperative patient?

1. Administer pharmacologic agents, such as serotonin receptor antagonists: ondansetron (Zofran), granisetron (Kytril), and dolasetron.
2. Place the patient in an upright position, unless contraindicated (prevents aspiration of vomitus).
3. Encourage slow, deep breathing.
4. Provide mouth care.
5. Apply cool washcloths to the patient's forehead.

What respiratory complications can occur postoperatively?

Pneumonia, atelectasis, and pulmonary embolism

Which patients are at the greatest risk for respiratory complications postoperatively?

Smokers (sixfold increased risk), thoracic or abdominal surgical patients, older patients, and those who underwent intubation and general anesthesia

What are important considerations when assessing for respiratory complications?

1. Patency of airway
2. Respiratory rate
3. Oxygen saturation
4. Breath sounds
5. Skin color
6. Ability to cough
7. Use of accessory muscles
8. Arterial blood gas results

What nursing actions are important in preventing respiratory complications postoperatively?

1. Place the patient in a side-lying position to prevent aspiration until he's fully conscious.
2. Protect the patient's airway if the gag reflex is absent.
3. Encourage early ambulation.
4. Instruct the patient on the appropriate use of incentive spirometry and turning, coughing, and deep-breathing exercises.
5. Suction the oral cavity and airways as needed.
6. Titrate opioids and sedatives to reduce pain while avoiding respiratory depression.

How are deep-breathing exercises performed?

Ten deep abdominal breaths, in which the breath is held for 3 to 5 seconds at least every 2 hours

Instruct the patient to splint abdominal or thoracic incisions with a pillow during deep-breathing exercises.

What circulatory complications can occur postoperatively?

Hemorrhage, hypovolemic shock, thrombophlebitis, development of a thrombus and embolus, and myocardial infarction as well as vasodilation and hypotension from continuous epidural anesthesia

What are important factors in the assessment for circulatory problems?

1. Blood pressure
2. Heart rate and rhythm
3. Heart sounds
4. Peripheral pulses and temperature of extremities
5. Capillary refill
6. Homans' sign (pain with dorsiflexion of the foot)
7. Type, amount, color, and character of drainage from tubes, drains, or the incision

What nursing actions are important in preventing circulatory problems postoperatively?

1. Assess for blood pooling underneath the patient or on the bed linens.
2. Assess dressings, tubes, catheters, and drains for blood.
3. Monitor heart rate and blood pressure at frequent intervals.

4. Encourage leg exercises every hour while awake.
5. Encourage fluid intake.
6. Position the patient in bed to facilitate blood flow to the extremities (no pillows under knees).
7. Encourage early ambulation.
8. Apply compression stockings and sequential compression device as ordered.
9. Administer anticoagulants as ordered.

✎ When should sequential compression devices be worn?

At all times other than when ambulating, bathing, or during skin assessment; sequential compression devices are discontinued when the patient is ambulating regularly

▐ *Time without sequential compression devices should be limited to 1 hour in the postoperative period, unless the patient has been ambulating during that time.*

What urinary complications can occur postoperatively?

Urine retention and urinary tract infection

What are important considerations when assessing for urinary complications?

1. Intake and output
2. Bladder distention
3. Amount, color, and character of urine from indwelling catheter (if present)

✎ What nursing actions are important in the prevention of urinary complications postoperatively?

1. Encourage frequent voiding.
2. Catheterize as needed per physician's order.
3. Assist to normal position when voiding.
4. Monitor intake and output.
5. Report hematuria, cloudy urine, or a urine output less than 30 ml/hour immediately.

✎ What's the minimum acceptable urine output postoperatively?

30 ml/hour in an adult (or 0.5 mg/kg/hour)

✎ When should the surgeon be notified regarding a patient's urinary status?

If the (noncatheterized) patient hasn't urinated within 8 hours after surgery or after the removal of a urinary catheter, if the urine output of any patient is less than 30 ml/hour, or as otherwise ordered by the surgeon

▐ *Anesthetics temporarily decrease urinary bladder tone, but the tone typically normalizes within 8 hours after surgery.*

What GI complications can occur postoperatively?

Nausea, vomiting, tympanites (retention of gas within the intestines), constipation, and the development of an ileus

What are important factors in assessing for GI complications?	1. Bowel sounds 2. Passage of flatus 3. Type, amount, and character of nasogastric tube drainage 4. Abdominal distention 5. Presence of nausea, vomiting, or anorexia
✎ **What nursing actions are important in preventing GI complications postoperatively?**	1. Progress diet as ordered and tolerated. 2. Encourage early ambulation. 3. Promote adequate fluid intake. 4. Administer fiber supplements, stool softeners, enemas, and rectal suppositories as ordered. 5. Assist the patient to a normal position during defecation.
What wound complications can occur postoperatively?	Infection, dehiscence, and evisceration

Dehiscence

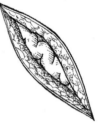

Evisceration

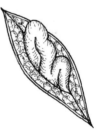

🔖 *Dehiscence is a separation of the fascial suture line, and evisceration is the extrusion of internal organs through the incision.*

What are important factors in assessing wound complications?	1. Intact suture line 2. Amount and character of drainage on dressing 3. Warmth, swelling, tenderness, or pain around the incision 4. Body temperature
✎ **What nursing actions are important in preventing wound complications postoperatively?**	1. Instruct the patient to splint the incision with a pillow when coughing or sneezing. 2. Reinforce or change dressings as necessary. 3. Maintain adequate nutrition to promote wound healing.

✎ **What factors can assess for neurologic complications?**

1. Level of consciousness and mental status
2. Movement, sensation, and strength in the extremities
3. Presence of gag reflex
4. Cranial nerve function
5. Intracranial pressure

✎ **What nursing actions are important in preventing neurologic complications postoperatively?**

1. Orient the patient to environment.
2. Protect the patient's airway if the gag reflex is absent.
3. Perform neurologic checks at frequent intervals.

What psychologic complications can occur postoperatively?

Postoperative depression due to altered body image or poor prognosis based on surgical findings; sundowning (especially in the elderly)

Surgical drain management

What are the purposes of surgical drains?

1. *Prophylactic:* prevents development of fluid collection or abscess (infected fluid collection) by maintaining drainage of the operative space
2. *Therapeutic:* facilitates healing

What are the two primary types of drains?

1. *Passive:* work by gravity or capillary action (Penrose, Foley, Malecot, Word catheters)
2. *Active:* work by suction from bulb device or suction pump (Hemovac, Jackson-Pratt)

What are other methods of classifying drains?

1. *Open:* external end is left unattached (drainage may cause skin irritation); used when drainage of short duration is anticipated, or if the area being drained was severely infected at the time of surgery
2. *Closed:* external end attached to collection device, which may use vacuum effect or suction; results in a decreased risk of infection, prevents skin irritation from drainage and enables accurate measurement of drainage

✎ **What complications most commonly occur with surgical drains?**

Blockage, dislodgement of drain, and skin irritation or infection

✎ **What nursing actions are important when caring for a patient with surgical drains?**

1. Observe and record drainage color, odor, and volume; assess for presence of clots.
2. Empty collection bulb every 8 hours or when it's two-thirds full.

3. Maintain separate output totals for each drain every shift.
4. Keep skin dry; change dressing and provide skin and drain care daily.
5. Assess the insertion site for secure anchor (intact suture) as well as for signs of infection.
6. Obtain a culture if a new infection is suspected (foul odor, purulent drainage, or sudden increase in drainage volume).
7. Assess the position of Penrose drains with each dressing change.

▶ *Remember to compress the bulb and close the cap after emptying Jackson-Pratt, Davol, or Hemovac drains.*

What are potential causes of increased bloody drainage?

Vessel leakage, catheter erosion into a vessel, or liquefaction of a hematoma

What are potential causes of increased serous drainage?

Increased lymphatic drainage (from increased activity) or fat breakdown (necrosis)

What might cause urine to be found in a surgical drain?

Fistula formation from the urinary tract

✎ What might cause a sudden cessation of drainage?

Tissue debris or clot formation

✎ What might cause increased purulent drainage?

Infection

What might cause increased drainage from a mediastinal tube on a cardiac surgery patient?

Bleeding is almost always the cause

✎ What might cause decreased drainage from a mediastinal tube on a cardiac surgery patient?

Clot in the tube, which can lead to cardiac tamponade

When are drains removed?	When drainage has ceased or is considered insignificant, typically within a few days after the surgical procedure; may also be removed when imaging studies (ultrasound or computed tomography scan) demonstrate resolution of fluid collection being drained
How are drains removed?	By the minimally painful removal of a stitch that secures the drain to the patient's skin, followed by pulling the tube quickly through the exit site

> *A small amount of fluid may leak from the drain site for a few days after removal. A dry gauze dressing should be placed over this site.*

Discharge teaching for the postsurgical patient

What standard discharge instructions should be given to a postsurgical patient?	1. Avoid strenuous activities and lifting heavy objects (greater than 10 lb [4.5 kg]) for 6 weeks, if open procedure was performed. 2. Avoid driving until cleared by surgeon. 3. Avoid tub bathing for 2 weeks (may sponge bathe or shower with water running over incision). 4. Avoid direct sunlight to incision (prevents hyperpigmentation).
What wound care instructions should be given to a patient at the time of discharge?	1. Don't remove adhesive strips for 2 weeks; however they may fall off on their own before that time. 2. Gently wash off dried material around the incision. 3. Inform the patient that he may see a small amount of clear or light red drainage for the first several days. 4. Have normal expectation of wound healing (incision may be slightly red where staples or stitches insert; may feel a ridge along the incision that is normal, which will go away with time).
For what conditions should a patient notify the surgeon after discharge?	1. Fever greater than 101° F (38.3° C) 2. Severe diarrhea, vomiting, or abdominal pain 3. Worsening pain at operative site 4. Spreading erythema and edema around the incision 5. Cloudy or foul-smelling drainage or bright red blood from the incision

Nursing skills

Putting on and removing sterile gloves (open method)

When should sterile gloves be worn?

When the hands may introduce microorganisms into a body orifice or open wound

What's the proper technique for putting on sterile gloves using the open method?

1. Wash your hands thoroughly for at least 10 seconds.
2. Select a pair of gloves of proper size and place the package on a clean, dry surface.
3. Open the outer wrap and remove the inner package.
4. Fold open the inner package and carefully open the flaps to expose the gloves. Be careful not to touch the inner surface of the wrap because it's considered sterile.
5. Grasp the dominant hand's glove by the folded cuff using the thumb and index finger of the nondominant hand, as shown. Use skin-to-skin technique, being careful not to touch the outside of the glove with your bare hand.

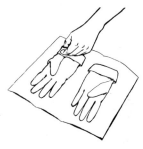

6. Insert your hand into the glove and pull it up, leaving the cuff turned down over the hand; be sure to keep the thumb of the dominant hand against the palm (minimizes risk of thumb contaminating outside of glove).

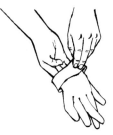

7. Pick up the glove and carefully insert your hand by slipping the fingers of the gloved hand under the cuff of the nondominant glove (glove-to-glove technique).

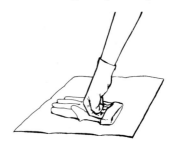

8. Adjust both gloves for a smooth fit.
9. Pull up the cuff (glove-to-glove technique) by carefully sliding gloved fingers under everted cuff of dominant glove. Repeat for nondominant glove cuff.

What's the proper technique for removing sterile gloves using the open method?

1. Remove first glove by rolling it inside out.
2. While holding the removed glove with the gloved hand, place the first two fingers of the nongloved hand inside the cuff of the gloved hand and remove it by turning it inside out.
3. Discard both gloves (the first glove should be inside the second, with the inside portion being outermost).
4. Wash your hands thoroughly for at least 10 seconds.

⚡ *Use the open method of putting on sterile gloves when only sterile gloves are required (insertion of indwelling urinary catheters, surgical preps). The closed method requires using a sterile gown and is typically used only in operating or delivery rooms.*

Establishing a sterile field

What nursing actions should be performed before establishing a sterile field?

1. Inspect the expiration date and integrity of sterile kit or supplies to be used within the sterile field.
2. Prepare the work area that is clean, dry, and above waist level.

Opening sterile wrapped packages

How should sterile wrapped packages be opened?

1. Place the package in the center of clean a work area and position it to allow the top flap of the wrapper to open away from you (prevents subsequent reaching over exposed sterile items).
2. Reach around the kit and open the first flap by grasping it with the thumb and index finger. Be sure to touch only the outside of the wrapper.
3. Repeat the procedure for the side flaps, being sure to use the right hand for the right flap and left hand for the left flap to avoid reaching over exposed sterile items.
4. Grasp the turned-down corner of the fourth flap and open it toward you.

◤ *If the inner surface of a sterile wrapper touches any nonsterile item, it becomes contaminated and must be discarded.*

Using a drape in a sterile field

What's the proper technique for establishing a sterile drape?

1. Open the drape package.
2. Grasp the folded corner on top of the drape using only one hand.
3. Lift the drape out of its packaging and allow it to open freely. To avoid contaminating the drape, don't allow it to contact any nonsterile surface. Discard packaging.
4. Use the other hand to carefully grasp another corner of the drape and place on work surface. The side that's hanging freely (bottom) should be placed farthest from you to avoid leaning over it.

Introducing sterile supplies onto a sterile field

What's the proper technique for introducing sterile supplies onto a sterile field?

1. Open packages in a manner that preserves sterility of contents.
2. Hold the package 6″ (15.2 cm) above the sterile field and allow contents to drop onto the center of the field (inside 1″ [2.5 cm] margins).

Pouring sterile solutions

What's the proper technique for pouring a sterile solution?

1. Obtain the correct solution (read the label three times before opening) and verify the expiration date.
2. Remove the container cap and invert it (maintains its sterility by avoiding contact with nonsterile surface).
3. Hold the bottle with label facing up and 6″ (15.2 cm) above the sterile field, and carefully pour solution into a sterile bowl in corner of the field. Avoid splashing to prevent contamination of the sterile field (moisture facilitates passage of microorganisms through sterile drape).
4. Discard any unused solution, or replace the cap and label the bottle with date and time of opening (according to your facility's policy).

◤ *The outside of a bottle is considered contaminated, while the inside is considered sterile.*

7

Principles of emergency management

Emergency management

✎ What are the three primary patient assessments for any emergency situation?

1. Check the airway.
2. Check breathing.
3. Check circulation.

During a primary survey, what are indications that a patient's airway is patent?

1. Airway doesn't appear narrowed or obstructed (stridor).
2. Speech is clear.
3. Skin is acyanotic.

◤ *The tongue is the most common cause of airway obstructions in unconscious patients.*

✎ What nursing interventions are appropriate if a patient's airway isn't patent?

1. Clear the mouth of any obstructions (foreign objects, food).
2. Perform chin-lift maneuver (or jaw-thrust maneuver if neck injury is suspected) to open airway.
3. Administer supplemental oxygen via nasal cannula or face mask.
4. Assess vital signs, lung sounds, and oxygen saturation level.
5. Prepare for placement of an artificial airway (endotracheal [ET] tube).

During a primary survey, what are indications that a patient's breathing is effective?

1. Skin is acyanotic.
2. Capillary refill time is less than 3 seconds.
3. Oxygen saturation is greater than 94%.

✎ What nursing interventions are appropriate if a patient's breathing isn't adequate?

1. Administer supplemental oxygen (2 to 4 L/minute via nasal cannula if the patient is awake with spontaneous breathing; 12 to 15 L/minute via nonrebreather mask if unstable; 12 to 15 L/minute via bag-valve-mask if conscious with respiratory failure).

2. Place the patient in Fowler's position.
3. Assess vital signs, lung sounds, and oxygen saturation level.
4. Aid in placement of an ET tube, if the patient isn't responding to other measures.

✎ **During a primary survey, what are indications that a patient's circulation is effective?**

1. Adequate organ perfusion (awake and alert; warm, dry skin without mottling or cyanosis; urine output greater than 30 ml/hour)
2. Pulses are palpable (particularly central pulses such as carotid or femoral)
3. Capillary refill time less than 3 seconds

✎ **What nursing interventions are appropriate if a patient's circulation isn't effective?**

1. Place the patient in a recumbent position and maintain a patent airway.
2. Establish I.V. access (2 large-bore I.V. lines).
3. Infuse a fluid bolus as ordered by the physician (typically 250 to 500 ml bolus of normal saline or lactated Ringer's).
4. Obtain electrocardiogram or place on cardiac monitor, if available.

Code situations

What's a "code"?

A team response initiated for patients experiencing cardiac and respiratory arrest or other emergent conditions

✎ **What are the indications for calling a code?**

1. Respiratory and cardiac arrest (actual or impending)
2. Acute, massive hemorrhage
3. Rapid deterioration in patient medical condition
4. Falls (in some hospitals)

When is it appropriate to call the patient's physician STAT as opposed to calling a code?

When the patient experiences an acute change, but remains clinically stable (alert, stable vital signs)

◤ *No code should be called for a patient who has a proper do-not-resuscitate order in the chart.*

✎ **Who's responsible for calling a code?**

The person who locates a patient who isn't responsive or who meets the criteria for a code alerts unit staff to a code situation. The unit clerk typically makes the appropriate institutional phone calls to activate the code team.

Who's responsible for initiating basic life support and calling for help?

Trained health care professionals caring for or in the vicinity of the coding patient

What are the responsibilities of the first responder?

1. Place the patient in supine position, open the airway, and check for breathing; if absent, initiate rescue breathing with barrier resuscitation mask.
2. Assess pulses; if absent, initiate chest compressions.
3. Designate others to obtain additional supplies as well as the code cart.
4. Remain in the patient's room to provide information about the patient and assist the code team, if necessary.

What are the typical responsibilities of the second responder?

1. Make sure the unit secretary has notified the hospital switchboard of the code location.
2. Obtain code cart as well as I.V. pole and suction equipment.
3. Assist the primary nurse to place the patient on a backboard and administer oxygen at 15 L/minute.
4. Assist with cardiopulmonary resuscitation (CPR) until the code team arrives.

What are the responsibilities of other staff nurses during a code?

1. Clear the area of excess equipment to facilitate access of code team.
2. Remove the patient's roommate and any visitors.
3. Set up extra trash cans in area of code.
4. Serve as a runner for the code team.
5. Take the patient chart and medication list to the code team.
6. Assume care for code nurse's other patients.

What nursing actions are appropriate once the code cart arrives?

1. Begin ventilating with bag-valve-mask device (hand-held resuscitation bag).
2. Set up oxygen flowmeter and ventilate with 100% oxygen.
3. Place the patient on a backboard (if he isn't already on one) and continue chest compressions.
4. Set up suction and intubation equipment.
5. Initiate I.V. infusion of normal saline or lactated Ringer's solution.
6. Place patient on a cardiac monitor.

What departments in the hospital typically manage their own codes (no code calls)?

Emergency department, intensive care unit (ICU), operating room, and postanesthesia care unit

What equipment is commonly used in a code?

Oxygen, handheld resuscitation bag, code cart, backboard, suction equipment, intubation equipment, and I.V. pole and supplies

Who's typically on the code team?	Anesthesiologist or nurse anesthetist, critical care physicians, critical care nurse, respiratory therapist, and electrocardiography technician
Who might be additional responders?	Pharmacist, surgeon, and hospital or nursing administrators
Who's usually the code team leader?	Medical physician or resident
What's the code team leader's primary responsibility?	The leader "runs" the code by giving orders to code team members.

> *The code team leader is the only person who should be giving orders during a code.*

What are the documentation nurse's responsibilities?	1. Record all events that occur during the code (time of event, interventions, patient response). 2. Ensure appropriate signatures are obtained on the code record.
What important factors should be documented in the code record?	1. Patient's name 2. Time of arrest and patient's activities at time of arrest 3. Time of CPR initiation 4. Time of code cart arrival 5. I.V. line established (size, location, time) 6. Cardiac rhythms (initial and after interventions) 7. Procedures (defibrillations, intubation) and patient response with exact times 8. Medications and fluids administered and patient response with exact times 9. Names of all participating staff 10. Time of code termination and patient's condition
When is it appropriate to terminate a code?	When a patient has been stabilized to warrant cessation of resuscitative efforts and transfer to the ICU, or if resuscitative efforts have been deemed unsuccessful by the code team leader
Who's responsible for informing the patient's family about the code and the condition of the patient?	The attending physician
What are the responsibilities of the primary nurse once the patient has been transferred into the ICU?	Obtain updates on other patients, including what medications were given

Medications commonly used in a code

✎ **What route is preferable for administering emergency medications?**

I.V. route (preferably central) due to rapid rate of action; some emergency medications may be given via an endotracheal tube during an emergency, particularly if no I.V. access is available

Sympathetic agonists

EPINEPHRINE

✎ **What are the actions of epinephrine?**

Enhances coronary and cerebral perfusion by increasing cardiac contractility, heart rate, and vascular resistance; increases blood pressure and reroutes blood to the heart and brain; may also increase automaticity and make ventricular fibrillation more susceptible to defibrillation

⚡ *Small doses of epinephrine cause vasoconstriction, whereas larger doses can cause vasodilation.*

For what conditions is epinephrine most commonly used in a code?

1. Ventricular fibrillation
2. Pulseless ventricular tachycardia
3. Asystole
4. Pulseless electrical activity

⚡ *Epinephrine is the drug of choice when a patient is pulseless.*

⚡ *Epinephrine is commonly supplied in 10 ml prefilled syringes on code carts.*

What are common adverse effects of epinephrine?

Dizziness, anxiety, tremors, palpitations, tachycardia, nausea, and dyspnea; may also worsen myocardial ischemia and cause premature ventricular contractions (PVCs) or ventricular tachycardia

VASOPRESSIN (PITRESSIN)

What are the actions of vasopressin?

Stimulates vasoconstriction, which increases the effectiveness of CPR and increases responsiveness of the myocardium to resuscitative interventions; also increases blood flow to the brain and heart during CPR

What are the uses of vasopressin during a code?	Ventricular fibrillation and pulseless ventricular tachycardia; used as an alternative to epinephrine
What are common adverse effects of vasopressin?	Diaphoresis, abdominal cramps, nausea, and vomiting

NOREPINEPHRINE (LEVOPHED)

What are the actions of norepinephrine?	Increases cardiac output by increasing cardiac contractility and heart rate as well as by causing peripheral vasoconstriction
✎ **For what conditions is norepinephrine most commonly used in a code?**	Acute hypotension unrelated to volume and cardiogenic shock
What are common adverse effects of norepinephrine?	Headache, palpitations, tachycardia, hypertension, ectopy, and angina; may worsen myocardial ischemia and cause PVCs or ventricular tachycardia

DOPAMINE

✎ **What are the actions of dopamine?**	Enhances perfusion by increasing cardiac output
For what conditions is dopamine most commonly used in a code?	Mild hypotension that's unrelated to hypovolemia; also used to treat bradycardia
What are common adverse effects of dopamine?	Headache, palpitations, tachycardia, hypertension, ectopic beats, and angina

DOBUTAMINE

✎ **What are the actions of dobutamine?**	Improves cardiac output by increasing myocardial contractility, coronary blood flow, and heart rate
For what conditions is dobutamine most commonly used in a code?	Heart failure related to poor cardiac output

What are common adverse effects of dobutamine?	Hypotension, light-headedness, anxiety, leg cramps, tachycardia, and palpitations

ISOPROTERENOL (ISUPREL)

What are the actions of isoproterenol?	Increases myocardial contractility and heart rate
For what conditions is isoproterenol most commonly used in a code?	Heart blocks and ventricular arrhythmias (although transcutaneous pacing is now the treatment of choice); may also be of benefit in the treatment of torsades de pointes (a type of ventricular tachycardia in which a ventricular rate greater than 200 typically occurs in short episodes lasting less than 90 seconds)
✎ **What are common adverse effects of isoproterenol?**	Tremors, anxiety, palpitations, tachycardia, hypertension; may also worsen myocardial ischemia and cause PVCs or ventricular tachycardia

Antiarrhythmics

AMIODARONE (CORDARONE)

What are the actions of amiodarone?	1. Slows atrioventricular (AV) nodal conduction and prolongs its refractoriness by blocking myocardium potassium channels 2. Decreases cardiac workload and resultant myocardial oxygen consumption due to its vasodilatory actions
For what conditions is amiodarone most commonly used in a code?	Life-threatening ventricular arrhythmias, such as recurrent ventricular fibrillation and recurrent ventricular tachycardia in a hemodynamically unstable patient
What are common adverse effects of amiodarone?	Light-headedness, facial flushing, diaphoresis, headache, paresthesia, hypotension, chest pain, nausea, metallic taste, and dyspnea

LIDOCAINE (XYLOCAINE HCL IV)

✎ **What are the actions of lidocaine?**	Increases cardiac electrical stimulation threshold, which stabilizes the cardiac membrane and decreases automaticity

▧ *Lidocaine is the drug of choice if amiodarone isn't available. It shouldn't be administered to a patient who has already received amiodarone.*

For what conditions is lidocaine most commonly used in a code?

Ventricular tachycardia and ventricular fibrillation as well as suppression of ventricular ectopy (PVCs)

What are common adverse effects of lidocaine?

Dizziness, headaches, bradycardia, hypotension, and seizures (if toxic)

ADENOSINE (ADENOCARD)

What are the actions of adenosine?

Slows conduction through the AV node and reduces SA node automaticity; restores normal sinus rhythm in patients with tachycardias associated with the AV node

For what condition is adenosine commonly used in a code?

Paroxysmal supraventricular tachycardia (PSVT)

What are common adverse effects of adenosine?

Light-headedness, facial flushing, headache, diaphoresis, paresthesia, palpitations, chest pain, hypotension, nausea, metallic taste, dyspnea, heart block and, possibly, asystole

DILTIAZEM (CARDIZEM)

What are the actions of diltiazem?

Blocks calcium channels, which reduces cardiac tissue automaticity (impulse formation) and excitability, as well as slows conduction; also dilates peripheral arteries

For what conditions is diltiazem most commonly used in a code?

Premature supraventricular tachycardia; also slows the ventricular rate in atrial flutter and atrial fibrillation

What are common adverse effects of diltiazem?

Headache, drowsiness, dizziness, nausea, hypotension, peripheral edema, bradycardia, and AV block

MAGNESIUM SULFATE

What are the actions of magnesium sulfate?

Stabilizes cell membranes, resulting in the suppression of cardiac irritability; also produces peripheral vasodilation

For what conditions is magnesium sulfate commonly used in a code?

Torsades de pointes (a type of ventricular tachycardia) and severe refractory ventricular fibrillation with suspected hypomagnesemia

What are common adverse effects of magnesium sulfate?

Facial flushing and diaphoresis with low doses; moderate doses may result in hypotension, bradycardia, decreased reflexes, and respiratory depression (if toxic) due to vasodilatory effects.

What is the antidote for magnesium toxicity?

Calcium chloride

Anticholinergics

ATROPINE

What are the actions of atropine?

Increases heart rate, systemic vascular resistance, and blood pressure

For what conditions is atropine commonly used?

1. Sinus bradycardia (symptomatic)
2. AV blocks
3. Asystole (after epinephrine)

Atropine doses less than 0.5 mg may actually enhance bradycardia.

What are common adverse effects of atropine?

Dry mouth, urinary retention, headache, light-headedness, tachycardia, facial flushing; may also cause worsening of myocardial ischemia and AV blocks as well as cause PVCs or ventricular tachycardia

Alkalinizing agents

SODIUM BICARBONATE

What are the actions of sodium bicarbonate?

Buffers hydrogen ion concentration to reverse acidosis

For what conditions is sodium bicarbonate most commonly used in a code?

Metabolic or respiratory acidosis

Hyperventilation is the treatment of choice for both metabolic and respiratory acidosis in a code situation.

What are common adverse effects of sodium bicarbonate?

Metabolic alkalosis, twitching, hyperreflexia, tetany, and seizures

Common emergency interventions

Oxygen therapy

What devices deliver a low oxygen flow?

1. Nasal cannula
2. Face shield
3. Face tent
4. Oxygen mask

What devices deliver a moderate oxygen flow?

1. Partial rebreather mask
2. Venturi mask

What devices deliver a high oxygen flow?

1. Nonrebreather mask
2. Oxygen hood
3. Endotracheal tube

✎ At what flow rate should oxygen therapy be initiated for a patient in respiratory arrest?

15 L/minute

Rescue breathing

✎ How is rescue breathing administered?

1. Place the patient in a supine position.
2. Clear the patient's mouth and open the airway by using either the head-tilt–chin-lift or jaw-thrust (with or without head tilt) maneuvers.

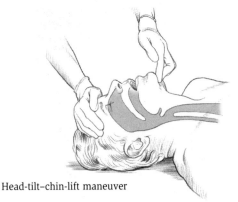

Head-tilt–chin-lift maneuver

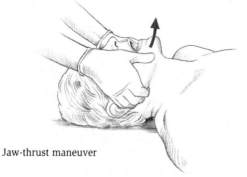

Jaw-thrust maneuver

3. Place your ear and cheek next to the patient's mouth and nose to listen for air escaping, while watching for a rising and falling motion of the chest.

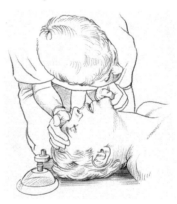

4. If no sign of breathing is detected, begin rescue breathing (a pocket face mask may be used).

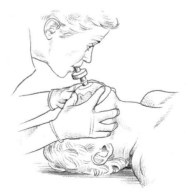

5. Alternatively, a resuscitation bag may be used. Place the resuscitation bag snugly over the patient's mouth and nose with one hand while placing the thumb and index finger of the other hand on the seal positioning middle fingers to support the jaw.

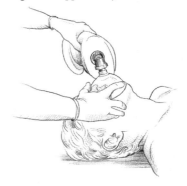

Avoid submental pressure; it may obstruct the airway. Compress the handheld resuscitation bag until adequate elevation of the patient's chest is observed (comparable to a normal breath), then release the bag. Make sure oxygen is attached to the resuscitation bag.

6. Auscultate lung or tracheal sounds for air entering the lungs. Mask condensation indicates ventilation is occurring within the lungs.
7. Assess for restoration of breathing.
8. Reposition airway before resuming rescue breathing if ventilation is unsuccessful. If subsequent ventilations are unsuccessful, reevaluate technique and prepare for possible intubation.
9. Assess for a carotid pulse to determine the need for chest compressions.

■ *Check for the carotid pulse by first locating the trachea and slide the fingers slightly to the side.*

■ *Use the jaw-thrust maneuver for any patient with a suspected head or neck injury.*

✎ What's the venti-lation rate for an adult?

12 breaths/minute

How long should each ventilation last?

1 to 1½ seconds

Why is hyperventila-tion sometimes useful?

It corrects acidosis and lowers intracranial pressure (ICP).

Chest compressions

✎ What's the indication for initiation of chest compressions?

Absence of a pulse

How are chest compressions administered on an adult when only one rescuer is available?

1. Position the patient supine on a firm surface.
2. Place the heel of one hand along the patient's sternum above the xiphoid, and place the other hand on top of the second hand so that they are parallel.

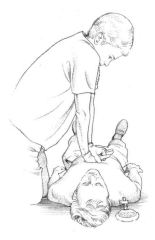

3. Administer cardiac compressions by thrusting straight downward 1$^1/_2$" to 2" (3.5 to 5 cm) with your arms straight and your shoulders directly over your hands.
4. Completely release the compression without lifting your hands from the chest.
5. Deliver compressions at a rate of 100 per minute.
6. Coordinate compressions with two rescue breaths.
7. Reassess every four cycles.

⚡ *CPR is considered a life-sustaining measure rather than a life-saving one. It should be considered an interim measure to support life until defibrillation can occur.*

✎ What is the ratio of compressions to breaths?

15 compressions:2 breaths

How does the performance of chest compressions differ when two rescuers are available?

Until the airway is secured, 15 compressions should be given for every two breaths. However, once the airway is secured five compressions should be given for every one breath, and patient reassessment is performed every ten cycles.

Defibrillation or cardioversion

What's defibrillation?

Delivery of a direct electrical current (measured in joules) in order to terminate ventricular fibrillation

What's the most common indication for defibrillation?

Ventricular fibrillation

> **◤** *In ventricular fibrillation, the electrical activity of the heart becomes scrambled, resulting in the replacement of normal cardiac pumping by an ineffective quivering motion.*

> **◤** *For each minute ventricular fibrillation persists, the likelihood of successful resuscitation decreases by 10%.*

◥ Where should the paddles be placed for defibrillation?

One in the upper right sternum, just beneath the right clavicle and another one to the left of the nipple in the midaxillary line

Where should the electrodes be placed for hands-off defibrillation?

One anteriorly over the precordium (left of the lower sternal border) and the other behind the heart

◥ What's the typical strength of the initial shock for ventricular fibrillation?

200 joules

What's the typical strength of the second shock?

200 to 300 joules

What's the maximum amount of energy that can be delivered?

360 joules

◥ What's the proper technique for defibrillation?

1. Ensure proper placement of electrodes and paddles.
2. Turn on defibrillator.
3. Select the energy level to be delivered.
4. Charge capacitors.
5. State "Clear," and make sure all persons are out of direct and indirect contact with the patient (including bed frame).
6. Apply approximately 25 lb of pressure on each paddle, and depress discharge buttons simultaneously.
7. Reassess the patient's cardiac rhythm.
8. If no response, consider increasing joules and prepare to administer a second shock.

◤ *Continue to perform CPR until a defibrillator is connected to the patient. Don't delay CPR to search for a defibrillator if one isn't immediately available.*

◣ What's an automatic external defibrillator?

A defibrillator device with a microprocessor that senses and analyzes cardiac rhythms and then determines the need for defibrillation based on the rhythm

◤ *CPR should be performed for 1 minute between shock attempts (after the first three shocks have been delivered in rapid sequence), if the heart rhythm doesn't respond.*

◤ *Don't use an automatic external defibrillator for rhythm analysis during CPR because this may result in accidental shocking.*

◤ *Minimize motion of the patient to ensure accurate analysis (don't use if the patient is having a seizure).*

What's a precordial thump?

A technique of delivering a blow to the center of the sternum with the hypothenar aspect from a height of less than or equal to 12″ (30.5 cm); used in an attempt to convert an abnormal cardiac rhythm when a defibrillator is unavailable; same concept can be accomplished in the event of ventricular tachycardia by asking the alert patient to cough

◤ *Administer a precordial thump only in the event of a witnessed cardiac arrest.*

Fluid resuscitation

What's the primary goal of fluid resuscitation?

Volume expansion to maintain adequate perfusion to vital organs

◣ What types of fluids are commonly used for fluid resuscitation?

1. *Colloid solutions:* albumin, fresh frozen plasma, Hetastarch, Dextran, Plasmanate, Hespan
2. *Crystalloid solutions:* normal saline, lactated Ringer's solution
3. *Blood products:* packed red blood cells (PRBCs)

What are the advantages of colloid solutions?

Colloid solutions remain in the intravascular space much longer (several hours) than crystalloid solutions

What are the disadvantages of colloid solutions?	Allergic reactions may occur; they're more expensive than alternatives
What are the advantages of crystalloid solutions?	Crystalloid solutions are readily available, inexpensive, and don't cause allergic reactions.
What are the disadvantages of crystalloid solutions?	Crystalloid solutions remain in the intravascular space only temporarily; infusions of up to five times the fluid deficit may be required, which may lead to pulmonary edema.
When are blood products typically used for fluid resuscitation?	If no improvement after two crystalloid boluses, or for coagulopathy

✎ What adverse reactions are associated with blood product infusions?

1. Transfusion reactions
2. Hypocalcemia (due to citrate)
3. Hypothermia (blood products should be warmed prior to infusion whenever possible)

🔋 *1 to 2 units of fresh frozen plasma should be given for every 5 units of blood transfused to correct dilutional coagulation.*

✎ How quickly should fluid boluses be infused?

Typically less than 20 minutes or as otherwise ordered by the physician

✎ Why shouldn't dextrose solutions be used for fluid resuscitation?

May worsen ischemic brain injury and causes hypokalemia, osmotic diuresis, and hyperglycemia

✎ What are important nursing actions for a patient receiving fluid boluses?

1. Monitor vital signs, especially blood pressure and pulses.
2. Assess for volume overload (crackles on auscultation, shortness of breath, peripheral edema).
3. Reassess the patient after each bolus.

Endotracheal intubation

What's endotracheal (ET) intubation?

An invasive procedure that involves the insertion of a tube into the trachea for management of the airway

What are common uses of ET intubation?	1. Provision of a patent airway during surgical procedures or emergency situations 2. Prevention of aspiration in an unconscious or paralyzed patient 3. Administration of positive-pressure ventilation 4. Provision of sterile route for suctioning of secretions 5. Administration of medications in an emergency situation
What are the different routes in which an ET tube may be inserted?	1. *Nasotracheal:* used for patients with jaw fractures, trauma to mouth or lower face, or recent oral surgery 2. *Orotracheal (using direct laryngoscopy):* preferred route for easier insertion and use of larger tube

⊠ *Dental appliances, such as dentures or bridges, should be removed before orotracheal intubation.*

✎ **What risks are associated with ET intubation?**	Injury to teeth or gums, tracheal rupture, aspiration, intubation of either esophagus or right mainstem bronchus with subsequent hypoxia, and pneumothorax
What medications can be administered via an ET tube?	Use the mnemonic "NAVEL": 1. Naloxone (Narcan) 2. Atropine 3. Versed 4. Epinephrine 5. Lidocaine
What's the proper technique for administering medications via an ET tube?	1. Disconnect artificial ventilation. 2. Discontinue chest compressions (if being performed). 3. Dilute appropriate medication in 10 ml normal saline, and inject into the ET tube. 4. Reattach appropriate ventilation device to ventilate patient. 5. Resume CPR, if indicated.
✎ **What are important nursing interventions when providing care for a patient with an ET tube?**	1. Monitor vital signs, and assess respiratory effort at frequent intervals. 2. Maintain airway patency by suctioning secretions (assess need every 2 hours) and providing oral and nasal care every 2 hours, or as needed. 3. Assess the amount of air in the cuff every 8 hours (usually 20 mm Hg, but no greater than 30 mm Hg). 4. Reposition the tube every 8 hours to prevent tissue damage from continuous pressure. 5. Assess oral and nasal skin for breakdown. Each day, remove tape from one side of face and reposition on the opposite side. 6. Reassess respiratory status, and reconfirm proper tube placement after each episode of ET tube care.

How should proper ET tube position be determined after tube care is provided?

Measure (in centimeters) from the tip of tube to the patient's teeth or gums; observe chest movement, and auscultate chest and stomach. A chest X-ray is another means of tube position verification but isn't performed after each episode of tube care.

Patients with ET tubes can't speak because the tube passes through the vocal cords. Alternative means of communication must be instituted to alleviate patient anxiety.

What's the proper technique for suctioning a patient with an ET tube?

1. Place the patient in the proper position (semi-Fowler's if conscious, lateral position if unconscious).
2. Preoxygenate the patient with 100% oxygen for 2 minutes before suctioning.
3. Obtain the proper supplies, and turn on the wall suction pressure to an appropriate setting (100 to 120 mm Hg for adults). Inform the patient that suctioning may stimulate coughing or gagging.
4. Open the packages containing the sterile gloves and suction catheter. Place a sterile glove on your dominant hand, and connect the suction catheter to the suction tubing. Use only the hand with the sterile glove to handle the suction catheter. Test suction pressure by applying your gloved thumb over the port.
5. Pull the patient's tongue forward and use aseptic technique to pass the catheter down into the ET tube 4″ to 6″ (10 to 15 cm) or until the patient coughs. Suction shouldn't be used before this point.
6. Initiate suctioning (less than 10 seconds at a time) while slowly withdrawing the suction catheter with a rotating motion. If repeat suctioning is necessary, clean the catheter with sterile gauze and flush with sterile water or saline. Allow the patient to rest 30 seconds between suctioning efforts, and limit total suctioning time to 2 minutes. One-hundred-percent oxygen should be administered if the patient becomes distressed or drops the oxygen saturation during suctioning.
7. Instruct the patient to cough and breathe deeply between suctioning efforts to facilitate removal of secretions.
8. Using either a suction catheter or a Yankauer catheter, clean the oropharyngeal airway. Don't place a suction catheter back into the ET tube once it has been used in the mouth or nasal passages.
9. Assess the patient's respiratory effort after the procedure, and document characteristics of secretions removed.
10. Reconfirm proper tube placement by measuring from the tip of tube to the patient's teeth or gums.

◤ *Use aseptic technique when suctioning is performed.*

◤ *Suction catheters should be less than half the size of the ET tube.*

◤ *Suctioning should be performed while withdrawing the catheter with a rotating motion for less than 10 seconds at a time with a 30-second rest period between suctioning efforts. Total suctioning time shouldn't exceed 2 minutes.*

◤ *Total suctioning time should not exceed 2 minutes. Over-suctioning can cause airway damage.*

What are important nursing actions in the event of accidental extubation?

1. Open the airway by using the chin-lift–jaw-thrust maneuver.
2. Assess the patient's respiratory effort.
3. Perform mechanical ventilation using a handheld resuscitation bag, if necessary.
4. Notify the physician.

Common hospital emergencies

Anaphylaxis

✎ **What's an anaphylactic reaction?**

An acute systemic allergic reaction involving bronchial constriction and edema that obstructs the airway and causes generalized vasodilation in response to exposure to an allergen; histamine is released and antibodies are produced.

✎ **What are the clinical manifestations of anaphylaxis?**

Dyspnea, wheezing, or high-pitched breath sounds; cough; abdominal pain and cramps; vomiting; hives or generalized itching; dizziness; confusion; tachycardia and palpitations; cyanosis (late)

What complications may be prevented with early intervention?

Shock, pulmonary edema, angioedema, and arrhythmias as well as cardiac and respiratory arrests if prolonged

✎ **What are important nursing interventions for a patient experiencing an anaphylactic reaction?**

1. Establish patent airway.
2. Administer supplemental oxygen at 5 L/minute via nasal cannula.
3. Establish I.V. access for administration of medications and fluids.
4. Instruct another person to notify the physician.
5. Administer medications (epinephrine, diphenhydramine, steroids) as ordered by the physician.

6. Monitor vital signs and respiratory status, including oxygen saturation level, at least every 15 minutes until stable.

Transfusion reaction

What's a transfusion reaction?

Activation of an immune response against antigens or preservatives in the transfused blood cells, which can result in hypotension, lung injury, shock, or hemolysis

What are the causes of transfusion reactions?

Blood transfusions between incompatible blood groups; may occur also with minor red cell antigens, platelets, and other blood products, such as plasma proteins or preservatives added to the blood products

✎ What types of transfusion reactions may occur?

Hemolytic reaction, febrile reaction, or allergic reaction

✎ What are the clinical manifestations of a hemolytic reaction?

Shivering, headache, lower back pain, tachycardia and tachypnea, hemoglobinuria, oliguria, and hypotension; typically occurs within the first 15 to 20 minutes of the transfusion

✎ What are the clinical manifestations of a febrile reaction?

Fever, rigors, back pain, headache, and mild confusion; typically occurs within the first 30 minutes of the transfusion and is self-limited

✎ What are the clinical manifestations of an allergic reaction?

Hives, wheezing, pruritus, and joint pain

What complications may be prevented with early intervention?

Anemia, kidney failure, and shock

✎ What are important nursing interventions for a patient experiencing a transfusion reaction?

1. Stop the infusion immediately.
2. Notify the physician.
3. Monitor vital signs and respiratory status every 15 minutes for 1 hour, then every hour for 2 hours, and then every 4 hours for 8 hours after that.
4. Administer antihistamines as ordered by the physician.
5. Save the remaining blood product for testing.
6. Send blood to the laboratory to confirm that the clinical findings were caused by the transfusion.
7. Send urine if a hemolytic reaction is suspected.

Respiratory distress or hypoxia

What are common causes of respiratory distress?

Asthma or airway obstruction; pneumothorax; heart failure; pulmonary embolus; drug overdose; fluid overload or pulmonary edema; sepsis or shock; pain, especially from chest or abdominal incision or trauma; anemia

What are early clinical manifestations of hypoxia?

1. Tachycardia
2. Tachypnea
3. Mild elevation of systolic blood pressure
4. Dizziness
5. Confusion, memory loss, irritability, anxiety
6. Cold, clammy skin

What are late clinical manifestations of hypoxia?

1. Use of accessory muscles
2. Bradycardia
3. Hypotension
4. Dyspnea
5. Cyanosis
6. Unresponsiveness

What diagnostic tests should be anticipated in the event of respiratory distress?

Arterial blood gas (ABG), blood and sputum cultures (if febrile), and chest X-ray; electrocardiogram (ECG) and ventilation/perfusion ($\dot{V}/\dot{Q}$) scan may also be performed

What complication can be prevented with early intervention?

Respiratory arrest

What are important nursing interventions for a patient in respiratory distress?

1. Administer supplemental oxygen to maintain oxygen saturation greater than 94%.
2. Place the patient in high Fowler's position.
3. Notify the physician.
4. Establish I.V. access for administration of medications and fluids.
5. Monitor vital signs and assess respiratory status (dyspnea, oxygen saturation level) at least every 15 minutes until stable.
6. Administer medications (diuretics if fluid overloaded; bronchodilators if asthmatic) as ordered by the physician.
7. Monitor intake and output every hour. Prepare to place an indwelling urinary catheter if none present.
8. Assess pain level.
9. Make sure intubation equipment is readily available.

Chest pain and myocardial infarction

What are potential causes of chest pain?

Pleural inflammation, pericarditis, gastric ulcer, cholelithiasis, anxiety, pneumonia, pneumothorax, pulmonary embolism, costochondritis, rib fractures, herpes zoster, indigestion, esophageal spasm, trauma, asthma, and cardiac events, such as unstable angina or an acute myocardial infarction (AMI)

What are the clinical manifestations of cardiac-related chest pain?

Pain, heaviness, pressure, squeezing, or discomfort in the chest (usually in the center under the breastbone) that may radiate to the neck, jaw, shoulder, or left arm; may be associated with shortness of breath, nausea, vomiting, and diaphoresis

What diagnostic tests should be anticipated in the event of a suspected AMI?

12-lead ECG and blood studies to include electrolytes, complete blood count (CBC), coagulation studies, and cardiac markers (troponin, creatine kinase, CK-MB, myoglobin, lactate dehydrogenase); chest X-ray and echocardiogram may also be obtained

What are important nursing interventions for a patient suspected of having an AMI?

1. Administer supplemental oxygen at 4 L/minute via nasal cannula and place the patient in an upright position.
2. Notify the physician and ECG technician.
3. Administer morphine (2 to 4 mg I.V. push), nitroglycerin (sublingual or I.V.), and aspirin as ordered by the physician.
4. Establish I.V. access for administration of fluids and medications (heparin and thrombolytic agents).
5. Monitor vital signs and respiratory status (oxygen saturation level) at least every 15 minutes until stable, and place on continuous cardiac monitor if available.
6. Make sure the code cart is readily available.
7. Maintain nothing-by-mouth status.

The primary goal of therapy is to minimize the patient's oxygen needs.

What arrhythmia most commonly occurs in a patient having an MI?

Ventricular fibrillation from electrical instability of the ischemic heart; atrial fibrillation, atrial flutter, and ventricular tachycardia may also occur

What complications of an AMI may be prevented with early intervention?

Arrhythmias, heart failure, formation of thrombus and ventricular aneurysm, permanent cardiac and brain damage, and death

| **What's the optimal time frame for reperfusion to the heart using thrombolytic agents?** | Thrombolytic agents should be administered within 4 to 6 hours after an MI to prevent further cardiac muscle damage. |

Cardiopulmonary arrest

✎ **What are the common causes of cardiac arrest?**	MI, respiratory failure, extensive hemorrhage, brain injury, sepsis, massive aspiration, arrhythmias, pulmonary embolus, drug overdose, and anaphylactic reaction
✎ **What are the cardinal signs of cardiac arrest?**	Absence of a carotid or femoral pulse, apnea, and unobtainable blood pressure
✎ **How long after a full cardiac arrest is a patient at risk for brain damage?**	4 to 6 minutes
✎ **What are the common causes of respiratory arrest?**	An obstructed airway, cardiac failure or arrest, drug overdose, pulmonary embolus, pneumothorax, and sepsis
What are important nursing actions in the event of cardiopulmonary arrest?	Activate the hospital code team, and intervene in the same manner as for code situations

Deep vein thrombosis

What's a deep vein thrombosis (DVT)?	A blood clot in a deep vein, typically involving the lower leg, thigh, or pelvis
✎ **What are common causes of a DVT?**	Recent major surgery and immobilization, fracture or trauma, malignancy, thrombophlebitis, obesity, smoking, and estrogen therapy
	Fifty percent of all DVTs related to surgery occur within 24 hours of the procedure.
✎ **What are the clinical manifestations of a DVT?**	Pain isolated to one leg, unilateral edema, warmth and erythema of the affected area, pain on calf flexion (Homans' sign), palpable cord, and possibly a low-grade fever

✎ What diagnostic tests should be anticipated in the event of a suspected DVT?

Venous duplex Doppler or contrast venogram; other diagnostic tests include the cuff pain test of Löwenberg (lower threshold for pain occurs when blood pressure cuff inflated around affected extremity) and impedance plethysmography (based on electrical conduction of the blood); baseline coagulation studies should also be obtained prior to administering antithrombotic agents

✎ What complications may be prevented with early intervention?

Pulmonary embolus (breaking off of a clot) that becomes lodged in the lungs or chronic leg swelling and pain

✎ What are important nursing interventions for a patient with a DVT?

1. Elevate the affected extremity above the level of the heart.
2. Avoid any unnecessary activity involving the affected extremity.
3. Notify the physician.
4. Administer anticoagulants as ordered (heparin initially) to maintain partial thromboplastin time (PTT) $1\frac{1}{2}$ to $2\frac{1}{2}$ times the control.
5. Monitor vital signs at frequent intervals, and assess for signs of pulmonary embolus, including sudden respiratory distress.
6. Monitor intake and output, and ensure adequate hydration.
7. Prepare the patient for possible radiologic studies and thrombolytic therapy.

Pulmonary embolism

What's a pulmonary embolism (PE)?

A blood clot that travels from a thrombosed vein (most commonly in the pelvis or a lower extremity) to the lungs, where it obstructs pulmonary artery blood flow. This obstruction causes ischemia and infarction of lung tissue as well as cardiac dysfunction; less commonly caused by air or fat entering the venous system

✎ What are common causes of a PE?

1. DVT
2. Central venous catheterization (air embolus)
3. Long bone fracture (fat embolus)

✎ What are the clinical manifestations of a PE?

Classical clinical triad includes sudden dyspnea, pleuritic chest pain, and hemoptysis; anxiety, restlessness, diaphoresis, cough, tachycardia, tachypnea (greater than 16), wheezing, hypotension, pleural friction rub, syncope, and cyanosis may also occur

✎ What diagnostic tests should be anticipated in the event of a PE?

Arterial blood gas (ABG) analysis, ECG, and chest X-ray are typically done first to rule out other causes, although ventilation-perfusion ($\dot{V}/\dot{Q}$) scans, pulmonary angiography, and spiral computed tomography (CT) scans of the chest are more definitive tests for PE

✎ What complications may be prevented with early intervention?

Right ventricular ischemia that can progress to MI, heart failure, cardiovascular collapse, and possible pulseless electrical activity

✎ What are important nursing interventions for a patient with a PE?

1. Administer 100% oxygen via face mask.
2. Place the patient in high Fowler's position.
3. Notify the physician.
4. Establish I.V. access for possible infusion of crystalloid solutions, vasopressors, and heparin.
5. Monitor vital signs and respiratory status (oxygen saturation level) at least every 15 minutes until stable.
6. Administer medication (analgesics; heparin bolus; thrombolytic agents, such as streptokinase; urokinase; or tissue plasminogen activator, such as alteplase [Activase]) as ordered by the physician.

◤ *Obtain baseline coagulation studies (prothrombin time [PT], PTT) prior to administration of antithrombotic medications.*

Pulmonary edema

What's pulmonary edema?

Abnormal and rapid accumulation of serous fluid in the alveolar spaces and interstitial tissues of the lungs

✎ What are common causes of pulmonary edema?

1. Left-sided heart failure (most common) as a result of MI or acute left ventricular dysfunction
2. Valvular disease
3. Circulatory volume overload
4. Inhalation injuries
5. Near-drowning event
6. Sepsis
7. Acute respiratory distress syndrome (ARDS)

✎ Who's at risk for pulmonary edema?

People with hypertension, coronary artery disease, burns, sepsis, massive transfusions or volume replacement, or those who abuse I.V. opioids

✎ What are the clinical manifestations of pulmonary edema?

Tachypnea, tachycardia, dyspnea, intercostal retractions, crackles, wheezes, pink and frothy sputum, decreased oxygen saturation level, decreased level of consciousness (LOC), anxiousness, restlessness, and jugular vein distention

What diagnostic tests should be anticipated in the event of pulmonary edema?

Chest X-ray confirms the diagnosis, but ABG analysis reveals the degree of the hypoxia; an ECG may reveal cardiac ischemia or infarction

What complications may be prevented with early intervention?

ARDS, respiratory arrest, and ventilatory dependence

✎ What are important nursing interventions for a patient with pulmonary edema?

1. Administer 100% oxygen by face mask.
2. Place the patient in an upright position to maximize lung expansion.
3. Monitor oxygen saturation level and vital signs at least every 15 minutes until patient is stable.
4. Establish I.V. line for administration of medications (diuretics, morphine, dobutamine, nitroglycerin) as ordered by the physician.
5. Make sure chest X-ray has been ordered.
6. Monitor intake and output every hour, and maintain strict fluid restriction. Prepare for insertion of an indwelling urinary catheter if one isn't present.

Pneumothorax

✎ What's pneumothorax?

Accumulation of air in the pleural space; a partial or complete lung collapse occurs due to a disruption of the negative pressure that exists normally within the intrapleural space

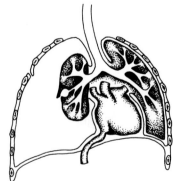

✎ What are common causes of pneumothorax?

May occur spontaneously (high rate of recurrence) or as a result of trauma or a medical procedure, such as subclavian line insertion, thoracentesis, percutaneous lung biopsy, or bronchoscopy

✎ What's the most life-threatening type of pneumothorax?

Tension pneumothorax, in which the pressure builds up causing a mediastinal shift in the heart, trachea, esophagus, and great vessels toward the *uninjured* side

✎ What are the clinical manifestations of pneumothorax?

1. Sudden and sharp, pleuritic chest pain that occurs at rest
2. Dyspnea
3. Cough, possibly associated with mild hemoptysis
4. Stabbing sensation in the back
5. Tachycardia
6. Tachypnea
7. Diminished breath sounds on the affected side
8. Hypotension

What diagnostic tests should be anticipated in the event of spontaneous pneumothorax?

Chest X-ray (during inspiration and expiration) is the standard, although computed CT scan is more sensitive. ABGs are helpful in determining the extent of hypoxia but aren't used to diagnose a pneumothorax.

What complications may be prevented with early intervention?

Hypoxia, retention of carbon dioxide (hypercarbia), and cardiovascular collapse.

✎ What are important nursing interventions for a patient with spontaneous pneumothorax?

1. Administer 100% oxygen via face mask.
2. Place the patient in high Fowler's position.
3. Monitor vital signs, respiratory status, and pain level (to determine if pneumothorax is expanding) at least every 15 minutes until stable.
4. Establish I.V. access for administration of fluids and medications.
5. Prepare the patient for chest tube insertion to allow the air to be evacuated and the lung to reexpand. If extent of collapse of one lung is less than 20%, observation alone may be all that's necessary.
6. Administer medications (analgesics) as ordered by the physician.
7. Ensure bed rest.
8. Make sure a chest X-ray has been ordered.

Gastrointestinal bleeding

What are the potential sources of GI bleeding?	1. Ruptured esophageal varices (from hepatic disease) 2. Gastroduodenal ulcers 3. Esophageal perforation 4. Mucosal tears in the gastroesophageal tract 5. Malignancy
✎ **What are the clinical manifestations of GI bleeding?**	1. Hematemesis or "coffee ground" emesis 2. Black, tarry stools (melena) 3. Hypotension 4. Decreased LOC
✎ **What tests should be anticipated in the event of upper GI bleeding?**	ECG and blood studies, including CBC with platelets, coagulation studies (PT and PTT), blood type, and crossmatch; endoscopic procedures may be performed for diagnosis and treatment; angiography may sometimes be necessary
What complications may be prevented with early intervention?	Aspiration, hypovolemic shock, and respiratory and cardiovascular failure
✎ **What are important nursing interventions for a patient experiencing GI bleeding?**	1. Elevate the head of the bed, and place the patient in a lateral position to prevent aspiration. 2. Provide supplemental oxygen at 2 to 3 L/minute. 3. Monitor vital signs (blood pressure and pulse) and oxygen saturation level at least every 15 minutes until stable. Place the patient on continuous cardiac monitor if available. 4. Establish two large-bore I.V. lines (18 to 14 gauge) for administration of fluids and possible blood products to maintain hematocrit greater than 25%. 5. Administer medications (acid suppressors, vitamin K, vasopressin) and fluid boluses as ordered by the physician. 6. Insert a nasogastric tube, and prepare for possible gastric lavage. 7. Monitor intake and output every hour. Monitor volume of blood loss. Prepare for placement of an indwelling urinary catheter. 8. Maintain nothing-by-mouth status and prepare for potential esophagogastroduodenoscopy (EGD) and balloon tamponade.

Shock

What's shock?

Inadequate tissue perfusion and oxygenation that can progress to end organ dysfunction if not corrected

▨ *A mean arterial pressure (MAP) of 70 to 100 mm Hg is necessary to maintain adequate tissue perfusion. If the MAP decreases, blood is shunted to vital organs (brain, heart) and away from less critical organs (GI system, kidneys).*

What types of shock may occur?

1. *Hypovolemic:* hemorrhage, burns, dehydration
2. *Cardiogenic:* MI, heart failure, arrhythmias
3. *Distributive:* anaphylactic, neurogenic, septic; blood vessels dilate without a compensatory increase in circulating blood volume

What are the clinical manifestations of shock?

Agitation, restlessness, diaphoresis, pallor, cold and clammy or mottled skin, oliguria, weak and thready pulse, tachycardia, hypotension, eventual confusion, and coma; a widening pulse pressure (decreasing diastolic pressure without significant change in systolic pressure) is seen in the early stages of shock syndrome

▨ *Manifestations of hypovolemic shock occur when 500 to 1,500 ml of the total circulating blood volume is lost.*

▨ *Decreasing hourly urine output is the best indicator of impending shock. A gradual increase in respiratory rate and a decrease in the depth of respirations are also good indicators.*

What are the compensatory mechanisms for shock?

1. Heart rate increases
2. Vasoconstriction occurs
3. Fluids shift from tissues to vascular bed
4. Respiratory rate increases

What complications of shock may be prevented with early intervention?

Shock can progress rapidly and may result in brain or organ damage, cardiac arrest, and death. Metabolic acidosis may also occur due to the production of lactic acid in the setting of tissue hypoxia. Disseminated intravascular coagulation may occur as the blood becomes more acidic (and therefore hypercoagulable).

What are important nursing interventions for a patient in shock?

1. Administer supplemental oxygen at 15 L/minute via nonrebreather mask.
2. Place the patient in modified Trendelenburg position (torso flat, legs elevated), unless respiratory compromise is suspected.

3. Notify the physician.
4. Monitor vital signs and respiratory status (oxygen saturation level) at least every 15 minutes until stable. Place the patient on continuous cardiac monitor if available.
5. Establish two large-bore I.V. lines for fluids and blood replacement and administration of medications: vasoconstricting drugs such as dopamine for hypovolemic shock, antihistamines or epinephrine for anaphylactic shock, inotropes for cardiogenic shock, antibiotics and fluid for septic shock.
6. Monitor intake and output every hour. Anticipate the placement of an indwelling urinary catheter.
7. Place warm blankets on the patient to prevent hypothermia (if hypovolemic).
8. Maintain nothing-by-mouth status.
9. Prepare for possible intubation and insertion of pulmonary artery catheter (Swan-Ganz).

 Make sure blood cultures are obtained prior to administration of antibiotics.

Seizures

What's a seizure?	Sudden, violent, and uncontrollable contractions of a group of muscles as a result of a massive electrical discharge from neurons in the brain
What are common causes of seizures?	Idiopathic epilepsy (most common), noncompliance with anticonvulsant regimen, hypoglycemia, head trauma, vascular disorders, strokes, infection, electrolyte abnormalities, drug or alcohol withdrawal, overdose, and structural brain disorders such as tumors
What are the clinical manifestations of a seizure?	Clinical findings may be dramatic or subtle, but common findings include an aura or sense of warning, momentary unresponsiveness, tonic and clonic movement of the muscles, brief or prolonged loss of consciousness, fixed and dilated pupils, bowel or bladder incontinence, and lethargy in the postictal state.
What tests should be anticipated in the event of a seizure?	Blood studies to include electrolytes, renal function, CBC, blood cultures (if febrile), toxicology screen and serum levels of anticonvulsants; brain CT scan should be obtained for new onset seizures; X-rays may be indicated if injury is suspected

✎ **What complications may be prevented with early intervention?**

Injury, aspiration of vomitus, and coma

✎ **What are important nursing interventions for a patient experiencing a seizure?**

1. Protect the patient from injury during the seizure activity by moving dangerous objects out of the way.
2. Secure the patient's airway as the opportunity arises.
3. Position the patient on his *right* side to prevent aspiration if vomiting occurs.
4. Notify the physician.
5. Assess vital signs, oxygen saturation level, blood glucose level, and LOC.
6. Provide supplemental oxygen at 2 to 3 L/minute if oxygen saturation level is less than 94%.
7. Establish I.V. access for administration of fluids (dextrose solution if hypoglycemic) and medications (lorazepam, diazepam, phenytoin, midazolam).
8. Inspect for injuries. Raise side rails and place the bed in the lowest position.
9. Maintain nothing-by-mouth status.
10. Make sure appropriate blood studies have been obtained.

◤ *Never restrain a patient or place anything between the teeth of a patient during a seizure.*

Substance withdrawal

What's the cause of substance withdrawal?

Sudden cessation of alcohol or opioid ingestion after chronic use

✎ **When does substance withdrawal typically occur?**

1. *Alcohol:* within 12 to 72 hours after the last drink, but up to 7 days
2. *Opioids:* within 2 to 48 hours of last use

✎ **What are the clinical manifestations of withdrawal?**

Anxiety, nervousness, disorientation, shakiness, irritability, emotional volatility, confusion, muscle tremors, tachycardia, headache, sweating, nausea and vomiting, anorexia, insomnia, and hallucinations

What complications may be prevented with early intervention?

Alcohol withdrawal delirium and seizures

✎ **What's alcohol withdrawal?**	An acute, hypermetabolic response to alcohol withdrawal that may include seizures, hallucinations, violent tremors, and disorientation; potentially fatal if not treated with hypnotics, tranquilizers, and nutritive therapy to restore normal metabolism
✎ **What are important nursing interventions for a patient going through withdrawal?**	1. Monitor vital signs and mental status frequently. 2. Maintain patient safety (may include restraints). 3. Monitor intake and output. 4. Monitor serum electrolytes. 5. Administer sedatives (benzodiazepines) as ordered by the physician. 6. Involve a social worker and substance abuse expert.

Wound dehiscence or evisceration

What's dehiscence?	Acute separation of fascia prior to skin incision healing after an operation
What's evisceration?	Extrusion of bowel or other abdominal structures through a wound separation
✎ **What are the clinical manifestations of dehiscence and evisceration?**	Separation of the incisional line, popping sensation, and sudden pain at insertion site
What complications can be prevented with early intervention?	Hypothermia, infection, and organ ischemia
✎ **What are important nursing interventions for a patient with wound evisceration?**	1. Cover exposed organs with warm gauze or towels soaked in normal saline to keep moist. 2. Place the patient in a supine position with his knees bent. 3. Instruct another person to notify the surgeon. 4. Assess vital signs at frequent intervals until the surgeon arrives. 5. Establish I.V. access for administration of fluids and medications (analgesics). 6. Cover the patient with warm blankets to prevent hypothermia. 7. Prepare for surgery; maintain nothing-by-mouth status.

⚡ *Don't attempt to reinsert exposed organs because this may result in ischemia of the organs.*

Compartment syndrome

What's compartment syndrome?

A condition in which circulation in a closed compartment is compromised due to rising pressure in that space; normal intercompartmental pressure is 0 mm Hg; in compartment syndrome, the pressure in the space within the muscle is usually greater than or equal to 25 mm Hg.

What are common causes of compartment syndrome?

1. Extremity fractures (commonly tibial)
2. Open reduction and internal fixation of fractures
3. Surgical osteotomies
4. Muscle ischemia and reperfusion

What are the risk factors for developing compartment syndrome?

1. History of recent trauma (particularly crushing injuries), surgery, or extravasation
2. History of diabetes, poor neurovascular status, or infection
3. Revascularization of an ischemic extremity

✎ What are the clinical manifestations (five P's) of compartment syndrome?

1. Pain (disproportionate to extent of injury; refractory to opioids)
2. Pallor
3. Paresthesia
4. Paresis
5. Pulselessness

What complications may be prevented with early intervention?

1. Tissue ischemia and necrosis
2. Irreversible nerve damage or permanent muscle contractures
3. Loss of function of the affected extremity
4. Need for amputation of affected extremity

✎ What are important nursing interventions for a patient with compartment syndrome?

1. Position the affected extremity at heart level, *not above*, because this may further compromise circulation.
2. Notify the surgeon immediately.
3. Establish I.V. access for administration of medications (analgesics).
4. Prepare the patient for cast removal (if present) and fasciotomy (if pressure is greater than 30 mm Hg).

⚡ *Don't apply heat or cold to an extremity with compartment syndrome. Heat may cause edema, and cold may worsen ischemia.*

Cardiac tamponade

What's cardiac tamponade?	A life-threatening condition in which blood accumulates between the heart and the pericardial sac
	In normal conditions, the pericardial sac contains 25 ml of serous fluid that acts as a cushion to protect the heart. However, in the event of cardiac tamponade, the ventricles become compressed and cardiac output decreases as more blood accumulates (hemopericardium).

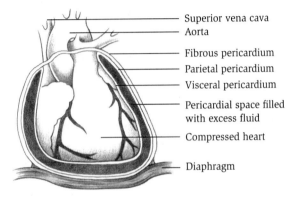

Superior vena cava
Aorta
Fibrous pericardium
Parietal pericardium
Visceral pericardium
Pericardial space filled with excess fluid
Compressed heart
Diaphragm

In determining the severity of cardiac tamponade, the rate at which blood accumulates is more important than the volume that accumulates. Slower bleeding is better tolerated by the patient.

What clinical manifestations comprise Beck's triad in cardiac tamponade?	Jugular vein distention, hypotension, and distant heart sounds
What other clinical manifestations are associated with cardiac tamponade?	1. Pallor and diaphoresis 2. Tachycardia and a thready pulse 3. Dyspnea, tachypnea, and hypoxia 4. Narrowed pulse pressure (difference between systolic and diastolic blood pressures) 5. Pulsus paradoxus (loss of peripheral pulses during inspiration or loss of audible heart beat upon inspiration during manual blood pressure monitoring) 6. Sudden cessation of mediastinal drainage (after cardiac surgery) 7. Pulseless electrical activity
What diagnostic tests should be anticipated?	ABG analysis, echocardiogram, ECG, and chest X-ray

What complications may be prevented with early intervention?	Shock, cardiac arrhythmias, and death

✎ **What are important nursing interventions for a patient with cardiac tamponade?**	1. Provide supplemental high-flow oxygen via a nonrebreather mask, and elevate the head of the bed 45 degrees to minimize work of breathing. 2. Notify the physician. 3. Establish 2 large bore I.V. lines for administering fluids and medications (diuretics, analgesics). Administer fluids to maintain systolic blood pressure 90 to 100 mm Hg (higher pressures worsen tamponade). 4. Assess vital signs and respiratory status (oxygen saturation level) at least every 15 minutes until stable. 5. Monitor intake and output every hour. 6. Prepare for pericardiocentesis (removal of some or all of the fluid trapped within the pericardial sac).

Nursing skills

Mechanical ventilation

✎ **What's mechanical ventilation?**	Use of a machine to maintain ventilation when a patient can't do so independently; a ventilator can completely regulate a patient's breathing or it can support the patient's own respiratory efforts (decreases the work of breathing)
How does a ventilator work?	The ventilator generates positive pressure, which forces air into the lungs through an artificial airway.
✎ **In what situations would a patient benefit from mechanical ventilation?**	1. Respiratory failure or arrest (impaired gas exchange or labored breathing) 2. Cardiopulmonary failure (decreases myocardial and systemic oxygen consumption) 3. Brain injuries (decreased ICP results from decreased work of breathing; decreases metabolism and oxygen consumption by the brain) 4. Chest trauma involving broken ribs (mechanical ventilation provides stability to chest wall) 5. Recovery from extensive surgery
What's neuromuscular blockade?	Pharmacologic blockader of motor neuron transmissions resulting in paralysis; commonly used for patients who require mechanical ventilation

What paralytic agents are commonly used in neuromuscular blockade?

Pancuronium, succinylcholine (Anectine), atracurium (Tracrium), cisatracurium (Nimbex), and vecuronium (Norcuron)

What factors enhance neuromuscular blockade?

1. Respiratory acidosis
2. Hypothermia
3. Electrolyte imbalances
4. Muscular disorders such as myasthenia gravis

What are important nursing interventions for a patient requiring neuromuscular blockade?

1. Assess vital signs (core body temperature) and neurologic status (pupillary response) every hour.
2. Assess level of paralysis via peripheral nerve stimulator every 4 hours once stabilized (every 15 minutes during initial blockade or during any bolus infusion of paralytic agent).
3. Change body position every 2 hours. Three people should assist in patient repositioning.
4. Assess the effectiveness of analgesia and sedation every hour.
5. Monitor ventilatory status, including peak inspiratory pressure and fraction of inspired oxygen (F_{IO_2}).
6. Reorient the patient every hour.
7. Apply lubricants and artificial tears every hour to prevent injury to sclera and conjunctiva.
8. Provide mouth care and oral suctioning every 2 hours.
9. Apply sequential compression devices as ordered.
10. Initiate physical therapy consult for patients with prolonged neuromuscular blockade.
11. Consider daily neuromuscular blockade holidays.

◥ *Neuromuscular blockade induces paralysis, but the patient may remain fully awake unless sedatives and opioids are used in conjunction with the paralytic agent.*

What's the Train of Four?

A type of peripheral nerve stimulation involving the delivery of four consecutive electrical stimuli used to determine the level of paralysis; the number of twitches corresponds to the level of paralysis; typically, the desired goal is one twitch, or 90% blockade.

What are commonly used ventilator settings?

1. *Respiratory rate:* number of breaths the ventilator delivers per minute
2. *Tidal volume:* volume of gas delivered with each ventilator breath
3. *F_{IO_2}:* amount of oxygen delivered to the patient by the ventilator; usually 30% to 100%
4. *Inspiratory: expiratory ratio (I:E ratio):* inspiration length in comparison to expiration length
5. *Pressure limit:* maximum amount of pressure that can be generated by the ventilator to deliver a breath

6. *Flow rate:* speed with which the tidal volume is delivered
7. *Sensitivity or trigger:* determines the amount of patient effort required to initiate inspiration; pressure or flow can act as the trigger

What are commonly used ventilator modes?

1. *Control ventilation:* preset volume or pressure is delivered regardless of patient's own inspiratory efforts
2. *Assist-control ventilation:* preset volume or pressure is delivered in response to patient's own inspiratory attempt; however, breath is initiated by ventilator if patient can't do so independently within a set period of time
3. *Synchronous intermittent mandatory ventilation (SIMV):* preset volume or pressure and rate are delivered simultaneously while the patient is allowed to breathe spontaneously between ventilator breaths; commonly used during ventilator weaning because the patient completely controls the spontaneous breaths
4. *Pressure support ventilation (PSV):* present pressure that supplements the spontaneous inspiratory efforts of the patient and reduces the work of breathing
5. *Positive end-expiratory pressure (PEEP):* positive pressure applied by the ventilator at the end of expiration; it improves oxygenation by maintaining open alveoli at the end of expiration, but may result in pneumothorax, decreased cardiac output, and increased ICP
6. *Independent lung ventilation:* ventilates each lung separately in patients with unilateral lung disease
7. *High-frequency ventilation:* small amount of gas is delivered at a rapid rate (60 to 100 breaths/minute); useful if the patient is at risk for pneumothorax, is hemodynamically unstable, or is undergoing a procedure of short duration; requires sedation and paralysis
8. *Inverse ratio ventilation (IRV):* I:E ratio is reversed to facilitate longer inspiration; shorter expiratory time prevents alveolar collapse and improves oxygenation in patients who are still hypoxic despite PEEP; normal I:E ratio is 1:2, but in IRV, the ratio is 2:1 or greater; requires sedation and paralysis

What types of positive pressure ventilators exist?

1. *Volume-cycled:* preset tidal volume is delivered regardless of the amount of airway resistance; passive expiration allowed; ideal use for bronchospasm, most common type used in critical care
2. *Pressure-cycled:* gases delivered at preset pressure, with passive expiration allowed; used for short-term therapy (less than 24 hours) because patients may not receive complete tidal volume if poor lung compliance or increased airway resistance are present; decreases risk of lung damage from high inspiratory pressures

3. *Flow-cycled:* breath delivered until a preset flow rate is achieved during inspiration
4. *Time-cycled:* breath delivered over a preset period

What are typical responsibilities of the respiratory therapist when mechanical ventilation is used?

1. Setting up ventilator
2. Changing settings based on the physician's orders
3. Performing a daily maintenance check of the ventilator
4. Assessing the patient's respiratory status
5. Administering aerosol treatments (breathing and respiratory) via the ventilator
6. Performing suctioning periodically
7. Changing ventilator tubing as well as cleaning filters
8. Checking the air temperature and level of sterile water in humidifier every hour, if humidification is provided
9. Performing weaning criteria

What are important nursing actions for a patient requiring mechanical ventilation?

1. Assess and document appropriate ventilatory settings at least every 4 hours (mode, tidal volume, rate, PEEP, alarm parameters).
2. Assess and document adequacy of ventilatory support at least every 4 hours (ABG analysis, pulse oximetry, peak inspiratory pressures, exhaled tidal volumes).
3. Monitor and document vital signs, intake and output, breath sounds, and ET or tracheostomy tube position (cm marking at teeth/gums) at least every 4 hours.
4. Determine the need for suctioning.
5. Turn the patient every 2 hours.
6. Provide chest physiotherapy (postural drainage, gentle percussion) at least every 4 hours.
7. Provide the patient with an alternative means of communicating (pen and paper, communication board).
8. Administer paralytics, analgesics, and antianxiety medications as ordered by the physician.

When is weaning from mechanical ventilation appropriate?

When the patient is alert, has a strong cough reflex, has required minimal ventilatory support with a spontaneous respiratory rate less than 24, and can maintain own airway

During the weaning process, the modes of mechanical ventilation are gradually altered so that the ventilator provides less support while the patient is allowed to initiate more breaths.

When is extubation appropriate?

When the patient demonstrates stable hemodynamic parameters, vital signs, blood gas levels, and oxygen saturation levels as well as exhibits a good spontaneous cough

What are important nursing actions immediately following extubation?

1. Place the patient on supplemental, humidified oxygen via mask.
2. Monitor vital signs every 15 minutes for 2 hours and then at least hourly for 2 hours.

3. Observe respiratory effort, oxygen saturation level, and breath sounds every 15 minutes for 2 hours and then at least hourly for 2 hours.
4. Obtain ABG analysis 1 hour after extubation (sooner for dyspnea, diaphoresis, hypoxemia, or decreased LOC).
5. Observe for breathing difficulties (dyspnea, tachypnea, paradoxical breathing pattern, oxygen saturation less than 92%), aspiration, laryngospasm, bronchospasm, or stridor.
6. Encourage deep-breathing and coughing exercises along with incentive spirometry (splint any abdominal or chest incisions).
7. Make sure the call bell is within reach.
8. Make sure nebulizer treatment is readily available.

What's the indication for the use of noninvasive (no artificial airway) mechanical ventilation?

Sleep apnea

What types of noninvasive mechanical ventilation exist?

1. *Continuous positive airway pressure* (CPAP): maintains constant airway pressure and decreases the work of breathing; nasal mask or full face masks are commonly used, although CPAP may be administered by a ventilator through an ET tube or tracheostomy
2. *Bilevel positive airway pressure (BiPAP):* maintains positive airway pressure during both inspiration and expiration; typically administered via a nasal mask, which allows exhalation through the mouth
3. *Intermittent positive-pressure breathing (IPPB):* delivers compressed gas under positive pressure into the patient's airway during inhalation; allows passive exhalation, and aids patient in taking deeper breaths; applied on a scheduled basis

Tracheotomy

✎ What's a tracheotomy?

A surgical incision in the trachea just below the second and third tracheal ring for the purpose of establishing an airway; the tracheotomy site — or the tube that keeps it open — is called a tracheostomy, which may be temporary or permanent and emergent or prophylactic

✎ Why is a tracheotomy performed?

1. To bypass an upper airway obstruction (surgical edema, tumors, traumatic injuries)

2. To permit long-term positive pressure ventilation (respiratory failure, high lesion spinal cord injury, prolonged coma)
3. To facilitate removal of secretions (paralysis of chest muscles and diaphragm, neuromuscular disease)

✎ When is a tracheostomy considered appropriate?

If a patient is expected to require (or has required) intubation for more than 2 weeks

✎ What complications are associated with a tracheostomy?

1. Bleeding
2. Tracheal or laryngeal damage
3. Swallowing impairment and aspiration (secretions)
4. Airway obstruction (secretions, overinflated cuff)
5. Infection
6. Trapping of air in surrounding tissues or the chest (subcutaneous or mediastinal emphysema)
7. Pneumothorax
8. Tube dislodgment

✎ What are the various parts of a tracheostomy?

1. *Obturator:* guides tube into position and is removed once tube is in place; should remain at bedside at all times for patients with a tracheostomy
2. *Inner cannula:* removable sleeve that fits inside the tracheostomy tube; can be removed for cleaning
3. *Flange:* prevents pressure points and movement; holds ties
4. *Cuff:* encircles the outer cannula and is inflated with air inside the trachea to prevent aspiration and to seal the tracheal wall for more efficient air exchange
5. *Ties:* cotton ties worn around the neck and attached to the flange to decrease movement of tracheostomy tube

What types of tracheostomy tubes exist?

1. Disposable versus permanent
2. Short-term versus long-term
3. Single cannula versus double cannula
4. Cuffed versus uncuffed
5. Metal (Jackson) versus plastic (Portex, Shiley)
6. Fenestrated (has hole for speaking) versus nonfenestrated

✎ What equipment should always be kept at the bedside of a patient with a tracheostomy?

1. Handheld resuscitation bag
2. Scissors (postlaryngectomy patient)
3. Replacement tracheostomy tube (one size smaller than the one in use)
4. Syringe (10 ml) for inflation or deflation of cuff
5. Suction equipment
6. Obturator for tube currently in use

✎ What are important nursing actions for a patient with a tracheostomy?

1. Assess vital signs (temperature), breath sounds and oxygen saturation level every hour during the first postoperative day, every 2 to 4 hours during the second postoperative day, every 4 hours until first dressing change, and every 8 hours thereafter.
2. Assess the condition of stoma (erythema, edema) and type of secretions (purulent, colored, odorous) at frequent intervals.
3. Assess the patient's ability to swallow and to cough independently to clear secretions every 4 hours for 24 hours and every 8 hours thereafter.
4. Ensure accurate cuff inflation volume; deflate cuff at frequency and duration specified in the physician's order.
5. Perform tracheostomy suctioning as needed.
6. Perform tracheostomy care as directed (strict aseptic technique).
7. Perform tracheostomy dressing change every 8 hours for new tracheostomy, or as needed.
8. Provide a means of communication (pen and paper, communication board, call bell) for patients with non-fenestrated tracheostomies.
9. Verify that an emergency tracheostomy kit is available at the bedside.

Why is suctioning a patient with a tracheostomy important?

Suctioning removes secretions that have accumulated, which might otherwise interfer with airway patency, respiratory efficiency, and result in the development of an infection.

▎ *Suctioning should be performed based on the amount of secretions being produced, the oxygen saturation level (if decreasing), and the ability of the patient to clear secretions by coughing.*

✎ What complications are associated with suctioning a patient with a tracheostomy?

Hypoxia, hypotension, atelectasis or lung collapse, arrhythmia, and cardiac arrest

How is tracheostomy suctioning performed?

1. Obtain equipment and supplies, and wash your hands.
2. Position the patient's bed at a comfortable working level.
3. Open one end of the suction catheter package, but leave the catheter inside.
4. Ensure suction setting is appropriate (maximum of 80 to 120 mm Hg), and connect catheter and suction tubing while the catheter remains in the package.

5. Open sterile suction kit, and set up the sterile container, filling it with saline. Be sure to touch only the outside of the container.

6. Ventilate with a handheld resuscitation bag before suctioning.

7. Put on sterile gloves and withdraw suction catheter from package using the nondominant hand (which is considered nonsterile hand). Grasp the remainder of the catheter as it's removed from the package with the dominant hand (considered the sterile hand).

8. Suction the sterile saline to moisten the catheter, and occlude the suction port several times to assess suction pressure.

9. Cover the suction port with the thumb and insert the catheter, rotating it between the thumb and forefinger, to a depth of 2″ to 3″ (5 to 7.5 cm) beyond the distal end of the tracheostomy tube. Don't exceed a total suction time of 10 seconds with each suctioning.

10. Encourage the patient to breathe and cough between suctioning, and replace oxygen source between each suctioning. Assess the patient's response and respiratory effort.

11. Flush the suction catheter with sterile saline solution and repeat suctioning procedure as necessary. Turn off the suction and disconnect the catheter from the suction tubing.

12. Document the time of suctioning, type of secretions (color, quantity, consistency, odor, and patient response).

⚡ *Performing suctioning with pressure that exceeds 80 to 120 mm Hg may cause a lung collapse or tracheal tissue damage.*

✎ **What's the proper technique for providing tracheostomy care?**

1. Assess the need for analgesic or sedative.

2. Elevate the head of the bed 45 degrees (unless contraindicated), and preoxygenate the patient with 100% oxygen.

3. Obtain supplies and prepare dressing tray.

4. Wash your hands thoroughly.

5. Suction the patient orally and via the tracheostomy (sterile technique) to ensure patency of airway.

6. Put on clean gloves and remove the inner cannula from the tracheostomy tube. Immerse in hydrogen peroxide, rinse in normal saline, and replace. If disposable inner cannula is used, discard and replace with new, sterile inner cannula using sterile technique. Return the patient to oxygen therapy or ventilator.

7. Remove old gauze dressing and loosen ties. Note characteristics of drainage.
8. Clean the stoma and external portion of the tracheostomy tube with cotton-tipped applicator (one sweep per applicator) and normal saline. Move from the stoma outward (clean-to-dirty technique). If significant crusting is present, a half-and-half solution of normal saline and hydrogen peroxide may be used. Dry the area with sterile gauze.
9. Change the tracheostomy ties if they're soiled or according to the physician's order. The previous ties should be left secured to the flange and patient while a new tie is attached. Ties should be loose enough to allow two fingers between the ties and neck. Remove the old tie and discard.
10. Apply a new tracheostomy dressing using clean technique.
11. Reassess respiratory status and suction as necessary.

◤ *Another nurse should be available to hold the tracheostomy tube during dressing changes in order to minimize its movement and to prevent its expulsion due to coughing.*

✎ How often should tracheostomy care be provided?

Every 8 hours, or when dressings are wet or stoma isn't clean and dry

◤ *The surgeon generally performs the first tracheostomy dressing change 4 to 10 days after the operation.*

✎ What are the appropriate nursing actions in the event of accidental decannulation?

1. Maintain patency of stoma with hemostat.
2. If ventilated, attempt to reinsert the tracheostomy tube immediately. Remove the inner cannula and put obturator in place. If reinsertion is successful, remove the obturator and replace with a sterile inner cannula. If reinsertion attempt is unsuccessful but the patient can breathe spontaneously, elevate the head of the bed. Anticipate the need for artificial respiration.
3. Notify the physician.

8

Neoplastic disorders and basic concepts of oncology nursing

Basic concepts of neoplastic disorders

What's a neoplasm?
"New growth;" an abnormal mass of tissue with progressive and uncontrolled growth that serves no physiologic function; also called a *tumor;* can be benign or malignant

What's cancer?
A disease of the cell characterized by uncontrolled growth, invasiveness, and the ability to develop new blood vessels; if the spread of cancer isn't controlled it can result in the host's death

What two major dysfunctions are present in cancer?
1. Uncontrolled cell proliferation and growth (loss of contact inhibition)
2. Defective cellular differentiation

▶ *Cancer cells don't always grow at a faster rate than normal cells, but their growth is continuous and indiscriminate.*

✎ What's metastasis?
The processes by which malignant cells leave the original tumor site and spread to distant sites in the body

What's cellular differentiation?
An orderly cellular process that involves progression from an immature state (stem cells) to a mature state in which a cell has specific functions and properties

▶ *Cancers that exhibit undifferentiated cells (bear little resemblance to their tissue of origin) are typically more aggressive in their growth and behavior than those with differentiated cells.*

What's a carcinogen?
A substance or agent that has the potential to cause cancer

What's carcinogenesis?	The process in which a normal cell undergoes progressive changes and becomes malignant
What's an oncogene?	A tumor-inducing gene that results from mutations
What are tumor cell markers?	Substances in the body that may indicate the presence of cancer cells; tumor markers may be secreted by the tumor itself or may be produced in the body in response to cancer Typically, tumor markers may be specific for a certain type of cancer (prostate specific antigen [PSA] for prostate cancer). Tumor markers may also be used to monitor for cancer recurrence or to evaluate the response to cancer treatments.
What's anaplasia?	Loss of structural organization and useful function of a cell
What's dysplasia?	Disturbance in size, shape, and organization of cells and tissues
What's hyperplasia?	An increase in the number of cells in a tissue or organ
What's myelodysplasia?	Abnormal bone marrow production and development of blood cells; it commonly results in deficiencies of red blood cells (RBCs), white blood cells (WBCs), or platelets
What's cancer in situ?	Malignant cell changes that are localized, confined to one area, and haven't invaded normal surrounding tissues
What's palliative therapy?	Treatment that relieves symptoms and pain; it isn't curative and therefore doesn't alter survival
What's a remission?	The state of having no evidence of cancer
What's a relapse?	The state when a disease process recurs following a period of remission

Biology of neoplastic disorders

How do normal cells become cancerous?	External factors, internal factors, or a combination can cause cancer. These factors disrupt normal cellular homeostasis, and a mutation or malfunction occurs within the genes that regulate division and proliferation. Several theories of carcinogenesis exist; however, the precise biochemical cause of cancer is unknown.

▶ *The cause of cancer is likely multifactorial, including environmental, genetic, immunologic, chemical, or viral origins.*

What are the stages involved in cancer development?

1. *Initiation:* permanent alteration occurs in the cell's genetic structure
2. *Promotion:* reversible proliferation of the altered cell occurs
3. *Progression:* the tumor's growth rate increases with resultant increased potential for metastasis

What external factors can lead to carcinogenesis?

Tobacco and alcohol use, diet, air pollution, occupational exposure, and ultraviolet and ionizing radiation as well as certain medications

What internal factors can lead to carcinogenesis?

1. Genetics
2. Viruses: hepatitis B and C and hepatocellular carcinoma; Epstein-Barr virus and lymphoma; human papillomavirus, herpes simplex II virus, and cervical cancer
3. Bacteria: *Helicobacter pylori* and mucosa-associated lymphoid tissue
4. Hormones

What are common characteristics of cancer cells?

1. Increased number of cells locally
2. Loss of normal arrangement of cells
3. Change in cell size and shape
4. Increased nuclear size
5. Increased mitotic activity
6. Abnormal chromosomes
7. Can divide indefinitely
8. Require fewer growth factors for survival

How do cancer cells kill normal cells?

By competing with normal cells for nutrients and blood supply

How do cancer cells metastasize?

By vascular spread, by lymphatic spread, by diffusion within a body cavity (seeding), and by direct extension into adjacent tissues

What's angiogenesis?

The formation of blood vessels; tumor angiogenesis is the formation of blood vessels within the tumor itself, enabling it to create its own blood supply, which in turn allows the tumor to grow and metastasize

What are the most common sites of metastasis?

Liver, lungs, brain, and bones

✎ **What are the common sites of metastasis for the following types of cancer?**

1. *Lung:* brain, liver, lymph nodes, and bone
2. *Breast:* lymph nodes, lung, bone, liver, skin, and chest wall
3. *Prostate:* bone, lymph nodes, lung, and liver
4. *Head and neck:* lymph nodes, lung, liver, and bone
5. *Colon, pancreas, and stomach:* liver, lung, and lymph nodes
6. *Ovary:* intraperitoneal, lung, and liver
7. *Bone, kidney, uterus, and testicle:* lung
8. *Melanoma:* liver, brain, and lung

What role does the immune system play in cancer control?

Through the lymphatic system and specialized surveillance cells (lymphocytes, natural killer cells, and macrophages), the immune system monitors for "foreign" cells or antigens and destroys them.

How do cancer cells evade the immune system?

By metabolic changes, increased growth rates, and changes on the cell surface; in addition, tumor cells can secrete immunosuppressive substances, which weaken the immune response to the tumor

Is cancer preventable?

It's estimated that about one-third of cancer deaths each year could be prevented through behavioral and lifestyle changes as well as the use of vaccines and antibiotics.

✎ **What are the seven warning signs of cancer?**

1. **C**hange in bowel or bladder habits
2. **A** sore that doesn't heal
3. **U**nusual bleeding or discharge from a body orifice
4. **T**hickening or a lump in the breast or elsewhere
5. **I**ndigestion or difficulty swallowing
6. **O**bvious change in wart or mole
7. **N**agging cough or hoarseness

Diagnosing cancer

✎ **What methods are used to diagnose cancer?**

1. *Laboratory studies or blood tests:* complete blood count (CBC), stools for occult blood
2. *Tumor cell markers in blood:* PSA, alpha-fetoprotein, carcinoembryonic antigen, cancer antigen (CA) 125, CA 19-9; not definitive, but suggestive of cancerous process
3. *Imaging studies:* ultrasound, magnetic resonance imaging (MRI), computed tomography (CT) scan, angiography, and positron emission tomography scan
4. *Biopsies:* surgical or needle
5. *Cytology:* Papanicolaou smear

What types of surgical biopsies can be performed to diagnose cancer?

1. *Excisional:* removal of the entire tumor with clean margins (distance from the edge of the lesion into normal tissue) if possible; generally performed as an outpatient or day surgery procedure
2. *Incisional:* removal of small portion of a large tumor for diagnosis, which will later require major surgery for complete removal
3. *Endoscopic:* removal of a tissue specimen of the tumor from accessible lumens (respiratory, GI, and genitourinary tracts)

What types of needle biopsies can be performed to diagnose cancer?

1. *Fine needle aspiration:* aspiration of individual cells through a small-bore needle
2. *Core needle biopsy:* removal of a piece of tissue with a large needle; tissue architecture is preserved

Tumor grading and staging

What's histological grading?

As cancer cells continue to grow and mutate, they appear less like the normal tissue, thus becoming more undifferentiated or anaplastic. Tumor grading is a gauge of the tumor's degree of malignancy, or level of differentiation.

How are tumors graded?

1. *Grade I* (well differentiated): tumor closely resembles the tissue of origin and retains some specialized functions
2. *Grade II* (moderately differentiated): tumor has less resemblance to tissue of origin; more variation in size and shape; increased mitosis
3. *Grade III* (poorly differentiated): tumor has minimal resemblance to tissue of origin; much variation in size and shape of tumor cells; greatly increased mitosis
4. *Grade IV* (very poorly differentiated): tumor has no resemblance to tissue of origin; great variation in size and shape

What's tumor staging?

A measure of the extent of disease based on the size of the primary tumor, the degree of lymph node involvement, and the presence or absence of metastasis; the tumor stage determines the appropriate care plan, which is individualized

Staging is based on clinical, radiologic (CT scan, ultrasound, MRI, bone scan), and pathologic findings.

When is staging performed?

At the time of diagnosis to determine the most effective treatment; it also may be performed at several subsequent intervals to evaluate the response to treatment

What two clinical staging classification systems are commonly used?

1. *Clinical staging:* commonly used for cervical cancer and non-Hodgkin's lymphoma
2. *TNM classification system:* commonly used for breast cancer, head and neck cancer, lung cancer, colorectal cancer, urinary tract cancer, and skin cancer

What's the clinical staging classification system?

1. *Stage 0:* carcinoma in situ (lesion containing all histologic features of cancer with the exception of invasion; will eventually become invasive if untreated)
2. *Stage I:* tumor limited to tissue of origin; localized tumor growth
3. *Stage II:* limited local spread
4. *Stage III:* extensive local and regional spread
5. *Stage IV:* metastasis

What's the TNM classification system?

T = primary tumor size, N = nodal involvement, and M = metastasis

A combination of the TNM and numerical staging systems provides a profile of the disease for prognosis and treatment recommendations.

Benign and malignant tumors

What's the difference between the structure and differentiation of benign and malignant tumors?

Benign tumors resemble the tissue of origin; malignant tumors are atypical of the tissues of origin.

What's the difference in rate of growth between a benign and malignant tumor?

Benign tumors usually grow slowly, whereas malignant tumors usually have a rapid rate of growth.

What's the difference in progression between a benign and malignant tumor?

Benign tumors are slowly progressive and may remain stationary or they may regress. They're rarely fatal if treated. Malignant tumors are progressive and almost always fatal if untreated.

What's the difference in the mode of growth between benign and malignant tumors?

Benign tumors grow by expansion within a capsule. Malignant tumors grow by local infiltration or metastasis to distant sites.

✎ **What's the differ-ence in tissue destruc-tion between benign and malignant tumors?**

No tissue destruction occurs in benign tumors. Tissue destruction is common in malignant tumors, involving ulceration and necrosis.

✎ **What's the differ-ence in recurrence between benign and malignant tumors?**

Recurrence of benign tumors is rare; recurrence of malignant tumors is common.

Tumor nomenclature

How are tumors named?

Malignant tumors are generally named based on the type of tissue from which the cancer arises

✎ **What are the two broad classifications of malignant tumors?**

1. *Carcinomas:* tumors arising in epithelial tissue (skin, glands, and mucous membranes of the respiratory, GI, and genitourinary tracts)
2. *Sarcomas:* tumors arising in connective (bone and fat) and muscular tissues

✎ **What other nomenclature may be used to name tumors?**

1. *Adeno:* glandular epithelium
2. *Fibro:* fibrous tissue
3. *Chondro:* cartilage
4. *Rhabdo:* striated muscle
5. *Osteo:* bone
6. *Mening:* meninges
7. *Neuro* or *ganglio*: nerve cells
8. *Lympho:* lymphoid tissue
9. *Myelo:* bone marrow

Cancer treatments

✎ **What treatment modalities are used to treat cancer?**

Pharmacologic therapy (chemotherapy, biotherapy, hor-monal therapy, retinoid therapy), radiation therapy, surgi-cal therapy, and bone marrow transplantation

What are some import-ant nursing considera-tions regarding cancer treatment?

1. Only nurses familiar with adverse effects and toxici-ties of chemotherapy and biotherapy should adminis-ter these drugs.
2. Anticancer agents are considered mutagenic, terato-genic, and carcinogenic and should be handled, ad-ministered, and disposed of accordingly.
3. Patients should be encouraged to keep all appoint-ments because results typically depend on specific time intervals between treatments.

4. Patients should be encouraged to report unusual symptoms and adverse effects.

Pharmacologic therapy

How are pharmacologic anticancer agents administered?

Topically, orally, subcutaneously (S.C.), I.M., intra-arterially, intravesicularly, intraperitoneally, intrapleurally, intrathecally or intraventricularly, and I.V. (as an I.V. push or continuous infusion); when I.V. chemotherapy is planned, it's important to establish a venous access for future treatments

✎ What types of vascular access devices are used to administer chemotherapeutic or biotherapeutic agents?

1. *Nontunneled central venous catheters:* peripherally inserted central catheter, multilumen subclavian catheter
2. *Tunneled central venous catheters:* Groshong catheter, Hickman catheter
3. *Implantable ports:* central catheter placed S.C., which is accessed percutaneously using a special needle; an Ommaya reservoir (placed under the scalp) is an example; peripheral implantable ports are also now available commercially

Chemotherapy

What's chemotherapy?

The use of drugs to treat cancer; chemotherapy may: produce a regression of the tumor or metastasis, slow the appearance of secondary growths, relieve pain or other symptoms, or debulk tumors in preparation for surgical removal

✎ How do chemotherapeutic agents work?

By destroying young, rapidly multiplying cells such as cancer cells; they function at a cellular level by interrupting the cell life cycle (usually by interfering with deoxyribonucleic acid [DNA] synthesis) so that cellular growth and replication are inhibited

Aside from direct cytotoxic effects, how else are chemotherapeutic agents used in cancer treatment?

To enhance the effects of radiation therapy in conjunction with certain types of chemotherapy (fluorouracil, cisplatin); they may also be used in conjunction with transplantation of peripheral blood stem cells to restore hematopoiesis through autologous rescue

What's a growth fraction?

The portion of cells actively dividing relative to the entire population of cells

▨ *Cells with a rapid cycling time and tumors with a large growth fraction are typically the most responsive to chemotherapy.*

What's dose intensity?

The total amount of chemotherapeutic drug delivered per unit of time (usually a week)

✎ Why do chemotherapeutic agents have so many adverse effects?

Because many normal cells in the body also grow and divide rapidly and have short life spans (GI tract, bone marrow, hair follicles), many chemotherapeutic agents directly attack these normal cells

✎ What's the major life-threatening adverse effect of chemotherapeutic agents?

Pancytopenia (neutropenia, anemia, thrombocytopenia) from chemotherapy's depressive effect on the bone marrow

✎ What toxicities are associated with various types of chemotherapy?

1. *Cardiotoxicity* (anthracyclines such as doxorubicin [Rubex] as well as cyclophosphamide [Cytoxan], trastuzumab [Herceptin] and paclitaxel [Taxol]): nonreversible cardiomyopathy
2. *Neurotoxicity* (vincristine, cisplatin): peripheral neuropathy, hand and feet paresthesia
3. *Pulmonary toxicity* (bleomycin [Blenoxane], cytarabine [Cytosar], mitomycin-C [Mutamycin], cyclophosphamide, carmustine [Gliadel], methotrexate [Trexall]): irreversible "honeycombing" of the lungs, caused by dilation of air spaces and obliteration of alveoli; leads to the development of restrictive lung disease
4. *Hepatotoxicity* (methotrexate, cytarabine, 6-mercaptopurine [6-MP]): fatty changes of the liver, cholestasis, hepatitis, hepatocellular necrosis, and veno-occlusive disease may result
5. *Nephrotoxicity* (cisplatin [Platinol-AQ], mitomycin-C, carmustine): direct renal cell damage, or obstructive nephropathy from precipitate formation (uric acid); mannitol (Osmitrol) and amifostine (Ethyol) may be used to prevent or minimize nephrotoxicity

✎ What other complications are associated with chemotherapy?

1. *Bone marrow suppression* (myelosuppression): neutropenia, thrombocytopenia, anemia; most common dose-limiting complication of chemotherapy
2. *GI problems:* nausea, vomiting, mucositis (stomatitis, esophagitis), diarrhea, constipation, altered taste sensation (dysgeusia)
3. *Skin disorders:* hyperpigmentation (discoloration of skin, tongue, nails, and mucous membranes due to increased production of melanin; occurs more common-

ly in dark-skinned individuals), hypersensitivity, photosensitivity, pruritus, alopecia

4. *Hemorrhagic cystitis* (cyclophosphamide, ifosfamide [IFEX]): metabolic by-product (acrolein) is deposited in the bladder mucosa, which causes inflammation and ulceration; mesna may be given to protect the bladder from acrolein

5. *Drug resistance:* alterations in topoisomerase enzyme systems and overexpression of the *MDR-1* gene

6. *Extravasation of a vesicant* (doxorubicin): potentially leading to tissue necrosis

What are important nursing actions when caring for a patient receiving chemotherapeutic agents?

1. Implement infection prevention precautions and encourage importance of good hygiene and hand hygiene (neutropenia). Monitor for signs of infection, such as swelling or erythema of a body part, especially the rectal area.

2. Implement bleeding precautions. Instruct the patient to avoid cuts, bruises, or trauma, and to avoid shaving with a straightedge razor. Administer injections only if necessary and apply pressure to prevent bleeding (thrombocytopenia).

3. Anticipate symptoms of anemia. Avoid overexertion. Encourage frequent rest periods and instruct the patient to change positions slowly to avoid orthostatic hypotension.

4. Monitor CBC and platelet count at least weekly during treatment.

5. Explain to the patient that blood and blood product transfusions (packed RBCs, platelets) are a part of therapy, and aren't necessarily a setback.

6. Explain to the patient the importance of not skipping doses. Some patients skip doses in an attempt to minimize adverse effects.

What safety precautions should be observed when providing care for a patient receiving chemotherapy?

1. Avoid direct exposure to chemotherapeutic agents during preparation, administration, and disposal. Exposure can occur through inhalation, ingestion, and absorption. Disposable latex gloves should be worn during administration of a chemotherapeutic agent; a gown and mask may be worn as well.

2. Put on latex gloves as well as a gown and mask when handling vomitus and excreta.

3. Avoid administering chemotherapeutic agents while pregnant. The Occupational Safety and Health Administration recommends assigning pregnant women to other duties while they're pregnant.

4. Clean up spills with a special cytotoxic drug spill kit, while wearing latex gloves and a disposable gown with elastic cuffs.

What medications may be given to prevent or minimize hypersensitivity reactions in patients receiving taxanes?	Corticosteroids (dexamethasone), antihistamines (diphenhydramine), and histamine-2 blocker (ranitidine, cimetidine)
What adverse reactions are associated with epipodophyllins?	Myelosuppression, hypersensitivity reactions, and hypotension related to infusion rate (etoposide)
What adverse effects are associated with camptothecins?	Myelosuppression (topotecan), diarrhea (irinotecan), and alopecia

Antitumor antibiotics

What are examples of antitumor antibiotics?	1. *Anthracyclines:* daunorubicin (Cerubidine), doxorubicin, mitoxantrone (Novantrone), idarubicin, epirubicin
	2. *Other antibiotics:* Bleomycin (Blenoxane), plicamycin (Mithracin), dactinomycin (Cosmegen), mitomycin-C (Mutamycin)
How do antitumor antibiotics work?	By interfering with nucleic acid synthesis and function
What adverse effects are associated with antitumor antibiotics?	Cardiotoxicity (from doxorubicin-induced cardiomegaly), myelosuppression, nausea, vomiting, stomatitis, sperm and ovarian suppression, discoloration of urine (red or blue), hyperpigmentation, alopecia, severe extravasation injury, and renal failure (from mitomycin-C–induced hemolytic-uremic syndrome)
What drugs require a multiple-gated acquisition scan to be performed before use?	Daunorubicin, doxorubicin, and mitoxantrone (because of their cardiotoxic effects)
What drug may be administered to minimize cardiotoxicity?	Dexrazoxane (Zinecard)
Use of which drug necessitates obtaining baseline pulmonary function test results?	Bleomycin, because of the risk of pulmonary toxicity

What are other uses of bleomycin in cancer therapy?	1. Synchronization of cells into the G_2 and S phases to increase sensitivity to antineoplastic agents, which work in those phases 2. Combination use with other chemotherapeutic agents because of its less dramatic myelosuppressive effects

Miscellaneous agents

What miscellaneous agents are used in cancer treatment?	L-asparaginase (Elspar), hydroxyurea (Hydrea), imatinib (Gleevec)

Hormonal therapy

What are examples of hormonal therapies used in the treatment of cancer?	1. *Antiestrogens:* tamoxifen (Nolvadex), megestrol (Megace) 2. *Antiandrogens:* flutamide (Euflex), nilutamide (Nilandron), bicalutamide (Casodex) 3. *Gonadotropin-releasing hormone analogues:* leuprolide (Lupron), goserelin (Zoladex) 4. *Aromatase inhibitors:* anastrozole (Arimidex), letrozole (Femara), exemestane (Aromasin) 5. *Glucocorticoids:* prednisone, dexamethasone (Decadron) 6. *Estrogens:* diethylstilbestrol, estradiol 7. *Progestins:* medroxyprogesterone (Depo-Provera)
How do hormonal therapies work?	Although their mechanism is incompletely understood, their action likely involves the inhibition of steroid-specific receptors on cell surfaces, which ultimately decreases the tumor growth fraction of cells that are dependent on the hormone for division
How do hormonal therapies differ in relation to other anti-cancer medications?	They aren't cytotoxic drugs; they're usually administered orally
✎ **What adverse effects are associated with hormonal therapy?**	Hot flashes (tamoxifen), thromboembolic events (tamoxifen), fluid retention, diarrhea (antiandrogens), libido changes, menstrual irregularities, and gynecomastia (antiandrogens)

Retinoid agents

What retinoids are used in the treatment of cancer?	Isotretinoin (Accutane) and tretinoin (Vesanoid)
	⚡ *Retinoids are teratogenic and should never be administered to pregnant females or those who plan to conceive during therapy.*
How do retinoids work?	By influencing the proliferation and differentiation of tumor cells
What adverse reactions are commonly associated with retinoids?	Dry mucous membranes, photosensitivity, brittle nails, headache, nausea, vomiting, elevations of triglycerides and liver enzymes, arthralgia, and bone pain

Biotherapy

What's biotherapy?	The use of substances (natural or synthetic) that stimulate the body's immune system to fight disease by affecting biological responses in host-tumor interactions
What are examples of biotherapeutic agents?	Interferons and interleukins
How do biotherapeutic agents work?	1. Have a direct cytotoxic effect on cancer cells 2. Initiate or augment the host's tumor-immune rejection response 3. Affect the tumor's ability to metastasize, and affect cell transformation
What classifications of biotherapeutic agents exist?	Immunomodulating agents, interferons, antigens, lymphokines, monoclonal antibodies, and growth factors
What are monoclonal antibodies?	Antibodies directed against a specific antigen
What are colony-stimulating factors?	Substances that encourage the production of bone marrow stem cells

⬥ What growth factor is commonly used to accelerate neutrophil recovery within the bone marrow?

Granulocyte-colony stimulating factor (G-CSF), also known as filgrastim (Neupogen)

What are the adverse effects of G-CSF?

Bone pain and pain at injection site

⬥ What growth factor is commonly used to treat anemia?

Epoetin (Epogen, Procrit) administered subcutaneously once weekly

What adverse reactions are associated with epoetin?

Flulike symptoms (fever, chills, rigors, nausea, vomiting, headache, malaise, arthralgias), urticaria, skin rashes, and hypertension

What life-threatening reaction is associated with interleukin-2?

Cardiovascular and pulmonary adverse effects due to capillary-leak syndrome

⬥ What are important nursing actions when caring for a patient receiving biotherapeutic agents?

1. Inform the patient and his family of anticipated adverse effects (flulike symptoms).
2. Premedicate the patient for therapies with known sensitivity reactions. Make sure emergency medications (epinephrine) are readily available in the event of hypersensitivity reactions.
3. Monitor vital signs and assess for allergic responses.
4. Encourage increased fluid intake.
5. Administer pharmacologic agents (antipyretics) as ordered by the physician.

What are tumor-infiltrating lymphocytes?

Special cancer-fighting cells of the immune system that target tumor cells

Radiation therapy

What's radiation therapy?

The use of a focused, high-energy ionizing radiation to destroy cancer cells by damaging the cancer cells' DNA and inhibiting their ability to divide and proliferate

How does radiation therapy work?

Ionizing radiation penetrates tissue cells and deposits intense energy within them, which causes breakage in chromosomes within the cell. Replication of the cell is then prevented.

✎ What's the purpose of radiation therapy?

1. Used to eliminate or shrink localized tumors; it can be curative or palliative, and it may help to control cancer
2. Used commonly in conjunction with surgery; surgery focuses on removing the bulk of the disease using tissue-sparing techniques, which inevitably leaves behind microscopic cancer cells that radiation can then destroy
3. Used in combination with chemotherapy, which sensitizes cells to the effects of the radiation treatment

✎ What cells are the most radiosensitive?

Cells that are in the G and M phases of the cell cycle; in contrast, cells in the S phase are the most resistant to radiation therapy

✎ Why is it important to maintain a patient's hemoglobin (Hb) greater than 12 g/dl during radiation therapy?

Cells that are the most radiosensitive are undifferentiated, dividing and well oxygenated; as a result, maintaining an Hb greater than 12% will increase sensitivity to the radiation treatment

◥ *Oxygenated cells are more radiosensitive than hypoxic cells.*

What's fractionation?

The process of dividing total radiation dose into single sessions or "fractions" to reduce the risk of adverse reactions; because the repair rate of normal cells exceeds the repair rate of cancer cells, spacing treatments over time allows greater destruction of cancer cells with less overall damage to the surrounding normal cells

What's protraction?

The overall time it takes to deliver the entire treatment

What techniques exist for delivering radiation therapy?

1. *External beam:* beam passes through body tissues in its path before and after it reaches the tumor being treated
2. *Brachytherapy:* internal radiation; a form of radiation therapy in which radioactive substances are placed in direct contact with the tissue being treated; commonly used in the treatment of cancers of the rectum, bladder, brain, tongue, lip, and vagina
3. *Radioimmunotherapy:* experimental treatment in which antibodies bind specific cancer cells, which are then killed by gamma rays

How is a patient prepared for radiation therapy?

1. Imaging studies, such as an MRI or CT scan, are obtained to determine the exact size and location of the tumor as well as the nature of the surrounding tissue.
2. A determination is made of the radiation dose, number of sessions, and the time interval between sessions.
3. Shields may be made to protect specific parts of a patient's body from the radiation.
4. Markings are made on the patient's skin showing where the radiation beam should be focused.

5. Simulation is performed to ensure optimal delivery of radiation to site of tumor.

What's simulation?

An imitation of how a patient's treatment will be set up; it involves marking a patient's body where radiation treatment will be delivered and using laser beams to record the target area; positioning the patient is very important (he should be positioned in the same manner for each treatment); molds may be made to fit the specific area to be treated in order to prevent movement during therapy

Markings for radiation therapy shouldn't be removed from the patient's skin until the entire treatment course is completed.

What acute complications (occurring within 6 months) are associated with radiation therapy?

1. *Skin reactions:* alopecia (hair loss), erythema, hyperpigmentation, pruritus, loss of perspiration or sebaceous excretion, desquamation; appositional skin found in the axillae, groin, perineum, inframammary, and other skin folds is at increased risk for reactions
2. *Mucous membrane alterations:* mucositis (stomatitis, esophagitis, enteritis, cystitis, urethritis, vaginitis, proctitis) and xerostomia (decreased salivation)
3. *Bone marrow suppression:* neutropenia (first week of treatment), thrombocytopenia (2 to 3 weeks of treatment), and anemia (2 to 3 months of treatment) because of the effects on myeloblasts, megakaryoblasts, and erythroblasts

Skin care products, such as powders, perfumes, and deodorants shouldn't be applied in the treatment field.

The degree of bone marrow suppression depends on the amount of bone marrow included in the treatment field. The greatest amount of bone marrow suppression is associated with total body, total lymphatic, whole abdomen, craniospinal, and large area pelvic (iliac crest and fossa) irradiation.

The immune and hematologic systems should be monitored weekly using a CBC with differential and platelet count during radiation therapy.

What late complications are associated with radiation therapy?

Subcutaneous fibrosis, pigmentation changes, and necrosis; fistula formation; nonhealing ulcerations; and damage to specific organs

What's radiation enteritis?

A disorder of the large and small bowel that may occur during or following a course of radiation therapy to the abdomen, pelvis, or rectum

✎ What are important nursing actions when caring for a patient receiving radiation therapy?

1. Instruct the patient to avoid skin care products (deodorants, powders, perfumes) in the treatment field, sun exposure, and temperature extremes.
2. Encourage the use of a mild soap and an electric razor; encourage allowing hair to dry naturally, avoiding hairdryers.
3. Encourage a balanced diet that's high in protein, and the consumption of plenty of fluids.
4. Apply skin products (hydrous lanolin, aloe vera gel, ointments, moisturizing lotions, and topical steroids) as ordered by the physician for treatment of acute skin reactions.
5. Instruct the patient to avoid activities and clothing that increase skin friction and the risk of skin breakdown (nylon increases skin moisture and tight fitting clothes increase friction).
6. Encourage the use of a soft-bristle toothbrush.
7. Assess oral mucosa and skin for breaks in integrity weekly during radiation treatment.
8. Monitor CBC with differential and platelet count weekly during radiation treatment.
9. Monitor for signs of infection; instruct patient to notify the oncologist immediately of signs of infection (fever). Obtain a culture of any suspicious infectious process.

Surgical treatments

✎ What types of surgery may be used to treat a patient with cancer?

1. *Resection:* local excision of the lesion when there are no other identifiable lesions seen or when the primary lesion is believed to have been eradicated; radical surgical resection is performed for local control or palliation of symptoms
2. *Debulking:* removal of as much of a tumor as possible when removal of the entire tumor isn't feasible (when attached to a vital organ); used when the size of the tumor has grown large enough to cause symptoms that affect quality of life; adjuvant therapy is more effective after this type of surgery
3. *Shunting:* used to divert body fluids to another area capable of managing it
4. *Bone stabilization procedures:* used to decrease pain and improve function
5. *Tube placements:* used to bypass obstructions, decrease pain, and give nutritional supplementation (percutaneous endoscopic gastrostomy tube placement)

| **What factors are considered when deciding if surgical treatment of cancer is the best option?** | Physical status of patient, tumor growth rate, invasiveness, and metastatic potential |

| **What types of tumors are most amenable to surgical resection?** | Those that arise from a tissue with a slow rate of cell growth or replication |

Bone marrow transplantation

✎ What types of bone marrow transplants are performed?

1. *Allogeneic:* a transplant from a donor who's a match
2. *Autologous:* the patient receives his own bone marrow that has been purged before receiving high-dose chemotherapy and radiation therapy to eliminate any remaining tumor
3. *Peripheral stem cell:* a transplant that involves obtaining and infusing true pluripotent stem cells
4. *Umbilical stem cell:* a transplant that's still an emerging technique

What's the basic concept of bone marrow transplantation?

The dose of most chemotherapeutic agents is limited by subsequent dose-related marrow toxicity. The availability of donor marrow makes it possible to administer chemotherapy in supralethal doses in an effort to kill malignant cells. The patient is then rescued with marrow to prevent iatrogenic death.

What complications are associated with bone marrow transplantation?

Adverse effects of high-dose chemotherapy and radiation therapy, graft-versus-host disease (GVHD), rejection, and relapse

✎ What's GVHD?

A condition that occurs after bone marrow transplantation in which the donor's immune cells in the transplanted bone marrow produce antibodies against the host's tissues, resulting in the attack of vital organs; the process may be acute or chronic, mild, or severe

✎ What clinical manifestations are associated with GVHD?

1. *Acute:* skin rash, diarrhea, elevated liver function tests, increased susceptibility to infections
2. *Chronic:* skin rash, dry eyes and mouth, alopecia, elevated liver function tests, increased susceptibility to infections

What's the typical treatment for GVHD?

Immune suppression with high-dose corticosteroids or other immunosuppressive agents

Oncology complications

Complications related to disease process

HEMORRHAGE

✎ **What causes hemorrhage in a patient with cancer?**

Thrombocytopenia or altered platelet function, tumor invasion of bone marrow or a blood vessel, medications that interfere with hemostasis, or the development of an ulcer; disseminated intravascular coagulation may also occur due to the release of thromboplastic substances from cancer cells, or in the setting of sepsis

▧ *Hematologic neoplasms such as leukemia are associated with a higher rate of bleeding complications than are solid tumors.*

✎ **Where are the most common sites for hemorrhage in a patient with cancer?**

Gingiva, nose, bladder, brain, and GI tract

✎ **What are important nursing actions in the care of a patient with cancer who's at risk for hemorrhaging?**

1. Monitor vital signs (especially blood pressure and pulse) at frequent intervals.
2. Monitor CBC with platelet count.
3. Assess for overt bleeding as well as for signs of anemia from prolonged blood loss.
4. Minimize venipuncture sticks and use smallest gauge needle. Maintain direct pressure if bleeding occurs from venipuncture sites, incisions, or catheter insertion sites. Application of cold compresses may be of benefit due to vasoconstrictive effect.
5. Establish two large-bore I.V. accesses.
6. Anticipate the need for blood or blood product transfusions.
7. Use electric razors on the patient and avoid straight-edge razors.
8. Encourage the patient to avoid forceful nose blowing.

PARANEOPLASTIC SYNDROME

What's paraneoplastic syndrome?

A condition that results from the release of hormones by cancer cells in the primary or metastatic sites. It may occur at all stages of the cancer process, but most commonly occurs with advanced disease.

What's the pathophysiologic process of paraneoplastic syndrome?

Hormones are secreted from cancer cells that arise from tissues that don't typically release the hormone.

What are the most common paraneoplastic syndromes?

1. Parathormone-like substance or calcitonin secretion by tumors involving the lung, breast, kidney, colon, or thyroid; hypercalcemia is the end result
2. Antidiuretic hormone (ADH) production by tumors involving the lung, pancreas, or prostate gland; syndrome of inappropriate antidiuretic hormone (SIADH) is the end result
3. Corticotropin secretion by tumor involving the lung, thyroid, thymus, stomach, pancreas, or ovary
4. Insulin secretion by tumor involving the pancreas, liver, adrenal glands, stomach, or ovary

HYPERCALCEMIA

Which types of cancers are most likely to be associated with hypercalcemia?

Lung and breast cancer (related to their overall incidence); however, multiple myeloma, which isn't as common, is the underlying cause in 10% of malignancy-induced hypercalcemia

◥ *Hypercalcemia is the most common oncologic emergency, occurring in 10% to 20% of patients with cancer.*

What's the pathophysiology of hypercalcemia in a patient with cancer?

Results from paraneoplastic syndrome or from tumors with extensive bone involvement (including bony metastasis) that cause a release of calcium secondary to osteolytic activity

✎ **What are the clinical manifestations of hypercalcemia?**

Early symptoms can include nausea, vomiting, anorexia, and constipation. Other symptoms may include headaches, lethargy, polyuria, and bradycardia. A serum calcium value greater than 11 mg/dl is diagnostic of hypercalcemia. A more common finding is hypoalbuminemia.

✎ **What complications can result from hypercalcemia?**

Pathologic fractures, renal calculi with impairment of renal function, ileus, arrhythmias, cardiac arrest, and coma

✎ **What are important nursing actions when caring for a patient with cancer who's experiencing hypercalcemia?**

1. Maintain vigorous I.V. hydration with normal saline. Encourage fluid intake by mouth.
2. Monitor intake and output (input goal of 3 L/day).
3. Administer medications (diuretics to increase urine flow, calcitonin and bisphosphonates, such as pamidronate, to prevent bone resorption, and cortico-

steroids to reduce calcium resorption from the GI tract) as ordered by the physician.

4. Monitor electrocardiographs.
5. Monitor laboratory values (serum calcium level).
6. Encourage mobilization and weight-bearing activities.
7. Exercise safety precautions because of patient's confusion, weakness, and susceptibility to fractures.
8. Anticipate need for plicamycin (Mithracin) to lower calcium levels if severe symptoms are present.

Dietary intake of calcium has very little effect on serum calcium levels in cancer patients.

SYNDROME OF INAPPROPRIATE ANTIDIURETIC HORMONE

What causes syndrome of inappropriate antidiuretic hormone (SIADH) in a patient with cancer?

ADH may be abnormally produced by tumor cells, resulting in water retention and dilutional hyponatremia (due to inappropriate reabsorption of water by the kidney); water intoxication may also result

What type of cancer is most commonly associated with SIADH?

Small-cell lung cancer

What are the clinical manifestations of SIADH?

Early symptoms of SIADH can include nausea, weakness, anorexia, or fatigue. As the hyponatremia worsens, symptoms may progress to confusion, irritability, seizures, and lethargy.

How is the diagnosis made?

1. Decreased serum sodium (less than 130 mEq/L)
2. Decreased serum osmolality (less than 280 mOsm/kg)
3. Increased urine sodium greater than 20 mEq/L

What are important nursing actions when caring for a patient with cancer who's experiencing SIADH?

1. Monitor intake and output carefully. Enforce water restriction of less than 1 L/24 hours.
2. Administer pharmacologic agents (diuretics to eliminate excess water, demeclocycline to interfere with action of ADH) as ordered by the physician.
3. Obtain daily weight.
4. Monitor for development of heart failure and pulmonary edema secondary to fluid overload.
5. Implement seizure precautions if serum sodium less than 120 mEq/L.
6. Anticipate the need for hypertonic saline (3% to 5% sodium chloride) for severe cases.

SUPERIOR VENA CAVA SYNDROME

What's superior vena cava syndrome?

A condition in which blood flow through the superior vena cava to the right atrium is impaired, which interferes with venous drainage above the blockage; superior vena cava syndrome may occur as a result of tumor compression or as a complication of a central venous access device, involving thrombus formation

✎ What are the clinical manifestations of superior vena cava syndrome?

Edema of the face (especially periorbital), neck, upper trunk, and extremities; jugular vein distention; dyspnea; tachypnea; nonproductive cough; hoarseness; headache; chest pain; confusion; and visual disturbances

Chest X-ray or CT scan may reveal a mediastinal mass, cardiomegaly, pleural effusion, or lobar collapse.

■ *The severity of superior vena cava syndrome depends on how quickly the obstruction occurs. Symptoms are typically more severe if the obstruction develops rapidly, because collateral veins of the neck and chest don't have adequate time to distend to accommodate the increased blood flow.*

What types of cancer are most commonly associated with superior vena cava syndrome?

Advanced lung cancer and non-Hodgkin's lymphoma

What's the typical treatment for superior vena cava syndrome?

1. *Tumor-related:* chemotherapy, radiation therapy, or both at the site of obstruction
2. *Thrombus-related:* thrombolytic therapy (streptokinase, urokinase, alteplase, heparin), catheter removal, stent placement, balloon dilatation, or surgical intervention (thrombectomy, surgical bypass)

What complications are associated with superior vena cava syndrome?

Central edema, airway compromise (tracheal obstruction), and cerebral edema

✎ What are important nursing actions when caring for a patient with cancer who's experiencing superior vena cava syndrome?

1. Elevate the head of the bed (Fowler's position) to facilitate venous drainage, but maintain the lower extremities in a dependent position.
2. Administer supplemental oxygen if ordered by the physician.
3. Monitor intake and output. Maintain adequate hydration, but avoid overhydration (exacerbates symptoms).

4. Avoid invasive procedures involving the upper body, including blood draws and I.V. therapy, because pooling of medications may occur in the upper torso or arms, and because of the potential for venous stasis, phlebitis, and thrombosis
5. Avoid constrictive procedures, including obtaining blood pressures in the arms.
6. Administer pharmacologic agents (corticosteroids, diuretics, thrombolytics) as ordered by the physician.
7. Provide a calm, restful environment.

SPINAL CORD COMPRESSION

What's spinal cord compression?

Direct pressure on the spinal cord caused by the extension of adjacent bony or soft-tissue lesions: those involving the spinal cord (intramedullary) or those of tissues that surround the spinal cord (extramedullary) lesions; tumors of the spinal cord and surrounding areas may be primary or metastatic

What malignancies are commonly associated with spinal cord compression?

Lung, breast, and prostate cancers as well as lymphoma and multiple myeloma; other types of tumors that can cause spinal cord compression are colorectal cancer, melanoma, sarcoma, and renal cell carcinoma

What are the clinical manifestations of spinal cord compression?

Severe pain that worsens with movement, straining, coughing, or leg raising is the most common presenting symptom; other symptoms depend on the level involved (cervical, thoracic, or sacral), but all symptoms will appear below the tumor; examples include lower extremity weakness, paralysis, numbness, tingling, and a loss of bowel or bladder control

What radiologic studies are performed to evaluate for spinal cord compression?

MRI is the diagnostic test of choice to confirm and diagnose spinal cord compression. However, an X-ray of the affected area is usually performed first to rule out other causes.

What's the treatment for spinal cord compression?

Radiation therapy can be used to shrink the tumor, and chemotherapy may be ordered as adjuvant treatment if the tumor is chemosensitive. High-dose steroids (dexamethasone) may be used to decompress the spinal cord, reduce local edema, and improve neurologic function. Removal of the tumor is usually desired, but not always feasible with surgery.

What complications are associated with the development of spinal cord compression?	Permanent neurologic impairment and paralysis

📘 *Rapid onset and quick progression of symptoms are worse prognostic factors for full recovery from spinal cord compression.*

What are important nursing actions when caring for a patient with spinal cord compression?

1. Administer pharmacologic agents (dexamethasone, analgesics) as ordered by the physician.
2. Perform neurologic assessments at frequent intervals.
3. Institute safety measures if motor-sensory loss is present.

PAIN

🖋 **What causes pain in a patient with cancer?**

1. Inflammation, ulceration, or necrosis of affected tissues
2. Compression of blood vessels, lymphatic vessels, and nerves
3. Obstruction of genitourinary or GI tract

🖋 **What are important nursing actions when caring for a patient with cancer who's experiencing pain?**

1. Facilitate reduction of fatigue, fear, and anxiety (all lower the pain threshold).
2. Promote nonpharmacologic methods of pain relief (relaxation, guided imagery, massage, change of position, biofeedback, music, transcutaneous electrical nerve stimulation).
3. Administer analgesics as ordered by the physician.
4. Use valid pain assessment tool to monitor pain intensity and effectiveness of interventions.
5. Consult the appropriate health care professional (physician, pharmacist, or pain management team) for refractory pain.

FATIGUE

🖋 **What causes fatigue in a patient with cancer?**

Increased metabolic rate in the presence of cancer, the release of cellular waste products into the bloodstream as a result of cancer therapy, anemia, poor nutrition, or infection secondary to cancer therapy; it generally occurs after the second week of radiation therapy

📘 *Fatigue is the most common symptom related to cancer and cancer treatments; it impacts quality of life significantly.*

✎ What are important nursing actions when caring for a patient with cancer who's experiencing fatigue?

1. Encourage frequent rest periods throughout the day and additional hours of sleep at night.
2. Instruct the patient to go to bed at the same time each evening to maintain circadian rhythms.
3. Encourage low-intensity exercises such as walking.
4. Encourage good nutritional intake as well as adequate fluid intake.
5. Assist with activities of daily living as necessary.
6. Educate the patient about energy-saving techniques (sitting to comb hair or brush teeth, using a shower chair).
7. Instruct the patient to prioritize activities and to consider reducing work hours or taking time off from work during therapy.
8. Administer pharmacologic agents (iron or folate supplements, epoetin) as ordered by the physician.
9. Assess for depression and consult the appropriate health care professional (social worker, physician, or psychiatrist).

Complications related to cancer therapy

NAUSEA AND VOMITING

What are the causes of nausea and vomiting in patients with cancer?

Stimulation of the vomiting center by chemotherapeutic agents or waste products of cellular breakdown that results from chemotherapy or radiation therapy; may also be caused by obstruction of the GI tract by tumor growth or by severe constipation; may be acute (within a few minutes to several hours following drug administration) or delayed (occurs more than 24 hours following drug administration)

✎ What medication is most commonly used to prevent nausea and vomiting in patients undergoing chemotherapy?

Ondansetron (Zofran)

✎ What other medications may be used to treat nausea and vomiting associated with cancer therapy?

1. *Serotonin inhibitors:* granisetron (Kytril) and dolasetron (Anzemet)
2. *Dopamine antagonists:* metoclopramide (Reglan); phenothiazines such as prochlorperazine (Compazine); butyrophenones such as droperidol (Inapsine)
3. *Corticosteroids:* dexamethasone
4. *Benzodiazepines:* lorazepam (Ativan)
5. *Cannabinoids:* dronabinol (Marinol)

6. *Histamine antagonists:* diphenhydramine, promethazine; minimal effect on chemotherapy-induced nausea and vomiting

❧ What are therapeutic interventions for a patient with cancer who's experiencing nausea and vomiting?

1. Eliminate noxious odors from the environment.
2. Promote oral hygiene after each episode of emesis and before each meal. Use frequent mouthwash rinses of diluted saline.
3. Instruct the patient to breathe slowly and deeply as well as change positions slowly during episodes of nausea.
4. Instruct the patient to eat small, frequent meals (with low-roughage foods), to eat and drink slowly, and to avoid highly seasoned foods. Discourage food ingestion within 3 hours of chemotherapy administration.
5. Encourage fluid intake and administer I.V. fluids as ordered by the physician.
6. Monitor intake and output. Assess for dehydration (skin turgor for tenting, blood pressure for hypotension). Monitor electrolytes with prolonged vomiting (hypokalemia and metabolic alkalosis can occur).
7. Administer I.V. cytotoxic agents slowly to minimize stimulation of the vomiting center. Consider administering these agents at night so that sleep may prevent nausea.
8. Encourage nonpharmacologic interventions (guided imagery, relaxation, distraction, music, and biofeedback).
9. Administer antiemetics as ordered by the physician.

ANOREXIA AND CACHEXIA

What causes anorexia in a patient with cancer?

May occur secondary to nausea, vomiting, altered taste sensation, pain, psychological stress, fatigue, and depression

What's cachexia?

Physical wasting due to problems with ingestion, digestion, or absorption; may result from increased nutrient needs related to increased metabolic demands

❧ What are important nursing actions when caring for a patient with cancer who has anorexia or cachexia?

1. Offer foods that the patient prefers, and encourage patient participation with menu selection. Encourage small, frequent meals high in carbohydrates and protein.
2. Perform calorie counts and nutritional assessments. Implement nutrition consultation.
3. Encourage the use of seasonings or flavorings to enhance the taste of foods.

4. Encourage light exercise for appetite stimulation.
5. Encourage good oral hygiene.
6. Obtain daily weight.
7. Monitor intake and output.
8. Monitor serum albumin (and prealbumin) levels to assess nutritional status.
9. Administer appetite stimulants or megestrol as ordered by the physician.
10. Increase intake of calories and protein with oral supplementation, enteral feedings, or parenteral feedings to maintain nitrogen balance for severe malnutrition.

ALTERED TASTE SENSATION

What causes altered taste sensation in a patient with cancer?

1. Radiation-induced destruction of taste buds
2. Chemotherapy or radiation therapy-induced release of cellular waste products
3. Decreased saliva production

What's dysgeusia?

An unpleasant taste sensation; a metallic taste is sometimes described by a patient receiving certain chemotherapeutic agents

What's ageusia?

The absence of taste sensations

What are important nursing actions when caring for a patient with cancer who's experiencing altered taste sensation?

1. Promote good oral hygiene.
2. Eliminate noxious odors from the environment (smell and taste sensations are closely related).
3. Encourage the use of mouth rinses with warm saline and provide saliva substitutes to prevent mouth dryness.
4. Discourage the use of tobacco products.

MUCOSITIS

✎ **What causes mucositis in a patient with cancer?**

Chemotherapy or radiation therapy-induced destruction of epithelial cells of mucosa along the GI tract; due to the rapid turnover of cells in the outer epithelial layer (1 to 2 weeks), these cells are particularly susceptible to the effects of cancer therapies; disruptions in the mucosal lining may serve as a portal for microorganisms to cause infection or enter the bloodstream

What's stomatitis?

Inflammation of the mucosa of the oral cavity; commonly caused by radiation to the head and neck as well as use of certain chemotherapeutic agents

What's xerostomia?

Dry mouth caused by destruction of salivary glands; may be progressive and irreversible

What's esophagitis?

Inflammation of the esophageal mucosa; esophagitis may result in difficulty swallowing (dysphagia) or pain with swallowing (odynophagia)

What's enteritis?

Inflammation of the intestinal mucosa that can result in diarrhea

What are important nursing actions in the care of a patient with cancer who's experiencing mucositis?

1. Encourage meticulous oral care (brushing, rinsing, flossing) after each meal and at bedtime, including the use of mouth rinses, such as warm saline, baking soda, or chlorhexidine (Peridex). Encourage the use of a narrow, soft-bristle toothbrush or a sponge-tipped swab. For severe stomatitis, the patient should remove dentures at all times except during meals.
2. Encourage small, frequent meals of soft and moist foods. Encourage good oral fluid intake, including the use of liquid dietary supplements or high-calorie milkshakes. Instruct the patient to avoid food temperature extremes and spicy foods.
3. Encourage the use of sugarless candy or chewing gum to stimulate salivation. Administer pharmacologic agents for xerostomia (pilocarpine, saliva substitutes, mucin-based preparations, or carboxymethyl cellulose preparations) as ordered by the physician.
4. Assess oral cavity at regular intervals; instruct the patient on self-assessment.
5. Lubricate the patient's lips frequently.
6. Encourage the use of ice chips during chemotherapy administration.
7. Instruct the patient to avoid tobacco and alcohol, products containing glycerin or lemon, and mouthwashes containing alcohol because of their irritating and drying effects.
8. Administer pharmacologic agents (sucralfate suspension, viscous lidocaine, benzocaine, tetracaine, capsaicin, or a mucosa-adhesive water-soluble polymer; analgesics if topical anesthetics unsuccessful) for stomatitis and esophagitis as ordered by the physician.
9. Consider crushing non–enteric-coated tablets to facilitate swallowing.

DIARRHEA AND CONSTIPATION

What causes diarrhea and constipation in a patient with cancer?

Diarrhea may result from chemotherapy or radiation-induced inflammation and damage to the GI mucosa. Constipation may result from the disease process itself in which mechanical pressure or obstruction of the bowel occurs. Constipation may also occur from impairment of peristalsis by neurotoxic chemotherapy, the use of opioid analgesics, alterations in eating habits, or as a result of immobility.

✎ What are important nursing actions when caring for a patient with cancer who's experiencing constipation or diarrhea?

1. Encourage adequate fluid intake.
2. Encourage appropriate dietary modifications: low-residue, high-calorie, and high-protein diet for diarrhea; high-fiber diet for constipation.
3. Promote regular toileting schedule to prevent constipation.
4. Assess chemistry panel for serum electrolyte abnormalities (potassium, magnesium).
5. Administer pharmacologic agents (anticholinergics, loperamide for diarrhea; stool softener, laxative for constipation) as ordered by the physician.
6. Obtain stool cultures (*Clostridium difficile* as well as ova and parasites) for persistent diarrhea.

▶ *Antidiarrheal agents should be avoided if the cause of diarrhea is infectious because they would prolong the mucosal exposure to the toxins produced by the organism.*

SKIN REACTIONS

What types of skin reactions can occur as a result of cancer therapy?

Hyperpigmentation of mucous membranes, tongue, and nails; photosensitivity; pruritus and allergic dermatitis; desquamation (dry or wet); and alopecia (hair loss from scalp, eyebrows, axillae, or pubic area) that's reversible with possible changes in texture and pigmentation with regrowth

✎ What are important nursing actions when caring for a patient with cancer who has a skin reaction?

1. Gently clean the affected area with a mild, hypoallergenic soap and lukewarm water. Pat skin with a soft towel to dry.
2. Apply skin products (moisturizing lotions; emollient creams) for treatment of acute skin reactions as directed by the physician. Apply dry cornstarch, aloe vera gel, oatmeal colloid soap or lotion, and topical steroid for pruritus and desquamation as directed by the physician.

3. Encourage the use of cotton sheets and clothing.
4. Encourage avoidance of sun exposure or the use of tanning beds to prevent increased hyperpigmentation and photosensitivity reactions. Encourage use of sunscreen.
5. Initiate physical therapy for gentle massage or myofascial release to minimize fibrosis and scar formation.
6. For alopecia, discourage daily shampooing as well as use of hairdryers, permanents, or color processing. Encourage the use of mild, protein-based shampoos with lukewarm water and a wide-tooth comb or soft-bristle brush. Reassure the patient that hair loss is only temporary. Encourage him to consider getting a short haircut to prevent distress at watching large quantities of hair fall out.
7. Promote preservation of self-image by encouraging the use of makeup, wigs, scarves, and false eyelashes and eyebrows if desired. Assist with grooming and make-up application if necessary, but encourage and support patient's independence to enhance self-esteem.

NEUTROPENIA AND INFECTION

What's neutropenia?

An absolute neutrophil count (ANC) less than 1500 μl. Neutropenia generally occurs 6 to 12 days after chemotherapy and can result from cancer therapy or from the disease process itself (ulceration and necrosis of the tumor, compression of vital organs by tumor). Recovery from neutropenia generally occurs in 3 to 4 weeks.

Chemotherapy is generally withheld if the WBC count is less than 1000 to 3000 μl or the ANC is less than 1500/μl.

Neutropenia can occur in the setting of a normal WBC count.

What's the life span of a granulocyte?

6 to 8 hours after it's released from the bone marrow

What's a nadir?

The lowest WBC count after treatment; usually occurs 10 to 14 days after cancer therapy

What causes neutropenia in a patient with cancer?

Involvement of bone marrow in tumors or treatment with chemotherapy or radiation therapy (bone marrow depression)

Why is neutropenia dangerous?

A neutropenic patient is at risk for infection, because the body's defense mechanism of phagocytosis is drastically reduced. An immunocompromised patient can become infected with minimal exposure to nonpathogens.

What life-threatening condition can occur in a patient with neutropenia who develops an infection?

Septic shock with organ failure

Infection is the most common cause of morbidity and mortality in a patient with cancer.

What organisms most commonly cause infections in a patient with cancer?

Gram-negative bacteria and fungi

The classic manifestations of infection, such as fever, may not always be present in the setting of neutropenia.

What are the most common sites of infection in a patient with cancer?

Venous access exit sites, sinuses, periodontium, oral cavity, pharynx, lower esophagus, lung, skin, anus, and perineum

What's the most common oral cavity infection in an immunocompromised patient?

Candida albicans (oral thrush), nystatin oral rinses, or clotrimazole troches are the usual treatments. Other common infectious agents of the oral cavity include streptococcal and herpes infections.

If a patient with neutropenia develops a fever without other symptoms, what tests should be ordered to determine the source of infection?

Blood cultures, chest X-ray, and urinalysis; stool and sputum cultures may also be obtained

What measures should be instituted to prevent infections in a patient with cancer?

1. Implement neutropenic precautions (place in a private room, maintain strict hand hygiene, restrict flowers or live plants, restrict *unpeeled* fresh fruits or vegetables, and restrict sick visitors or contact with small children).
2. Instruct the patient on proper personal hygiene (mouth care protocols, bathing, hand washing, and perineal care, including routine care and after each bowel movement).
3. Limit exposure to crowds and avoid contact with persons who have known or suspected infectious diseases or who have recently received vaccinations (because of possible subclinical infection). Avoid administering any immunizations.
4. Maintain sterile technique when caring for open wounds and I.V. care.

5. Assess for signs of infection. Assess temperature frequently (every 4 hours if hospitalized and at least daily if outpatient).
6. Encourage a low-microbial diet (no raw, unwashed vegetables or fruits).
7. Avoid invasive procedures unless absolutely necessary. Avoid rectal temperatures, rectal tubes, enemas, and suppositories.
8. Encourage deep-breathing and coughing exercises to prevent stasis of respiratory secretions.
9. Prevent urine retention (frequent voiding and intermittent urinary catheterization rather than placing an indwelling catheter).
10. Administer pharmacologic agents (antibiotics or CSFs) as ordered by the physician.

ANEMIA

What causes anemia in a patient with cancer?

The effects of chemotherapy or radiation therapy, tumor infiltration of bone marrow, or anemia of chronic disease; it occurs less frequently than neutropenia or thrombocytopenia because RBCs have a life span of 120 days — therefore, bone marrow tends to recover before a significant decrease in circulating RBCs occurs

What are important nursing actions in the care of a patient with cancer who has anemia?

1. Assess vital signs (tachycardia) and respiratory status (tachypnea) including oxygen saturation at least every shift.
2. Encourage additional rest periods and consolidation of tasks if significant activity intolerance occurs secondary to fatigue.
3. Instruct the patient to change positions slowly because of the possibility of light-headedness, dizziness, and syncope.
4. Monitor CBC (Hb levels, hematocrit [HCT]) and reticulocyte count (reticulocytes are immature RBCs; if the reticulocyte count is low, the bone marrow isn't actively producing RBCs). Anticipate the need for a possible blood transfusion if HCT is less than 25% or Hb level is less than 8 g/dl.
5. Administer iron, folate, or vitamin B_{12} supplements, as ordered by the physician (iron stores are necessary to support erythropoiesis).
6. Administer pharmacologic agents (epoetin) as ordered by the physician.

THROMBOCYTOPENIA

What causes thrombo-cytopenia in a patient with cancer?

Chemotherapy or radiation-induced myelosuppression; may also occur as a result of malignant infiltration of the bone marrow or as a result of abnormal destruction of circulating platelets; platelet life span is 7 to 10 days
Thrombocytopenia occurs 8 to 14 days following chemo-therapy, and tends to occur concomitantly with neutro-penia.

✎ What life-threatening condition can occur with throm-bocytopenia?

Hemorrhage

✎ When would spontaneous bleeding be expected?

Platelet count less than 20,000 cells/µl; a platelet trans-fusion may be necessary if the platelet count falls below this level; the use of interleukin-2 may also be used to in-duce megakaryocyte maturation

✎ What are important nursing actions in the care of a patient with cancer who has thrombocy-topenia?

1. Implement bleeding precautions, including avoidance of straightedge razors, dental floss, and contact sports.
2. Assess for overt bleeding, easy bruising, or petechiae.
3. Monitor for hematuria and hematemesis. Perform stool guaiac analysis.
4. Assess for headaches and altered mental status.
5. Avoid invasive procedures (including venipuncture and rectal invasion) and injections, unless absolutely necessary. Anticipate the need for a platelet transfu-sion before invasive procedures. Apply gentle, pro-longed pressure on insertion sites following invasive procedures.
6. Administer pharmacologic agents, such as oprelvekin (Neumega), or blood products (platelets) as ordered by the physician.

HEMORRHAGIC CYSTITIS

What causes hemor-rhagic cystitis in a patient with cancer?

Chemotherapy (cyclophosphamide) or radiation-induced destruction of the epithelial cells lining the bladder

What are the clinical manifestations of hemorrhagic cystitis?

Hematuria, frequency, and urgency

✎ What are important nursing actions in the care of a cancer patient with hemorrhagic cystitis?

1. Administer diuretics, as ordered by the physician, to promote diuresis.
2. Encourage adequate fluid intake and frequent voiding.
3. Monitor intake and output.
4. Monitor urine for blood (direct observation and dipstick); assess the patient for suprapubic pain, dysuria, and urinary frequency and urgency.
5. Anticipate the need for bladder irrigation with saline solution to prevent clot formation and the possible need for cystoscopy to cauterize bleeding vessels. Continuous bladder irrigation with silver nitrate or alum may be necessary to stop bleeding.
6. Administer pharmacologic agents (mesna), as ordered by the physician, to inactivate toxic metabolites.

TUMOR LYSIS SYNDROME

What's tumor lysis syndrome?

A complication of cancer therapy characterized by hyperuricemia, hyperkalemia, hyperphosphatemia, and hypocalcemia, which may lead to acute renal failure; the destruction of tumor cells causes a rapid release of cell components (uric acid, potassium, phosphorus) that leads to metabolic imbalances due to the kidneys' inability to clear these waste products

Which malignancies are most commonly associated with tumor lysis?

Tumors with a high growth fraction and that are highly sensitive to chemotherapy; lymphomas and leukemias are most commonly associated with tumor lysis syndrome

What are the clinical manifestations of tumor lysis syndrome?

Hematuria, oliguria, anuria, urine crystals, flank pain, neuromuscular cramps, tetany due to hypocalcemia (caused by inverse relationship with hyperphosphatemia), confusion, and cardiac arrhythmias

When is tumor lysis syndrome most likely to occur?

Within 48 hours of cancer therapy

What medication is typically used prophylactically against tumor lysis syndrome?

Allopurinol, which decreases uric acid concentration

What are important nursing actions in the treatment and prevention of tumor lysis syndrome?

1. Administer I.V. fluids with sodium bicarbonate to increase diuresis and to alkalinize urine (promotes solubility of uric acid and prevents formation of renal calculi).
2. Monitor intake and output carefully. Maintain urine output greater than 30 ml/hour, maintain urine pH greater than 7.0. Obtain daily weight and assess for fluid overload.
3. Administer allopurinol (300 to 800 mg/day), as ordered by the physician, to lower uric acid.
4. Monitor renal function and serum electrolytes and assess for abnormalities.
5. Administer phosphate-binding antacids or aluminum antacid gels to decrease serum phosphate levels. Calcium supplements may be used to correct hypocalcemia, although their use remains controversial in this setting.
6. Anticipate the possible need for hemodialysis (to lower uric acid, phosphorus, and potassium levels).

Supportive care and palliation of symptoms

What's grief?

A reaction to a significant loss, such as the death of a loved one, or the end of a familiar pattern or behavior, such as the result of divorce; grief is a natural response to the loss of someone or something of value; it's a universal phenomenon, and at the same time it's an intensely personal experience

What's bereavement?

The manner in which grief is processed

What's mourning?

The state of feeling sorrow over the loss of a loved one

✎ What are the five stages of grieving as defined by Dr. Elisabeth Kübler-Ross in *On Death and Dying*?

1. *Denial:* disbelief, sense of unreality
2. *Anger:* sense of rage or loss of control, blaming others
3. *Bargaining:* makes promises to God or promises to change life if allowed to live
4. *Depression:* crying, withdrawal from others, sleep disturbances, altered eating habits, inability to concentrate
5. *Acceptance:* coming to terms with a loss; resolution

The stages of grieving don't necessarily occur in any particular order, and two or more stages may occur simultaneously.

✎ **What are important nursing actions in the care of someone who's grieving?**

1. Encourage the patient to express his feelings (verbalization, crying) and provide an atmosphere of care and concern (provide privacy, display empathy).
2. Promote trust in the patient by answering his questions truthfully and completely.
3. Identify and encourage the use of coping techniques that have worked in previous situations; encourage the use of available support systems.
4. Promote communication between the patient and his family or significant other.
5. Provide information about grief counseling and encourage participation in a support group.
6. Encourage good nutrition, adequate sleep, and exercise.
7. Reassure the patient and his family that feelings experienced are normal and that there's no right or wrong way to grieve, nor is there a set timeframe for healing.
8. Offer to arrange a visit by someone who has experienced the same situation, such as the same medical diagnosis or treatment regimen, or the loss of loved one.
9. Consult the appropriate health care professional (social worker, psychiatrist) if concerned about dysfunctional grieving. Administer antidepressants if ordered.
10. Discourage the use of nonprescription drugs or alcohol to dull painful emotions.

What's suffering?

Physical, psychological (emotional), social, or spiritual pain

What's palliative care?

The care of patients whose disease is refractory to curative treatment; goal is to relieve suffering and provide the best possible quality of life for patients and their families across the illness spectrum; control of pain and other symptoms is provided, and psychological, social, and spiritual support may be integrated as well

What's hospice?

A term that may describe places where dying persons are cared for, such as a freestanding facility or a dedicated unit within a hospital; may also describe an organization that provides end-of-life care in various settings, but generally focuses on the patient's home

Hospice is currently the most widely available program for the delivery of multidisciplinary palliative care for those with a terminal illness (cancer, acquired immunodeficiency syndrome, Alzheimer's disease) and their families. Nurses, physicians, chaplains, social workers, therapists (physical and occupational), counselors, and volunteers may all participate in hospice care.

When is admission to a hospice program appropriate?

When efforts to control the biological disease are ineffective and the primary care focus becomes symptom control and maintaining quality of life. The Medicare Hospice Benefit requires the patient be diagnosed with a terminal illness with a life expectancy of less than 6 months, if the disease runs its typical course.

What factors are generally included in a patient assessment in end-of-life care?

1. Disease history
2. Physical symptoms: fatigue, weakness
3. Psychological symptoms: anxiety and depression
4. Decision-making capacity: mental competence
5. Communication skills and information sharing: accurate understanding of information
6. Social circumstances: financial resources, care-giving needs
7. Spiritual needs: personal meaning, religious beliefs
8. Practical needs: availability of human and financial resources to assist with daily living activities
9. Anticipatory planning for death

✎ **What symptoms do patients with a terminal, advanced illness commonly experience?**

Pain, dyspnea, weakness, fatigue, nausea, vomiting, constipation, diarrhea, anorexia or cachexia, edema, and insomnia

What medications might be used to manage dyspnea?

Oxygen, opioids, and anxiolytics are most commonly used, typically in combination with nonpharmacologic interventions

What medications might be used to assist in the management of fatigue and weakness?

Corticosteroids and psychostimulants

✎ **What are the most important factors in a psychological assessment in a patient with advanced illness?**

Cognition (confusion, hallucinations) and mood (anxiety, sadness)

✎ **What psychological conditions commonly occur in a patient with a terminal illness?**

Fear, anxiety, confusion (delirium), and depression

⚡ *Depression and anxiety are among the most prevalent and most underdiagnosed symptoms in patients facing end of life.*

What are important nursing actions when caring for a patient with a terminal illness who expresses psychological conditions?

1. Orient the patient to the environment, care providers, and routines.
2. Encourage verbalization of feelings.
3. Provide a calm, restful environment and maintain a quiet, supportive, and confident demeanor when interacting with the patient.
4. Facilitate the identification of specific stressors and means of coping with them. Encourage active participation in activities of daily living.
5. Provide information based on the patient's current needs, and reinforce explanations provided by the physicians. Explain all tests and treatments ahead of time.
6. Encourage questions and clarify any misconceptions.
7. Encourage the participation of significant others in teaching sessions.
8. Assist with relaxation techniques (guided imagery).
9. Consult the appropriate health care professional (social worker, physician, or psychiatrist) for significant psychological conditions.
10. Administer pharmacologic agents (anxiolytics, antidepressants) as ordered by the physician.

What are some of the most important roles of the nurse during the last hours of life for the patient and family?

1. Manage the patient's distress (feeding and hydration, changes in consciousness and pain).
2. Prepare and educate the patient and his family.

When might end-of-life sedation be an alternative?

For the rare patient with refractory pain, or other intractable symptoms, who's approaching the last hours or days of life; this intervention is intended to relieve suffering without hastening death, and is usually a collaboration of the entire health care team (including several physicians), the patient, and his family

9

The immune system and infectious diseases

Basic concepts of the immune system and microbiology

Fundamentals of the immune system

✎ The immune system is composed of what types of cells?

1. *Lymphocyte:* a type of white blood cell (WBC) that develops into B and T cells, which are critical factors in humoral immunity and cell-mediated immunity, respectively
2. *Macrophage, monocyte:* a large, phagocytic WBC that stimulates antibody production
3. *Neutrophil:* a type of WBC with phagocytotic and antimicrobial action
4. *Other:* mast cells, basophils, eosinophils, natural killer cells

What are the different types of leukocytes (WBCs) and how are they classified?

1. *Granulocytes:* polymorphonuclear leukocytes, eosinophils, basophils, and neutrophils
2. *Agranulocytes:* lymphocytes and monocytes or macrophages

▎ *Granulocytes (particularly neutrophils) are the body's first line of defense against microorganisms because of their phagocytic activity. The number of these cells in the circulation helps determine susceptibility to infection. The lower the granulocyte count, the higher the risk of infection.*

✎ What are the types of lymphocytes?

T lymphocytes: mature in the **t**hymus; responsible for cell-mediated immunity and immune response regulation
B lymphocytes: mature in **b**one marrow; responsible for antibody production and humoral immunity

Humoral immunity

✎ **What's an antibody?**

A protein (immunoglobulin) produced by B lymphocytes that reacts with a specific antigen, usually targeting it for an immune response

✎ **What's an antigen?**

A molecule against which an immune response is raised

✎ **What's the function of humoral immunity?**

Fighting extracellular viruses and bacteria as well as respiratory and GI pathogens

⚑ *Humoral immunity can produce immediate and delayed responses.*

✎ **What are the types of immunoglobulins (Ig)?**

Placenta

1. *IgG:* secondary antibody response caused by subsequent exposure to the same antigen; binds the active protein in the serum to an antigen-antibody complex (fixes complement) to destroy bacteria by creating holes in them and rid the body of antigen-antibody complexes by producing an inflammatory response; only immunoglobulin that crosses the placenta and provides the neonate with passive acquired immunity for 3 months or more
2. *IgM:* primary antibody response because it's the first antibody produced following exposure to an antigen; responsible for antibody production to ABO blood antigens
3. *IgA:* lines mucous membranes; found in body secretions (saliva, tears, breast milk)
4. *IgE:* responsible for allergic response; fixes to mast cells and basophils; offers some protection against parasitic infections
5. *IgD:* functions as an antigen receptor for B lymphocytes and participates in their differentiation

Why is a secondary antibody response faster and stronger than a primary antibody response?

Memory cells are produced after the first exposure, which remain in circulation and cause a more rapid production of antibodies on subsequent exposures.

Cell-mediated immunity

✎ **What cell types are involved in cell-mediated immunity?**

1. *T lymphocytes:* regulate the immune response, usually via the production of cytokines or other proteins; produce some anticellular proteins

2. *Macrophages:* ingest bacteria, which breaks down their proteins (antigens) which are then displayed on the macrophage surface to mark them for destruction by T-cells; regulate immune response via the production of cytokines

3. *Natural killer (NK) cells:* involved in nonspecific killing of virus-containing cells and transplanted grafts; seek out cancerous cells and destroy them; doesn't need to have been exposed to the same or similar antigens in order to respond

◥ *Cell-mediated immunity results in a delayed response.*

What's the difference between a monocyte and a macrophage?

A monocyte is a cell of the immune system that circulates in the bloodstream. A monocyte becomes a macrophage after it has entered an organ or tissue and becomes differentiated. Both play a role in phagocytosis.

✎ How are T cells classified?

1. *T-cytotoxic:* killer cell
2. *T-helper (CD4⁺):* stimulate or enhance the immune response by secreting interleukins, which promote the proliferation and maturation of B cells
3. *T-suppressor (CD8⁺):* control the immune response and prevent overactivity of the immune system

✎ What are cytokines?

Soluble factors secreted primarily by T cells, B cells, and monocytes or macrophages that act as messengers between cell types; cytokines can be classified as lymphokines (secreted from lymphocytes) or monokines (secreted from monocytes or macrophages)

What function does cell-mediated immunity serve?

Fighting intracellular viruses and fungi, chronic infectious agents, and cancer cells

What mediators are involved in cellular immunity?

1. *Interleukins, tumor necrosis factor (TNF), lymphotoxin:* major regulators of the immune response
2. *Interferons:* stimulates activity of macrophages, lymphocytes, and NK cells; antiviral action
3. *Colony-stimulating factors (granulocyte, granulocyte-macrophage):* attract and activate leukocytes; regulate growth and differentiation of hematopoietic cells
4. *Lymphocyte-derived chemotactic factor:* recruits macrophages and neutrophils to the area of an antigen
5. *Macrophage-activating and inhibiting factors:* increase tumoricidal and antimicrobial effects of macrophages; inhibit macrophage migration
6. *Chemokines:* attract WBCs to areas of inflammation or infection

Processes

What's phagocytosis?

Ingestion and destruction of microbes or particles by cells (usually macrophages and neutrophils)

✎ What are the steps involved in the process of phagocytosis?

1. *Chemotaxis:* movement of WBCs (macrophages) toward an attractor
2. *Opsonization:* modification of microbes (antibodies coat the surface) by the host to enhance macrophage binding
3. *Ingestion:* extension of macrophage cell membranes around the opsonized microbe to engulf it within a vacuole (phagosome)
4. *Digestion:* digestion of microbe by phagosomes, which then bind with liposomes to form phagolysosomes that release microbe-destroying enzymes
5. *Release:* release of digestive debris by the macrophage

Fundamentals of microbiology and infections

Classifications of microorganisms

How are microorganisms classified?

Bacteria, viruses, fungi, protozoa, helminths

▶ *Microorganisms can behave as nonpathogens, pathogens, or opportunists depending on the condition of the host environment.*

How can bacteria be classified?

Bacteria may be classified in many ways, including by shape (cocci, rods, spirals), morphology, chemical reactions, and response to various staining techniques (gram-positive or gram-negative).

What's a pathogen?

Any microorganism that can cause disease

✎ What's an infection?

The entry and replication of an infectious agent in host tissues; may be subclinical (no obvious symptoms, although an immune response *is* initiated) or clinical (symptoms develop as a result of an immune response)

✎ How are infections classified?

1. *Nosocomial or health care associated:* acquired as a result of contact with a health care facility; mostly bacterial; urinary tract infections and pneumonia are the most prevalent
2. *Community-acquired:* acquired before contact with a health care facility
3. *Idiopathic:* acquired from an unknown source

✎ **What's an opportunistic infection?**

One that results from the introduction of a potential pathogen into an immunocompromised individual that wouldn't typically cause an infection in an immunocompetent host

Antibiotic resistance

What's an antibiotic-resistant bacterium?

One that has undergone genetic alterations (changes in cell wall and cell wall proteins; changes in enzyme secretion) that allow it to evade the effects of specific antibiotics and continue to replicate, causing more harm to the host

How does a patient develop a drug resistant infection?

1. Contracting a resistant microbe from another patient, commonly through contact with persons in the health care system
2. The resistant microbe emerges in the body after antibiotic treatment has begun

What are some common causes of antibiotic resistance?

Overuse of antibiotics (routine prophylaxis over long duration of treatment), incomplete or ineffective treatment of bacterial infections (noncompliance, subtherapeutic levels), and misuse of antibiotics (for viral infections)

What are important measures that can be taken to reduce the incidence of antibiotic resistance?

1. Use antibiotics only when necessary.
2. Use the narrowest spectrum antibiotic to which bacteria are susceptible.
3. Take antibiotics at the prescribed dosage and until the medication is finished. Many patients stop taking antibiotics when the clinical condition improves, even though the infection hasn't completely resolved.
4. Adhere to infection-control guidelines.
5. Use symptomatic care for viral infections and avoid use of antibiotics for viral conditions, unless a secondary bacterial infection is diagnosed.
6. Encourage vaccinations.
7. Avoid taking antibiotics prescribed for someone else or those that were prescribed for another illness.

What are the three most common antibiotic-resistant bacteria?

1. *Methicillin resistant* Staphylococcus aureus *(MRSA):* currently treated with vancomycin or linezolid (Zyvox)
2. *Vancomycin resistant enterococci (VRE):* Zyvox or a combination antibiotic such as quinupristin and dalfopristin (Synercid) may be useful
3. *Multi-drug resistant* Pseudomonas aeruginosa

What's the difference between colonization and infection?

Colonization indicates the presence and growth of a microorganism, although no tissue invasion or damage occurs. Infection is the presence and growth of a microorganism as well as the invasion or destruction of tissues with possible clinical manifestations.

Which patients are at the highest risk for VRE and MRSA colonization?

1. Immunocompromised patients such as those with human immunodeficiency virus (HIV) or burns and organ transplant recipients
2. Patients in the intensive care unit
3. Patients who are admitted to the hospital from a long-term care facility
4. Patients who have previously been treated with antimicrobials
5. Surgical patients

▎ *Patients on isolation precautions should have equipment, such as thermometers, stethoscopes, and blood pressure cuffs, dedicated for their exclusive use, or the equipment must be disinfected according to facility policy between patients.*

Isolation precautions

✎ What are standard precautions?

Safety measures that emphasize consistent use of blood and body fluid precautions for all patients because the infectious potential for blood and body fluid isn't always known. Barrier protection should be used routinely to prevent skin and mucous membrane exposure to blood and body fluids. Standard precautions were previously known as *universal precautions.*

✎ What's the single most important measure in reducing the risks of transmitting organisms from one patient to another or from one site to another on the same patient?

Hand hygiene, performed either through use of alcoholic hand gels or by washing with soap and water

What types of personal protective equipment should be utilized to provide barrier protection?

A mask, goggles, face shields, gloves, and gowns, as appropriate for the task or situation

How should soiled linen be handled?	Linen soiled with blood, body fluids, secretions, and excretions should be handled in a manner that prevents skin and mucous membrane exposure and contamination of clothing
What's the purpose of isolation precautions?	To prevent the transmission of pathogens

▰ *Standard precautions should be used in all situations. Additional transmission-based precautions are implemented as appropriate.*

▰ *Patients with the same infection or disease may share a room when private rooms aren't available.*

Needlestick and sharps injury precautions

What are the infection rates for hepatitis B (HBV), hepatitis C (HCV), and HIV from a needlestick?	1. *HBV:* 6% to 30% infection rate for needlestick with HBV-infected blood to a susceptible (no HBV antibodies; nonvaccinated) health care worker 2. *HCV:* 2% infection rate for needlestick with HCV-infected blood 3. *HIV:* 0.3% infection rate for needlestick with infected blood and delayed or absent antiretroviral therapy

▰ *Postexposure prophylaxis (PEP) for HIV-suspected needlestick should be initiated within 2 hours of exposure because it may reduce the risk of infection by as much as 80%.*

What's the typical PEP for the blood-borne pathogens in HBV, HCV, and HIV?	1. *HBV:* dose of HBV immune globulin, preferably within 2 days of exposure, and HBV vaccination series, if source blood is antigen-positive or unknown and health care worker isn't immune (no antibodies); follow-up blood tests generally at 3 and 6 months to monitor for seroconversion (becoming HBV-positive) 2. *HCV:* no prophylaxis currently available; follow-up blood tests at 3 and 6 months to monitor for seroconversion (becoming HCV-positive) 3. *HIV:* lamivudine and zidovudine (Combivir), lamivudine (Epivir), indinavir (Crixivan); follow-up blood tests at 3 and 6 months to monitor for seroconversion (becoming HIV-positive)
What are appropriate actions if a needlestick or sharps injury occurs?	1. Wash needlestick site and any cuts with soap and water. Splashes to the nose, mouth, or skin should be flushed with water and eye splashes should be irrigated with water or saline. 2. Notify your supervisor and occupational health immediately to evaluate need for postexposure prophylaxis.

3. Complete an incident or injury report.
4. With the patient's permission, test source individual's blood for blood-borne infection with HIV, HBV, and HCV. If permission is denied by source individual, follow the procedure outlined by local or state laws and regulations.
5. Undergo follow-up blood tests at 6 weeks, 3 months, and 6 months following exposure.

✎ **How can needle-sticks and sharps injuries be prevented?**

1. Avoid unnecessary use of needles and other sharps when other devices are available.
2. Use sharps devices with safety features provided by the hospital.
3. Activate safety mechanisms as soon as possible after use.
4. Avoid recapping needles.
5. Promptly dispose of used needles in puncture-resistant sharps containers.

Types of immunity

✎ **What types of immunity exist?**

1. *Active natural:* contact with antigen through clinical or subclinical case (chickenpox)
2. *Active acquired:* immunization with antigen (live or killed vaccines)
3. *Passive natural:* transfer of immunoglobulins from a mother to a child via placenta or breast-feeding
4. *Passive acquired:* injection of serum from immune human or animal

Immunizations

What's an immunization?

Vaccines — containing either a live but weakened virus or an inactivated bacteria, virus, or toxoid — cause the body to produce antibodies that, along with memory B cells that produce them, remain in the body preventing further illness.

What are the four types of vaccines?

1. *Attenuated (weakened) live virus vaccines:* measles, mumps, and rubella (MMR); yellow fever; oral polio vaccine (OPV)
2. *Killed (inactivated) viruses or bacteria:* inactivated polio vaccine (IPV), influenza, cholera, hepatitis A (HAV), plague

3. *Toxoid:* contain a toxoid produced by the bacterium, such as tetanus diphtheria (Td)
4. *Biosynthetic vaccines: Haemophilus influenzae*

What's the primary concern with administration of a live, attenuated vaccine?

A remote possibility exists that the organism may revert to a virulent form and cause disease, particularly in immunocompromised persons or pregnant women.

At what age are most of the childhood vaccines given?

Most vaccines should be complete by age 18 months.

At what age are booster vaccines given?

1. *Varicella and HBV:* before age 24 months
2. *Diptheria and tetanus toxoids and acellular pertussis (DtaP), polio, and MMR:* between ages 4 and 6
3. *Td:* between ages 11 and 16

What's the vaccine for poliomyelitis?

IPV: a killed vaccine administered by injection; currently the recommended form of polio vaccine in the United States

⚡ *Live vaccines shouldn't be administered to immunocompromised persons or pregnant women. Women receiving live vaccines should be advised to defer pregnancy for 3 months.*

✎ What symptoms should be reported to a physician after a child has received an immunization?

1. High fever (103° F [39.4° C] or above)
2. Constant crying; inconsolable
3. Listless behavior
4. Severe swelling or redness at the injection site

What three immunizations are recommended for those older than age 65?

1. *Influenza vaccine:* given yearly
2. *Pneumococcal vaccine:* typically given once, but may be repeated every 5 to 10 years
3. *Tetanus booster:* given every 10 years, or at time of exposure if last tetanus shot was more than 5 years before

✎ Why should the flu shot be repeated every year?

Because the vaccine changes every year, depending on the type of virus that's predicted to cause the most influenza cases that year

How long does the protection from the flu shot last?

Approximately 6 months

When is the best time of year to receive the flu shot?	October or November is the best time to receive the flu shot, although the influenza vaccine may be given throughout the influenza season. Antibodies from the flu shot may take up to 2 weeks to develop; flu season generally runs from December to April.
What vaccines should be given to a patient before an elective splenectomy or following emergent splenectomy?	*Haemophilus influenzae* type B vaccine, pneumococcal vaccine, and meningococcal vaccine
✎ **Why is the varicella (chickenpox) vaccine also recommended for adults who haven't had the disease?**	It helps prevent chickenpox, which is associated with more severe disease in adults, and shingles.
What routes are most commonly used to administer vaccines?	Oral, intradermal, I.M., and subcutaneous (S.C.)

Common clinical manifestations of infections

FEVER

What's the body's systemic response to an infection?	Fever (pyrexia), or a rise in body temperature caused by the upward displacement of the hypothalamic set point for temperature control; fever is produced in response to a pyrogen (viruses, bacteria, inflammatory products, antibody complexes, and some drugs) and signals the presence of an inflammatory stimulus such as an infection
	It may also enhance the function of the immune system by increasing motility and activity of WBCs as well as stimulate the production of interferon and T cell activation. Fever may also inhibit the growth of some microbial agents that grow best at normal body temperatures.
✎ **What are the potential complications of a fever?**	1. *Fever greater than 104° F (40° C):* delirium, seizures
	2. *Fever greater than 106° F (41.1° C):* damage to the hypothalamic temperature control center, resulting in the inability to lower body temperature

✎ **What interventions can be used to lower a patient's body temperature?**

Antipyretic administration, hypothermia blanket, tepid bath, removal of excess clothing or bedding, fluids, environmental temperature adjustment, and ice packs

What diagnostic tests are used to evaluate the patient with a significant fever?

1. Cultures (blood, urine, vascular access, wound, sputum)
2. Chest X-ray
3. Lumbar puncture (if meningitis is suspected)
4. Additional tests, which may be performed based upon the patient's clinical presentation, history, and physical examination

LEUKOCYTOSIS

✎ **What's the significance of an increased WBC count?**

A high WBC count may indicate an inflammatory process, an infection, leukemia, or tissue damage.

What's a WBC differential?

A blood test that determines the percentage of each type of WBC in a sample; multiplying the percentage by the total count of WBCs indicates the actual number of each type in the sample

What's a left shift in the WBC count?

An increased percentage of neutrophils and bands (immature cells being released into circulation by the bone marrow in response to an infection); commonly indicative of a bacterial infection rather than an infection caused by other types of microbes

What blood tests may be performed for a patient with an infection?

Complete blood count (CBC), WBC differential, blood cultures, peripheral blood smear, erythrocyte sedimentation rate, and C-reactive protein (protein produced by the liver only in the presence of acute inflammation)

Physical assessment of the immune system

Normal findings

What are the most important questions to ask the patient during examination of the lymph nodes?

Are you aware of any lumps? How long have they been present?

What technique is used to examine the superficial lymph nodes?

Gentle palpation with a rotary motion using the pads of the index and middle fingers

✎ What characteristics of a lymph node should be assessed?

Size and shape, mobility, tenderness, warmth, consistency (soft, hard, or spongy), and border definition

How are a blood vessel and a lymph node differentiated on a physical examination?

A blood vessel exhibits a pulsation and a bruit when auscultated with a stethoscope, whereas a lymph node exhibits neither of these features.

In what areas of the body should lymph nodes be assessed?

1. *Head and neck region:* parotid, preauricular, mastoid, occipital, submandibular, submental, supraclavicular, superficial anterior cervical and superficial posterior cervical
2. *Axillary region:* subclavian, subscapular, central and lateral axillary nodes
3. *Epitrochlear region*
4. *Inguinal region:* superior and inferior superficial inguinal nodes
5. *Popliteal region*

In what positions should the patient be placed for optimal palpation of the lymph nodes?

1. *Sitting:* head, neck, axillary, and epitrochlear lymph nodes
2. *Lying in a supine position:* inguinal and popliteal lymph nodes, although popliteal nodes may also be palpated with the patient in a standing position

What accessory organs are involved in the immune process?

Tonsils, adenoids, thymus, appendix, and Peyer's patches (lymphoid tissue in the intestines)

What organ should be percussed and palpated during an examination of the lymph system?

Spleen; size estimated with percussion and enlargement and tenderness detected with palpation

What role does the spleen play in preventing infections?

The spleen is a source for antibody production and helps remove bacteria from the bloodstream through mononuclear phagocytic cells.

What type of sound is associated with percussion of a normal spleen?

Tympanic dullness on inspiration would indicate enlargement

What are important considerations for palpation of the spleen?

1. Apply gentle pressure to avoid rupturing an enlarged spleen.
2. Palpate with fingers below the left costal margin so the lower edge of an enlarged spleen isn't missed.

▧ *The spleen isn't usually palpable in adults. In fact, it must be enlarged to nearly three times its normal size to be palpated.*

Abnormal findings

◥ What's lymphadenopathy?

Enlargement of a lymph node, which suggests a current or recent inflammatory process; tenderness is associated with lymphadenopathy and may indicate an infectious process

What are important assessment factors during visual inspection of the lymph nodes?

Edema, erythema, and red streaking

How does lymphadenopathy differ in acute and chronic conditions?

Acute infections usually cause large, discrete, tender nodes, whereas chronic infections typically cause the lymph nodes to run together (become confluent).

What's the next appropriate step if an enlarged lymph node is detected?

Examine the adjacent area drained by the enlarged node for signs of infection or malignancy.

◥ What might red-streaked skin located over a lymph node indicate?

Acute lymphadenitis

What might unilateral lymphadenopathy that's nontender, hard, and immobile indicate?

Cancer metastasis

What might nontender splenomegaly indicate?

An immune disorder or liver disease

What might a tender, enlarged spleen indicate?

An infectious process

Major disorders of the immune system

Hypersensitivity reactions

✎ What are the four types of hypersensitivity reactions?

1. *Type I (anaphylactoid):* immediate (humoral) response that involves the IgE antibody predominantly; for example, allergic rhinitis and asthma
2. *Type II (cytotoxic and cytolytic):* immediate (humoral) response that involves direct binding of IgM, IgG, or IgA to an antigen on the cell surface leading to tissue destruction; for example, blood transfusion (hemolytic) reactions
3. *Type III (immune-complex):* immediate (humoral) response that involves large antigen-antibody complexes, which become lodged in small blood vessels or tissues, resulting in inflammation and phagocytosis of the affected tissue; for example, Arthus reactions and serum sickness
4. *Type IV (delayed hypersensitivity):* cell-mediated response; macrophages (attracted by lymphokines from T lymphocytes) and their enzymes cause tissue destruction; contact dermatitis and organ transplant rejection are examples

Allergies and atopic reactions

What's an allergy?

The immune system's hypersensitive response to an environmental allergen (antigen) that may manifest as a rash, hives, sneezing, and red, itchy eyes

What's the pathophysiologic process of an allergy?

Exposure to an allergen for which sensitization has occurred results in the release of chemical mediators that produce tissue damage.

What chemical mediators may be involved in an allergic reaction?

1. *Histamine:* increased vascular permeability; smooth-muscle constriction
2. *Leukotrienes:* increased vascular permeability; bronchial smooth-muscle constriction
3. *Prostaglandins:* vasodilation; smooth-muscle constriction
4. *Kinins:* increased vascular permeability; slow, sustained smooth-muscle constriction; mucus secretion; pain
5. *Platelet-activating factor:* platelet aggregation; vasodilation

6. *Serotonin:* increased vascular permeability; contraction of smooth muscles
7. *Eosinophil chemotactic factor:* influx of eosinophils
8. *Anaphylatoxins:* histamine release

What are some of the clinical manifestations of allergies?

Rhinitis, tearing, allergic shiners (dark circles under eyes), sneezing, boggy mucous membranes, urticaria, rash, wheezing, and stridor

What complications are associated with allergies?

Anaphylaxis, involving respiratory distress and hypovolemic shock

What's a skin test?

A test used to confirm sensitivity to a specific allergen that involves either a scratch or prick method to introduce an allergen extract to the skin

⚡ *Anaphylaxis is possible in highly sensitized patients following a skin test. Resuscitative equipment and epinephrine must be readily available.*

What's the typical treatment for chronic allergies?

1. Avoidance of allergen
2. Antihistamines, such as diphenhydramine (Benadryl), which also has antipruritic activity
3. Antipruritics, such as calamine lotion, coal tar solutions, and methdilazine (Tacaryl)
4. Bronchodilators such as theophylline (Accurbron)
5. Sympathomimetics such as epinephrine for severe reactions

What are important nursing actions in the care of a patient with allergies?

1. Educate the patient about avoiding known allergens.
2. Administer allergy medications as ordered by the physician.
3. Monitor for signs of respiratory distress and anaphylactic shock after exposure to allergen.
4. Educate the patient about proper use of allergy medications.

Autoimmune disorders

What's autoimmunity?

A state in which the immune system can't differentiate between self and nonself, causing an immune response to self-antigens

What's the patho-physiologic process involved in the development of an autoimmune disorder?	Although the cause is unknown, B cells, T cells, or both become activated to produce autoantibodies and auto-sensitized T cells, which damage specific tissues.
What are examples of autoimmune disorders?	1. *Systemic lupus erythematosus, scleroderma, and rheumatoid arthritis:* affecting connective tissues and joints 2. *Multiple sclerosis:* affecting nervous system 3. *Myasthenia gravis:* affecting muscles and thymus cells 4. *Addison's disease:* affecting adrenal glands 5. *Thyroiditis and hypothyroidism:* affecting the thyroid gland 6. *Type 1 diabetes:* affecting pancreatic islet cells 7. *Inflammatory bowel disease:* affecting GI tract 8. *Primary biliary cirrhosis:* affecting mitochondria in liver 9. *Goodpasture's syndrome:* affecting glomerular basement membrane of kidneys

> *The specific autoimmune disorder that's manifested depends on which self-antigen is recognized.*

How are autoimmune disorders typically treated?	1. *Immunosuppressants:* prednisone, azathioprine (Imuran), methotrexate (Folex), cyclosporine (Neorol), tacrolimus (Prograf), and mycophenolate (CellCept) 2. *Anti-tumor necrosis factor (TNF) antibodies:* agents, such as infliximab (Remicade) and etanercept (Enbrel) 3. *Plasmapheresis:* removal of circulating autoantibodies, antigen-antibody complexes, and inflammatory mediators
How does plasmapheresis work?	Whole blood is removed and circulated through a cell separator. The plasma containing the antibodies is discarded, while the platelets, red blood cells (RBCs), and WBCs are returned to the patient. Plasmapheresis enables plasma, platelets, RBCs, and WBCs to be selectively separated.
What adverse reactions are commonly associated with plasmapheresis?	Hypotension and citrate toxicity
What are important nursing actions when providing care for a patient with an autoimmune disorder?	1. Administer medications as ordered by the physician. 2. Encourage the patient to take immunosuppressants exactly as directed.

Human immunodeficiency virus and acquired immunodeficiency syndrome

What's human immunodeficiency virus (HIV)?

A virus that gradually destroys the immune system

What's the pathophysiologic process in the contraction of HIV?

The virus enters the bloodstream and binds to CD4$^+$ antigens on the surfaces of T-helper (T4) lymphocytes. The virus can then enter (infect) the T4 cells where it can replicate. This replicative process eventually leads to the cell's death. In addition, antibodies are made against HIV, and because infected T4 cells display the viral protein on their surface, those T4 cells are lysed by activation of the complement system. These processes cause the low T4 counts and immunocompromised state in patients with active, replicating HIV.

🔑 **What are the risk factors for acquiring HIV?**

1. Having sexual intercourse with an infected partner
2. Sharing needles with someone who's infected
3. Being born to a mother who's infected or drinking the breast milk of an infected woman (Although, if the mother is receiving antiviral therapy for HIV, the risk to the breast-feeding infant is decreased.)
4. Receiving a blood transfusion, tissue, or organ for transplantation from an infected person

📑 *Although HIV has been detected in nearly all body fluids, only blood, semen, breast milk, and vaginal and cervical secretions have been proven to cause HIV infection.*

🔑 **What's acquired immunodeficiency syndrome (AIDS)?**

A condition in which an opportunistic infection occurs in an HIV-infected person; an HIV-positive person who hasn't had any serious infections can also have an AIDS diagnosis on the basis of low or decreasing CD4$^+$ counts

🔑 **What are the clinical manifestations of an HIV infection?**

Most HIV-positive persons are asymptomatic for 5 or more years after infection, but early clinical signs include those that resemble a flulike illness (fever, fatigue, myalgias, arthralgias, lymphadenopathy, sore throat). Other symptoms may include profuse night sweats, cyclical fevers, diarrhea, anorexia, and unexplained weight loss.

🔑 **What are the potential complications of an HIV infection?**

1. *Opportunistic infections:* Pneumocystis carinii pneumonia, tuberculosis, *Mycobacterium avium* complex, cytomegalovirus (CMV) infection usually affecting the eyes, and fungal infections such as esophageal candidiasis
2. *Malignancies:* Kaposi's sarcoma, skin cancer

What's CMV?

A herpes virus transmitted through direct contact with mucous membranes or via blood transfusion or tissue transplants; although it typically results in a benign, chronic infection in immunocompetent people, it may result in CMV-related retinitis, encephalitis, esophagitis, gastritis, or colitis in immunocompromised individuals; prophylaxis and treatment with antiviral agents, such as ganciclovir (Cytovene), valganciclovir (Valcyte), and foscarnet (Foscavir), may be used in susceptible individuals

What laboratory tests are commonly used to diagnose an HIV infection?

1. *Enzyme-linked immunosorbent assay (ELISA):* blood test used to screen for antibodies to HIV
2. *Western blot:* more specific than ELISA; used to confirm all positive ELISA tests
3. *Rapid HIV tests:* recently approved for HIV testing, with results available in less than 30 minutes; must be confirmed by standard testing measures before the final diagnosis of HIV infection is made

✎ How long after infection with HIV does the ELISA test become positive (seroconverts from negative to positive)?

Seroconversion typically occurs within 3 months of infection.

What laboratory tests are commonly ordered in the management of a patient with HIV infection?

1. $CD4^+$ (T4 or T-helper) counts every 3 to 6 months
2. HIV viral load by polymerase chain reaction (PCR) every 3 to 6 months and 1 month after a change in therapy (measures the amount of HIV ribonucleic acid (RNA) in the blood)
3. CBC to monitor for anemia, leukopenia, and thrombocytopenia

When is antiviral therapy typically initiated to treat an HIV infection?

When the $CD4^+$ count is less than 350/μl or when the viral load is greater than 55,000 copies/μl by PCR

✎ What categories of antiviral medications are used to treat HIV infection?

1. *Nucleoside/nucleotide reverse transcriptase inhibitors (NRTIs):* abacavir (Ziagen), zidovudine or AZT (Retrovir), stavudine (Zerit), tenofovir (Viread), lamivudine, and AZT plus lamivudine (Combivir)
2. *Nonnucleoside reverse transcriptase inhibitors (NNRTIs):* delavirdine (Rescriptor), efavirenz (Sustiva), and nevirapine (Viramune)
3. *Protease inhibitors:* nelfinavir (VIRACEPT), indinavir, ritonavir (Norvir), and saquinavir (Invirase, Fortovase)

What's HAART?

Highly Active Anti-Retroviral Therapy, a combination of drugs (usually two nucleoside analogues and a protease inhibitor) used in the treatment of HIV infections

What are the benefits of HAART?

1. Suppression of viremia and virus shedding in semen and vaginal secretions
2. Increased CD4$^+$ T-cell counts
3. Prolonged survival
4. Clinical improvement, including fewer opportunistic infections or HIV-associated malignancies
5. Ability to discontinue prophylaxis for opportunistic infections and maintenance therapy

What are important nursing actions in the care of a patient who's HIV-positive?

1. Encourage consistent administration of antiviral agents, even if the patient is feeling well.
2. Promote good nutritional habits, including high-calorie, high-protein foods.
3. Monitor for development of opportunistic infections.
4. Monitor blood test results (CBC, lymphocyte counts, viral load) for complications.
5. Encourage the patient to stop smoking and to avoid alcohol (depress immune system).
6. Educate the patient about the use of latex condoms for sexual contact (anal, oral, and vaginal) from start to finish, and discuss with him how to reveal his HIV status with current and past sexual partners.
7. Discuss the use of illicit drugs and the risk of spreading HIV through needle sharing.
8. Advise the patient not to share toothbrushes or razors.
9. Instruct the patient not to donate blood, tissue, organs, or semen.
10. With the patient's permission, educate his family about how HIV is and isn't transmitted.
11. Instruct the patient to prevent opportunistic infections with good hand hygiene, proper food handling, and avoiding exposure to persons who are obviously ill. If the patient has no history of chickenpox or shingles and is varicella antibody negative, advise him to avoid any person with these illnesses. In the event of exposure, prophylaxis with varicella zoster immune globulin (VZIG) should be administered within 96 hours.
12. Encourage stress reduction, sufficient rest, and attention to emotional and spiritual needs.
13. Assess for the presence of other sexually transmitted diseases (STDs), such as syphilis, gonorrhea, herpes, and chlamydia as well as HAV, HBV, and HCV.

◤ *Although HAV is transmitted by the fecal-oral route and isn't generally considered an STD, sexual transmission is possible in some populations such as homosexual men.*

Major infectious diseases

Influenza

What's influenza?
A contagious viral infection of the respiratory tract

What's the pathophysiologic process of influenza?
The influenza virus is transmitted by contact with droplets that are generated from an infected person's cough. The virus then enters the body, producing illness.

What are the common clinical manifestations of influenza?
Nonproductive cough, sneezing, sore throat, rhinitis (watery nasal discharge), malaise, myalgias, headache, fever, fatigue, and anorexia

✎ How do influenza and the common cold differ in their clinical presentation?
High fevers (102° to 104° F [38.9° to 40° C]) for several days, headaches, myalgias, and profound fatigue are more typical manifestations of the flu. Rhinitis, sneezing, and a sore throat are more typical manifestations of the common cold. Chest discomfort and a cough typically accompany the flu and the common cold.

What complications are associated with influenza?
Bacterial or viral pneumonia, tracheobronchitis, and death

◤ *Death from influenza can be reduced through yearly vaccinations, particularly for people over age 65, health care workers, and those with a chronic disease process.*

✎ What's the typical treatment for a patient with influenza?
1. Hydration (oral or I.V.)
2. Symptomatic treatment (antipyretics, antihistamines, decongestants)
3. Antivirals (amantadine, rimantadine, oseltamivir); only useful if administered within the first 36 hours of symptom development or within 48 hours of exposure

◤ *Antibiotics should not be used to treat influenza unless a secondary bacterial infection has been diagnosed.*

What are important nursing actions in the care of a patient with influenza?
1. Encourage increased fluid intake.
2. Administer medications (antipyretics, antihistamines, decongestants) as ordered by the physician.

3. Assess vital signs and respiratory status every 4 hours or as directed by the physician. Humidify air when appropriate.
4. Monitor intake and output.
5. Encourage bed rest and decreased physical activity. Instruct the patient to refrain from aerobic exercise during the flu, because of risk (low) of cardiac involvement.
6. Monitor for development of complications (respiratory distress, pneumonia).
7. Encourage annual influenza vaccination.

Mononucleosis

What's mono-nucleosis?

A self-limiting viral infection characterized by fever, lymphadenopathy, and lymphocytosis. Epstein-Barr virus (EBV) and CMV can cause mononucleosis.

What's the patho-physiologic process of mononucleosis?

EBV and CMV are found in secretions from mucous membranes of the mouth, respiratory tract, and GI tract. These viruses are usually passed through kissing, although they may rarely be passed in other ways, such as coughing and hand contact.

✎ What are the common clinical manifestations of mononucleosis?

Profound fatigue, fever, sore throat, tender cervical lymphadenopathy (neck), headaches, anorexia, white patches on the back of the throat, and splenomegaly

What are the potential complications of mononucleosis?

Pneumonia, neurologic changes, thrombocytopenia, hemolytic anemia, splenic rupture, and cardiac involvement, as well as the possible development of chronic fatigue syndrome

Patients with mononucleosis should avoid contact sports because of the risk of splenic rupture.

What are the most useful diagnostic studies?

1. CBC with differential: leukocytosis (WBC greater than 20,000/µl) with increased lymphocytes (particularly atypical lymphocytes) and monocytes
2. Monospot test

What are important nursing considerations in the care of a patient with mononucleosis?

1. Encourage rest and avoidance of contact sports.
2. Encourage increased fluid intake and good nutritional intake.
3. Monitor intake and output.
4. Provide salt-water gargles, throat lozenges, hard candy, or flavored frozen desserts such as popsicles for sore throat.

5. Administer medications (antipyretics, analgesics) as ordered by the physician.
6. Inform the patient that it may take several weeks to recuperate enough to return to his previous activity level.

Infection from a bite

How are bites categorized?

Human or animal; human bites are more serious than animal bites because of the presence of multiple aerobic and anaerobic bacterial species

⚡ *Cat bites more commonly result in infections than dog bites.*

What's the pathophysiologic process of a bite?

Bites of any nature may introduce bacteria into deep tissues through puncture wounds or lacerations, causing an infection

What are the clinical manifestations of a bite?

Symptoms vary greatly, but crushing-type wounds can result from humans or large animals, resulting in damage to deep structures, including nerves, muscles, tendons, blood vessels, and bones. Small animals typically produce puncture wounds and lacerations of the skin.

What complications are associated with bites?

Infections, such as cellulitis, septic arthritis, tetanus, and rabies

How are bites typically treated?

1. Copious irrigation with saline
2. Antibiotics for high-risk wounds (deep puncture wounds or a patient with history of diabetes, prosthetic heart valves, or immunocompromised state), preceded by wound cultures and Gram stains
3. No suturing, to allow for drainage of infectious material

What are important nursing actions in the care of a patient with a bite?

1. Irrigate fresh bites with large amounts of saline.
2. Elevate the affected extremity.
3. Obtain wound cultures if indicated.
4. Administer antibiotics as ordered by physician.
5. Determine the date of last tetanus booster; if more than 5 years, revaccinate.
6. Instruct the patient to report fever, foul-smelling wound drainage, or increased pain to physician immediately.

Rabies

What's rabies?

An infection capable of producing respiratory paralysis that results from the introduction of the rabies virus into a bite or other open wound of a mammal

What's the pathophysiologic process of rabies?

The rabies virus travels from the site of entry by peripheral nerves to the spinal cord and brain where it multiplies. The virus then continues to travel through nerves to the salivary glands and into saliva. The disease progresses to paresis or paralysis and ultimately, death, usually due to respiratory paralysis.

What are the common clinical manifestations of rabies?

Mental depression, malaise, fever, restlessness that progresses to uncontrollable excitement, excessive salivation, severe spasm of the laryngeal and pharyngeal muscles, delirium, and seizures

What complications are associated with rabies?

Respiratory paralysis and death

What's the typical treatment for rabies?

1. Thorough washing of the wound with soap and water
2. Postexposure prophylaxis (one dose of immune globulin and five doses of rabies vaccine directly into the wound over 28-day period) for unknown animal or suspected rabid animal
3. No treatment after symptoms of the disease appear

What are important nursing actions in the care of a patient with rabies?

1. Wash the wound with soap and water.
2. Administer immune globulin and rabies vaccine as ordered by the physician.
3. Monitor for complications (respiratory distress and seizures) and notify the physician immediately if they develop.

Tetanus (lockjaw)

What's tetanus?

An acute infection affecting spinal and cranial nerves that's caused by a neurotoxin produced by *Clostridium tetani;* spores may be found in soil, animal feces, or dust and are introduced into the body through a wound; wounds more than 1 cm deep and crush injuries are most prone to tetanus

What's the patho-physiologic process of tetanus?	The endotoxin (tetanospasmin) enters the central nervous system (CNS) where it interferes with neurotransmitter release and causes tonic rigidity
What clinical manifestations are associated with tetanus?	1. Excessive yawning due to prickly sensation in jaw muscles, which eventually causes stiffening of the jaw muscles (lockjaw) 2. Progressive stiffening of the neck, back, and extremity muscles 3. Dysphagia 4. Laryngeal and respiratory spasms 5. Rigidity of abdominal muscles 6. Diaphoresis and fever 7. Generalized tonic spasms
What complications are associated with tetanus?	Anoxia from respiratory involvement, asphyxial seizures, hemorrhage of striated muscles, vertebral fractures, and brain damage
What's the treatment for tetanus?	Tetanus immune globulin (TIG) or antitoxin may be given. However, they're only effective at neutralizing circulating toxins before the onset of neurologic symptoms. Antibiotics for infection, sedatives to control spasms, and analgesics for pain control may also be provided. ◥ *Anaphylaxis is possible if the antitoxin treatment is of animal origin.*
What are the important nursing actions in the care of a patient with tetanus?	1. Maintain a calm, quiet environment. Subtle noises, bright lights, and jarring motions may trigger a seizure. 2. Administer medications (TIG, antibiotics, sedatives, analgesics) as ordered by the physician. 3. Administer tetanus toxoid booster after the patient's condition has stabilized if last booster was given 5 or more years before. 4. Monitor for complications and anticipate the need for mechanical ventilation.

Lyme disease

What's Lyme disease?	A spirochetal infection that's spread by a bite from an infected deer tick; peak incidence occurs during summer months
What's the patho-physiologic process of Lyme disease?	Immature deer ticks feed on small mammals that are infected with the bacterium *Borrelia burgdorferi*. In later stages, these ticks transmit the Lyme disease bacterium to humans.

✎ **What are the common clinical manifestations of Lyme disease?**

"Bull's-eye" rash or lesion (alternating light and dark rings with a pale center; known as erythema migrans) and flulike symptoms, including headache, sore throat, stiff neck, fever, migratory arthralgias, fatigue, and general malaise

What complications are associated with untreated Lyme disease?

Arthritis, neurologic symptoms (facial palsy, seizures), and cardiac damage

What's the typical treatment for Lyme disease?

Antibiotic treatment for 3 to 4 weeks, usually doxycycline or tetracycline

What are important nursing actions in the prevention of Lyme disease?

1. Instruct the patient to wear long pants tucked into boots or socks and light-colored clothing (to detect ticks more easily). Check for ticks periodically, but especially after coming in from outdoors.
2. Educate the patient about the use of insect repellant containing DEET, particularly on lower extremities.
3. Instruct the patient to avoid walking through tall grass or low brush.
4. Educate the patient about the use of tick collars for pets.
5. Instruct the patient to remove any ticks, wash the bite area with soap and water, and apply an antibiotic ointment. The patient should notify a physician if a bull's-eye rash develops within 1 month of tick removal.

Toxoplasmosis

What's toxoplasmosis?

Toxoplasmosis is a parasitic infection that results from ingestion of *Toxoplasma gondii* eggs on contaminated surfaces, most commonly soil and cat feces. Most persons who acquire toxoplasmosis don't become ill. However, immunocompromised persons (patients with HIV/AIDS, and chemotherapy or organ transplant recipients) are at increased risk for infection and may develop severe illness.

What's the pathophysiologic process of toxoplasmosis?

The eggs (oocysts) of the parasite *T. gondii* live only in cats' intestines. The eggs are excreted by cats and then undergo a 1- to 3-week period of development in soil. During development, the eggs become infectious and ultimately make their way into the food chain.

What are the common clinical manifestations of toxoplasmosis?

Flulike symptoms (fever, headache, myalgias, lymphadenopathy), confusion, headache, disorientation, personality changes, tremors, and seizures

| **What complications are associated with toxoplasmosis?** | Encephalitis, coma, death, eye or brain damage with severe illness (especially in immunocompromised people), and mental retardation or physical disabilities for unborn babies whose mothers were first exposed to the parasite shortly before or during pregnancy (although most exposed infants don't develop symptoms) |

| **What's the typical treatment for toxoplasmosis?** | No treatment is necessary for an otherwise healthy (immunocompetent), nonpregnant individual. Treatment for immunocompromised or pregnant persons should be coordinated by the appropriate specialists. |

What are the important nursing actions when caring for a patient who's at risk for toxoplasmosis?

1. Instruct the patient to wear gloves when handling soil, changing litter boxes, or handling raw meats.
2. Instruct the patient to wash his hands with soap and water after handling soil or emptying cat litter boxes, especially before eating or preparing foods.
3. Encourage the patient to keep cats indoors and use only dry or canned foods to prevent cats from becoming infected.
4. Instruct the patient to eat only thoroughly cooked meats.

Clostridial myonecrosis (gas gangrene)

| **What's myonecrosis?** | A severe type of gangrene (tissue necrosis) that results from toxins produced by *Clostridium perfringens* |

| **What's the pathophysiologic process of myonecrosis?** | Clostridial cellulitis occurs as a localized infection in a superficial or surgical wound, particularly in a patient with occlusive vascular disease. Myositis progresses to myonecrosis (gas gangrene). |

| **What are the common clinical manifestations of myonecrosis?** | Bullae at wound site; foul-smelling, serous brown exudates; bubbling of gas; subcutaneous emphysema (air under skin); crepitations under the skin (gas bubbles in tissues); edema; and pain |

| **What complications are associated with myonecrosis?** | Secondary infections, loss of a limb, systemic toxemia, and death |

What's the treatment for myonecrosis?

1. Drainage and debridement of the wound
2. Early use of broad-spectrum antibiotics to treat secondary infections
3. Hyperbaric oxygen
4. Analgesics

What are important nursing actions in the care of a patient with myonecrosis?	1. Provide meticulous wound care as ordered by the physician. 2. Obtain wound cultures for anaerobic and aerobic pathogens. 3. Administer antibiotics and analgesics as ordered by the physician.

West Nile virus

What's West Nile virus?	West Nile virus is an infection with an arbovirus transmitted from certain types of mosquitoes (Northern house mosquitoes, primarily) that get the virus from feeding on infected birds. Most persons are asymptomatic or develop a flulike illness; however, those who are immunocompromised may develop a more severe febrile illness, encephalitis, or death.
How is West Nile virus transmitted?	By infected mosquitoes ⚡ *West Nile virus isn't transmitted from person to person.*
What groups are at increased risk if they become infected with West Nile virus?	Elderly people and those who are immunocompromised are at risk for fatal infections. Children are *not* at an increased risk.
What's the typical treatment for West Nile virus?	Supportive care including adequate hydration
What preventive actions can be taken?	1. Apply mosquito repellent to exposed skin when outdoors. 2. Minimize time outdoors, particularly during the early evening. 3. Wear long pants and long sleeve shirts when outdoors. 4. Reduce mosquito-breeding sites by eliminating standing water, particularly if it contains decaying organic matter (leaves, animal wastes). 5. Spray insecticides to kill larvae and adult mosquitoes. ⚡ *Preventive measures should be continued until two hard frosts occur.*
What are important nursing actions in the care of a patient with West Nile virus?	1. Encourage bed rest or minimal exertion with adequate rest periods. 2. Encourage increased fluid intake. 3. Monitor for complications such as encephalitis.

4. Administer medications (antipyretics) as ordered by the physician.

Anthrax

What's anthrax?

Anthrax is an infection caused by the bacterium *Bacillus anthracis,* which can cause either cutaneous or pulmonary disease, and may result in sepsis or death. Persons who are most susceptible are those who come in contact with infected animals, animal hair or hides, and bone products.

What's the pathophysiologic process of anthrax?

B. anthracis is contracted primarily through direct inoculation through a break in the skin when contact is made with an infected animal. Toxins are produced, resulting in extensive tissue necrosis.

What clinical manifestations are associated with anthrax?

1. *Cutaneous* (95% of cases): itchy skin lesion that eventually blisters and breaks down, resulting in a painless, black ulceration with edema of surrounding skin
2. *Pulmonary* (inhalation): biphasic presentation with a brief period of improvement followed by rapid deterioration; initial presentation as a flulike illness with low-grade fever, malaise, myalgia, and headache; later manifestations of respiratory distress evidenced by dyspnea, stridor, and cyanosis without evidence of pneumonia

What's the typical treatment for anthrax?

Antibiotics (penicillin, ciprofloxacin, doxycycline) for 60 days (allows all spores time to germinate)

What are important nursing actions in the care of a patient with anthrax?

1. Administer medications (antibiotics, analgesics, antipyretics) as ordered by the physician.
2. Encourage bed rest and monitor for respiratory complications, such as dyspnea or stridor, with pulmonary anthrax.

Smallpox

What's smallpox?

Smallpox is a highly contagious viral disease caused by the variola virus, which is most commonly characterized by a pustular rash on the face, back, chest, and extremities. It's transmitted through respiratory droplets of an infected person as well as by direct contact with lesions. The smallpox rash is predominantly located on the face and extremities, and all lesions are in the same stage of development.

▧ *The rash associated with smallpox is distinct from the rash associated with chickenpox. The latter is primarily concentrated on the trunk and has lesions that appear in successive crops.*

What clinical manifestations are associated with smallpox?

High fever, malaise, severe headache, and a rash of small, red spots involving the tongue, mouth, face, and forearms that spreads to the trunk and lower extremities, becomes vesicular and pustular (occurs in mouth and pharynx first), and usually begins scabbing after 1 week

▧ *People with smallpox are most contagious for the first 7 to 10 days after rash develops and remain contagious until all scabs fall off (approximately 3 weeks).*

What potential complications are associated with smallpox?

Encephalitis and death (30% mortality); permanent scarring common in survivors

What's the typical treatment for smallpox?

1. Airborne and contact precautions until all scabs fall off
2. Supportive care, including hydration and antipyretics
3. Administration of the antiviral agent cidofovir (Vistide)

How can smallpox be prevented?

Vaccination

Infectious diseases of the GI system

Gastroenteritis

What's gastroenteritis?

Gastroenteritis is a typically self-limited condition (resolving on its own in several days) involving an infection or irritation of the digestive tract (frequently the stomach and intestines) caused by bacteria, a virus, or parasites contracted by ingesting contaminated food or water or, less commonly, fecal-oral transmission.

What's the pathophysiologic process of gastroenteritis?

Diarrhea results from the adherence of infectious agents by invasion of the intestinal mucosa or production of enterotoxins and cytotoxins.

What pathogens typically cause gastroenteritis?

Campylobacter, Escherichia coli, Shigella, Salmonella, Norwalk virus, adenoviruses, rotaviruses, and parasites

| **What are the common clinical manifestations of gastroenteritis?** | Watery or bloody diarrhea, nausea, vomiting, abdominal pain, fever, myalgias, and headache |

How is gastroenteritis treated?

1. *Bacterial:* hydration and antibiotics, depending on causative agent and severity of illness
2. *Viral:* hydration and symptomatic care
3. *Parasitic:* hydration and medication specific to the parasite

What are the potential complications?

Dehydration, electrolyte imbalances, and oliguria can result from profuse or persistent diarrhea, and organ failure and death can occur after infection with certain strains of *E. coli.* Persons who are very old or very young are at greatest risk for severe dehydration.

⚡ *Agents that suppress intestinal motility are not given for diarrhea that's associated with a high fever or has persisted for more than 48 hours because of concern for bacterial gastroenteritis. Antiperistaltic agents (loperamide, opiates) may increase the risk of intestinal pathogen colonization.*

What are the important nursing actions in the care of a patient with bacterial or viral gastroenteritis?

1. Monitor intake and output. Encourage increased fluid intake and administer I.V. fluids as ordered by physician to maintain adequate hydration. Oral rehydration solution may be indicated for infants or young children with severe or prolonged diarrhea.
2. Administer antibiotics as ordered by the physician.
3. Follow standard precautions during hospitalization.

Infectious diseases of the respiratory system

Legionellosis (legionnaires' disease)

What's legionellosis?

Legionellosis is a bacterial disease that may cause respiratory illness or pneumonia.

What's the pathophysiologic process of legionellosis?

Inhalation of *Legionella pneumophila* causes pathologic changes in the lung consistent with lobar pneumonia. This disease progresses rapidly within the first 4 to 6 days.

What clinical manifestations are associated with legionellosis?

High fever, malaise, myalgia, nonproductive cough, and patchy pulmonary infiltrate and consolidation on chest X-ray

| What complications are associated with legionellosis? | Respiratory failure and death |

| What's the typical treatment for legioncl-losis? | Antibiotics, most commonly erythromycin |

| What are the most important nursing actions in the care of a patient with legionellosis? | 1. Monitor respiratory status closely.
2. Implement measures to reduce hyperthermia.
3. Administer medications (antibiotics, antipyretics) as ordered by the physician.
4. Explain to the patient that legionellosis isn't communicable from person-to-person contact. |

Sexually transmitted diseases

| What are examples of diseases that can be transmitted sexually? | Gonorrhea, syphilis, chlamydia, trichomoniasis, genital herpes, genital warts (human papilloma virus), HBV, and HIV |

| What adverse outcomes can occur in a pregnant woman with a sexually transmitted disease (STD)? | Spontaneous abortion, low birth weight and prematurity, congenital or perinatal infections, pneumonia, eye infections, and permanent neurologic damage |

| ✎ What education should be given to a patient diagnosed with an STD? | 1. Get treatment to prevent transmission to others.
2. Notify all recent sex partners and urge them to be examined.
3. Complete the full course of medicine as prescribed.
4. Return to the facility for a follow-up examination to ensure the STD has resolved.
5. Avoid all sexual activity while being treated for the STD. |

| ✎ How can STDs be prevented? | Abstinence or participation in a mutually monogamous sexual relationship with an uninfected partner as well as correct and consistent use of a condom |

| ✎ What are important nursing actions in the care of a patient at risk for developing an STD? | 1. Encourage the use of a latex condom for oral, genital, or anal sex. Explain that condoms don't offer complete protection from STDs.
2. Tell the patient to notify the physician immediately if sores or unusual discharge develops. Abstain from all forms of sexual contact until evaluated by the physician, treated with appropriate antibiotics, and free from all syphilis or herpes lesions. |

3. Explain to the patient that urinating, douching, or washing the genitals following sexual intercourse doesn't protect against STDs.
4. Administer medications (antibiotics, antivirals) as ordered by the physician.
5. Encourage the patient to notify recent sexual partners so that proper testing is performed and treatment can be initiated, if indicated.
6. Notify the public health department in accordance with state policy.
7. Inform the patient that it's possible to get gonorrhea, syphilis, chlamydia, and trichomoniasis again if reexposed to an infected partner.

Gonorrhea

What's gonorrhea?

Gonorrhea is an STD caused by the bacterium *Neisseria gonorrhoeae* that may cause urethritis, cervicitis, epididymitis, pharyngitis, proctitis, and pelvic inflammatory disease (PID).

What's the patho-physiologic process of gonorrhea?

The bacterium is introduced into the columnar mucosal cells of the lower genital tract via sexual contact. Localized or disseminated disease may result.

✎ What are the clinical manifestations of gonorrhea?

1. *Women:* painful or burning sensation when urinating and yellow or bloody vaginal discharge
2. *Men:* pain and pus from the penis and a burning sensation during urination

What complications are associated with untreated gonorrhea in women?

PID, scar tissue in the fallopian tubes, which may eventually cause an ectopic pregnancy or infertility, and joint inflammation and pain

How is gonorrhea treated?

Antibiotic therapy, typically with cefixime (Suprax), ceftriaxone (Rocephin), cefotaxime (Claforan), ciprofloxacin (Cipro), levofloxacin (Levaquin), or ofloxacin (Floxin)

Syphilis

What's syphilis?

Syphilis is an STD caused by the bacterium *Treponema pallidum;* it's characterized by a primary lesion, a secondary eruption involving the skin and mucous membranes, a long latency period, and late disabling lesions of the skin, bone, viscera, central nervous system (CNS), and cardiovascular system.

What's the patho-physiologic process of syphilis?

The spiral-shaped bacterium (spirochete) burrows into the mucosal cells of the mouth or genitals, producing a chancre.

What's a chancre?

A small, round, firm, painless sore that develops during the primary stage of syphilis at the location where the syphilis-causing bacterium entered the body

✎ What are the four stages of syphilis?

1. *Primary:* appearance of the chancre 10 days to 3 months after exposure
2. *Secondary:* development of a skin rash with rough, reddish-brown spots on the palms of the hands and soles of the feet, which may clear on its own without treatment, although the individual still has syphilis
3. *Latent:* possibly years of latency in untreated syphilis during which time it's noncontagious and produces no symptoms but damages internal organs (CNS, cardiovascular system, liver, bones, and joints)
4. *Tertiary:* clinical evidence of degenerative lesions of the cardiovascular system, CNS, skin, and viscera

✎ At what stages can syphilis be transmitted to a sexual partner?

During the primary and secondary stages

⚡ *Because syphilis sores may be hidden in the mouth, vagina, or rectum, it isn't always obvious that a person has syphilis.*

What complications are associated with untreated syphilis?

Neurosyphilis (seizures, personality changes, psychosis, ataxia, or paresis), stillbirths or infected infants born to infected mothers (congenital syphilis), and death

What diagnostic tests are used to determine if a patient has syphilis?

1. *Microscopic examination:* examination of material from infectious sores for characteristic appearance, dark field examination, and direct fluorescent antibody test
2. *Blood and serum:* rapid plasma reagin, microhemagglutination-*T. pallidum*, *T. pallidum* particle agglutination, and fluorescent treponemal antibody absorption
3. *Cerebrospinal fluid (CSF):* Venereal Disease Research Laboratory (VDRL)-CSF

⚡ *Low amounts of antibodies may remain in the blood for years in a previously infected individual, even if adequate treatment was provided.*

How is syphilis treated?

Antibiotics, typically penicillin or tetracycline

Chlamydia

What's a chlamydial infection?	Chlamydia is an STD caused by the bacterium *Chlamydia trachomatis.* Genital chlamydial infection can occur during oral, vaginal, or anal sexual contact.
What's the pathophysiologic process of a chlamydial infection?	The bacterium *C. trachomatis* enters mucosal cells and can infect the vagina, cervix, anus, penis, and eyes.
✎ **What are the clinical manifestations of a chlamydial infection?**	Although the symptoms may be mild, mucus or pus from the vagina or penis as well as pain with urination typically develop 1 to 3 weeks following exposure or infection. Infected men may also be asymptomatic.
✎ **What are the long-term complications of untreated chlamydial infections?**	PID in women, epididymitis in men, and infertility in men and women
What's the typical treatment for a chlamydial infection?	Antibiotics, such as azithromycin, doxycycline, and erythromycin

Trichomoniasis

What's trichomoniasis?	Trichomoniasis is a parasitic infection spread through sexual activity. It affects women more commonly than men.
What's the pathophysiologic process of trichomoniasis?	The parasite is transmitted during sexual contact with an infected person. It has a whiplike tail that it uses to propel itself through the vaginal and urethral mucosa.
✎ **What are the clinical manifestations of trichomoniasis?**	1. *Women:* possibly asymptomatic; foul-smelling, green vaginal discharge; vaginal itching; painful sexual intercourse (dyspareunia); and urinary urgency 2. *Men:* usually asymptomatic; urethral discharge and urinary symptoms of urgency and burning
How is the diagnosis of trichomoniasis made?	Culture of the vaginal or penile secretions and microscopic examination of these secretions for visualization of the parasite
What complications are associated with untreated trichomoniasis?	Infection of infants during birth

What's the typical treatment for trichomoniasis?	Metronidazole (Flagyl) by mouth

Genital herpes

What's genital herpes?	Genital herpes is an STD caused by the herpes simplex virus (HSV) that manifests as blisters in the genital or anal areas. These lesions break open and form ulcerations that eventually crust over. HSV is characterized by a localized primary lesion, latency (resides in sensory ganglion), and a tendency for localized recurrence, although future outbreaks are typically less severe and tend to decrease in frequency over time.
What's the patho-physiologic process of genital herpes?	HSV enters the body and resides in the nerves at the base of the spine. When activated, the virus travels to the surface of the infected skin or mucous membranes where it replicates, producing open lesions.
✎ **What are the two types of HSV?**	1. *HSV-1:* usually affects oral, labial, or ocular skin; commonly causes sores (fever blisters) 2. *HSV-2:* most commonly causes genital herpes but can also infect the mouth during oral sex
✎ **What are the clinical manifestations of genital herpes?**	1. Possibly produces no symptoms or only mild symptoms, such as tingling and itching 2. Itching or burning sensation in the genital or anal area 3. Painful lesions or ulcerations that appear near the area of viral entry into the body, such as the mouth, anus, vagina, and penis 4. Lesions that become crusty then heal over 7 to 12 days without leaving a scar 5. Pain in the legs, buttocks, or genital area 6. Discharge of fluid from the vagina or penis
What complications are associated with an HSV infection?	Neuralgias, encephalitis, spontaneous abortion or congenital herpes infection in neonate (rare), cervical cancer, and hepatitis
✎ **Is it possible to spread genital herpes when an infected person is asymptomatic (no sores)?**	Yes; the virus can be shed from skin that isn't broken or open from a sore.
✎ **What factors may cause HSV reactivation?**	Emotional stress, immunosuppression, menstruation, and the presence of another infection

What's the typical treatment for genital herpes?	Although no cure for HSV is known, antiviral therapy, such as acyclovir (Zovirax), famciclovir (Famvir), and valacyclovir (Valtrex), may prevent future outbreaks or lessen the severity or duration of outbreaks. ◧ *Sexual contact should be avoided from the time the symptoms are first noticed (tingling, burning, itching, and ulcerations) until the sores are completely healed.*

Genital warts

What are genital warts?	Genital warts are an STD in which the human papilloma virus (HPV) produces single or clustered soft, cauliflower-like growths in the genital region (internally or externally). Genital warts may also be referred to as condylomata acuminate and are associated with cervical cancer.
What's the pathophysiologic process of genital warts?	Certain types of HPV can infect the genital tissue through sexual contact, resulting in the formation of fleshy growths (warts).
What are the clinical manifestations of genital warts?	Small, painless, flesh-colored bumps in the vaginal area, on the penis, or around the anus that may have a cauliflower-like appearance
✎ **What complications are associated with genital warts?**	Cervical and other genital cancers
How are genital warts typically treated?	Topical antiviral agents, cryotherapy (freezing), surgical removal, and laser therapy

Pharmacology related to the immune system

Systemic antibiotics

How do antibiotics work?	1. *Inhibition of bacterial cell-wall synthesis:* penicillins, monobactams, cephalosporins, carbapenems 2. *Inhibition of bacterial protein synthesis:* tetracyclines, aminoglycosides, macrolides, clindamycin, linezolid, chloramphenicol, quinupristin and dalfopristin 3. *Decrease in bacterial synthesis of folic acid:* sulfonamides 4. *Inhibition of bacterial deoxyribonucleic acid (DNA) synthesis:* quinolones and metronidazole

5. *Inhibition of bacterial cell-wall synthesis and disruption of RNA synthesis:* vancomycin
6. *Disruption of bacterial enzyme systems:* nitrofurantoin

What are examples of antibiotics?

1. *Penicillins:* penicillin G, penicillin V, amoxicillin, ampicillin, mezlocillin (Mezlin), nafcillin (Unipen), oxacillin (Bactocill), piperacillin and tazobactam (Zosyn), ticarcillin (Ticar)
2. *Monobactams:* aztreonam (Azactam)
3. *Tetracyclines:* tetracycline, doxycycline (Vibramycin), minocycline
4. *Sulfonamides:* co-trimoxazole (Bactrim, Septra, SMZ-TMP)
5. *Cephalosporins:* cefaclor (Ceclor), cefadroxil (Duricef), cephalexin (Keflex), cefazolin (Ancef, Kefzol), cefuroxime (Ceftin), cefoxitin (Mefoxin), cefotetan (Cefotan), cefotaxime (Claforan), ceftriaxone (Rocephin), ceftazidime (Fortaz, Tazicef, Tazidime), cefepime (Maxipime), cefprozil (Cefzil), loracarbef (Lorabid)
6. *Aminoglycosides:* neomycin, gentamicin (Garamycin), amikacin (Amikin), streptomycin, tobramycin
7. *Macrolides:* erythromycin, azithromycin (Zithromax), clarithromycin (Biaxin)
8. *Iminostilbene derivatives:* carbapenem, imipenem, meropenem
9. *Lincomycin derivative:* clindamycin (Cleocin)
10. *Quinolones:* ciprofloxacin (Cipro), gatifloxacin (Tequin), moxifloxacin (Avelox), trovafloxacin (Trovan), levofloxacin (Levaquin), ofloxacin, nalidixic acid, enoxacin (Penetrex), norfloxacin (Noroxin)
11. *Nitroimidazole:* metronidazole (Flagyl)
12. *Tricyclic glycopeptide:* vancomycin
13. *Oxozolidinone:* linezolid (Zyvox)
14. *Nitrofuran:* nitrofurantoin (Macrobid, Macrodantin, Furadantin)
15. *Streptogramin:* quinupristin and dalfopristin

What adverse reactions are associated with antibiotics?

1. *Penicillins:* nausea, diarrhea, rash, pseudomembranous colitis, nephritis
2. *Monobactams:* nausea, vomiting, diarrhea
3. *Tetracyclines:* epigastric distress, nausea, diarrhea, bone and tooth malformation and discoloration, superinfections (candidiasis), photosensitivity, interference with oral contraceptive effectiveness
4. *Sulfonamides:* nausea, vomiting, diarrhea, fever, rash, photosensitivity
5. *Cephalosporins:* nausea, diarrhea, pseudomembranous colitis, rash, local irritation and thrombophlebitis at injection sites
6. *Aminoglycosides:* ototoxicity, azotemia

7. *Macrolides:* GI upset (nausea, vomiting, diarrhea, abdominal pain), ototoxicity with high I.V. doses (erythromycin)
8. *Carbapenems:* nausea, vomiting, diarrhea
9. *Clindamycin:* nausea, rash
10. *Quinolones:* nausea, altered taste, diarrhea, photosensitivity, pruritus, rash, headache, dizziness, interference with cartilage growth, myalgias, arthralgias, CNS stimulation
11. *Metronidazole:* headaches, dizziness, ataxia, metallic taste, nausea, vomiting, diarrhea
12. *Vancomycin:* angioedema, flushing, and hypotension due to histamine release (especially with rapid infusion), ototoxicity, dyspnea
13. *Linezolid:* rash, headache, fever, nausea, vomiting, diarrhea, constipation, hypertension (with certain medications)
14. *Nitrofurantoin:* nausea, vomiting, diarrhea
15. *Chloramphenicol:* headache, nausea, vomiting, diarrhea
16. *Quinupristin and dalfopristin:* arthralgias, myalgias, rash, pruritus, headache, nausea, vomiting, diarrhea

> *Cross sensitivity may occur between penicillins and cephalosporins.*

What life-threatening reactions are associated with antibiotics?

1. *Penicillins:* anaphylaxis and hypersensitivity reactions, hyperkalemia, seizures, hematologic disorders (thrombocytopenia, agranulocytosis, leukopenia)
2. *Monobactams:* hypersensitivity reactions, pseudomembranous colitis, seizures, hematologic disorders (neutropenia, thrombocytopenia, pancytopenia)
3. *Tetracyclines:* anaphylaxis, intracranial hypertension, neutropenia, thrombocytopenia
4. *Sulfonamides:* anaphylaxis, hematologic disorders (agranulocytosis, leukopenia, aplastic or hemolytic anemia), Stevens-Johnson syndrome, toxic epidermal necrolysis, hyponatremia, hepatitis, pancreatitis, seizures
5. *Cephalosporins:* disulfiram (Antabuse)-like reaction with alcohol (some cephalosporins), anaphylaxis, acute renal failure, hematologic disorders (thrombocytopenia, neutropenia)
6. *Aminoglycosides:* neuromuscular paralysis, apnea, bronchospasm (tobramycin), nephrotoxicity
7. *Macrolides:* anaphylaxis, angioedema (azithromycin), ventricular arrhythmias, pseudomembranous colitis, cholestatic jaundice, hematologic disorders (thrombocytopenia, leukopenia), Stevens-Johnson syndrome

8. *Carbapenems:* anaphylaxis, seizures, pseudomembranous colitis, hematologic disorders (thrombocytopenia, leukopenia)
9. *Clindamycin:* anaphylaxis, pseudomembranous colitis, hematologic disorders (thrombocytopenia, leukopenia)
10. *Quinolones:* hypersensitivity reactions, seizures, prolongation of QT interval (with antipsychotics or antiarrhythmics), hematologic disorders (thrombocytopenia, neutropenia, leukopenia), Stevens-Johnson syndrome, toxic epidermal necrolysis, pseudomembranous colitis
11. *Metronidazole:* disulfiram-like effect with alcohol
12. *Vancomycin:* anaphylaxis, pseudomembranous colitis, nephrotoxicity, hematologic disorders (neutropenia, leukopenia)
13. *Linezolid:* thrombocytopenia, myelosuppression
14. *Nitrofurantoin:* anaphylaxis, hepatitis, asthmatic attacks, Stevens-Johnson syndrome, hematologic disorders (thrombocytopenia, agranulocytosis)
15. *Chloramphenicol:* anaphylaxis, hematologic disorders (aplastic or hypoplastic anemia, thrombocytopenia, granulocytopenia)

✎ What are important nursing actions when administering an antibiotic?

1. Assess the patient for known or suspected previous allergic reactions to antibiotics.
2. Obtain specimens for culture and sensitivity before administration of first antibiotic dose.
3. Administer antibiotics on time to maintain therapeutic levels.
4. Instruct the patient not to share antibiotics with anyone.
5. Instruct the patient to finish the prescribed antibiotic, even if he feels better after a few doses.
6. Monitor the patient for development of superinfections due to alterations of normal flora.
7. Monitor the patient for development of hypersensitivity reactions.

What nursing considerations are specific to penicillins?

1. Inquire about overall allergies (cross sensitivities) or prior allergic reactions to penicillins or cephalosporins.
2. Instruct the patient to take the medication with food to minimize GI upset (except ampicillin).
3. Inform female patients taking hormonal contraceptives that penicillins may make the pills less effective. Encourage the patient to use an additional form of contraception during penicillin therapy.
4. Instruct the patient to notify the physician immediately if a rash or adverse reaction develops.

5. Inform the patient that probenecid increases serum levels of penicillins.
6. Monitor CBC, potassium, and sodium levels as well as liver enzymes during therapy.

What nursing considerations are specific to monobactams?

1. Prepare I.M. injection by adding 3 ml of sterile water or normal saline.
2. Monitor for local reactions at injection site.
3. Monitor CBC and platelet count periodically during long-term therapy.

What nursing considerations are specific to tetracyclines?

1. Tell the patient that taking medication on an empty stomach is preferable, although it may be taken with food if GI problems occur.
2. Instruct the patient to increase fluid intake during therapy.
3. Instruct the patient to avoid exposure to sun or artificial ultraviolet light, to use sunscreen, and to wear protective clothing.
4. Instruct the patient to take tetracyclines 1 hour before or 2 hours after dairy products, antacids, and iron supplements (decrease absorption of tetracyclines).
5. Inform the patient that tetracyclines decrease the effectiveness of hormonal contraceptives. Instruct her to use a second form of contraception during tetracycline therapy.
6. Inform the patient that carbamazepine and phenobarbital decrease the effectiveness of tetracyclines.
7. Inform the patient that tetracyclines may enhance the effects of oral anticoagulants. Dosage adjustments may be required.
8. Monitor renal and liver function as well as CBC with long-term use.

 Tetracyclines shouldn't be used by children younger than age 8 or by women in the last half of pregnancy because of risk of bone growth retardation and permanent teeth discoloration.

What nursing considerations are specific to sulfonamides?

1. Assess for known or suspected allergies to sulfa drugs.
2. Instruct the patient to take the medication with a full glass of water on an empty stomach (minimizes crystal formation and other renal complications).
3. Instruct the patient to increase fluid intake during sulfonamide therapy.
4. Instruct the patient to avoid exposure to the sun or artificial ultraviolet light, to use sunscreen, and to wear protective clothing.
5. Inform the patient that sulfonamides may decrease the effectiveness of hormonal contraceptives. Instruct her

to use a second form of contraception during sulfonamide therapy.

6. Inform the patient that sulfonamides may increase the
effects of oral antidiabetic agents, oral anticoagulants,
and phenytoin. Dosage adjustments may be required
during sulfonamide therapy.

7. Monitor renal and hepatic function as well as CBC
with long-term sulfonamide therapy.

8. Instruct the patient to notify the physician immediately if a fever, sore throat, or rash develop.

What nursing considerations are specific to cephalosporins?

1. Inquire about overall allergies (cross sensitivities) or
prior allergic reactions to penicillins or cephalosporins.

2. Encourage the patient to take the medication with
food to minimize GI upset.

3. Tell the patient to avoid alcohol with cefmetazole and
cefotetan because of the risk of a disulfiram-like reaction.

4. Monitor CBC, renal function, liver enzymes, and prothrombin time (PT) and international normalized ratio
(INR) during therapy.

5. Instruct the patient to notify the physician immediately if a rash or fever develops.

6. Inform the patient that probenecid may increase
serum levels of cephalosporins.

What nursing considerations are specific to amino-glycosides?

1. Assess hearing before initiation of aminoglycosides
and throughout therapy. Instruct the patient to notify
the physician if tinnitus or hearing loss occurs.

2. Encourage the patient to increase fluid intake during
therapy.

3. Monitor renal function (output, blood urea nitrogen,
creatinine, urinalysis, creatinine clearance) throughout
therapy.

4. Obtain peak levels within 1 hour of end of infusion or
1 hour after I.M. injection. Obtain trough levels just
before next dose.

5. Monitor peak and trough levels to ensure therapeutic
dosing.

What nursing considerations are specific to macrolides?

1. Instruct the patient to take the medication on an empty stomach (1 hour before or 2 hours after meals).

2. Instruct the patient to take aluminum and magnesium-
containing antacids 2 hours apart from macrolides.

3. Inform the patient that macrolides may increase levels
of theophylline, phenytoin, carbamazepine, digoxin,
and cyclosporine. They may also enhance the effects
of oral anticoagulants (increase PT/INR). Dosage adjustments of these agents may be required.

4. Monitor for ototoxicity in patients receiving I.V. erythromycin.

What nursing considerations are specific to carbapenems?

1. Assess for known or suspected allergies to penicillins or cephalosporins (cross sensitivity is possible).
2. Monitor CBC and platelet count periodically during therapy.

What nursing considerations are specific to clindamycin?

1. Instruct the patient to take the oral formulation with a full glass of water to prevent esophageal irritation.
2. Monitor CBC and platelet count periodically during long-term therapy.
3. Instruct the patient to notify the physician immediately if he develops diarrhea.

What nursing considerations are specific to quinolones?

1. Instruct the patient to take the medication on an empty stomach.
2. Instruct the patient to increase fluid intake during therapy to prevent crystalluria.
3. Instruct the patient to take quinolones at least 2 hours before or 6 hours after antacids, iron, or zinc supplements and sucralfate.
4. Instruct the patient to avoid or minimize use of caffeine during quinolone therapy because of enhanced effects of CNS stimulation.
5. Instruct the patient to avoid exposure to the sun or artificial ultraviolet light, to use sunscreen, and to wear protective clothing.
6. Inform the patient that quinolones may increase theophylline levels and may enhance the effects of oral anticoagulants. Dosage adjustments may be required.
7. Inform the patient that probenecid increases the serum quinolone level, increasing the risk of toxicity. Therefore, he should avoid concomitant use.
8. Monitor renal and hepatic function as well as CBC during long-term therapy.
9. Instruct the patient to notify the physician immediately if rash, fever, or severe diarrhea occurs.

What nursing considerations are specific to metronidazole?

1. Instruct the patient to avoid alcohol consumption during therapy and for 3 days afterward because of risk of a disulfiram-like reaction.
2. Instruct the patient to take the oral formulation with meals.
3. Inform the patient that increased metronidazole levels may occur with concurrent use of cimetidine, and that decreased metronidazole levels may occur with concurrent use with phenytoin and phenobarbital.

4. Explain that metronidazole may enhance effects of oral anticoagulants and may increase lithium levels. Dosage adjustments may be required.

What nursing considerations are specific to vancomycin?

1. Monitor renal function and CBC periodically during therapy.
2. Monitor for complications, such as ototoxicity and angioedema, flushing, and hypotension.

What nursing considerations are specific to linezolid?

1. Inform the patient that linezolid may be taken with or without meals.
2. Instruct the patient to consume a low-tyramine diet during therapy to prevent hypertension. Red wines, aged cheeses, sauerkraut, tap beers, and soy sauce should be avoided.
3. Inform the patient that hypertension may occur with linezolid in combination with pseudoephedrine, epinephrine, and dopamine.
4. Monitor CBC and platelet count weekly during therapy.

What nursing considerations are specific to nitrofurantoin?

1. Instruct the patient to take the medication with food or milk to enhance absorption and minimize gastric distress.
2. Inform the patient that nitrofurantoin may cause brown or dark yellow discoloration of urine.
3. Monitor respiratory status during therapy as well as CBC.

What nursing considerations are specific to chloramphenicol?

1. Monitor CBC and platelet count every 2 days during therapy.
2. Obtain plasma levels daily during therapy to ensure therapeutic dose.
3. Inform the patient that chloramphenicol increases levels of anticoagulants, barbiturates, iron salts, and sulfonylureas. Dosage adjustments may be required.

What nursing considerations are specific to quinupristin and dalfopristin?

1. Monitor liver function weekly throughout therapy.
2. Inform the patient that levels of carbamazepine, cyclosporine, diltiazem, midazolam, nifedipine, verapamil, and others metabolized by the cytochrome P-450 enzyme system may be increased with the use of this antibiotic.

Antivirals

Treatment of influenza

How do antiviral agents work in the treatment of influenza?

1. *Amantadine (Symmetrel):* inhibits penetration of the host cell by the influenza virus
2. *Rimantadine (Flumadine):* inhibits viral replication
3. *Oseltamivir (Tamiflu):* blocks viral enzyme, which decreases the release of virus from cells and decreases its spread

 Anti-influenza agents only minimize symptoms and duration of the flu. They don't cure it.

 Anti-influenza agents are only effective if therapy is initiated within 36 hours of symptom onset. Prophylactic use of these agents should be initiated within 48 hours of exposure.

What adverse reactions are commonly associated with antivirals used in the treatment of influenza?

1. *Amantadine:* dizziness, insomnia, nausea, irritability, mood changes
2. *Rimantadine:* dizziness, insomnia, irritability, mood changes, nausea
3. *Oseltamivir:* nausea, diarrhea, headache, rhinitis

What are important nursing actions when administering antiviral agents for the treatment of influenza?

1. Encourage the patient to take the full course of therapy.
2. Inform the patient that anti-influenza agents don't decrease the risk of transmission of the flu to others.
3. Instruct the patient to take anti-influenza agents several hours before bedtime to prevent insomnia.
4. Instruct the patient to avoid alcohol consumption during amantadine therapy because of increased CNS effects.
5. Instruct the patient to avoid activities that require mental alertness until the effects of anti-influenza agents are known.
6. Inform the patient that concomitant use of anticholinergic agents and amantadine increases atropine-like adverse effects.

Treatment of herpes simplex virus

How do antiviral agents used in the treatment of herpes simplex virus (HSV) work?

1. *Acyclovir (Zovirax):* inhibits viral replication by interfering with DNA synthesis
2. *Valacyclovir (Valtrex):* inhibits viral replication by becoming incorporated in the viral DNA after conversion to acyclovir

What adverse reactions are associated with antiviral agents used in the treatment of HSV?

1. *Acyclovir:* nausea, vomiting, malaise, headache
2. *Valacyclovir:* headache, nausea, vomiting

What life-threatening reactions may be associated with antiviral agents used in the treatment of HSV?

Renal failure, seizure, hematologic disorders (thrombocytopenia, leukopenia)

What are important nursing actions when administering antiviral agents in the treatment of HSV?

1. Instruct the patient to take antiherpetic agents at the earliest signs of recurrence (tingling, burning, itching).
2. Monitor renal function and CBC periodically during therapy.
3. Inform the patient that antiherpetic agents will *not* prevent the spread of HSV to others.

Treatment of cytomegalovirus

How do antiviral agents used in the treatment of cytomegalovirus (CMV) work?

1. *Ganciclovir (Cytovene):* inhibits DNA synthesis and therefore viral replication
2. *Valganciclovir (Valcyte):* inhibits DNA synthesis (through conversion to ganciclovir) and therefore viral replication
3. *Foscarnet (Foscavir):* inhibits replication of all known herpes viruses by binding to pyrophosphate binding site

What adverse reactions are commonly associated with antiviral agents used in the treatment of CMV?

1. *Ganciclovir:* nausea, vomiting, diarrhea, fever, rash, diaphoresis
2. *Valganciclovir:* headache, insomnia, diarrhea, nausea, vomiting, abdominal pain, retinal detachment (with CMV retinitis)
3. *Foscarnet:* cardiovascular disorders (hypotension, hypertension, palpitations, tachycardia), metabolic disturbances (hypokalemia, hypomagnesemia, hypophosphatemia, hyperphosphatemia, hypocalcemia, hyponatremia), CNS disorders (headache, dizziness, neuropathy, asthenia, paresthesia), GI disorders (nausea, vomiting, diarrhea, abdominal pain), rash, fever, diaphoresis, flushing, cough, dyspnea, renal impairment

What life-threatening reactions are associated with antiviral agents used in the treatment of CMV?

1. *Ganciclovir:* seizures, leukopenia, agranulocytosis, thrombocytopenia
2. *Valganciclovir:* neutropenia, aplastic anemia, thrombocytopenia, pancytopenia, seizures
3. *Foscarnet:* acute renal failure, pancreatitis, hematologic disorders (leukopenia, thrombocytopenia, anemia, granulocytopenia), bronchospasm, seizures

◢ *Cell counts typically return to normal within 1 week of drug discontinuation.*

What are important nursing actions when administering antiviral agents for the treatment of CMV?

1. Instruct the patient to take with food to enhance absorption and to minimize gastric distress.
2. Encourage adequate fluid intake during therapy.
3. Monitor renal and hepatic function as well as CBC and platelet count every 48 hours with twice daily dosing and at least weekly with daily dosing. Discontinue if absolute neutrophil count is less than 500/µl, platelet count is less than 25,000/µl, or hemoglobin level is less than 8g/dl. Monitor for metabolic alterations with foscarnet use, and obtain baseline creatinine clearance level.
4. Inform the patient that a reliable form of birth control should be used during and for 3 months after treatment for CMV because birth defects are associated with the use of these medications.

Treatment of human immunodeficiency virus

How do antiviral agents used in the treatment of human immunodeficiency virus (HIV) work?

1. *NRTIs:* inhibit HIV replication by blocking DNA synthesis
2. *NNRTIs:* inhibit HIV replication by binding to reverse transcriptase, which inhibits HIV transcription from RNA to DNA
3. *Protease inhibitors (PIs):* block the action of an enzyme (protease) required for HIV replication

✎ **What are examples of antiviral agents used in the treatment of HIV?**

1. *NRTIs:* abacavir (Ziagen), zidovudine, AZT (Retrovir), stavudine (Zerit), tenofovir (Virend), lamivudine (Epivir), AZT plus lamivudine (Combivir), didanosine (Videx)
2. *NNRTIs:* delavirdine (Rescriptor), efavirenz (Sustiva), nevirapine (Viramune)
3. *PIs:* nelfinavir (VIRACEPT), indinavir (Crixivan), ritonavir (Norvir), saquinavir (Invirase, Fortovase)

What adverse reactions are commonly associated with antiviral agents used in the treatment of HIV?

1. *NRTIs:* nausea, abdominal discomfort, diarrhea
2. *NNRTIs:* rash, headache
3. *PIs:* diarrhea, abdominal discomfort, nausea, mouth sores, headache, rash, worsening diabetes or hypertension, nephrolithiasis (indinavir), lipodystrophy (diffuse fat deposits) with long-term use

What life-threatening reactions are associated with antiviral agents used in the treatment of HIV?

1. *NRTIs:* pancreatitis (some NRTIs), leukopenia, thrombocytopenia
2. *NNRTIs:* hepatitis, neutropenia, Stevens-Johnson syndrome
3. *PIs:* hepatitis, pancreatitis, seizures, leukopenia, thrombocytopenia

✎ **What toxicities are associated with HAART?**

Insulin resistance, hyperlipidemia, lipoatrophy and lipodystrophy, bone loss, marrow suppression, pancreatitis, hepatitis, nephropathy, and neuropathy

✎ **What are important nursing actions when administering antiviral agents for treatment of HIV?**

1. Instruct the patient to take antiviral agents at same time each day to maintain therapeutic levels.
2. Inform the patient that antiviral agents for the treatment of HIV don't necessarily decrease the risk of viral transmission to others.
3. Inform the patient that several weeks or months of antiviral therapy may be necessary before the effects are apparent.
4. Monitor viral load periodically during therapy.
5. Monitor CBC and liver enzymes.
6. Instruct the female patient to notify the physician immediately if she becomes pregnant during therapy.

Treatment of viral hepatitis (HBV and HCV)

How do antiviral agents used in the treatment of viral hepatitis work?

1. *Lamivudine (Epivir):* inhibits viral (HIV and HBV reverse transcription
2. *Ribavirin (Virazole):* inhibits RNA and DNA synthesis and therefore viral replication; commonly used in the treatment of HCV
3. *Adefovir (Hepsera):* inhibits DNA polymerase for HBV
4. *Interferons:* regulate cytokine expression, enhance phagocyte activity of macrophages, and augment lymphocyte cytoxicity for specific cells

What adverse reactions are commonly associated with antiviral agents used in the treatment of viral hepatitis?

1. *Lamivudine:* headache, fatigue, dizziness, neuropathy, insomnia, nausea, diarrhea, myalgias, arthralgias, fever, cough
2. *Ribavirin:* conjunctivitis, rash
3. *Adefovir:* weakness, headache, abdominal pain, nausea, renal insufficiency, pruritus

What life-threatening reactions are associated with antiviral agents used in the treatment of viral hepatitis?	1. *Lamivudine:* pancreatitis, neutropenia, thrombocytopenia 2. *Ribavirin:* bradycardia, cardiac arrest, bronchospasm, apnea, pulmonary edema 3. *Adefovir:* nephrotoxicity, lactic acidosis, hepatotoxicity, HIV resistance
What are important nursing actions when administering antiviral agents for the treatment of viral hepatitis?	1. Monitor liver enzymes and CBC periodically during therapy. 2. Monitor respiratory status carefully with ribavirin therapy. 3. Instruct the patient to avoid abrupt discontinuation of adefovir. Severe hepatitis exacerbations may occur. 4. Instruct the patient to notify the physician immediately if pregnancy occurs during therapy.

Systemic antifungals

How do antifungal agents work?	1. *Ketoconazole (Nizoral):* destroys fungal cells by altering cell-wall permeability 2. *Itraconazole (Sporanox):* destroys fungal cells by altering cell-wall permeability 3. *Fluconazole (Diflucan):* destroys fungal cells by altering cell-wall permeability 4. *Terbinafine (Lamisil):* inhibits enzyme necessary for fungal sterol synthesis 5. *Griseofulvin (Grivulvin V, Grisovin, Fulvicin, Grisactin):* stops fungal (tinea) cell activity by disruption of mitotic spindles 6. *Nystatin:* alters fungal-cell-wall permeability 7. *Amphotericin (Amphocin) and liposomal amphotericin (AmBisome and lipid complex amphotericin:* destroys fungal cells by altering cell-wall permeability 8. *Caspofungin (Cancidas):* inhibits synthesis in Aspergillus species 9. *Voriconazole (Vfend):* destroys fungal cells by altering cell-wall permeability
✎ **What adverse reactions are commonly associated with antifungal agents?**	1. *Ketoconazole:* nausea, vomiting, diarrhea, photophobia, depression, hyperlipidemia, gynecomastia 2. *Itraconazole:* nausea, headache, dizziness, rash, abdominal pain 3. *Fluconazole:* rash, nausea, vomiting, altered taste sensation, diarrhea, abdominal pain 4. *Terbinafine:* headache, visual and taste disturbances, diarrhea 5. *Griseofulvin:* headache, nausea, vomiting, diarrhea, transient hearing deficit, rash, photosensitivity 6. *Nystatin:* transient nausea, vomiting, diarrhea

7. *Amphotericin and liposomal amphotericin:* irreversible renal impairment (significantly less nephrotoxicity with liposomal formulation), nausea, vomiting, diarrhea, headache, tinnitus, ototoxicity, blurred vision, diplopia, dyspnea, tachypnea, fever, chills
8. *Caspofungin:* tachycardia, tachypnea, paresthesias, myalgias, histamine-mediated symptoms, including flushing, sweating, rash, pruritus
9. *Voriconazole:* mild confusion, altered color perception

✎ **What life-threatening reactions are associated with antifungal agents?**

1. *Ketoconazole:* suicidal tendencies, hepatic failure, leukopenia, thrombocytopenia
2. *Itraconazole:* hepatotoxicity
3. *Fluconazole:* anaphylaxis, hepatotoxicity, leukopenia, thrombocytopenia
4. *Terbinafine:* anaphylaxis, Stevens-Johnson syndrome, neutropenia
5. *Griseofulvin:* hepatotoxicity, angioedema, leukopenia, agranulocytosis
6. *Amphotericin and liposomal amphotericin:* anaphylaxis, renal or hepatic failure, hemorrhagic gastroenteritis, seizures, arrhythmias (due to hypokalemia, hypomagnesemia), bronchospasm, hematologic disorders (thrombocytopenia, leukopenia, agranulocytosis)
7. *Voriconazole:* anaphylaxis, hepatotoxicity, leukopenia, thrombocytopenia

✎ **What are important nursing actions when administering antifungal agents?**

1. Administer premedications, such as antihistamines, antipyretics, antiemetics, and low doses of corticosteroids, to minimize serious adverse reactions, if ordered.
2. Monitor intake and output and encourage increased fluid intake to reduce the risk of nephrotoxicity, unless contraindicated by the patient's condition.
3. Monitor for enhanced hypoglycemic effect with concomitant use of oral antidiabetic agents and fluconazole.
4. Monitor respiratory status during I.V. administration of amphotericin.
5. Monitor CBC, renal and hepatic function as well as serum potassium and magnesium levels periodically during therapy.
6. Instruct the patient to wear sunscreen and protective clothing when exposed to sunlight with griseofulvin use.
7. Instruct the patient to avoid alcohol consumption during griseofulvin therapy.
8. Instruct the patient to take griseofulvin with a high-fat diet for optimal absorption.

9. Inform the patient that long-term therapy may be necessary before effects appear. Encourage the patient to take the full course of antifungal agents.

Immunomodulatory agents

Interferons

How do interferons work?	Through various modifications of the biological response to viruses, including regulation of cytokine expression, enhancement of phagocytic activity of macrophages, and augmentation of lymphocyte cytotoxicity for specific cells
What are examples of interferons?	Interferon alfa-2a (Roferon-A), interferon alfa-2b (Intron A), and pegylated interferon alfa-2b (PEG-Intron)
What adverse reactions are commonly associated with interferons?	Flulike symptoms (malaise, myalgias, fatigue, fever, rigors), dizziness, depression, nausea, insomnia, hypothyroidism, and hyperthyroidism
What life-threatening reactions are associated with interferons?	Neutropenia, thrombocytopenia, and suicidal tendencies

What are important nursing actions when administering an interferon to a patient?

1. Instruct the patient to take interferons at night with an antipyretic to minimize flulike effects.
2. Monitor CBC, platelet count, and thyroid function periodically during therapy.
3. Monitor for depression and suicidal ideations.
4. Inform the patient that interferon doesn't necessarily reduce the risk of viral transmission to others.
5. Inform the patient that benefits of therapy may take several weeks to months.

Nursing skills

Hand hygiene

What's the goal of hand hygiene?	To remove microorganisms from the hands to prevent transmission to others

When must hand hygiene be performed?

1. Before and after any direct patient contact
2. After using the toilet or a bedpan

3. After contact with body fluids (sputum, wound drainage)
4. Before eating

What hand hygiene methods are commonly used in a hospital setting?

Hand washing with antimicrobial soap and alcohol hand gels

What's the proper technique for hand washing?

1. Remove all jewelry.
2. Inspect your hands for cuts or open sores (if present, may need to wear gloves or possibly be given a different work assignment).
3. Turn on the water and allow it to reach a warm temperature.
4. Hold your hands under running water to wet thoroughly.
5. Apply soap and rub hands firmly for at least 10 seconds.
6. Use circular rubbing motion to clean wrists, palms, and backs of hands. Interlock fingers and thumbs to clean interdigital spaces.
7. Thoroughly dry your hands and arms with paper towels.
8. Using a paper towel, turn off the water.

▧ *For clean technique, the hands should be held lower than the elbows so that water flows from the least contaminated area (elbows) to the most contaminated area (hands) during hand washing.*

▧ *Before a sterile procedure, the hands should be held higher than the elbows (hands become cleaner than the forearms and elbows) so that water flows from the least contaminated area to the most contaminated area during hand washing.*

Personal protective equipment

What are examples of personal protective equipment?

Gloves, a mask, face shields, goggles, and gowns

In what order should gloves, a mask, and a gown be applied when all are required?

Mask, gown, and then gloves

When a mask, a gown, and gloves are all worn, in what order should they be removed?

Mask, gown, and gloves

A properly worn mask covers the mouth and nose.

PUTTING ON AND REMOVING DISPOSABLE CLEAN GLOVES

What's the proper technique for putting on disposable clean gloves?

1. Assess the patient for latex allergies.
2. Wash your hands thoroughly for at least 10 seconds.
3. Select the appropriate size and type of glove.
4. Apply the gloves so that wrists are covered. If a gown is worn, gloves should be pulled up to cover the cuffs of the gown.
5. Inspect for any breaks in integrity of gloves (punctures).
6. Interlock fingers to ensure a proper fit.

When should clean gloves be replaced?

If they become torn or punctured, or if they become grossly contaminated

What's the proper technique for removing disposable clean gloves?

1. Remove the first glove by rolling it inside out.
2. While holding the removed glove with the gloved hand, place the first two fingers of the nongloved hand inside the cuff of the gloved hand and remove it by turning it inside out.
3. Discard both gloves (first glove should be inside the second glove, with inside portion being outermost).
4. Wash hands thoroughly for at least 10 seconds.

10

The integumentary system

Basic concepts of the integumentary system

Skin

What are the primary functions of skin, the largest body organ?

1. *Protection:* protects against fluid loss and serves as a physical barrier against potentially harmful external agents
2. *Thermoregulation:* regulates body temperature through sweating and circulation
3. *Sensation:* nerve receptors located in the skin are sensitive to touch, pain, pressure, and temperature
4. *Metabolism:* vitamin D synthesis occurs in the presence of sunlight, which activates minerals essential for bone formation
5. *Communication:* facial skin can form expressions, such as smiling, frowning, and blushing; it also plays cosmetic and identification roles

✎ What are the three layers of the skin?

1. *Epidermis:* thin, outer layer in which keratin is produced
2. *Dermis:* makes up the bulk of the skin; provides strength, blood, and oxygen to the epidermis
3. *Hypodermis:* subcutaneous fat and connective tissue; provides insulation for the body, calorie storage, and additional cushioning

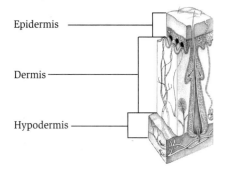

Epidermis

Dermis

Hypodermis

What types of cells are contained within the epidermis?	1. *Keratinocytes:* produce keratin, which serves to protect and waterproof the skin
	2. *Melanocytes:* produce melanin, which protects against ultraviolet light
	3. *Merkel cells:* sensory receptors
	4. *Langerhans' cells:* participate in the cutaneous immune response by presenting antigens to T or B cells
What structures are contained within the dermis?	Blood vessels, nerves, lymph glands, hair follicles, sweat glands, and sebaceous glands
✎ **What two major proteins are found in the dermis?**	1. *Collagen:* primary supportive protein of skin, which provides its strength and resilience
	2. *Elastin:* provides elastic recoil of skin, preventing it from being permanently reshaped
What structures make up the skin appendages?	Hair, nails, sweat glands, and sebaceous glands
What's a dermatome?	A specific area of skin that's supplied with sensory nerve fibers from a single spinal nerve root

Physical assessment of the integumentary system

Normal findings

What are important considerations before beginning a skin inspection?	1. Ensure patient privacy, a good source of illumination, and a comfortable room temperature.
	2. Obtain a small magnifying glass to aid in the examination of individual lesions and a centimeter ruler to measure size of wounds or lesions.
	◆ *Expose areas of skin to be examined in a sequential manner to avoid chilling and violating the privacy of the patient.*
What patient information is important to obtain when examining the skin?	1. Previous skin problems (may provide clues to current skin problems)
	2. Family history (to identify predisposition to certain skin disorders)
	3. Onset, duration, and location of skin problem, as well as any noted changes
	4. Self-treatment

✎ What factors should be included in the head to toe assessment of skin?

Color and pigmentation, temperature and presence of moisture, texture and thickness, turgor, general hygiene, presence of edema, presence of lesions or wounds, and presence of skin tenting (dehydration)

What constitutes "normal" skin color?

"Normal" skin color varies depending on ethnic origin, and may therefore appear whitish-pink to an olive tone to deep brown. Sun-exposed areas may appear darker than unexposed areas. Vascular areas, such as the genitalia, may have a reddish purple hue.

What's the most important determinant of skin color?

Melanin; it's produced by melanocytes in the epidermis and serves to filter ultraviolet light; the number of melanocytes is fairly consistent from one person to another — however, people with darker skin produce more melanin, whereas albinos produce little to no melanin

What constitutes normal skin temperature and moisture?

Normal skin feels warm and dry, although moisture accumulation in skin folds is also normal. Anxiety may cause perspiration in the palms, axillae, scalp, and forehead.

What are normal characteristics of hair?

Hair should be shiny and soft, although the texture varies across ethnic groups. Genetics and age influence normal hair color. Gray hair represents normal aging and is secondary to loss of melanocytes. Hair quantity generally increases after puberty, but then decreases with age. Male balding is a genetic tendency and is considered normal.

What constitutes a normal nail examintion?

The normal nail is flat, slightly convex, adheres to the nail bed, and feels firm. The nail should be smooth and have uniform thickness. The normal angle of the nail base is 160 degrees.

Abnormal findings

✎ What lesion characteristics should be assessed during a physical examination?

Color, pattern (positioning of lesions [clustered, linear]), edges (regular or irregular), size, general characteristics (hard, soft, flat, raised, sunken, fluid-filled), and patient perception (changes in size, shape, or color of lesion)

What are primary skin lesions?

Those that involve color or texture variation that may have been present at birth or that may have been acquired at some time during a person's life

What are examples of primary skin lesions that may be found on examination?

1. *Macule:* a flat, circumscribed eruption of skin with thickened or discolored areas; examples include freckles, flat moles, petechiae, and measles

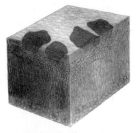

2. *Papule:* an elevated skin lesion that's typically less than 1 cm in diameter and solid; examples include warts, elevated moles, skin tags, and cherry angiomas

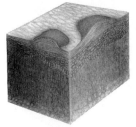

3. *Patch:* a flat, nonpalpable, irregular-shaped macule more than 1 cm in diameter; examples include vitiligo and port-wine stains

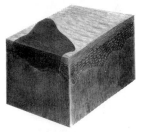

4. *Plaque:* an elevated, rough lesion with a flat top surface more than 1 cm in diameter; psoriasis is an example

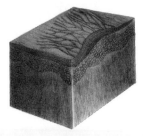

5. *Wheal:* an individual lesion of variable diameter that's irregularly shaped and has cutaneous edema; examples include urticaria, allergic reactions, and insect bites

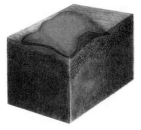

6. *Nodule:* a firm, circumscribed lesion that's deeper into the dermis than a papule; 1 to 2 cm in diameter; examples include lipomas, neurofibromas, and melanomas

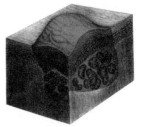

7. *Tumor:* an elevated, solid lesion that isn't clearly demarcated; deeper in the dermis and more than 2 cm in diameter; basal cell carcinoma is an example

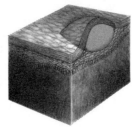

8. *Vesicle (blister):* a raised, circumscribed, superficial skin lesion containing serous fluid; less than 1 cm in diameter; examples include chickenpox (varicella), shingles (herpes zoster), and impetigo

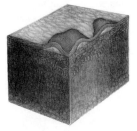

9. *Bulla:* a vesicle (blister) more than 1 cm in diameter; examples include pemphigus vulgaris, epidermolysis bullosa, lupus, and drug reactions

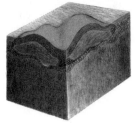

10. *Pustule:* a purulent, fluid-filled vesicle; impetigo is an example

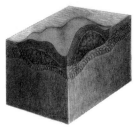

11. *Cyst:* an elevated, encapsulated lesion in the dermis or subcutaneous tissue; epidermoid cyst is an example

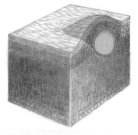

What are secondary skin lesions?

Those that result from primary lesions, either by a natural progression or from manipulation (scratching, picking) of a primary lesion

What are examples of secondary lesions that may be found on examination?

1. *Scale:* flaky skin; heaped up keratinized cells; eczema and flaking skin following a drug reaction are examples

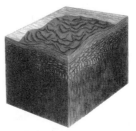

2. *Lichenification:* a thickening and hardening of the skin that's commonly due to persistent scratching of a pruritic lesion such as occurs with chronic dermatitis

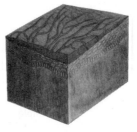

3. *Scar:* a thin to thick fibrous tissue that replaces normal skin following injury to the dermis

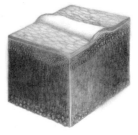

4. *Keloid:* an elevated, irregularly shaped scar that grows beyond the wound edges because of excessive collagen formation during healing; more common in blacks

5. *Excoriation:* an injury to the epidermis caused by scratching or an abrasion; atopic eczema is an example

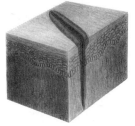

6. *Fissure:* a linear crack or break in the epidermis to the dermis, which can be moist or dry; athlete's foot, eczema, and intertrigo can result in fissure formation

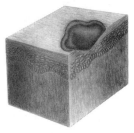

7. *Erosion:* a loss of part of the epidermis; appears moist and glistening; a ruptured vesicle or bulla, chemical burns from urinary or fecal incontinence, and candidiasis can cause erosion

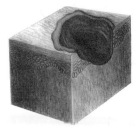

8. *Ulcer:* a loss of epidermis and dermis; concave and varies in size; pressure ulcers and venous insufficiency ulcers are examples

9. *Atrophy:* thinning of the skin surface; skin appears paperlike and translucent; aged skin and striae are examples

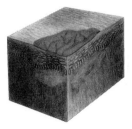

What's a lipoma?

A subcutaneous, benign tumor of adipose tissue

What's an exanthem?

A diffuse rash that's symmetrically distributed and is characteristic of an eruptive disease, such as varicella or rubeola

What's hirsutism?

Excessive body hair that can result from genetics, hormonal dysfunction, or certain medications

What's hyperhidrosis?

Excessive perspiration that can result secondary to heat, hyperthyroidism, menopause, or infection

What's intertrigo?

Erythematous irritation of skin folds (axillae, inner thighs, between fingers or toes, underneath breasts)

What are striae?

"Stretch marks" that appear silvery-white and are commonly associated with pregnancy or sudden weight gain or loss

What's cheilosis?

Dry, cracked lips

What's melasma?

A condition involving brown spots or patches on the face that are symmetrical and are most commonly seen in pregnant women or those who use hormonal contraceptives; because the areas darken upon sun exposure, sun avoidance should be encouraged in addition to the use of sunscreen

What's desquamation?

Scaling of the skin in which there's a rapid epithelial cell proliferation and the outer epidermal layer doesn't form

What might dry mucous membranes indicate?

Dehydration

❧ What might pale mucous membranes indicate?

Anemia

❧ What deviations in normal skin color may indicate local or systemic disease?

1. *Pallor:* unnatural paleness or absence of skin color, which may indicate anemia or vasoconstriction; easiest to see in the mucous membranes, lips, nail beds, and inner surface of the eyelids
2. *Cyanosis:* blue discoloration of the skin and mucous membranes; an excess of deoxygenated hemoglobin indicating hypoxemia causes this discoloration; in dark-skinned individuals, cyanosis will appear gray with loss of normal shine of well-oxygenated skin
3. *Jaundice:* yellow discoloration of the skin, mucous membranes, and sclerae, which is caused by an abnormal amount of bilirubin in the blood; is a symptom of many disorders including liver diseases and biliary obstruction
4. *Erythema:* reddish tone with evidence of increased skin temperature, which may indicate a local inflammatory response when confined to a specific area; widespread erythema indicates systemic vasodilation
5. *Mottling:* patchy discoloration of the skin that may indicate systemic hypoperfusion

What problems may be suggested when skin color deviates from the norm?

Deviations suggest compromises in metabolism, circulation, and oxygenation

What's vitiligo?

A noncontagious skin disorder involving white spots or patches that occur as a result of a progressive loss of melanin

What's albinism?

A group of rare genetic disorders that are characterized by the absence of pigmentation (melanin) of the skin, hair, and eyes from the time of birth

❧ What's an ecchymosis?

A large, bruiselike area that results from bleeding into the skin, subcutaneous tissues, or mucous membranes

❧ What are petechiae?

Small hemorrhagic spots that are red or purple, which may indicate a decreased platelet count or a vascular leak

❧ What are purpura?

Flattened areas in which blood has collected under the skin

❧ What's a hematoma?

A large subcutaneous collection of blood that creates a lump or gently raised area

What are telangiec-tasias?	Skin spots typically caused by superficial vasodilation
What's a nevus?	Also called a *mole* or a *birthmark;* a darkly pigmented skin growth made up of melanocytes, which is typically benign and usually grows as the individual does; certain nevi (large nevi or dysplastic nevi) are associated with the development of malignant changes and melanoma, particularly with repeated sun exposure
What are solar lenti-gines?	Brown spots greater than or equal to 1 cm in diameter that typically occur on the face and back of hands as a result of excessive sun exposure
What are café-au-lait spots?	Hyperpigmented oval patches that resemble coffee stains, which may be indicative of underlying disorders such as neurofibromatosis
What are port-wine stains?	Capillary malformations that appear as pink to dark red, irregularly shaped patches in the upper levels of the skin of some neonates, most commonly on the face, neck, and scalp; these lesions usually darken with age and may require laser treatments to lighten them for cosmetic reasons; also called nevus flammeus
What's xanthelasma and what might its presence indicate?	Raised yellow patches on the eyelids that represent oily deposits in the skin, which may be indicative of a high fat content in the blood
What might dia-phoresis that's associated with cold and clammy skin indicate?	Shock state
What may abnormally dry skin indicate?	Dehydration; dry or sensitive skin may make an individual more prone to itching or hives
What's urticaria?	A pruritic rash with localized swelling due to angioedema, which typically lasts several hours before fading; causes may include certain foods, medications, viruses, or physical agents such as cold, sunlight, or sweat
What's ichthyosis?	A congenital skin disease that causes excessive drying and scaling
What's a skin tag?	Soft lumps usually with a stalk (polypoid) that grow out of the skin and are harmless, although they may be removed with minor surgery for cosmetic reasons

| **What's a spider angioma?** | A red, central, raised area surrounded by a network of dilated capillaries that radiate out from the arteriole, resembling a spider's legs; they're commonly associated with pregnancy, birth control pills, estrogen therapy, or liver disease |

Hair and nails

| **What may be indicated if hair is dull, coarse, and brittle?** | Hair can be affected by several medical conditions including, but not limited to, malnutrition and thyroid disorders (hypothyroidism and hyperthyroidism). Hair changes can also be associated with overexposure to harsh hair products such as hair bleaching. |

| **What's alopecia and what might its presence indicate?** | Pathologic hair loss, which can occur for various reasons including, but not limited to, exposure to chemicals or harsh hair products, scarring, radiation, anemia, hypopituitarism, and chemotherapeutic agents |

| ✒ **What may hair loss on the lower extremities indicate?** | Poor peripheral perfusion |

| **What are examples of deviations in a normal nail examination that may indicate the presence of a medical problem?** | 1. *Abnormal shape:* malnutrition
2. *Concave or spooning nail plates:* iron deficiency anemia
3. *Clubbing:* respiratory or cardiovascular problems; may also occur with cirrhosis, colitis, and thyroid disease
4. *Thickening or hypertrophy of the nail:* repeated trauma, fungal infections, poor circulation, and diabetes
5. *Thinning of the nail:* malnutrition, poor peripheral circulation |

Major skin disorders

Acne vulgaris

| **What's acne?** | A common inflammatory disorder of the sebaceous glands and hair follicles; it appears in approximately 75% of adolescents but varies in severity and can continue into adulthood (particularly for women); hormone levels, genetics, and stress are known to exacerbate acne |

What's the pathophysiologic process in the development of acne?	Accumulation of sebum (oil composed of waxes, fatty acids, triglycerides, and cholesterol esters) and bacteria block the opening of hair follicles, forming comedones (open, blackheads; closed, whiteheads) and possibly pustules

What are the clinical manifestations of acne?

Formation of comedones, papules, pustules (pimples), nodules, and cysts of the face, neck, back, shoulders, and upper chest

What are common treatment modalities for acne?

1. *Mild acne:* usually managed with topical therapy, such as benzoyl peroxide and topical antibiotics (clindamycin, erythromycin, sulfa drugs)
2. *Moderate acne:* systemic antibiotic therapy (tetracyclines, such as minocycline, doxycycline, and erythromycin) and comedolytics such as tretinoin (Retin-A, Avita), adapalene (Differin), and tazarotene (Tazorac)
3. *Severe acne:* commonly treated with isotretinoin (Accutane)

What are other treatment options for acne?

1. *Acidic fruit solutions (salicylic and glycolic acids):* promote peeling of top layer of skin thereby opening blocked follicles
2. *Hormonal agents:* use of low-androgenic (low-dose estrogen) contraceptive pills (norgestimate and ethinyl estradiol [Ortho Tri-Cyclen], desogestrel and ethinyl estradiol [Ortho-Cept], ethynodiol diacetate and ethinyl estradiol [Demulen]), low-dose corticosteroids (prednisone, dexamethasone) or antiandrogenic agents, such as spironolactone for androgen suppression (androgens stimulate sebum production)
3. *Injections (cortisone, triamcinolone):* reduce inflammation of a deep nodule
4. *Light therapy (blue and red light wavelengths):* decreases inflammation

What are important nursing actions when caring for a patient with acne?

1. Instruct the patient to wash his face twice per day with warm water and soap or medicated cleansers to remove surface oils and to kill bacteria. Washing with hot water and scrubbing should be avoided because they cause irritation.
2. Instruct the patient not to pick, squeeze, or scratch lesions.
3. Encourage the use of water-based, oil-free cosmetics.
4. Encourage the patient to avoid environmental irritants (hot, humid weather) and pressure from hats, helmets, and tight collars.
5. Educate the patient on maintaining a healthy lifestyle including adequate rest, exercise, and diet.

6. Inform the patient that acne isn't caused by poor hygiene or food selections.

Dermatitis and eczema

What's dermatitis?

A skin disorder characterized by superficial inflammation that evolves into pruritic, red, and weeping crusted lesions

What's eczema?

A term used when referring to chronic forms of dermatitis

What's the pathophysiologic process of dermatitis and eczema?

Although the exact cause is unknown, inflammation of the skin occurs, which results in erythema, edema, papule formation, vesicles, crusting, and scaling. A genetic predisposition and a disordered immune response involving a cytokine imbalance are believed to play roles.

What are the clinical manifestations of dermatitis?

1. *Acute:* redness, inflammation, swelling, itching, blistering, and oozing, followed by formation of crusts and scales
2. *Chronic:* leathery, thickened skin with excess ridges

How is dermatitis classified?

1. *Atopic:* inherited condition consisting of sensitive, dry, and itchy skin; more common in infants and children
2. *Contact:* inflammatory reaction of the skin to external irritants
3. *Seborrheic:* more common in adult males; cause unknown
4. *Nummular:* coin-shaped eczema plaques on the legs; usually responds well to moisturizers

What types of contact dermatitis exist?

1. *Irritant:* caused by skin contact with potent irritants such as acids, alcohol, and some soaps; stinging and erythema are early manifestations; skin necrosis and ulceration may occur; diaper rash is an example
2. *Allergic:* caused by exposure to a substance to which a person has been sensitized; severe itching results; poison ivy is an example

What are common contact allergens that cause an inflammatory reaction of the skin?

Metals such as those found in fashionable jewelry, harsh chemical (detergents, insecticides), body substances (urine, stools), mechanical irritation (wool, glass, leather), and others (latex, dyes, poison, poison ivy)

What's the typical treatment for dermatitis?

Lubrication of skin, avoidance of irritants, elimination of contact allergens, application of topical corticosteroids, and application of topical immunomodulators such as tacrolimus (Protopic)

Why is petrolatum a good lubricant?	White petrolatum (Vaseline) is one of the blandest ointments and rarely causes skin irritation

✎ What are important nursing actions when caring for a patient with contact dermatitis?

1. Teach the patient to identify irritants.
2. Instruct the patient to use mild soaps and moisturizers.
3. Instruct the patient to use cool compresses, antipruritic lotions, and oatmeal baths (Aveeno baths) to relieve itching.
4. Encourage the patient to avoid overheating (may aggravate dermatitis) and to wear cotton clothing.
5. Inform the patient that corticosteroids or topical immunomodulators may be necessary in severe cases.

Psoriasis

What's psoriasis?

A chronic inflammatory, noninfectious disease of the skin that's characterized by periods of remission alternating with periods of active disease; the exact cause is unknown, however heredity is a factor; physical and emotional stressors are known to cause flare-ups

What's the pathophysiologic process of psoriasis?

An increased rate of epidermal cell turnover causes abnormal keratin production, resulting in dermal inflammation and red, thickened scales

✎ What are the clinical manifestations of psoriasis?

Round, red, raised plaques with sharply defined edges and overlying thick, silvery-white scales; commonly affected sites include the elbows, knees, lower back, scalp, and genitalia

What complications are associated with psoriasis?

Unpredictable flare-ups and psoriatic arthritis

What's the typical treatment for psoriasis?

1. *Topical therapies:* corticosteroid creams and foams (Olux and Luxiq); tar shampoos, bath additives, or tarlike (anthralin) creams; vitamin D-related ointments such as calcipotriene (Dovonex); retinoid gels such as tazarotene (Tazorac)
2. *Phototherapy:* moderate sunlight is usually helpful; ultraviolet light (UVB or UVA); photochemotherapy involves the use of an oral or topical medication (psoralen) to increase skin sensitivity to UVA rays; caution should be used because of increased risk of skin cancer with UV light exposure
3. *Oral agents:* acitretin (Soriatane); methotrexate; immunosuppressants, such as cyclosporine (Neoral) or

mycophenolate (CellCept); "biologic" drugs such as etanercept (Enbrel), Raptiva, infiximab, and Amevive

What are important nursing actions when caring for a patient with psoriasis?

1. Provide treatments as ordered by the physician.
2. Instruct the patient to keep his skin moist (Lac-Hydrin) to minimize itching and scaling.
3. Instruct the patient to protect his skin from scratches and cuts (may cause a flare-up at the injury site).
4. Provide emotional support because this patient may have low self-esteem due to the highly visible lesions. Monitor for depression.

Bacterial skin infections

What organisms most commonly cause bacterial skin infections?

Staphylococci or streptococci

What are common clinical manifestations of bacterial skin infections?

Redness, swelling, and pain at the site of infection

What are common bacterial skin disorders?

Folliculitis, furuncles (boils), carbuncles, impetigo, and cellulitis

What's folliculitis?

An infection or inflammation of hair follicles

What are the early clinical manifestations of folliculitis?

Formation of a small yellow or white pustule on an inflamed follicle; most commonly occurs on the scalp, thighs, buttocks, and legs

What's the typical treatment for folliculitis?

Antiseptic wash or topical antibiotics such as mupirocin (Bactroban); for chronic conditions, laser-assisted hair removal may be used to destroy the follicle and reduce scarring

What's a furuncle?

A deep infection (abscess) of several hair follicles and the adjacent tissue; usually occurs in hairy, sweaty body areas

What are the clinical manifestations of a furuncle?

A tender, reddened area that becomes hard and firm with a soft, pus-filled center or "head"; a fever and chills may also be present

What's the most common treatment for furuncles?

Hot compresses increase circulation to the area, which enables the body to better fight the infection. If the furuncle forms a head, minor surgery, such as an incision and drainage (I&D) may be needed to drain the pus. Antibiotics may be prescribed if the surrounding skin is infected, but they don't have much of an effect on the abscess itself.

What's a carbuncle?

A group of closely packed boils that create a larger lesion with a yellow core of pus; surgery (I&D) is typically required to drain pus and remove dead skin tissue; antibiotics are administered as well

What's impetigo?

Impetigo is a highly contagious bacterial infection of the skin caused by *Staphylococcus aureus* or group A streptococci that occurs most commonly in preschool or school-age children

What are the clinical manifestations of impetigo?

Rounded spots that ooze a honey-colored fluid, which form crusts that become progressively larger; most commonly affects the hands and face

What complications are associated with impetigo?

Because streptococci commonly cause impetigo, rheumatic fever or glomerulonephritis are possible complications

Impetigo is considered contagious when crusting and oozing are present. Infected persons should avoid close contact with others, and separate towels should be used for family members. Linens should be changed after the first treatment day, and clothing should be changed and laundered daily for at least the first 2 days.

What's the typical treatment for impetigo?

Antibiotic ointments, such as Bactroban, applied to each lesion several times per day for 5 to 7 days; thick crusts should be removed gently with warm soaks before ointment application; oral antibiotics may be necessary in more severe cases

What's cellulitis?

Cellulitis is an acute, noncontagious bacterial infection of the skin that can spread to the subcutaneous tissue. It can result from injury (including surgical wounds or puncture sites), insect or animal bites, ulcers, or for no apparent reason.

What are the clinical manifestations of cellulitis?

Blanching erythema, edema, tenderness, and warmth at the site of infection, commonly legs and arms. May exhibit fever, chills, lymphatic streaks, and lymphadenopathy with systemic involvement.

What complications are associated with cellulitis?

Thrombophlebitis, bacteremia or sepsis, and possibly gangrene or necrotizing fasciitis

What's the typical treatment for cellulitis?

1. Elevation of the affected extremity
2. Application of saline-soaked dressings to the area to promote healing and reduce pain
3. Application of hot compresses or a heating pad on low setting
4. Administration of antibiotics (oral, topical or I.V.), such as cephalexin (Keflex), penicillin, erythromycin, or vancomycin
5. I&D, if no improvement with medical management

What are important nursing actions in the care of a patient with cellulitis?

1. Elevate and immobilize the affected extremity.
2. Apply saline-soaked dressings to the affected area several times per day.
3. Apply hot compresses or a heating pad on low setting to the affected area several times per day.
4. Instruct the patient to take the entire course of prescribed antibiotics.
5. Encourage the patient to wear support stockings to prevent fluid buildup.
6. Instruct the patient to maintain good skin hygiene to minimize or prevent recurrences, especially if diabetes or circulatory problems are present.

What other bacterial skin infections pose significant complications?

1. *Staphylococcal scalded skin syndrome:* a superficial blistering disease that results in superficial necrosis; occurs most commonly in young, healthy children; debridement and antibiotics are essential in managing the infection
2. *Toxic shock syndrome:* widespread macular, erythematous eruptions with an acute onset; commonly affected sites include the fingertips and plantar surface of the palms; may be associated with irreversible shock and death
3. *Necrotizing fasciitis:* an uncommon, "flesh-eating" infection of the subcutaneous tissue; may be caused by a streptococcal or a mixed aerobic or anaerobic infection

What's erysipelas?

A skin infection caused by group A streptococcus

What are important nursing actions when providing care for a patient with a contagious skin infection?

1. Instruct the patient to wash his hands thoroughly and frequently, particularly after touching an infected body area.
2. Instruct the patient to avoid sharing towels, washcloths, clothing, and bedding.
3. Instruct the patient to avoid contact with others. Instruct parents to exclude the child from day care or

school until 24 hours after initiation of antibiotics. Instruct the patient to refrain from food handling until 24 hours after initiation of antibiotics.

Viral infections

What lesions can be produced by viral infections?

Rashes, macules, papules, vesicles, urticaria (hives), and warts

What are examples of viral skin infections?

1. *Herpes simplex viruses (HSV):* cause cold sores, fever blisters, genital sores
2. *Varicella zoster virus (VZV):* causes chickenpox (varicella) and shingles (herpes zoster)
3. *Human papillomavirus:* causes warts (verrucae) or benign growths of the skin or mucous membranes
4. *Poxvirus:* causes molluscum contagiosum, a benign viral infection of the skin

What are the clinical manifestations of varicella zoster infection (shingles)?

Formation of clusters of small vesicles over the course of a peripheral sensory nerve (dermatome); crusts form in several days; symptoms are mild to severe pain, itching, fever, and malaise; in older adults, pain can last for months to years.

Who's at risk for developing shingles (reactivation of varicella virus)?

Individuals with weakened immune systems or who take immunosuppressants, people with neoplasms, and elderly people are at an increased risk for reactivation VZV (development of shingles)

⚡ *Pregnant women should avoid contact with people with VZV (chickenpox or shingles) because of the risk of congenital anomalies.*

What's the typical treatment for shingles?

Antiviral agents (acyclovir) for patients in severe pain or who are immunosuppressed, analgesics for pain control, and antipruritic topical medications to relieve itching

How are warts typically treated?

No treatment is indicated for small, painless warts because they tend to disappear on their own. Larger warts can be removed with excision, laser therapy, or cryosurgery (freezing with liquid nitrogen).

Fungal infections

What are examples of fungal skin infections?

1. *Cutaneous candidiasis (yeast infection):* fungal skin infection commonly involving the perineal area or skin underneath large breasts, abdominal folds, or surgical dressings
2. *Tinea pedis (athlete's foot):* fungal infection of feet; occurs frequently between the toes
3. *Tinea corporis (ringworm):* raised, circular rash of fungal origin (not a worm as the name implies); commonly affects children
4. *Tinea cruris (jock itch):* fungal infection of groin
5. *Tinea capitis (ringworm of the scalp):* fungal infection of the scalp and hair; may cause patchy hair loss
6. *Onychomycosis:* fungal infection of the nails
7. *Tinea versicolor:* fungal infection of the outermost skin layer that causes discoloration (pink, white, or brown patches) with a powdery coating

▧ *All tineas are actually ringworms, and they're further named based on the location of growth.*

What are the clinical manifestations of candidiasis?

Red, pruritic rash with moist peeling

What are risk factors for the development of cutaneous fungal infections?

Presence of moisture; hot, humid environment; tight underclothing; history of diabetes; antibiotic therapy (current or recent); and depressed immune system from corticosteroid therapy and immunosuppressive agents

How are fungal infections diagnosed?

Physical examination, fungal cultures, and application of potassium hydroxide to specimens

What complications are associated with cutaneous fungal infections?

Hair loss and development of kerions (large oozing and crusting formations)

How are fungal infections typically treated?

1. *Antifungal creams, ointments, and powders:* nystatin
2. *Systemic antifungal agents:* ketoconazole (Nizoral), fluconazole (Diflucan), itraconazole (Sporanox), griseofulvin, terbinafine (Lamisil)
3. *Antifungal shampoos:* Nizoral, selenium (Selsun)

▧ *Fungal infections typically require long-term antifungal therapy and can recur; therefore, preventive measures should be taught.*

What are important nursing actions when caring for a patient with a cutaneous fungal infection?	1. Instruct the patient to complete the full course of the antifungal.
	2. Instruct the patient to reduce moisture and humidity by thoroughly drying skin and changing sweaty clothes and socks.
	3. Encourage the patient to wear cotton underclothes and to avoid tight-fitting clothing.
	4. Instruct the patient to avoid sharing hats, brushes, combs, pillows, and towels. Encourage the patient to disinfect hair care items periodically.
	5. Instruct the patient to wear flip-flops or shoes in public showers, locker rooms, and around swimming pools.
	6. Examine the patient's family members for signs of infection because they may also require treatment.

Infestations

What types of cutaneous infestations exist?	1. *Lice (pediculosis):* attach to hair; feed on blood; possible typhus transmission; spread by close contact with infected person or by sharing objects, such as combs, hats, towels, and brushes
	2. *Scabies (mites):* burrows, excoriations, and crusts associated with severe pruritus, which is typically worse at night
What are commonly used medications for treatment of various cutaneous infestations?	Lindane (G-well), permethrin (Nix, Elimite), pyrethrin (Tegrin-LT), crotamiton (Eurax)
What are important nursing actions when caring for a patient with an infestation?	1. Wash and dry clothing and bedding in hot temperatures.
	2. Instruct the patient to vacuum any affected areas (lice).
	3. Use a fine-toothed comb, and soak combs and brushes in hot water for at least 15 minutes (lice).
	4. Wet comb hair for 2 weeks for mechanical removal of nymphs (lice).

Skin cancers

What's skin cancer? The uncontrolled growth and division of skin cells; there are two general types of skin cancer: melanoma and non-melanoma; skin cancer is the most common form of cancer

What's the pathophysiologic process of skin cancer? Abnormal growth and proliferation of skin cells, resulting in the loss of their function and structure

What's the leading cause of skin cancer? Sun exposure; by age 20, most adults have experienced significant skin damage; however, it takes 10 to 20 years before unprotected sunbathing results in cancer

What are the most common sites for development of skin cancer? Sun-exposed areas such as the face, neck, back, forearms, and backs of hands

What are the three common types of skin cancers?

1. *Basal cell carcinoma:* most common type of skin cancer; commonly presents as a pink, translucent, or pearly papule with overlying small blood vessels; bleeds and scabs easily; painless and slow growing; surgical removal usually cures this type of cancer and it typically doesn't metastasize
2. *Squamous cell carcinoma:* typically presents as a rough, scaly, fleshy nodule that's firm; ulcerates with tumor growth and scabs; although it's usually localized, without treatment it can metastasize; also known as Bowen's disease when it's confined to the epidermis
3. *Malignant melanoma:* skin cancer involving the uncontrolled growth and division of melanocytes; typically presents as a dark brown, blue, or black skin lesion or ulcer that can begin in an existing mole, but can metastasize to every organ in the body; curable if caught early, but is potentially fatal if untreated or detected late

What's dysplastic nevus syndrome? An abnormal mole pattern, which suggests the person is at increased risk for melanoma

How is skin cancer diagnosed? Physical examination and skin biopsy for confirmation of diagnosis

What factors should be included in a mole assessment?

1. *Symmetry:* normal moles are round; suspicious moles are asymmetrical
2. *Border:* normal moles have a defined border; suspicious moles may have irregular edges

3. *Color:* normal moles are uniform in color (tan or brown); suspicious moles may contain various colors (purple, black, blue, red)
4. *Diameter:* normal moles are typically less than 5 mm in diameter; suspicious moles may be greater than 5 mm

What are common treatment modalities for skin cancer?

1. *Curettage and desiccation:* cancer cells are scraped out and burned; used for small, localized tumors such as squamous cell carcinoma in situ
2. *Cryosurgery:* lesion is frozen with liquid nitrogen causing a blister and scab formation, which then falls off leaving a smooth surface
3. *Surgical excision:* cancer cells are cut out along with a margin of normal appearing tissue to minimize the risk of recurrence; skin is sutured
4. *Chemotherapy and radiation therapy:* used when cancer cells have spread to the lymph nodes or distant sites
5. *Immunotherapy:* interferon stimulates immune system; used in treatment of melanoma

🔆 *Treatment of skin cancer is determined by the lesion's size and location, the patient's age, and the type of tumor.*

What's Moh's micrographic surgery?

A specialized type of surgical excision in which the tumor is sequentially shaved off with a very small margin of normal appearing tissue; the surgeon examines the tissue under a microscope while the patient waits to ensure no cancer cells appear in the margins of the excised tissue and that no further excision is necessary; advantages include maximum preservation of normal tissue and maximum cure rates relative to traditional excisions

What's actinic keratosis?

A common precancerous skin lesion that typically appears as a rough, red, blotchy patch on the face and head; the lesions are directly related to cumulative sun exposure and have the potential to develop into skin cancer; treatments commonly include cryosurgery, topical application of 5-FU, application of topical retinoids (Retin-A) or excision

What are important actions for a patient with skin cancer or for a patient who's at risk for skin cancer?

1. Perform monthly self-examinations in addition to having routine examinations performed by a dermatologist. Perform the examination in a brightly lit room with a full-length mirror and a handheld mirror.
2. Avoid unnecessary sun exposure, particularly between 10 a.m. and 2 p.m. when ultraviolet radiation peaks. Sunscreen products with sun protection factor (SPF)

greater than or equal to 15 should be applied liberally and frequently when skin will be exposed to sun. Encourage the use of protective clothing, such as long sleeved shirts, long pants, and broad-brimmed hats.

3. Avoid artificial sunlight (tanning beds).

Wounds

Basic principles of wound care

What's granulation tissue?	The development and growth of small blood vessels and connective tissue in a full-thickness wound; it should appear wet, red, and beefy
What's an exudate?	Production of pus, serum, or fibrinous material, or the production of fluid in a cavity
What's an induration?	Localized edema beneath the skin
What's maceration?	Tissue damage caused by water saturation
What's slough?	Necrotic yellow tissue that's commonly associated with venous wounds
What's tunneling?	The extension of a tract or sinus into tissue underlying a wound that's accompanied by an infection and inflammation
What's undermining?	A cavity beneath the periwound (area surrounding the wound opening) that occurs at the wound bed margin as a result of shearing forces

Tunneling extends more deeply into tissues, whereas undermining is less extensive.

What are the three phases of normal wound healing?	1. *Inflammatory phase:* characterized by edema, heat, and pain; involves hemostasis, inflammation, and epithelial cell migration; begins at the time of injury and lasts 4 to 6 days
	2. *Proliferative or reconstructive phase:* collagen tissue forms and granulation of the wound occurs; results in scar formation
	3. *Maturation phase:* scar tissue regains approximately 80% of the skin's original strength

◥ By what different methods do wounds heal?

1. *Primary intention:* wound edges are closely approximated; wound heals quickly with minimal scarring if no infection is present
2. *Secondary intention:* wound edges are uneven and tissue loss occurs, granulation tissue fills in the deficit, and the wound heals from the outer edges to the center; scarring results
3. *Tertiary intention (delayed or secondary closure):* surgical closure of the wound is delayed until more favorable conditions for wound healing exist; indicated when primary intention isn't possible; conditions that prevent primary closure include infection and poor circulation

◥ What factors can delay wound healing?

Age, presence of chronic diseases, poor nutritional status, poor oxygenation and perfusion, and immunosuppression and radiation

◥ What are important factors to include in a wound assessment?

1. *Location*
2. *Size:* width, length, and depth in centimeters; repeat measurements weekly
3. *Wound bed:* determines tissue viability; clean ulcers are red and necrotic ulcers may present as yellow, tan, or black
4. *Periwound skin:* observe for erythema, induration, maceration, blistering
5. *Exudate:* amount, color, and odor; can signal presence of wound infection
6. *Pain:* intermittent or constant; use pain scale
7. *Presence of undermining or sinus tract formation:* use sterile cotton-tipped applicator to gently probe wound margins for undermining (extension into surrounding tissue) or sinus tract formation (extension beyond wound base)

What's the function of wound exudate?

1. Transportation of leukocytes and plasma proteins (including antibodies) to the wound
2. Dilution of toxins produced by bacteria and dying cells
3. Transportation of bacterial toxins out of wound

What's serous exudate?

Pink-tinged watery fluid that's usually seen with mild inflammation

◥ What might the presence of purulent exudate (pus) suggest?

Severe inflammation and infection

What type of wound exudate is usually seen with a normal surgical wound?

Serosanguinous, which is clear with some blood tinge

What are the clinical manifestations of a wound infection?

1. Erythema, warmth, and swelling
2. Change in exudate amount, color, and odor
3. No change in wound size for 2 weeks or increase in size despite optimal wound care
4. Increased pain
5. Development of (or increase in) necrosis

What are important nursing actions when caring for a patient with a wound?

1. Administer pain medications 30 minutes before dressing changes, when appropriate.
2. Clean the wound and perform dressing changes as ordered by the physician.
3. Assess the wound with each dressing change. Obtain wound culture if infection is suspected.

Never massage a reddened area because it may result in tissue damage.

What are the basic principles of effective wound care?

1. Eliminate or control factors that inhibit wound healing (dry wound base, infection).
2. Remove devitalized tissue (debridement).
3. Clean the wound.
4. Control bacteria count and infection (bacteria compete with normal cells for oxygen and nutrients needed for healing, and their by-products adversely affect epithelialization and wound contraction).
5. Eliminate dead space.
6. Control odor and pain.
7. Protect the wound.

Nonviable (necrotic) tissue promotes bacterial growth and should be removed to prevent infection.

What types of debridement exist?

1. *Mechanical:* use of wet-to-dry dressings and whirlpools; nonselective removal of granulation tissue as well as nonviable tissue; should be discontinued when necrotic material is removed
2. *Surgical or sharp:* removal of nonviable (necrotic) tissue using a scalpel, scissors, or laser with sterile technique (surgical) or nonsterile technique (sharp)
3. *Autolytic:* use of moisture-retentive dressings to promote liquefaction of necrotic tissue
4. *Enzymatic:* use of prescription ointments whose sole purpose is to debride

▨ *Debridement doesn't make the wound worse, although the wound is larger following debridement.*

What factors determine the type of dressing selected?

1. Functions of the dressing (absorption, debridement, odor control)
2. Characteristics of the wound (noninfected, infected, necrotic, highly exudative)
3. Product availability and cost
4. Number of dressing changes required daily

✎ What's a wet-to-dry dressing?

A dressing that consists of gauze moistened with saline or antimicrobial solution that's placed in direct contact with the wound surface, but is allowed to dry between dressing changes; wet-to-dry dressings may be used for debridement of wounds with extensive tissue loss that heal by secondary intention, such as burns and pressure ulcers

What's a wet-to-wet dressing?

A variation of a wet-to-dry dressing, but the gauze is kept moist with a wetting agent between dressing changes; a layer of absorbent material saturated with the same solution is placed above the wet gauze; the moisture continuously bathes the wound bed and dilutes viscous exudates

What's the "no touch" technique used to perform dressing changes?

A method that uses sterile supplies for direct contact with the wound surface and clean supplies otherwise

What's the purpose of packing a wound?

Fills dead space, which promotes healing and prevents abscess formation caused by premature closure; packing prevents the wound from healing from the "outside in"; instead, healing occurs from the "inside out"

✎ What are common wound complications?

Infection, hemorrhage, dehiscence or evisceration, and fistula formation (abnormal passage between two organs or between organ and outside of body)

Wound care products

What are the characteristics of an appropriate wound care product?

1. Promotes moist wound healing (moisture promotes angiogenesis and tissue repair)
2. Is atraumatic to periwound skin and healthy granulation tissue
3. Prevents infection
4. Fills in dead space
5. Facilitates removal of exudate, slough, necrosis, eschar
6. Minimizes pain associated with dressing changes

What types of adjuvant wound therapies exist?

1. *Living skin equivalents:* produced from cultured skin tissue; used in the treatment of burns as well as venous and pressure ulcers
2. *Growth factors:* stimulate wound-healing activity; used for wounds refractory to more conventional therapy
3. *Hyperbaric oxygen (HBO):* exposure to 100% oxygen in a chamber at pressures that exceed those at sea level stimulates collagen synthesis and promotes angiogenesis; used for gas gangrene, thermal burns, necrotizing soft-tissue infections, refractory osteomyelitis as well as compromised skin grafts and flaps
4. *Electrical stimulation:* electric current is transferred through a surface electrode pad that's in wet contact with the wound bed to enhance blood flow, oxygen uptake, and synthesis of deoxyribonucleic acid (DNA) and protein; used for burns, surgical wounds, and ulcers of pressure, diabetic, or vascular etiologies
5. *Vacuum-assisted closure:* application of negative pressure by a device with a special dressing placed over the wound; assists wound closure by removing fluids and stimulating formation of granulation tissue; used for chronic wounds, meshed grafts, and flaps, as well as acute, traumatic wounds
6. *Warm-up therapy:* noncontact thermal therapy involving the use of an infrared heater and a bandage to stimulate the healing process; used for pressure ulcers as well as partial- or full-thickness ulcers of venous or diabetic etiology

Chronic wounds

What are the most common chronic wounds?

Pressure ulcers, venous insufficiency ulcers, arterial ulcers, diabetic ulcers, and other types, such as nonhealing surgical wounds, radiation wounds, vasculitis wounds, burns

Pressure ulcers

✎ What's a pressure ulcer?

An area of localized tissue destruction that results from sustained mechanical occlusion of the blood supply of soft tissues for an extended period of time; ischemia and cell death occur as a result

What's the patho-physiologic process of a pressure ulcer?

Tissue ischemia and destruction result from sustained mechanical occlusion of blood supply by compression, shearing, or friction.

What are the clinical manifestations of a pressure ulcer?

Depends on the stage, but may range from reactive hyper-emia to tissue necrosis or damage to muscle or bones

How are pressure ulcers classified?

1. *Stage I:* presents as nonblanchable erythema of intact skin; patients may experience warmth, edema, indura-tion, and hardness; dark-skinned individuals may ex-perience discoloration

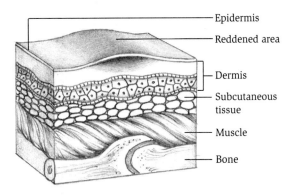

2. *Stage II:* partial-thickness skin loss in which the ulcer is superficial and presents as an erythematous abra-sion, blister, or shallow crater; wound base is pink, moist, and painful, but without necrotic tissue

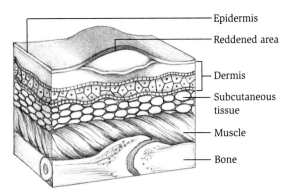

3. *Stage III:* full-thickness skin loss through the dermis that involves subcutaneous tissue; presents as a shallow crater with or without undermining of adjacent tissue; usually painless

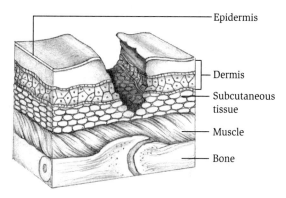

4. *Stage IV:* full-thickness skin loss with extensive destruction to muscle, bones, supporting structures; presents as a deep crater with or without undermining sinus tracts; usually painless

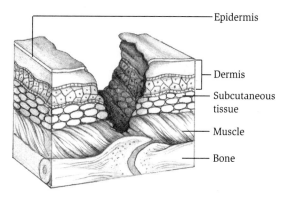

◪ *Only pressures ulcers are staged; all other wounds should be described as partial- or full-thickness wounds.*

◪ *Staging shouldn't be performed until the base is visible in a wound containing necrotic tissue.*

Why is down-staging (reverse staging) of wounds inappropriate?

Because the granulation tissue that fills in a wound space isn't equivalent to the tissue that was lost; therefore, a healing wound should be described as "a healing stage II," rather than as "reversed to stage I"

Where are pressure ulcers most likely to develop?

Over bony prominences, such as the sacrum, ischial tuberosity, trochanter, or heel

What factors increase the risk of pressure ulcer development?

Immobility, impaired neurologic functioning, decreased sensory perception, decreased circulation, presence of moisture, malnutrition, dehydration, and trauma from friction and shearing

How can patients at risk for pressure ulcers be identified?

By using screening tools such as the Braden or Norton scale; the most common parameters include sensory perception, activity, mobility, moisture or incontinence, fraction or shear, and nutritional status

What are important nursing actions in the prevention of pressure ulcers?

1. Turn and reposition the patient from side to side at least every 2 hours.
2. Use pressure-reducing devices (foam, air, and gel mattresses) to redistribute the pressure over bony prominences. Place pillows between the knees and ankles. Avoid donut-type devices as well as positioning patient directly on trochanter.
3. Avoid elevating the head of the bed more than 30 degrees.
4. Keep the patient's skin clean and dry. Avoid soaps and use moisturizing lotions.
5. Instruct the patient to use a trapeze to lift his body when moving up in bed. If the patient can't participate in the transfer, two people should use a bed sheet to lift the patient.

What's the typical treatment for pressure ulcers?

Debridement of necrotic tissue, cleaning the wound with each dressing change, and using a dressing that keeps the wound base continuously moist but the surrounding skin intact; advanced ulcers may require plastic surgery, including skin grafts or flaps

Prevention is the best treatment for pressure ulcers.

What are important nursing actions in the care of a patient with a pressure ulcer?

1. Implement preventive measures as outlined above to prevent additional ulcers or worsening of existing ones.
2. Clean and assess the wound with each dressing change. Obtain wound cultures if infection is suspected.
3. Ensure adequate nutrition to promote healing.

Venous insufficiency ulcers

What are venous insufficiency ulcers (venous stasis ulcers)?

Ulcerations of the skin caused by pooling or *stasis* of blood and swelling of leg veins due to improper functioning of the valves in the lower extremities; chronic wounds can result

What's the pathophysiologic process of venous insufficiency ulcers?

Because pooled blood has a lower oxygen concentration, ischemia of the skin and subcutaneous tissues occurs

What are the clinical manifestations of a venous insufficiency ulcer?

1. Large, shallow ulcers, usually near the medial malleolus
2. Typically painless
3. Edema and liposclerosis (thickening of skin) of surrounding tissue
4. Periwound hyperpigmentation (hemosiderin deposits)
5. Moderate to heavy serous exudate
6. "Bowling pin"-shaped leg
7. Pulses are present
8. Skin temperature is normal
9. Pain is relieved by elevation

What's liposclerosis and what's its significance?

Thickened, indurated skin that can occur before ulcers develop, and can therefore signal that preventive care should be implemented

Where do venous insufficiency ulcers most commonly occur?

Medial aspect of lower extremities and proximal to medial malleolus

What are associated risk factors?

Deep vein thrombosis, obesity, pregnancy, leg trauma, heart failure, vascular surgery, and family history

How are venous ulcers typically treated?

Wound care and compression therapy to optimize venous return (ace wraps, Unna's boots, gradient compression stockings)

What are Unna's boots?

A type of cast which uses dressing impregnated with zinc oxide, calamine lotion, glycerin, and gelatin to prevent infection and edema in the management of venous ulcers; Unna's boots should be changed every 7 to 10 days

✎ How can a patient with a venous insufficiency ulcer minimize or prevent a recurrence?	1. Wear antiembolism stockings everyday. 2. Elevate the legs several times during the day. 3. Avoid prolonged standing or sitting. 4. Maintain normal weight and exercise regularly. 5. Avoid smoking. 6. Avoid tight clothing that constricts circulation.
✎ What are important nursing actions in the care of a patient with a venous insufficiency ulcer?	1. Provide wound care as instructed. Assess wound with each dressing change and obtain wound cultures if infection is suspected. 2. Maintain elevation of the affected extremity 3. Implement the use of antiembolism stockings, Unna's boot, or elastic wraps to reduce edema. 4. Encourage adequate nutrition, smoking cessation, and maintenance of normal weight. 5. Instruct the patient to avoid prolonged sitting or standing as well as wearing tight-fitting clothing

Arterial ulcers

✎ What are arterial ulcers?	Ulcers that occur as a result of ischemia from arterial occlusion in the extremities
What's the pathophysiologic process of arterial ulcers?	Severe tissue ischemia and necrosis occur due to arterial insufficiency or occlusion
✎ What are the clinical manifestations of an arterial ulcer?	1. Painful, small, well-circumscribed ulcers that may be deep and may expose deep tendons, fascia, and bones 2. Wound bed may appear pale, dry, and necrotic with adherent eschar and minimal edema and exudates 3. Diminished or absent pulses and loss of hair of the affected extremity 4. Cool skin with possible loss of hair in the affected area 5. Increased capillary refill (greater than 3 seconds) of the affected extremity 6. Skin may appear shiny, thin, and dry 7. Dependent rubor, pallor on elevation of the affected extremity 8. Intermittent claudication (muscular cramping and pain in calf with activity, which improves with rest)
✎ What risk factors are associated with the development of arterial ulcers?	Diabetes, smoking, hypertension, and atherosclerosis

Where do arterial ulcers most commonly occur?

Toes and dorsal surface of foot or lateral malleolus

What's the typical treatment for arterial ulcers?

1. Wound care, bed rest, increase circulation to affected extremity (place in slightly dependent position), surgical revascularization, and hyperbaric oxyen
2. Protect affected extremity by padding all resting surfaces, placing cotton between toes, and use of pressure relief shoes for ambulation

◣ *Extremities with arterial ulcers should* not *be elevated because this would decrease blood flow to an ischemic area.*

✎ **What are important nursing actions in the care of a patient with an arterial ulcer?**

1. Provide wound care as instructed and assess the wound with each dressing change. Obtain wound culture if infection is suspected.
2. Encourage bed rest with the affected extremity placed in a slightly dependent position, to increase circulation.
3. Encourage adequate nutrition as well as good blood glucose and blood pressure control to promote wound healing and prevent recurrences.
4. Encourage smoking cessation.

Diabetic foot ulcers

What's a diabetic foot ulcer?

An ulceration that occurs on the foot of a patient with diabetes who has vascular disease; a patient is commonly unaware of the ulcer's presence because of impaired sensation

◣ *Foot ulcers in a patient with diabetes heal more slowly than ulcers in a patient who doesn't have diabetes. A foot ulcer in a patient with diabetes is at increased risk for infection.*

What's the typical treatment for diabetic foot ulcers?

Appropriate wound care, pressure reducing orthotics, topical or systemic antimicrobial therapy, and possibly reconstructive or vascular surgery

✎ **What are important preventive actions for a patient with diabetes at risk for developing a foot ulcer?**

1. Avoid cigarette smoking.
2. Inspect feet daily for blisters, cuts, and scratches. Also inspect the sides of shoes daily for foreign objects.
3. Wash feet daily and dry them thoroughly, especially between the toes. Avoid soaking feet.

4. Avoid temperature extremes to prevent burns or frost-bite.
5. Avoid the use of chemical agents to remove corns or calluses.
6. Avoid the use of adhesive tape on skin.
7. Wear properly fitting socks and shoes. Avoid walking barefoot.
8. Notify health care provider immediately if a blister or sore develops.

Burns

What are the most common causes of burns?

1. *Thermal:* fires, cooking or heating accidents, steaming or scalding accidents, playing with matches
2. *Chemical:* household or industrial substances
3. *Electrical:* high-voltage power lines, faulty electrical wiring, lightning
4. *Friction or abrasion:* carpet, roads, gym floors
5. *Radiation:* sun, tanning beds, X-rays

What's the Rule of Nines?

A method used to estimate a patient's burn percentage; this method divides the body into 11 areas, each of which represents 9% of the total body surface area (BSA); to calculate the burn percentage, count the number of areas burned and multiply by 9; burns greater than 30% BSA are extremely dangerous because the patient is more susceptible to infection and shock

How are burns classified?

1. *First-degree (superficial):* involves the epidermis only; causes painful erythema that blanches with mild pressure; usually heals in 3 to 4 days without scarring; not considered in estimating burn percentage; sunburn is an example
2. *Second-degree (partial-thickness):* involves the epidermis and dermis; causes blisters (vesications) as well as edema and pain; healing requires reepithelialization, which may result in scarring
3. *Third-degree (full-thickness):* involves the full thickness of the dermis and possibly underlying muscles and bones; causes necrosis through the entire skin and possible thrombosis of blood vessels; appears white and leathery to black charred; painless
4. *Fourth-degree:* involves muscle, bone, and interstitial tissues; bone is charred

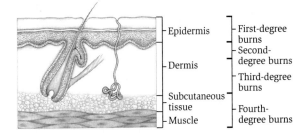

⚡ *Burns are classified according to the depth of the burn and the extent of skin damage, but it may take several days for burns to declare their true depth.*

✎ What are the two types of second-degree burns?

1. *Superficial partial-thickness:* involves injury to first two layers of skin; burn is moist and painful; blisters and swelling develop; sloughing of overlying skin may occur; usually heals in less than 2 weeks without surgical intervention and without scar formation
2. *Deep partial-thickness:* involves injury to deeper skin layers; burns are dry and white with red areas that don't blanch; skin may appear spotted; sensation is decreased; infection is a concern; healing takes longer than 2 weeks, with scarring and possible need for debriding and grafting

What factors can cause a second-degree burn to develop into a third-degree burn?

Inflammation, edema, ischemia, and infection

✎ What's the major concern with all burns?

Infection

How are burns treated?

1. *First-degree:* usually only minor care is needed, such as keeping wound clean and applying topical antibiotic ointments (Bacitracin, Neosporin)
2. *Second-degree:* superficial burns must be cleaned to remove foreign material and nonviable skin; a topical antibiotic ointment is also used (Bacitracin, Neosporin); debridement, early excision of eschar, and grafting are performed for a second-degree wound that hasn't healed within 2 to 3 weeks
3. *Third-degree:* escharotomy, debridement, skin grafting
4. *Fourth-degree:* escharotomy, debridement, skin grafting

▶ *Burns are treated according to their size, depth, and location, as well as the age and overall health of the patient.*

◆ What's eschar?

Black-brown necrotic tissue that resembles leather and is typically associated with arterial wounds and burns

What's an escharotomy?

An incision made through burn eschar to prevent or relieve compartment syndrome (compromised nerve or circulatory supply due to edema)

◆ What actions constitute standard treatment for any type of burn?

1. Elevation of affected area: minimizes swelling and pain
2. Topical agents such as silver sulfadiazine (Silvadene)
3. Gentle wound cleaning with disinfectant soap using sterile gauze

What are the advantages of early excision?

Early mobilization and rehabilitation, improved joint function, and a shorter hospitalization

What's skin grafting?

A surgical procedure in which skin from another area of a patient's body (or a skin substitute) is used to replace tissue lost in full-thickness burns or to cover nonhealing wounds; skin grafts can be temporary or permanent; skin grafting is essentially skin transplantation

What types of skin grafts exist?

1. *Autograft:* patient's own skin is applied to the wound
2. *Homograft (allograft):* skin is taken from a cadaver
3. *Heterograft (xenograft):* skin is taken from an animal such as a pig
4. *Synthetic skin substitutes:* man-made products with skinlike properties are applied to the wound; may be temporary or permanent; examples include TransCyte, Integra, AlloDerm, and graftskin (Apligraf)

▶ *A newly grafted area should be immobilized for 5 days to permit graft adherence and vascularization.*

◆ What are important treatment considerations in the care of a patient with extensive burns?

1. *Respiratory support:* administer supplemental oxygen to maintain saturation greater than 92%; intubate if inhalation injury or large percentage BSA; elevate head of bed 30 degrees if facial involvement and not in shock; assess for bronchospasm and need for bronchodilator
2. *Fluid resuscitation:* denuded skin causes a sixfold increase in evaporative fluid loss, which must be replaced; calculate fluid deficit from the time of injury; if percentage of BSA is greater than 20% in otherwise

healthy adult, administer one-half calculated volume in first 8 hours, followed by the remainder over the next 16 hours; then maintenance of 2 to 4 ml lactated Ringer's solution $\times$ BSA $\times$ kg body weight per 24 hours thereafter

3. *Neurovascular status:* eschar can function as a tourniquet for blood flow to distal sites; compartment syndrome can develop; neurovascular checks should be performed hourly for the first 48 hours
4. *Pain control:* repeated small boluses or continuous infusion of I.V. analgesics (morphine, fentanyl, benzodiazepines)
5. *Temperature regulation:* protect from hypothermia by warming I.V. fluids and avoiding wet dressings when possible
6. *Infection prevention:* sterile technique for all wound care
7. *Wound care:* cleaning, dressings, debriding
8. *Nutritional support:* 2,800 calories per day to meet protein and energy needs of hypermetabolic state; early tube feeding may be instituted; good nutrition decreases risk of infection and promotes wound healing

⚡ *Peripheral I.V. shouldn't be placed through burned skin when avoidable because of increased risk of infection.*

⚡ *Potassium shouldn't be added to I.V. fluids during the first 24 hours after a burn injury because large quantities are released into the extracellular fluid by injured cells.*

What types of pulmonary complications can occur in patients with extensive burns?

1. *Carbon monoxide poisoning:* competition for hemoglobin binding between carbon monoxide and oxygen; carboxyhemoglobin causes tissue hypoxia
2. *Smoke inhalation injury:* irritation and injury to tracheobronchial tree; loss of ciliary movement; decreased production of surfactant, edema of mucosa
3. *Inflammatory airway reaction:* can cause obstruction of airway
4. *Restrictive defects:* result from full-thickness burns around the neck or chest as well as from pulmonary edema as a result of fluid shifts; limits lung expansion

⚡ *Carbon monoxide's affinity for hemoglobin is 200 times greater than that of oxygen.*

What physical findings are indicative of airway or lung damage in a burn patient?

1. Obvious facial or neck burns
2. Singed nasal or facial hair
3. Presence of circumoral soot or carbonaceous sputum
4. Labored breathing, tachypnea, hoarseness, and stridor

5. Diagnostic tests, such as arterial blood gas (ABG) analysis, carboxyhemoglobin level, chest X-ray, and bronchoscopy

■ *Subcutaneous and I.M. routes of medication administration should be avoided in a patient with burns because absorption by these routes is affected by fluid shifts.*

What causes fluid shifts in burn patients?

Increased capillary permeability results in a loss of plasma proteins and electrolytes, which causes a reduction in intravascular volume and an increase in extracellular volume

How is adequacy of fluid resuscitation determined?

By assessing hourly urine output; adequate fluid resuscitation would be evidenced by a urine output of greater than or equal to 1 ml/kg/hour in adults; however, patients with electrical burns should maintain an hourly urine output of 1.5 to 2 ml/kg in order to prevent renal complications from urine myoglobin (myoglobinuria from muscle breakdown)

What are important nursing actions when caring for a patient with extensive burns?

1. Monitor vital signs at frequent intervals and assess for development of respiratory difficulties (particularly during the first 48 hours).
2. Monitor intake and output carefully. Administer I.V. fluids (maintenance plus replacement for burn losses) as ordered by the physician. Insert an indwelling urinary catheter.
3. Assess for pain and administer pain medications as ordered, especially before dressing changes.
4. Assess distal neurovascular status every hour for 48 hours. Monitor for development of limited movement and numbness of affected areas.
5. Provide dressing changes using sterile technique at least daily, or more frequently for excessive drainage.
6. Avoid chilling the patient and ensure water temperature lower than 98.6° F (37° C) for bathing because altered temperature regulation is common.
7. Monitor for development of complications, such as dehydration, hypovolemia, infection, and renal failure (from myoglobin released with breakdown of muscle).
8. Determine the date of most recent tetanus immunization; if it was more than 5 years before, reimmunize.

Pharmacology related to the integumentary system

Treatment of acne vulgaris

COMEDOLYTICS

How do comedolytics work?

By various methods including killing follicular bacteria, *Propionibacteria acnes* (benzoyl peroxide), breaking up oil and dead cell collections that block hair follicles, and increasing the rate of skin cell turnover (promotes extrusion of existing comedones), which helps to unclog pores (retinoids)

What are examples of comedolytics?

Benzoyl peroxide, salicylic acid, retinoids and Retin-A (Stieva-A, Avita), and adapalene (Differin)

What adverse reactions are commonly associated with comedolytics?

1. *Benzoyl peroxide:* skin dryness and irritation; may bleach hair, skin, and clothing
2. *Salicylic acid:* local irritation
3. *Retinoids:* photosensitivity, local irritation, temporary worsening of acne
4. *Adapalene:* skin irritation and dryness, although less than that experienced with retinoids

What are important actions when administering a comedolytic agent?

1. Wash your hands before and after each application.
2. Wash the patient's face and dry completely before application.
3. Apply a thin film (more isn't more effective). If retinoids are used in combination with a topical antibiotic, instruct the patient to apply one in the morning and the other at bedtime.
4. Slowly increase the amount of time agent is worn (initially only a few hours, but overnight as tolerated).
5. Avoid abrasive soaps or cleansers, alcohol-containing products or others that may cause excessive skin irritation and drying. Encourage the use of an oil-free moisturizer for dry skin.
6. Use topical agents regularly and inform that results may take weeks because acne may worsen for the first several weeks of therapy.
7. Encourage the patient to use sunscreen.

TOPICAL ANTIBIOTICS

How do topical antibiotic agents work?

Via penetration of comedones, which enhances bactericidal activity

What are examples of topical antibiotics used in the treatment of acne?	Clindamycin (Cleocin T), erythromycin (Erygel, Akne-Mycin), tetracycline (Topicycline), sulfur-containing products (Acne Lotion 10, Liquimat, Sulpho-Lac), and combination agents (erythromycin and benzoyl peroxide [Benzamycin], clindamycin with benzoyl peroxide, Triaz-benzoyl peroxide)
What adverse reactions are commonly associated with topical antibiotic agents?	Local skin irritation, dryness, diarrhea, photosensitivity, development of resistance over time

What are important nursing actions in the care of a patient using topical antibiotic agents?

1. Wash your hands before and after application.
2. Wash the patient's face and dry completely before application.
3. Apply a thin film (more isn't more effective).
4. Avoid use in or near the patient's eyes.
5. Encourage the patient to use sunscreen.
6. Avoid the use of harsh cleansers, alcohol-containing products, or other agents that may cause dry skin.
7. Encourage the use of an oil-free moisturizer for dry skin.

Systemic agents

ISOTRETINOIN (ACCUTANE)

How does isotretinoin work?	It reduces the size of oil glands, which decreases oil production and bacterial growth. A typical course is twice daily dosing over 15 to 20 weeks for refractory acne.

What are the indications for treatment of acne with isotretinoin?

1. Acne refractory to 6 months of systemic antibiotics
2. Acne controlled by more than 3 years of continuous systemic antibiotics
3. Males with moderate to severe acne (risk of pregnancy isn't a factor)

What adverse reactions are associated with isotretinoin?	Dry skin and mucous membranes (dry eyes, nosebleeds), peeling of the palms and soles, arthralgias and myalgias, hair shedding, elevated liver enzyme and serum triglyceride levels, photosensitivity, poor night vision, and depression or other alterations in mental health

◤ *Isotretinoin can cause significant birth defects (even one pill); therefore female patients of childbearing age should use two forms of birth control to avoid pregnancy during treatment.*

What are important nursing actions when providing care for a patient undergoing isotretinoin therapy?	1. Educate the female patient of childbearing age about the need for two reliable forms of birth control during therapy. 2. Inform the patient of the need for monthly blood studies (liver function tests, triglyceride and cholesterol levels) and urine pregnancy tests during therapy. Prescriptions are given for a 30-day supply only and can't be renewed without required blood and urine tests because of a program involving pharmaceutical company and the Food and Drug Administration. 3. Instruct the patient to avoid vitamin A supplementation during therapy to prevent toxicity (isotretinoin is a vitamin A derivative). 4. Encourage the use of moisturizers, artificial tears, and lip balms. 5. Inform the patient that acne may temporarily worsen for the first several weeks of therapy.

Treatment of dermatitis and eczema

TOPICAL CORTICOSTEROIDS

How do topical corticosteroids work in the treatment of dermatitis?	By initiating reactions that cause anti-inflammatory, antipruritic, and antiproliferative effects
What are examples of topical corticosteroids?	Hydrocortisone (Cortaid, Lanacort), triamcinolone (Aristocort, Triacet, Triderm), and betamethasone (Diprolene, Betacort)
✎ **What adverse reactions are associated with topical corticosteroids?**	1. *Local:* irritation, burning, striae, skin thinning, and secondary infection; glaucoma and cataracts may develop as a result of long-term periorbital use if drug enters eye 2. *Systemic:* hyperglycemia, Cushing's syndrome, and growth retardation in children ⚡ *Topical corticosteroids can be absorbed systemically with long-term use or with use over large body areas.*
What are important nursing actions in the care of a patient requiring a topical corticosteroid?	1. Wash your hands before and after medication application. 2. Gently clean the area before application to enhance its effect. 3. Apply a thin film two to three times per day and rub in gently.

4. Avoid applying the medication in or near the patient's eyes.
5. Avoid the use of occlusive dressings.
6. Discontinue topical corticosteroids if antibiotic or antifungal therapy is initiated, and don't reinitiate its use until the infection has cleared.

◤ *Topical corticosteroids shouldn't be applied to open lesions.*

◤ *Topical corticosteroids are best used two to three times per day for 2 to 3 days, followed by a period off the drug.*

Treatment of psoriasis

TOPICAL AGENTS

How do antipsoriatics work?	By regulating the production and development of keratinocytes; these skin cells contain vitamin D receptors, to which the antipsoriatics (vitamin D analogs) bind
What are examples of antipsoriatics?	Anthralin (Anthra-Derm) and calcipotriene (Dovonex)
What adverse reactions are associated with antipsoriatics?	1. *Anthralin:* staining of skin, hair, fingernails, and fabrics 2. *Calcipotriene:* local irritation, erythema, dry skin, thinning skin, hyperpigmentation
What are important nursing actions when administering antipsoriatics?	1. Wash your hands before and after applying this medication. 2. Avoid applying this medication to the patient's face or near his eyes. It's for external use only. Avoid applying anthralin to skin-fold areas (axillae, groin) because of the risk of severe soreness. 3. Apply very small amounts to affected area by gently rubbing it in. Anthralin should be left in contact with the skin for increasing amounts of time, up to 1 hour total as tolerated. 4. Monitor serum calcium levels with long-term use because of risk of rapid hypercalcemia (calcipotriene).

Treatment of bacterial skin infections

TOPICAL AGENTS

What are examples of topical agents used in the treatment of skin infections?

Mupirocin (Bactroban), neomycin, bacitracin, polymyxin B

What adverse reactions are associated with topical agents used to treat skin infections?

Burning, pruritus, rash, and the development of superinfections (due to fungal overgrowth)

What are important nursing actions when administering topical agents for a skin infection?

1. Wash your hands and put on gloves before applying the medication.
2. Avoid applying the medication over large areas of skin, to open wounds, or in or around the patient's eyes.
3. Avoid applying the medication more than three times per day, and avoid applying more than the recommended amount.
4. Monitor for signs of superinfection.

Treatment of viral skin infections

TOPICAL ANTIVIRALS

How do topical antivirals work?

By preventing the herpes simplex virus from adhering to cell membranes, thereby preventing its spread to healthy cells and shortening the duration of cold sores

What are examples of topical antivirals?

Acyclovir (Zovirax) and doconazole (Abreva)

What adverse reactions are associated with topical antivirals?

Acyclovir: local stinging and burning, rash, edema; doconazole: local skin irritation and pruritus, headache

What are important nursing actions when administering a topical antiviral?

1. Wash your hands before and after application (prevents spread to other areas of body).
2. Apply the medication only to the patient's lips and face. Avoid applying in or near his eyes.
3. Begin applying the medication at the first sign of a cold sore (tingling, burning), and continue applications until the lesion is completely healed.

4. Inform the patient that the medication doesn't cure the virus, but only shortens its duration and lessens its severity. A lesion is considered contagious until it's completely healed.
5. Notify the physician if the lesion doesn't heal within 10 to 14 days or if fever, rash, or lymphadenopathy develops.

Treatment of fungal skin infections

TOPICAL ANTIFUNGALS

How do topical antifungal agents work?	By altering fungal-cell-wall permeability
What are examples of topical antifungal agents?	Clotrimazole (Lotrimin, Mycelex), nystatin (Mycostatin), ketoconazole (Nizoral), econazole (Spectazole), ciclopirox (Loprox), butenafine (Mentax), and terbinafine (Lamisil)
What adverse reactions are commonly associated with topical antifungal agents?	Local skin irritation, erythema, burning, rash, peeling, and urticaria
What are important nursing actions when administering a topical antifungal agent?	1. Wash your hands before and after application. 2. Clean the affected area before application. 3. Avoid use in or near the patient's eyes. 4. Avoid contact with clothing because the medication may stain material. 5. Avoid the use of occlusive dressings in combination with topical antifungals. 6. Complete the full course of treatment (usually 2 weeks).

Treatment of infestations

TOPICAL AGENTS

How do topical antiinfestation agents work?	By various mechanisms, typically by disrupting the nervous systems of parasites and arthropods
What are examples of topical agents used to treat infestations?	Lindane (G-well), permethrin (Nix, Elimite), pyrethrin (Tegrin-LT), crotamiton (Eurax)

What adverse reactions are associated with the topical agents used to treat infestations?	Local skin irritation, tingling, edema, rash, and possibly seizures (lindane) ◤ *Seizures may occur with lindane if treatments are administered too closely together. Waiting 1 full week before beginning a second treatment is critical.*
What are important nursing actions when administering a topical anti-infestation agent?	1. Wash your hands and put on gloves before applying the medication. 2. Avoid use in or near the patient's eyes. 3. Avoid applying medications to open, weeping skin lesions.

Wound care

TOPICAL AGENTS

What are examples of topical agents commonly used in wound care?	1. *Silver sulfadiazine (Silvadene):* used to treat second- and third-degree burns; first-line agent for eschar because of its softening effects; not used for continuous treatment of deep burns because of adverse reactions 2. *Mafenide (Sulfamylon):* effective at eschar penetration
What adverse reactions are associated with topical agents used in the treatment of wounds?	1. *Silver sulfadiazine:* local burning, pruritus, rash; thrombocytopenia; leukopenia; allergy 2. *Mafenide:* pain on application and bicarbonate wasting ◤ *Because silver sulfadiazine and mafenide are sulfa derivatives and they can be absorbed systemically, allergic reactions are possible for persons with sulfa sensitivity.*
What are important nursing actions when administering a topical wound care agent?	1. Wash your hands and put on sterile gloves before administration. 2. Apply the medication to the wound using sterile technique to prevent wound contamination. 3. Apply cream to thickness of approximately one-sixteenth of an inch, and keep the wound covered with the cream at all times.

Nursing skills

Wound care

DRY DRESSINGS

✎ **What's the proper technique for changing a dry sterile dressing?**

1. Administer analgesics at least 30 minutes before dressing changes, when appropriate.
2. Obtain necessary supplies and equipment. Place pad underneath wound area and provide privacy.
3. Wash your hands and put on disposable gloves to remove the outer dressings. Discard the dressings and your gloves.
4. Open sterile dressing supplies and put on sterile gloves to remove and discard inner dressings. Assess the wound.
5. Clean the wound and periwound skin with gauze using strokes from top to bottom, beginning at the center working out (from least to most contaminated area; bottom is considered most contaminated). Use a separate swab for each stroke.
6. Clean any drains at the wound after the incision. Use circular strokes beginning with the area closest to the drain and then moving outwards.
7. Apply powders or ointments as ordered by the physician. Use sterile applicators for application of ointments.
8. Apply sterile dressings using sterile gloves or forceps.
9. After removing and discarding gloves, secure dressing with tape, Montgomery straps, or a binder, as appropriate.

⬧ *Remove tape or adhesive by pulling toward the wound or suture line.*

⬧ *If the dressing is attached to the wound base and debridement isn't the goal, the dressing can be moistened with water or saline to gently release tissue from dressing.*

WET-TO-DRY DRESSINGS

What's the proper technique for performing a wet-to-dry dressing change?

1. Administer analgesics at least 30 minutes before dressing changes, when appropriate.
2. Obtain the necessary supplies and equipment. Place a gauze pad underneath the wound area and provide privacy for the patient.

3. Wash your hands and put on disposable gloves to remove the outer dressings. Discard the dressings and your gloves.

4. Open sterile dressing supplies and put on sterile gloves to remove and discard inner dressings. Assess the wound.

5. Clean the wound and periwound skin with gauze using strokes from top to bottom, beginning at the center working out (from least to most contaminated area; bottom is considered most contaminated). Use a separate swab for each stroke.

6. Clean any drains at the wound after the incision. Use circular strokes beginning with the area closest to the drain and then moving outward.

7. Apply powders or ointments as ordered by the physician. Use sterile applicators for application of ointments.

8. Soak inner dressing material in sterile solution. Squeeze out excess solution to avoid over saturation.

9. Fanfold wet gauze dressing so that the wound base and all crevices are covered. Use enough gauze so that the packing material lies just above skin level.

10. Cover wet dressings with an abdominal pad.

11. After removing and discarding gloves, secure dressing with tape, Montgomery straps, or a binder, as appropriate.

▐ *Don't oversaturate gauze for a wet-to-dry dressing; dressings that are too wet won't dry completely before the next dressing change as they're intended to do.*

▐ *Avoid placing wet dressings in contact with intact skin as it will cause excoriation.*

▐ *Tight packing of a wound may produce excessive intrawound pressure, resulting in wound ischemia. Packing that's placed too loosely may cause abscess formation.*

WOUND IRRIGATIONS

What's the proper technique for performing a wound irrigation?

1. Obtain the necessary supplies and equipment.
2. Wash your hands.
3. Position the patient so that the irrigating solution will flow by gravity from the higher wound end to the lower wound end and drain into the basin.
4. Put on clean gloves and remove the old dressing. Discard the old dressing and gloves, and assess the wound.

5. Put on sterile gloves and clean the wound as directed by the physician. If ordered, apply a thin film of sterile petroleum jelly to the skin around the wound using a sterile tongue blade (protects intact skin from irrigating solution).

6. Irrigate the wound by gently instilling a steady stream of the irrigating solution into the wound through a syringe. Be sure to irrigate all areas of the wound, and continue irrigating until the solution becomes clear.

7. Dry the area around the wound with sterile forceps and sterile gauze to prevent skin irritation and microbial growth.

8. Assess the wound.

9. Apply sterile dressing to the wound according to physician's orders.

11

The musculoskeletal system

Basic concepts of the musculoskeletal system

What are the components of the musculoskeletal system?

1. *Muscles:* skeletal (voluntary, striated), visceral (involuntary, smooth), and cardiac
2. *Tendons:* strong non-elastic bands of collagen that hold muscles to bones
3. *Ligaments:* fibrous bands connecting one bone to another to strengthen the joint and either restrict or facilitate movement
4. *Bones:* hard connective tissue composed of bone cells, fat cells, blood vessels, water and minerals; form the frame (skeleton) of the body
5. *Cartilage:* dense connective tissue consisting of a strong gel-like material that cushions and absorbs shock
6. *Joints:* area where two or more bones meet
7. *Bursae:* enclosed sacs between muscles or tendons and bony prominences that are filled with viscous synovial fluid, which serve to cushion, separate, and lubricate tissue

What are synovial joints?

Freely movable joints with cartilage covering the surface of the opposing bones

What are nonsynovial joints?

Immovable (sutures of skull) or only slightly movable joints (vertebrae)

What's the purpose of synovial fluid?

Bathes articular cartilage to facilitate movement and to provide nutrients, phagocytes, and other immunologic functions within the joint

What's a meniscus?

A piece of cartilage located in certain joints that acts as a buffer between bones, lubricates the joint, and limits flexion and extension

What's muscle tone?

The degree of tension demonstrated by the resting muscle

✎ **What are the normal spinal curves?**

1. *Cervical:* concave
2. *Thoracic:* convex
3. *Lumbar:* concave
4. *Sacral:* convex

How many cervical, thoracic, lumbar, sacral, and coccygeal vertebrae are there?

7 cervical, 12 thoracic, 5 lumbar, 5 sacral, and 3 to 4 coccygeal vertebrae

What are intervertebral discs?

Fibrocartilaginous plates that cushion the spine and help it move; the elasticity of the discs provides compression on one side and expansion on the other side

Body movements

✎ **What's flexion?**

Bending a limb at a joint, thereby decreasing the joint angle

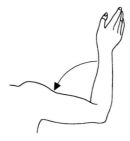

✎ **What's extension?**

Straightening a limb at a joint, thereby increasing the joint angle

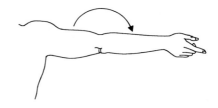

✎ **What's abduction?**

Moving a limb away from the midline of the body

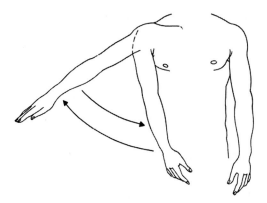

** What's adduction?**   Moving a limb toward the midline of the body

What's circumduction?   Moving in a circular manner; winding up to throw a ball is an example

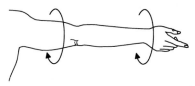

** What's supina-tion?**   Turning the forearm so that the palm is upward

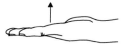

** What's pronation?**   Turning the forearm so that the palm is downward

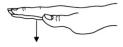

What's apposition?   Touching the thumb to the little finger

✎ What's inversion?   Turning the sole inward

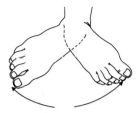

✎ What's eversion?   Turning the sole outward

✎ What's dorsi-flexion?   Pulling the foot and toes upward

✎ What's plantar flexion?   Pushing the foot and toes downward

What's internal rotation?   Turning toward midline around a central axis

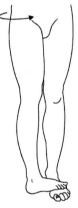

What's external rotation?   Turning away from midline around a central axis

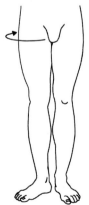

What's retraction?	Movement backward

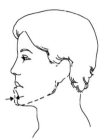

What's protraction?	Movement forward
🔖 **What are isometric exercises?**	Static movements in which muscle tension changes but no muscle or joint movement occurs and there's no change in muscle length; these types of exercises are commonly used to maintain muscle strength of a limb in a cast or traction
🔖 **What are isotonic exercises?**	Dynamic movements in which a muscle shortens to produce contraction and movement; examples include activities of daily living, active range-of-motion (ROM) exercises, and physical conditioning exercises, such as running or swimming
🔖 **What's active ROM?**	Isotonic exercise in which an individual moves a joint through its complete ROM; active ROM strengthens muscles and increases endurance
🔖 **What's passive ROM?**	An exercise in which another person moves a joint through its complete ROM in order to preserve joint mobility

Body positions

🔖 **What's Fowler's position?**	A semi-sitting position in bed in which the head of the bed is elevated 15 to 90 degrees; because it allows for greater lung expansion, Fowler's position is used for patients with respiratory or cardiovascular problems
🔖 **What's high Fowler's position?**	Fowler's position in which the head of the bed is raised 90 degrees
What's low or semi-Fowler's position?	Fowler's position in which the head of the bed is raised 15 to 45 degrees

What's the dorsal recumbent position?	A back-lying position in which the head and shoulders are slightly elevated on a pillow
What's the difference between supine and dorsal recumbent positions?	The head and shoulders aren't elevated in the supine position
✎ **What's the Trendelenburg position?**	A supine position in which the head is slightly lower than the feet; because this position distends the blood vessels in the neck and increases circulation to the brain, it's commonly used for central line placement and in the management of shock
✎ **What's the reverse Trendelenburg position?**	A supine position in which the feet are lower than the head
What's the prone position?	Face down in bed lying on the abdomen with arms in a flexed position level with the shoulders; the patient's head should be turned to one side and supported on a pillow; because it promotes mouth drainage, it's commonly used for mouth or throat postoperative patients; it may also be used for optimization of gas exchange in a patient with lung injury
What's the lateral position?	A side-lying position in which the upper hip and knee are flexed
What's the Sims' position?	A semi-prone, semi-lateral position in which the lower arm is positioned behind the patient, the upper arm is flexed at the shoulder and elbow, and the upper leg is more flexed at the hip and knee than the lower leg; it's commonly used for enema administration and for unconscious patients because it facilitates mouth drainage

Physical assessment

Normal findings

What are important considerations before beginning a musculoskeletal examination?	1. Ensure patient privacy and provide warmth. 2. Obtain the necessary equipment (tape measure, goniometer, protractor). 3. Position the table to allow complete range of motion for the patient as well as adequate access for the examiner.

What approach should be used for a musculo-skeletal examination?	Head to toe and proximal to distal examination; inspect the head and neck, spine and ribs, followed by the pelvis, upper extremities, and lower extremities
What observations should be made during a physical examination of the musculo-skeletal system?	Posture; gait (stance and swing) for foot position, balance, and coordination; and coordination of gross motor skills
How is gait assessed?	Instruct the patient to walk in a straight line for approximately 20′ (6.1 m), turn, and then return to the starting position. Evaluate for a limp, an abnormal motor pattern, or a loss of balance.
How is coordination of gait assessed?	Instruct the patient to walk in a straight line using a heel-to-toe method. Decreasing the base of support highlights problems with coordination and balance. Assess for staggering and loss of balance.
✎ **What factors should be assessed during inspection and palpation of the muscles?**	1. *Tone:* tension in a resting muscle 2. *Mass:* measure circumferences of muscles (typically thigh, calf, and upper arm) 3. *Strength:* measured on a 5-point scale (5 is normal, active range of motion against full resistance, 0 is paralysis)
What constitutes a normal muscle examination?	Firm with slight resistance during passive movement; muscle size should be almost equal bilaterally; the dominant side may be slightly larger (up to 1 cm larger)
Why are muscle groups assessed bilaterally?	To determine presence of muscle atrophy
✎ **How is muscle strength assessed?**	By applying resistance as the patient performs active range-of-motion (ROM) exercises; the applied force should be fully resisted and equal bilaterally ⚡ *Never force movement if resistance is met or if the patient reports pain or discomfort with movement.*
What factors should be assessed during inspection and palpation of the bones and joints?	1. Measurement of patient height as well as comparison of length of extremities 2. Characteristics of bones and joints 3. ROM of joints

How is ROM assessed?	Request active ROM; if ROM is limited, carefully attempt passive motion by supporting the joint with one hand and slowly moving the joint to its limit with the other hand. Note any pain, crepitation, or contractures.

▐ *If a patient can't perform active ROM, the joint should be moved through passive ROM.*

What factors should be assessed when inspecting a joint?	1. Size and contour of the joint, noting any swelling or deformity 2. Color of skin over the joint
What factors should be assessed during palpation of a joint?	1. Skin temperature 2. The joint, muscles, bony articulations, and joint capsule 3. Presence of heat, swelling, tenderness, or masses
Is the synovial membrane normally palpable?	No; a small amount of fluid is contained in a normal joint; however, it isn't palpable

Abstract findings

Abnormal findings

🔖 **What are examples of coordination abnormalities involving voluntary movement?**	1. *Ataxia:* impaired coordination, usually involving erratic muscular activity 2. *Tremor:* quivering of muscles 3. *Spasticity:* jerky, stiff movements
What's a fasciculation?	The localized, involuntary, visible twitching of a single muscle group innervated by a single motor nerve fiber
What's atony?	Loss of normal muscle tension
🔖 **What's a Parkinsonian gait?**	Shuffling, short gait in which the head and neck lean forward and arm swing is decreased
What gait changes commonly occur in elderly patients?	Shorter steps, slower speed, and decreased balance
🔖 **What's atrophy?**	Loss of muscle mass that may occur as a result of muscle disuse, muscle tissue damage, or lower motor neuron disease
🔖 **What's hypertrophy?**	Increase in muscle bulk

What's a contusion?	Disruption of soft tissue and muscle fibers that results from a blunt injury
🖎 **What's a contracture?**	The permanent tightening (and shortening) of a muscle, tendon, ligament, or skin, which prevents normal movement of the affected area; scarring, nerve damage, or lack of use due to immobility are common causes
What's an example of a pathologic contracture?	Burn scar tissue or Achilles tendon contractures
What's a Dupuytren's contracture?	A painless tightening of the tissue underneath the skin at the palm that causes difficulties extending the fingers; although the exact cause is unknown, it may be associated with alcoholism, diabetes, liver disease, and epilepsy
🖎 **What's footdrop?**	Plantar flexion of the foot caused by shortening of the Achilles tendon that occurs after the foot has assumed an unsupported position for a prolonged period of time; the foot of long-term injury patients should be supported in dorsiflexion through the use of a footboard, ankle splints, or high-top sneakers
🖎 **What's crepitation?**	A palpable or audible grating or crunching that occurs when irregular bone edges rub together
What's a ganglion?	A nontender, cystic nodule overlying a joint capsule or a tendon sheath that's caused by fluid leakage into a sac; repeated injuries to a particular area may cause irritation and tearing of the membrane overlying a tendon; ganglia are also known as synovial cysts and they most commonly occur on the dorsal surface of the hand
🖎 **What's scoliosis?**	Abnormal lateral (sideways) curvature of the spine; scoliosis should be suspected if the shoulders or the hips (hemlines of clothing) appear uneven; back braces (Milwaukee, Boston, and Wilmington braces) may be used to straighten the spine by application of asymmetric pressure
🖎 **What's kyphosis?**	Excessive curvature of the thoracic spine ("humpback" or "hunchback"), which may result from osteoarthritis, rheumatoid arthritis, osteoporosis, congenital anomalies, or some diseases of the spine
What's kyphoscoliosis?	An abnormally exaggerated front-to-back curvature of the spine that results in the appearance of a rounded back

✎ What's lordosis? An exaggerated curvature of the lumbar spine (dorsal concavity); pregnancy and morbid obesity increase the risk for lordosis

What's myositis? An inflammation of the skeletal (voluntary) muscles that commonly results from infection or injury

What's synovitis? Palpable bogginess of the synovial membrane

What might asymmetrical size of the same joints on the left and right sides of the body indicate? Bacterial arthritis; rheumatoid arthritis typically affects joints symmetrically

What might difficulty with arm abduction and pain in the deltoid muscle indicate? A rotator cuff tear; pain over the supraspinatus tendon insertion site may also be diagnostic

✎ What assessment descriptors are used in the evaluation of abnormal muscle tone or strength?

1. *Atrophy:* loss of muscle tissue from lack of use or from disease; "wasting"
2. *Flaccidity:* lack of tone; diminished resistance to passive movement
3. *Spasticity:* hypertonicity; rigid muscles with exaggerated deep tendon reflexes, which interfere with normal function; may be either sustained stiffness or intermittent spasms
4. *Contracture:* permanent tightening of muscles, tendons, ligaments, or skin that inhibits normal movement; may result in permanent deformity

What are shin splints? Pain that affects the front of the lower extremities that most commonly occurs as a result of strenuous activity following a period of inactivity

What are muscle spasms? Involuntary contractions of a muscle that occur from overuse or from an injury; stretching before an activity and maintaining hydration will help prevent spasms; application of ice packs, stretching, and massaging the affected muscle help alleviate the cramp

What's coccydynia? Pain of the coccyx most commonly caused by trauma to the area; donut-cushions and anti-inflammatory medications are common treatment measures

What's varus? An abnormal position involving the turning inward (toward midline) of part of an extremity

| **What's valgus?** | An abnormal position involving the bending or twisting outward (away from midline) of part of an extremity |

Major disorders of the muscles

Soft tissue injuries

STRAINS

✎ **What's a strain?**	Injury to a muscle or tendon from abnormal stretching or from tearing, which causes hemorrhage into the tissue; also known as *pulled muscles*
	⚡ *Strains involve tendons or muscles, whereas sprains involve ligaments.*
What's the patho-physiologic process of a strain?	Hemorrhage into nearby tissues occurs when a muscle or tendon is suddenly contracted or stretched abnormally far, which causes pain and possible loss of function.

How are strains classified?	1. *Grade I (mild):* indicates a slightly pulled muscle without significant disruption of the muscle tendon unit
	2. *Grade II (moderate):* indicates some disruption of the muscle tendon unit with loss of strength and limited movement
	3. *Grade III (severe):* indicates a complete rupture in the muscle tendon unit with bruising, pain, and obvious defect in the muscle on palpation

| **What are the clinical manifestations of a strain?** | Pain, muscle spasm or weakness, edema, cramping, and possible loss of muscle function |

| **What complications are associated with strains?** | Permanent decrease in muscle strength, increased susceptibility to reinjury, and muscle rupture with severe strain |

What's the typical treatment for a strain?	1. Rest the affected area by avoiding weight-bearing activities for 48 hours.
	2. Place an ice pack on the affected area 20 minutes at a time several times per day.
	3. Compress the affected area with elastic wraps, splints, or air casts.
	4. Elevate the affected area above the level of the heart whenever possible.

5. Use of anti-inflammatory medications, which may further reduce swelling and discomfort.
6. Seek surgery (if required) for some grade III strains.

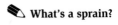 *Remember RICE for treatment of both sprains and strains in the first 48 hours: Rest, Ice, Compression, Elevation.*

What are important nursing actions in the care of a patient with a strain?

1. Instruct the patient to rest, elevate the affected extremity, and avoid weight bearing on the affected extremity for 48 hours.
2. Apply an ice pack to affected area for the acute phase (first 48 hours). Warm, moist heat should be applied after the acute phase.
3. Assess neurovascular status of the affected extremity.
4. Apply elastic wraps, splints, or air casts for compression of the affected area.
5. Administer anti-inflammatory medications as ordered by the physician.
6. Encourage slow stretching exercises before vigorous activities to minimize recurrence once able to return to normal function.

SPRAIN

What's a sprain?

Injury involving a ligament, joint capsule, or synovial membrane, which causes loss of functional stability (joint laxity) to the affected ligament

What's the pathophysiologic process of a sprain?

Ligaments are stretched or torn, which causes swelling and discomfort secondary to extravasation of blood into the surrounding tissues

How are sprains classified?

1. *Grade I (mild):* overstretching or partial tearing of ligaments without loss of joint stability
2. *Grade II (moderate):* partial tearing of a ligament with some loss of function and difficulty with weight bearing
3. *Grade III (severe):* complete tear or rupture of a ligament with inability to bear weight

What are the clinical manifestations of a sprain?

Pain (due to the large number of nerve endings in affected area), swelling, bruising, and loss of functional ability of the joint

What complications are associated with sprains?

Dislocation, hemarthrosis (blood in joint space), and avulsion fracture (fragment of bone pulled loose by severely sprained ligament)

What's the typical treatment for a sprain?

RICE (Rest, Ice, Compression, Elevation) treatment in the acute phase as well as nonsteroidal anti-inflammatory medications (NSAIDs)

What are important nursing actions in the care of a patient with a sprain?

1. Instruct the patient to rest, elevate the affected extremity, and avoid weight bearing on the affected extremity for 48 hours.
2. Apply an ice pack to the affected area for the acute phase (first 48 hours). Warm, moist heat should be applied after the acute phase.
3. Assess neurologic and circulatory status of the affected extremity.
4. Apply elastic wraps, splints, or air casts for compression of the affected area.
5. Administer medications (NSAIDs) as ordered by the physician.
6. Encourage slow stretching exercises before vigorous activities to minimize recurrence once the patient is able to return to normal function.

MENISCUS INJURY

What's a meniscus injury?

An injury (usually a tear) from rotational stress of the shock-absorbing cartilage (meniscus) of the knee that's commonly associated with ligament sprains

What's the pathophysiologic process of a meniscus injury?

Most commonly occurs when the knee is bent or twisted during weight bearing; swelling, discomfort, and loss of function may occur as a result of synovial effusions

What are the clinical manifestations of a meniscus injury?

Joint tenderness or pain that worsens when the area is palpated or swelling and locking or catching of the joint; the inability to fully extend the knee without discomfort is a strong indication that a meniscus tear has occurred

What physical tests are used to diagnose a meniscus injury?

1. *McMurray's test:* pain or a click over the knee joint when the leg is straightened and the foot turned inward is positive for a meniscus injury
2. *Ballottement test:* palpation technique to assess for synovial effusions; positive test indicates fluid and swelling around the joint

What conservative treatment may be used for a meniscus injury?

Application of ice, immobilization of the knee, protected weight bearing, and administration of NSAIDs as well as possible aspiration of fluid from the knee

What surgical procedures may be necessary for treatment of a meniscus injury?	Arthroscopy with meniscectomy is advised if persistent or recurrent locking, effusion, or disabling pain occurs
What complications are associated with a meniscus injury?	Atrophy of the quadriceps (if chronic injury) or degenerative joint disease
When can a patient with a meniscus injury resume exercising?	Physical activity is generally allowed as tolerated. Isometric quadriceps exercises (straight leg lifts) should be performed frequently throughout the day during the acute phase of injury. Once isometric quadriceps exercises can be done comfortably, graded resistance should be added as tolerated.
What are important nursing actions in the care of a patient with a meniscal injury?	1. Apply ice to minimize swelling during the acute phase of an injury. 2. Instruct the patient to avoid full weight bearing, if painful. Provide crutches or a knee immobilizer to prevent further injury. 3. Administer medications (NSAIDs) as ordered by the physician. 4. Encourage knee-strengthening exercises such as straight-leg raising.

BURSITIS

What's bursitis?	Inflammation of bursae (sacs of synovial fluid) that typically occurs over areas subject to friction, such as the elbow or shoulder; repeated or excessive injury, rheumatoid arthritis, gout, and infection are common causes
What's the pathophysiologic process of bursitis?	Inflammation of the bursae causes increased irritation with movement
What are the clinical manifestations of bursitis?	Pain with movement, restricted movement, and edema
What complications are associated with bursitis?	Chronic pain and freezing or locking of the affected area
What's the typical treatment for bursitis?	Rest or immobilization of the affected area, use of NSAIDs, and local application of cold packs; aspiration of the bursae and steroid injections are other treatment mea-

sures, and surgical procedures involving excision of the bursa or drainage of infectious material may be necessary

What are important nursing actions in the care of a patient with bursitis?

1. Instruct the patient to rest the affected area.
2. Apply cold packs or cool compresses to the affected area.
3. Administer medications (NSAIDs) as ordered by the physician.

TENDONITIS

What's tendonitis?

An inflammation of a tendon that can result from overuse or injury

What's the pathophysiologic process of tendonitis?

Inflammation or irritation of a tendon results in pain and tenderness, particularly with movement

What are the clinical manifestations of tendonitis?

Pain located near a joint that worsens with movement, inflamed and boggy tendon as well as warmth and erythema of overlying skin

What complications are associated with tendonitis?

Recurrent episodes of tendonitis and possible rupture of the tendon

What's the typical treatment for tendonitis?

1. Rest and immobilization of the affected tendon to reduce inflammation and relieve pain
2. Application of heat or cold to the affected area
3. Use of NSAIDs to reduce inflammation and relieve pain

What are important nursing actions in the care of a patient with tendonitis?

1. Instruct the patient to warm up prior to vigorous exercising.
2. Instruct the patient to avoid repetitive actions or overuse of extremities to prevent recurrence.
3. Administer medications (NSAIDs) as ordered by the physician.

DISLOCATION

What's a dislocation?

Separation or displacement of the articular surfaces of a joint as a result of injury to the ligamentous structures surrounding the joint

What's the patho- physiologic process of a dislocation?	The ends of the affected bones are forced from their nor- mal positions, which temporarily deform and immobilize the joint
✎ **What are the clin- ical manifestations of a dislocation?**	Asymmetrical changes in joint or musculoskeletal con- tour, pain, restricted movement, edema, and bruising

▷ *The affected extremity may appear shorter when it's dislocated.*

✎ **What complica- tions are associated with dislocations?**	Torn ligaments, nerve injury, open joint injuries, intra- articular fractures, increased susceptibility to reinjury (scar tissue is weaker than original tissue), and avascular necrosis if the dislocation remains unreduced (not re- aligned)

▷ *The risk for development of avascular necrosis increases the longer the joint remains unreduced.*

What's the typical treatment for a dislo- cation?	Open (surgical) or closed (nonsurgical) reduction and joint immobilization to permit healing of torn ligaments
What are important nursing actions in the care of a patient with a dislocation?	1. Immobilize or splint the affected area. Avoid attempts to straighten or change the position of the affected area.
	2. Apply ice or cool compresses to minimize swelling and discomfort.
	3. Maintain nothing-by-mouth status immediately fol- lowing dislocation.
	4. Assess circulatory status of the affected area but avoid assessment of function of any bone or joint that ap- pears misshapen or misaligned.
	5. Monitor for complications and notify the physician immediately if any develop.

SUBLUXATION

✎ **What's a sub- luxation?**	Partial dislocation of a bone in a joint
What's the patho- physiologic process of a subluxation?	Partial separation or displacement of the articular surfaces of a joint as a result of injury to the ligamentous struc- tures surrounding the joint
What are the clinical manifestations of a subluxation?	Pain and limitation of movement, although less severe than a dislocation

What complications are associated with a subluxation?

Similar to those that occur with a dislocation (torn ligaments, dislocations), although they generally occur less frequently and are less severe

Can subluxation become a chronic condition?

Yes; chronic glenohumeral instability is an example and occurs when a shoulder can voluntarily be dislocated

What's the typical treatment for a subluxation?

Immobilization or splinting of the affected area and application of ice or cool compresses are used in the acute phase. Chronic instability that can result from a subluxation is treated by strengthening the affected muscles through a rehabilitation program to compensate for the loose ligaments and to prevent further injuries. However, surgery may be necessary if the joint can't be stabilized sufficiently.

What are important nursing actions in the care of a patient with a subluxation?

1. Immobilize or splint the affected area. Avoid attempts to straighten or change the position of the affected area.
2. Apply ice or cool compresses to minimize swelling and discomfort.
3. Maintain nothing-by-mouth status immediately after dislocation.
4. Assess circulatory status of the affected area but avoid assessment of function of any bone or joint that appears misshapen or misaligned.
5. Monitor for complications such as nerve injury and notify the physician immediately if any develop.

CARPAL TUNNEL SYNDROME

✎ What's carpal tunnel syndrome?

Pain and weakness in the hands caused by median nerve compression at the wrist that occurs with inflammation and edema of a tendon, or with pressure from trauma; commonly associated with activities that involve repetitive wrist movements such as typing; also known as *median nerve dysfunction*

What's the pathophysiologic process of carpal tunnel syndrome?

Pressure is exerted on the median nerve, which causes numbness, tingling, and weakness of the hand

✎ What are the clinical manifestations of carpal tunnel syndrome?

Pain or weakness in one or both hands, weakened grip in one or both hands, uncoordinated fine finger movements in one or both hands, or numbness or tingling in the thumb and first fingers of one or both hands

What's Tinel's sign?

Shooting pain, tingling, or numbness from the wrist to the hand that occurs when the median nerve at the wrist is tapped in the presence of carpal tunnel syndrome

What's Phalen's test?

Pain, tingling, or numbness that occurs when the wrist is fully flexed in the presence of carpal tunnel syndrome

What complications are associated with carpal tunnel syndrome?

Permanent median nerve damage and atrophy of the thenar muscles, resulting in dysfunction of the hand

What's the typical treatment for carpal tunnel syndrome?

1. Use of wrist splints worn at night
2. Application of heat or cool compresses
3. Modifications of work environment, duties, and activities
4. Use of NSAIDs or injection of corticosteroids in carpal tunnel space

What type of surgery may be used to treat carpal tunnel syndrome?

Carpal tunnel release, in which a ligament is cut to relieve pressure on the median nerve; healing of the damaged nerve may take months

What are important nursing actions in the care of a patient with carpal tunnel syndrome?

1. Encourage the use of splints to protect the wrist.
2. Apply heat or cool compresses to decrease edema and pain.
3. Administer medications (NSAIDs) as ordered by the physician.
4. Assess neurovascular status of the hand, especially following surgical interventions.
5. Encourage modifications of activities and the work environment.

Major disorders of the spine

Back pain and strain

What's back pain?

Discomfort in any part of the back that can be caused by many factors, such as muscle strains, muscle spasms, osteoarthritis, or disc herniation

What's the pathophysiologic process of back pain?

A variety of factors may cause or exacerbate back pain; however, the source of discomfort may be muscular, skeletal, or neurologic in nature

What are some factors that may cause back pain?	Muscular strain, back overuse or injury, poor posture, excess weight, disc herniations, osteoarthritis, compression of a nerve root, and muscular disorders
How is chronic back pain defined?	Pain lasting 3 months or more, or repeated episodes of incapacitating back pain
🖎 **What's the most common cause of chronic back pain?**	Chronic instability of the posterior facets combined with a degeneration of the intervertebral disc that may be aggravated by weak abdominal and back muscles
🖎 **What life-threatening condition can present as lower back pain?**	Ruptured aortic aneurysm
What complications are associated with back pain?	Neurologic complications and disability
What's the typical treatment for chronic back pain?	Exercise, medications (NSAIDs, muscle relaxants, steroid injections), and use of transcutaneous electrical nerve stimulation unit; surgical intervention may be necessary depending on the underlying cause

🖎 **What are important nursing actions in the care of a patient with back pain?**	1. Encourage bed rest and inform the patient that walking, bending, and lifting may exacerbate pain and muscle spasms.
	2. Encourage the patient to sleep on a firm mattress.
	3. Instruct the patient to slowly increase activity once symptoms have resolved. Encourage exercises that strengthen the back, abdomen, and legs.
	4. Administer medications (NSAIDs, muscle relaxants, and steroids) as ordered by the physician.
	5. Apply moist heat to the affected area.
	6. Encourage the patient to maintain a healthy weight.
	7. Educate the patient regarding proper body mechanics, especially for lifting heavy objects (lift with legs while keeping back straight, keep object close to body).

Disc herniation

🖎 **What's a disc herniation?**	Also referred to as a *slipped disc;* a condition in which the nucleus pulposus (gel-like substance) is pushed out of the outer disc margin (annulus) of an intervertebral disc into the spinal canal, causing pressure on spinal nerves; it most commonly occurs in the lumbar spine because it carries the majority of the body's weight (See illustration, page 324)

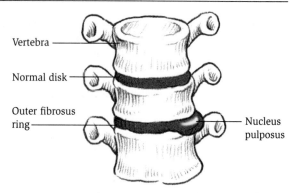

What's the patho-physologic process of a disc herniation?

Over time, the inner nucleus changes from a gel to a more fibrous material with decreased elasticity. When the interior disc material extrudes into the spinal canal, it compresses the spinal nerves, causing inflammation and pain associated with radiculopathy (neurologic deficit).

What are risk factors for the development of a herniated disc?

Weakened trunk musculature, frequent bending and twisting motions, lifting objects in combination with lateral bending and twisting, sudden movements and lifting while in a seated position

✎ What are the clinical manifestations of a herniated intervertebral disc?

1. *Pain and tenderness:* lower back tenderness, sciatica (sharp pain radiation from the low back through the buttock and down the leg); pain worsens with flexion and improves with extension and pain improves with rest
2. *Sensory changes:* paresthesia, numbness
3. *Motor changes:* weakness, decreased mobility, pain with knee extension and hip flexion in supine position (positive straight-leg raise test)

⚡ *The vertebral level of the disc herniation determines which extremities are affected.*

How is a herniated disc diagnosed?

Physical examination (including straight-leg raising test) or a magnetic resonance imaging of the lumbar spine

✎ What's the typical pattern of pain associated with disc herniation?

Unilateral pain that begins as an ache in the buttocks and radiates to the posterior thigh or calf

How does disc pain differ from a pinched nerve?

Pain from the disc itself produces referred or axial pain, whereas a pinched nerve produces radicular pain (nerve root or sciatica)

✎ What complications are associated with disc herniations?

Incapacitating lower back pain, permanent numbness, and cauda equine syndrome (bowel and bladder incontinence with perineal numbness)

What's the treatment for disc herniation?

1. Bed rest
2. Traction (especially with sciatic pain)
3. Medications including NSAIDs and muscle relaxants as well as possible epidural steroid injections
4. Local cold (first 48 hours) and heat (after first 48 hours) applications
5. Back supports
6. Lower back strengthening and stretching exercises
7. Therapeutic ultrasound (localized tissue heating to reduce chronic inflammation)
8. Treatment with transcutaneous electrical nerve stimulation unit inhibits pain perception

What types of surgery may be used in the treatment of disc herniation?

1. *Percutaneous endoscopic discectomy:* removal of extruded disc material under a microscope
2. *Laminectomy:* removal of a portion of a vertebra to relieve pressure on a spinal nerve (if the symptoms persist and become intolerable)
3. *Chemonucleolysis:* injection of a papaya extract (chymopapain) dissolves the extruded disc material and causes the disc to collapse
4. *Spinal fusion:* insertion of bone chips in the disc interspace to encourage new bone growth around the graft; the new bone growth fuses the vertebrae together and stabilizes the affected segment

✎ What are important nursing actions in the care of a patient with a disc herniation?

1. Encourage bed rest and a comfortable posture for several days (decreases inflammation of spinal nerve).
2. Administer medications (NSAIDs) as ordered by the physician.
3. Instruct the patient about proper body mechanics (lifting objects with his legs while holding object close to his body) and to avoid bending or twisting movements. Instruct him to avoid heavy lifting.
4. Instruct the patient to protect his back for at least 9 months after disc herniation.
5. Encourage lower back exercises once inflammation has subsided.
6. Anticipate physical therapy referral for back strengthening exercises.
7. Encourage frequent stretch breaks when sitting for a prolonged period (driving).
8. Encourage the use of lumbar supports to encourage proper alignment of the spine.

Degenerative disc disease

What's degenerative disc disease (DDD)?

A condition involving the deterioration of the discs between the vertebrae of the spine, which decreases the spine's ability to withstand mechanical stress

What's the pathophysiologic process of DDD?

Loss of disc height and water content cause the disc to collapse and possibly pinch a nerve root

What are the clinical manifestations of DDD?

1. Midline back pain that's worse with sitting, standing, bending, or lifting
2. Referred pain to buttocks, iliac crests, sacroiliac joints, and backs of thighs

What complications are associated with DDD?

Formation of osteophytes (bone spurs), disc herniation, and spinal stenosis

What's the typical treatment for DDD?

Conservative therapy includes bed rest, medications (NSAIDs, muscle relaxants, oral steroids), abdominal and trunk strengthening exercises, and braces to immobilize the disc space or to decrease the pressure on the degenerated disc.

Surgery (fusion procedures or those that involve heating catheters inserted through a disc to create new scar tissue around the disc for increased stability) may be attempted for those who fail at least 6 months of conservative measures.

What's spinal stenosis?

A narrowing of the spinal canal, nerve root canals, or intervertebral foramina caused by degenerative changes, trauma, or tumor of the spine

What are important nursing actions in the care of a patient with DDD?

1. Promote bed rest.
2. Encourage strengthening exercises for the trunk and abdomen.
3. Encourage the use of braces, if prescribed.
4. Administer medications (NSAIDs, muscle relaxants, oral steroids) as ordered by the physician.

Duchenne muscular dystrophy

What's muscular dystrophy?

An X-linked, progressive disorder involving skeletal muscle weakness and degeneration that ultimately leads to deformity and disability; there's no nerve involvement with muscular dystrophy; because it's X-linked, women are almost never affected

What's the patho-physiologic process of muscular dystrophy?

A genetic defect involving the production of muscle protein, dystrophin, which causes atrophy of muscle fibers; they are eventually replaced with fat and connective tissue, which can progress to fibrosis

What are the clinical manifestations of Duchenne muscular dystrophy?

Symmetrical muscle weakness and atrophy, which begins in the legs and pelvis

What complications are associated with Duchenne muscular dystrophy?

Progressive debilitation, contractures, fractures, obesity, respiratory infections, and cardiac decompensation

What's the typical treatment for Duchenne muscular dystrophy?

1. Although there's no cure, treatment includes performance of range-of-motion (ROM) exercises, use of orthotics and leg braces for support, and pharmacologic therapy with quinine, procainamide, and phenytoin for symptoms of myotonia.
2. Surgical intervention including fasciotomy or tendon lengthening may enhance ambulation.

What are important nursing actions in the care of a patient with muscular dystrophy?

1. Encourage independence with activities, but provide assistance as needed.
2. Perform ROM exercises to maintain the patient's joint flexibility.
3. Administer medications (quinine, procainamide, phenytoin) as ordered by the physician.

Arthritis and other rheumatic disorders

Degenerative arthritis

OSTEOARTHRITIS OR DEGENERATIVE JOINT DISEASE

What's osteoarthritis (degenerative joint disease)?

The most common form of arthritis, which involves the degeneration of cartilage and bones from "wear and tear" over time and possibly the formation of bone spurs (new bones) at the joint margins; primarily affects middle-aged and older adults; joints that have been previously injured or those subjected to prolonged heavy use are most susceptible

What's the patho-physiologic process of osteoarthritis?

Abnormal cartilage repair and remodeling, alterations in hyaluronic acid levels in synovial fluid, or the destruction of cartilage by proteolytic enzymes cause an asymmetric loss or degeneration of cartilage, resulting in bone rubbing on bone

✎ What clinical manifestations are associated with osteoarthritis?

1. Joint pain, aching, or swelling of gradual onset that worsens in humid (rainy) weather or with activity
2. Morning joint stiffness
3. Limited range of motion
4. Joint effusion, instability, or crepitation (grating sensation with movement)
5. Presence of Heberden's nodes (small, bony nodules of the fingertips)

⚡ *Unlike other arthritic conditions, osteoarthritis is not associated with systemic manifestations.*

✎ What joints are commonly affected?

Weight-bearing joints, such as the hips and knees, are the most susceptible, although the cervical and lumbar spine and joints of the hands and feet can also be affected.

⚡ *In contrast with rheumatoid arthritis, the wrist, elbow, and ankle joints are spared in osteoarthritis.*

How is osteoarthritis diagnosed?

Physical examination and possibly X-rays of the affected joints; blood tests including erythrocyte sedimentation rate and rheumatoid factor may be useful to exclude other causes

What complications are associated with osteoarthritis?

Chronic pain, limited range of motion, muscle contractures, and atrophy as well as disabilities

What's the typical treatment for osteoarthritis?

1. Low-impact aerobic exercise and strengthening exercises; physical therapy is usually of benefit
2. Weight reduction for overweight individuals (reduces pressure on knees and other weight-bearing joints)
3. Applications of heat and ice to decrease swelling and pain
4. Applications of topical capsaicin cream for refractory joint pain
5. Medications such as acetaminophen, NSAIDs, COX-2 inhibitors, oral glucosamine or chondroitin, and corticosteroid injections
6. Injection of artificial joint fluids such as sodium hyaluronate (Synvisc) into the knee for temporary pain relief (up to 6 months)
7. Surgery for severe, debilitating arthritis

⚡ *Corticosteroid injections should be avoided in the setting of infectious arthritis, a joint prosthesis, or* *unstable joints. No more than three steroid injections should be administered per year in a weight-bearing joint.*

What types of surgery may be used in the treatment of arthritis?

1. *Arthroscopy:* involves the use of a small camera located at the tip of a tube that's inserted into a joint for removal of torn or damaged cartilage and washing out of the joint
2. *Arthroplasty:* involves partial or total replacement of a damaged joint with an artificial one
3. *Osteostomy:* involves repositioning a bone that's close to a damaged joint to relieve pressure from the arthritic portion of the joint and transfer the pressure to an area with more normal cartilage
4. *Arthrodesis:* involves the surgical fusion of bones to reduce pain and improve stability

What are important nursing actions in the care of a patient with osteoarthritis?

1. Encourage the patient to avoid overuse of joints.
2. Encourage the use of assistive devices to support the joints during activities.
3. Encourage weight loss in overweight patients.
4. Encourage the patient to engage in appropriate exercises (low impact aerobic) such as swimming.
5. Encourage stretching prior to any exercise.
6. Encourage warm baths.

Pain associated with degenerative arthritis is typically worse at the end of the day or with activity, whereas the pain associated with inflammatory arthritis is typically worse in the morning and improves throughout the day.

Inflammatory arthritis

RHEUMATOID ARTHRITIS

What's rheumatoid arthritis (RA)?

A chronic, autoimmune-related disease characterized by recurrent inflammation of the lining of a joint (synovium), which causes destructive changes in the joint; most commonly affected areas include the small joints of the hands and feet as well as the wrists, and joints are typically *symmetrically* affected (both wrists, both knees); other affected areas may include the knees, shoulders, hips, spine, and neck; women are affected twice as often as men

What's the pathophysiologic process of RA?

Although the exact cause is unknown, an autoimmune mediated process is involved, which causes white blood cells to enter the synovial membrane, resulting in chronic inflammation

✎ What are the clinical manifestations of RA?

1. *Early stage:* fatigue, malaise, morning stiffness longer than 1 hour in duration, diffuse muscle aches, anorexia; low-grade fever; widened joint space on X-ray
2. *Later stage:* joint pain associated with edema, erythema, tenderness or stiffness (commonly symmetrical and bilateral); development of firm, nontender, mobile subcutaneous nodules, commonly at pressure points; destruction and fusion of joints on X-ray

What complications are associated with RA?

Because it's a systemic disease, almost every organ system can be affected. GI bleeding, pericarditis, heart failure, pleuritis, pulmonary fibrosis, anemia, thrombocytopenia, eye involvement, vasculitis, neuropathy, and joint deformities including instability of the cervical spine are all complications associated with rheumatoid arthritis.

▨ *Rheumatoid arthritis is generally more disabling than osteoarthritis.*

What's the typical treatment for RA?

1. Use of COX-2 inhibitors (rofecoxib, celecoxib), NSAIDs (ibuprofen, indomethacin, naproxen), disease-modifying antirheumatoid drugs (DMARDs) such as methotrexate, and antitumor necrosis factor (anti-TNF) agents, such as infliximab (Remicade) and etanercept (Enbrel); other medications may include hydrochloroquine (Plaquenil), sulfasalazine, and corticosteroids (low doses, short courses)
2. Performance of ROM and strengthening exercises with frequent rest periods
3. Heat and cold treatments as well as possible electrical stimulation
4. Use of splints and orthotic devices to support and align joints
5. Surgery such as a synovectomy (removal of synovial membrane) or possibly joint replacement in severe cases
6. Apheresis to remove inflammatory antibodies from the blood in persons with refractory RA

✎ What are important nursing actions in the care of a patient with RA?

1. Encourage ROM and strengthening exercises to maintain flexibility.
2. Encourage the use of splints or other orthotic devices, if prescribed.
3. Administer medications (COX-2 inhibitors, NSAIDs, DMARDs, anti-TNF agents) as ordered by the physician.
4. Obtain laboratory studies to monitor for adverse reactions (increased liver function tests).

SPONDYLITIS

What's spondylitis?

A form of arthritis that causes inflammation of the spinal joints and the peripheral joints of the extremities; it can also affect ligaments and tendons that attach to bones; the affected bones eventually fuse together as a result of chronic inflammation, damage to the joint and the joint's attempt to heal, and immovable joints or a rigid spine may occur

What's the patho-physiologic process of spondylitis?

Inflammation of one or more vertebrae causes pain and discomfort in the back and may result in the fusion of the affected vertebrae; although the exact mechanism of the disease isn't well understood, genetic factors are suspected

What's ankylosing spondylitis?

A form of inflammatory arthritis that typically affects the sacroiliac joints, the hips, and the spine

What clinical manifestations are associated with spondylitis?

Aches, pains, or stiffness in the lower back, buttocks, and hips that worsen after periods of inactivity are the most common early symptoms. However, fever, fatigue, and anorexia may also occur because the disease is systemic in nature. The eyes, lungs, and heart may also be affected.

What complications are associated with spondylitis?

Permanent immobility of affected joints, difficulty with deep breathing (if ribs are affected), poor posture, deformities, heart valve disease, uveitis (eye inflammation), and pulmonary fibrosis

What's the typical treatment for spondylitis?

1. Physical and occupational therapy as well as daily physical activities to maintain function and minimize deformity
2. Anti-inflammatory medications (NSAIDs), such as ibuprofen, naproxen, and piroxicam
3. Disease-modifying anti-rheumatic drugs (DMARDs), such as methotrexate and sulfasalazine
4. Corticosteroid injection
5. Artificial joint replacement surgery for severe joint disease of hips or knees

What are important nursing actions in the care of a patient with spondylitis?

1. Encourage the patient to sleep on a hard mattress to keep his back straight. Instruct him to avoid using multiple or large pillows to prevent neck flexion.
2. Advise the patient to select chairs that maintain good posture (armchairs are better than chairs without arms).
3. Encourage daily ROM exercises as well as physical activities, such as swimming, to maintain joint mobility.

4. Instruct the patient to avoid sudden impacts whenever possible due to risk of injury to rigid neck and back.
5. Encourage deep-breathing exercises to maintain flexibility of rib cage.
6. Administer medications to reduce inflammation (NSAIDs, DMARDs) as ordered by the physician.

GOUT

What's gout?

An arthritic condition of abnormal purine metabolism that causes the deposition of needle-like uric acid crystals in tissues, particularly the joints of the great toes, ankles, heels, and knees; heavy alcohol use, male gender, renal disease, diabetes, obesity, and sickle cell anemia are all associated with an increased incidence of gout

What's the pathophysiologic process of gout?

Uric acid is either overproduced due to a metabolic defect or is ineffectively excreted by the kidneys, which results in crystal formation and deposition in joints

Uric acid is a by-product of purine metabolism.

What are tophi?

Collections of uric acid crystals underneath the skin

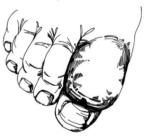

What are the clinical manifestations associated with gout?

Joint swelling, stiffness, pain of sudden onset, warmth, and erythema most commonly affecting the great toes, ankles, and knees; chalk-like drainage from a skin lump as well as a fever may also be present

What complications are associated with gout?

Development of chronic gout, joint deformities, renal calculi, or renal dysfunction

What's the typical treatment for acute gout attacks?

Colchicine (reduces the joint inflammation caused by uric acid crystals) and nonsteroidal anti-inflammatory drugs such as indomethacin

Colchicine does not decrease uric acid levels.

✎ What's the typical treatment for chronic gout?

1. Uric acid lowering agents, such as probenecid (helps kidneys eliminate uric acid), sulfinpyrazone, or allopurinol (blocks uric acid production)
2. Colchicine to prevent future acute attacks

✎ What are important nursing actions in the care of a patient with gout?

1. Encourage bed rest and immobilization of the affected extremity during an attack.
2. Administer medications (antigout agents and anti-inflammatory agents) as ordered by the physician.
3. Instruct the patient to increase fluid intake to prevent the development of renal calculi.
4. Encourage a low-purine diet (no organ meats, anchovies, herring, mackerel, dried peas, or beans) and avoidance of alcoholic beverages (may precipitate attacks).
5. Encourage weight loss to reduce stress on the patient's joints if he's overweight. Rapid weight loss and fasting should be discouraged because they increase uric acid levels.
6. Monitor serum uric acid levels.

What's pseudogout?

A condition similar to gout characterized by the abnormal production of calcium pyrophosphate crystals in cartilage and their eventual release into the synovial fluid; pseudogout most commonly affects the knees or wrists and occurs more commonly in people with thyroid or parathyroid disorders, renal failure, or conditions that affect the metabolism of calcium, phosphate, or iron.

What's the typical treatment for pseudogout?

Medications similar to gout treatment (NSAIDs, corticosteroids, and possibly colchicines), with the exception of uric acid lowering agents; no treatment is currently available to dissolve the calcium crystal deposits

FIBROMYALGIA

What's fibromyalgia?

An arthritis-related condition of generalized musculoskeletal aches and pains that persists longer than 3 months; the trapezius muscles of the neck and shoulders are the most commonly affected, and it's more prevalent in women

What's the pathophysiologic process of fibromyalgia?

Although the exact mechanism isn't known, an infectious process, hormonal changes, physical or emotional trauma, and function of neurotransmitters are speculated to amplify pain signals to and from the brain

What are the clinical manifestations of fibromyalgia?	Widespread musculoskeletal aches and pains associated with fatigue and stiffness, which is worse in the morning and is exacerbated by exertion or stress; multiple trigger points (tender spots) may be present
What other conditions are associated with fibromyalgia?	Sleep disturbances, depression, anxiety, migraines, dysmenorrhea, irritable bowel syndrome, restless leg syndrome, and temporomandibular joint disorder
How is fibromyalgia diagnosed?	By meeting certain criteria based on physical examination; pain must affect both the left and right side of the body, areas above and below the waist as well as the axial skeleton (chest, spine, low back); 11 of the 18 designated trigger points must also be present to confirm the diagnosis; laboratory tests may be performed to exclude other causes
What's the typical treatment for fibromyalgia?	1. Aerobic and stretching exercises 2. Relaxation techniques to reduce anxiety and muscle tension 3. Medications to promote sleep and reduce pain (antidepressants)
What are important nursing actions in the care of a patient with fibromyalgia?	1. Encourage aerobic and stretching exercises as well as relaxation techniques to minimize pain. 2. Administer medications (antidepressants) as ordered by the physician.

Other rheumatic disorders

SYSTEMIC LUPUS ERYTHEMATOSUS

What's systemic lupus erythematosus (SLE)?	A chronic autoimmune disorder that causes inflammatory changes in the skin, joints, and organ systems; it's nine times more common in women than men, and the underlying cause isn't known
What's the pathophysiologic process of SLE?	Auto-antibodies are produced, which attack the body's own blood cells, tissues, and organs, resulting in chronic disease of the involved area
What are the clinical manifestations of SLE?	1. Fever, fatigue, and malaise 2. "Butterfly" (malar) rash across nose and cheeks 3. Sun sensitivity 4. Joint pain and swelling 5. Muscle aches 6. Enlarged glands

What are clinical manifestations associated with internal organ involvement?	*Kidneys:* hematuria due to lupus nephritis, which may result in renal failure *Heart:* endocarditis, pericarditis, or myocarditis, causing arrhythmias and chest pain *Nervous system:* headaches, mild mental dysfunction, seizures, and psychosis *Lungs:* pleuritic chest pain, pleural effusions, dyspnea *Blood:* thrombocytopenia, hemolytic anemia, formation of blood clots, resulting in pulmonary embolism or stroke
What complications are associated with SLE?	Organ failure, complications from treatment and death
What's the typical treatment for SLE?	1. Because there's no cure, symptomatic treatment, such as NSAIDs for arthritis and corticosteroid creams for skin rashes, is used. 2. Severe disease may be treated with oral corticosteroid therapy to suppress the immune system.
What are important nursing actions for a patient with SLE?	1. Instruct the patient to wear sunscreen, sunglasses, and protective clothing when outdoors. 2. Administer medications (NSAIDs, corticosteroids) as ordered by the physician. 3. Educate the patient about the importance of taking medications regularly. 4. Monitor the patient for complications (hematuria, dyspnea, endocarditis, or hematologic disorders) and notify the physician if any develop.

SYSTEMIC SCLEROSIS (SCLERODERMA, CREST SYNDROME)

What's systemic sclerosis?	A connective tissue disorder involving fibrosis of the skin, blood vessels, skeletal muscles, and internal organs as a result of excess collagen deposits; cutaneous involvement may be limited or diffuse; women are more commonly affected, and individuals with occupational exposure to silica dust and polyvinyl chloride are at an increased risk for development of systemic sclerosis
What's the pathophysiologic process of systemic sclerosis?	Increased collagen deposition causes progressive fibrosis of tissues with subsequent loss of mobility and altered function
What's CREST syndrome?	A subtype of systemic sclerosis that involves limited cutaneous manifestations

✎ CREST is an acronym for what cardinal features of the syndrome?

1. **C**alcinosis: calcification of soft tissues
2. **R**aynaud phenomenon: bilateral pallor, cyanosis, and rubor of fingers and toes on exposure to cold; triphasic color changes due to vasoconstriction, sluggish blood flow, and reperfusion
3. **E**sophageal dysmotility: decreased or absent peristalsis
4. **S**clerodactyly: thickening of the skin in the hands and feet
5. **T**elangiectasia: collection of dilated blood vessels, usually on face, upper trunk or hands, but may also occur along the GI tract, resulting in bleeding

What are the clinical manifestations of systemic sclerosis?

1. Hardened, tight, and thickened skin with shiny hands and forearms
2. Masklike facial skin
3. Changes in skin pigmentation (abnormally dark or light)
4. Arthralgias or muscle weakness
5. Dyspnea or cough with pulmonary or cardiac involvement
6. Ulcerations on tips of fingers or toes
7. Burning, itching, or discharge involving the eyes

What complications are associated with systemic sclerosis?

Pulmonary fibrosis, malabsorption syndromes with intestinal involvement, hypertension, renal failure, arrhythmias, and cardiac failure

What's the typical treatment for systemic sclerosis?

1. Symptomatic treatment is used, primarily because there's no known cure for the condition and no known prevention for collagen deposition.
2. Calcium channel blockers may be used in the management of Raynaud's phenomenon.
3. Esophageal reflux may be treated with elevation of the head of the bed, antacids, histamine blockers, and proton pump inhibitors.
4. Joint symptoms may be treated with anti-inflammatories including NSAIDs and colchicine, DMARDs (penicillamine, hydroxychloroquine), or immunosuppressants, such as methotrexate and cyclophosphamide.

What are important nursing actions in the care of a patient with systemic sclerosis?

1. Encourage the patient to remain as active as possible to maintain flexibility and increase circulation.
2. Encourage smoking cessation to improve circulation.
3. Instruct the patient to apply skin moisturizers or topical corticosteroids.
4. Instruct the patient to wear gloves, a coat, and a hat when outdoors in cold weather.

5. Administer medications (NSAIDs, DMARDs, immuno-suppressants, calcium channel blockers) as ordered by the physician.

Major disorders of the bones

Osteoporosis

🔖 What's osteoporosis?

A metabolic bone disease characterized by the progressive loss of bone mass and density; affects the entire skeleton, but is most marked in the spine, pelvis, and wrist; women older than age 50 are most commonly affected

What's the pathophysiologic process of osteoporosis?

Failure of the body to produce adequate new bone (osteoblast underactivity), or excessive reabsorption of old bone (osteoclast overactivity) result in a loss of bone density

What's osteomalacia?

Softening of the bones due to inadequate mineralization of newly formed bone matrix secondary to insufficient vitamin D intake, hypophosphatemia, or defective nucleation of preformed bone matrix

What's osteopenia?

A condition of low bone density that may progress to osteoporosis if untreated

🔖 What two minerals are important in bone formation?

Calcium and phosphate

What vitamin aids in the absorption of calcium?

Vitamin D

🔖 What are the major causes of osteoporosis?

1. *Calcium deficiency:* inadequate dietary intake or lack of absorption
2. *Hormone deficiencies:* estrogen in females, testosterone in males
3. *Excess corticosteroids:* hyperthyroidism, hyperparathyroidism, prolonged steroid use, Cushing's syndrome
4. *Immobility:* non weight bearing

🔖 What risk factors are associated with the development of osteoporosis?

1. Advanced age
2. Prolonged inactivity
3. Eating disorders and low body weight
4. Smoking

5. Endocrine disorders involving the thyroid (Grave's disease, Cushing's disease) or parathyroid glands
6. Early menopause or amenorrhea
7. Prolonged use of certain medications, such as corticosteroids and some anticonvulsants (phenytoin)
8. Liver disease and alcoholism
9. Malignancies including leukemias, lymphomas, and multiple myeloma
10. Excessive caffeine consumption as well as excessive soda consumption (high phosphate content)

What are the clinical manifestations of osteoporosis?

Produces no symptoms in the early phase of the disease, although bone pain and tenderness, a stooped posture, loss of height over time, neck or lower back pain, and fractures may develop with advanced disease

What complications are associated with osteoporosis?

Fractures (even in the absence of trauma) and severe disability as a result of weakened bones

What are the most common osteoporosis-related fractures?

Compression fractures of the spine

What's the most reliable diagnostic testing method to determine the presence of osteoporosis?

Bone mineral density measurements using dual-energy X-ray absorptiometry

What's the typical treatment for a patient with osteoporosis?

1. Lifestyle modifications, including smoking cessation, increased weight-bearing activity, increased dietary intake of calcium, and reduced consumption of alcohol, sodas, and caffeine
2. Supplements of calcium (slows bone loss) and vitamin D (increases bone density)
3. Medications including bisphosphonates, such as alendronate (Fosamax), pamidronate, and risedronate (Actonel), as well as raloxifene (Evista), calcitonin (Miacalcin), and estrogen replacement therapy (if postmenopausal)

What are important nursing actions in the care of a patient with osteoporosis?

1. Encourage smoking cessation and limitation or avoidance of alcohol consumption.
2. Encourage routine weight-bearing exercises, such as walking, jogging, and riding stationary bicycles; avoid exercises that present a falling risk.

3. Administer medications (bisphosphonates, raloxifene, calcitonin, estrogen replacement) as ordered by the physician.
4. Encourage increased dietary intake of calcium and vitamin D.
5. Ensure a safe environment that prevents falls or other injuries.

Fractures

What's a fracture?

A disruption in the continuity of bone tissue caused by an injury or by a disease (pathologic) process

✎ What are primary descriptive terms for fractures?

1. *Closed:* indicates no break in the skin
2. *Open or compound:* indicates part of the bone is sticking out through the skin, or a break in the skin indicates a fracture

✎ What other descriptive terms may be used for fractures?

1. *Incomplete:* indicates bones are only partially broken or are cracked
2. *Complete:* indicates bones are broken apart
3. *Greenstick:* indicates an incomplete fracture in which bones are bent; most common in growing children

What's a pathologic fracture?

A disruption of bone tissue that occurs when the bone has become weakened due to a disease process, but is unrelated to trauma

✎ What types of complete fractures exist?

1. *Oblique:* involves a fracture line diagonally across the bone shaft
2. *Transverse:* involves a break straight across a bone (perpendicular to its long axis)
3. *Spiral:* involves a coil-like fracture in which the break runs around the bone
4. *Comminuted:* involves crushing or shattering of a bone resulting in multiple bone fragments

✎ What are the clinical manifestations of a fracture?

Obvious deformity of bone or joint, pain or tenderness, edema, ecchymosis, muscle spasms, and loss of function of affected area

What complications may be associated with fractures?

Hemorrhage, compartment syndrome, infection, venous thrombosis, fat or pulmonary embolism, arterial insufficiency, malunion, nonunion, or avascular necrosis

✎ What are key elements to assessing fractures?

Assess neurovascular status by palpating pulses and observe for classic signs of arterial insufficiency (5 P's: pulselessness, pallor, paresthesia, pain, and paralysis).

What's the immediate treatment for a fracture?

Immobilization; anatomical realignment of the bone fragments will be performed by a physician

✎ What are important nursing actions in the care of a patient with a fracture?

1. Immobilize the affected extremity. Elevate when possible.
2. Maintain nothing-by-mouth status in the immediate postinjury phase.
3. Refrain from straightening the affected extremity or changing its position.
4. Apply ice packs to minimize pain and swelling during the acute phase.
5. Administer medications (muscle relaxants, analgesics) as ordered by the physician.
6. Encourage a diet with adequate amounts of protein, vitamins, and calcium.
7. Monitor the patient for complications (hemorrhage, arterial insufficiency, compartment syndrome) and notify the physician immediately if any develop.

✎ What assessment parameters are appropriate when caring for a patient with a cast?

1. Evaluate neurovascular status every 1 to 2 hours for the first 24 hours after the cast is applied. Observe the temperature, color, and mobility of digits. Ensure nail beds are pink and capillary refill time is less than 3 seconds. Make sure the skin is warm and that the patient can move his digits.
2. Insert two fingers in the proximal and distal ends of the cast to ensure it isn't too tight.
3. Assess the skin adjacent to the cast and ensure there are no areas where the cast is rubbing.
4. Palpate pulse under the cast, if possible.
5. Compare extremity with cast to extremity without cast.
6. Assess for foul smell from the cast.

What measures may decrease swelling?

Elevating the extremity with cast on two pillows

✎ What are signs of decreased circulation?

A cool, pale, mottled extremity with diminished pulse or capillary refill time greater than 3 seconds is indicative of decreased circulation. Pain, tingling, numbness, or inability to wiggle digits may also be signs of decreased circulation.

What might be done to improve circulation?

The casted extremity can be elevated (to reduce edema) or the cast may need to be bivalved (cut) or removed to regain circulation

What's closed reduction (manipulation)?

Manual (nonsurgical) realignment of bones; local or general anesthesia and sedation may be used

What's open reduction?	Surgical correction of bone alignment; internal or external fixators, such as screws, rods, plates, or pins, may be used
What's traction?	Devices that apply a pulling force to align and immobilize bones into correct anatomical position as well as to minimize muscle spasms
How is traction classified?	Manual, skin, skeletal, plaster, and brace

What are commonly used types of traction?

1. *Buck's:* fractures of hips and femoral shaft
2. *Russell's:* fractures of hip, femur, and some knee conditions
3. *Bryant's:* fractures of femur; commonly used in children
4. *Overhead arm/Lateral arm:* fractures and dislocations of shoulder and upper arm
5. *Balanced suspension:* fractures of hip, acetabulum, femoral shaft, or lower leg

✎ What assessments should be made of a patient in traction?

Assess circulation and nerve of the extremity in traction, the condition of the skin for irritation or pressure, and body alignment and level of pain.

✎ What basic care applies to traction equipment?

1. Assess the traction cord for weakness.
2. Make sure the correct amount of weight is hanging.
3. Make sure the weights are hanging freely and aren't touching the floor.
4. Maintain continuous traction.

What might symptoms of pain, spasms, or muscular burning in a patient with traction indicate?

Misalignment of bones or increasing pressure on injured nerve endings

What nursing care is appropriate for a patient in traction?

1. Perform neurovascular assessments 15 minutes after application of traction and every 1 to 2 hours for the first 24 hours.
2. Inspect the skin around traction straps and pins for irritation and breakdown.
3. Perform pin care according to facility policy. Inspect for drainage or inflammation.
4. Assess for signs of infection, such as fever, elevated WBC count, pain, erythema, and warmth in extremity.
5. Monitor for signs of perineal nerve damage (footdrop with inability to dorsiflex or evert the foot).
6. Monitor for signs of radial or median nerve damage (inability to approximate fingers and thumb; numb-

ness and tingling of the thumb, index and middle fingers; and wristdrop).
7. Monitor for signs of deep vein thrombosis or embolism (restlessness, mental status changes, hypoxia, tachypnea, tachycardia, petechial rash over chest and neck).

What's halo skeletal traction?

Skeletal fixation by a stainless steel ring that's attached to the skull by four pins; steel rods are then attached to a body brace

What's the appropriate action if the halo pins loosen?

Tighten them with the wrench kept at the bedside and notify the physician.

What's counter-traction?

Pulling forces applied in the opposite direction to prevent a patient from sliding in the bed

What's an external fixator?

Metallic gear attached directly to bones by percutaneous pins to hold bone fragments in place

What's an internal fixation device?

A surgically inserted device used to stabilize fractured bones and to maintain their alignment during the healing process

✎ What are important considerations the nurse should explain to the patient after a hip replacement?

1. Maintain the hip in a straight, neutral position during lying, sitting, or ambulating.
2. Place a pillow between the knees when in a supine position for the first 8 postoperative weeks.
3. Use a raised toilet.
4. Don't force the hip into adduction, internal rotation, or more than 90 degrees of flexion, as these may cause dislocation of the prosthesis.
5. Don't cross the legs.
6. Notify dentist of prosthesis before any dental work (prophylactic antibiotics may be necessary).

Compartment syndrome

✎ What's compartment syndrome?

A condition in which the circulation or function of tissues within a closed space is compromised by increased pressure within that space caused by edema; it's commonly associated with fractures or extensive soft tissue injuries; the forearms and lower extremities are the most commonly affected sites

What's the pathophysiologic process of compartment syndrome?

Compression of nerves and blood vessels within a compartment impairs the blood flow, which results in nerve damage

✎ What clinical manifestations are associated with compartment syndrome?

Pain out of proportion to injury or refractory to analgesics, paresthesia, pallor, pulselessness, and edema

Does a palpable pulse rule out compartment syndrome?

No; pressure may be high enough to cause muscle and nerve ischemia without being high enough to occlude a major artery

What complications may develop if compartment syndrome isn't recognized and treated early?

Delay in diagnosis for 6 to 8 hours after onset of ischemia can lead to irreversible death of muscle and nerve

What's the typical treatment for compartment syndrome?

Fasciotomy

✎ What's a fasciotomy?

An incision into the fascia to relieve compression and to restore circulation

What pressure level would require treatment?

Compartments with pressures greater than 30 to 40 mm Hg should be considered for fasciotomy

How is intracompartmental pressure measured?

A large-bore catheter is placed into the compartment using sterile technique. The catheter is connected to a pressure monitor with I.V. tubing filled with sterile saline solution.

✎ What are important nursing actions in the care of a patient with compartment syndrome?

1. Elevate the extremity and apply ice to minimize edema and improve venous return. Notify the physician immediately and prepare the patient for fasciotomy.
2. Assess the need for removal of bandage or cast, or the need to decrease the amount of traction to relieve edema.
3. Assess neurovascular status of the affected extremity at frequent intervals.

Paget's disease (Osteitis deformans)

What's Paget's disease?	A condition involving hyperactive bone destruction and ineffective bone formation that predominately affects the long bones, pelvis, lumbar vertebrae, and skull; it's most commonly associated with malignant degeneration and osteoarthritis; a familial tendency is associated with the disease
What's the patho-physiologic process of Paget's disease?	Increased osteoclastic activity with ineffective mineralization of newly formed bone results in sclerotic, weakened bones
What are the clinical manifestations of Paget's disease?	Pain with weight bearing, which may be described as constant or intermittent, aching, or stabbing; when the bones of the skull are affected it may cause headaches, facial pain, and enlargement of the skull; progressive development of bowlegs may also occur, and elevation of serum alkaline phosphatase may be noted in laboratory studies
What complications are associated with Paget's disease?	Pathologic fractures and malignant tumors
What's the typical treatment for Paget's disease?	Calcium and vitamin D supplementation, low-impact exercises, and medications, such as analgesics, bisphosphonates (to retard bone resorption), and calcitonin; surgery may be indicated to treat fractures and correct deformities
What are important nursing actions in the care of a patient with Paget's disease?	1. Use extreme caution when moving or turning the patient (high risk of pathologic fractures). 2. Administer medications (analgesics, muscle relaxants, bisphosphonates, vitamin and mineral supplements) as ordered by the physician. 3. Encourage activity as tolerated to prevent demineralization of bone that occurs with prolonged immobility or disuse. 4. Encourage the use of a firm mattress to support the spine. 5. Instruct the patient about proper body mechanics and discourage twisting or lifting activities.

Osteomyelitis

What's osteomyelitis?	Inflammation of the bone, bone marrow, and surrounding soft tissue caused by pus-producing bacteria (most commonly *Staphylococcus aureus*)
What's the pathophysiologic process of osteomyelitis?	An infection in one part of the body spreads via the bloodstream to the bone tissue where it produces pus, and an abscess may develop; the abscess deprives the bone of its blood supply, and the bone tissue dies secondary to the ischemia
What are the clinical manifestations of acute osteomyelitis?	1. *Local:* sudden onset of severe pain with movement, erythema over infected bone, heat, edema, restricted movement of infected bone, wound drainage 2. *Systemic:* chills, high fever, headache, nausea, tachycardia, leukocytosis, positive blood cultures
What are the clinical manifestations of chronic osteomyelitis?	Exacerbation is characterized by fever, pain, and persistent drainage from a sinus
What complications are associated with osteomyelitis?	Septicemia, bacterial arthritis, pathologic fractures, nonunion of fractures, and chronic osteomyelitis
What's the typical treatment for osteomyelitis?	Extended antibiotic therapy and bed rest with immobilization of the infected bone is instituted until the acute infection is eliminated. Chronic infections may require surgical removal of poorly vascularized tissue and necrotic bone as well as extended antibiotic therapy. Amputation of the extremity may also be necessary to preserve life if infection and bone destruction is extensive.
What are important nursing actions in the care of a patient with osteomyelitis?	1. Use extreme caution when moving or turning the patient to prevent pathologic fractures. 2. Administer medications (antibiotics, analgesics) as ordered by the physician. 3. Change the patient's body position at frequent intervals maintaining proper body alignment to prevent contractures or other complications. 4. Perform meticulous wound care and dressing changes as ordered by the physician. Sterile technique is critical. 5. Monitor the patient for complications (septicemia, pathologic fractures) and notify the physician immediately if any develop.

Amputations

What are the indications for amputation?

Treatment of a limb severely affected by trauma, infection, tumor, or the end stages of ischemia from peripheral vascular disease

How is the appropriate level of amputation determined?

Amputation is performed at the level that will allow for the most complete healing and permit most efficient use of the limb

What's a disarticulation?

An amputation performed through a joint

What complications are associated with amputations?

Hemorrhage, infection, thromboembolism, and development of contractures, particularly hip flexion

✎ What's phantom pain?

A continuous pain sensation in the amputated limb

What medications are most effective at relieving phantom pain?

Tricyclic antidepressants and anticonvulsants such as gabapentin (Neurontin)

✎ What constitutes routine stump care?

1. Inspect skin daily for signs of irritation or skin breakdown.
2. Clean with warm water and an antibacterial soap each evening. Rinse thoroughly, pat dry, and expose to air for 20 to 30 minutes.
3. Avoid the use of powders, lotions, or oils on the stump, unless prescribed by a physician.
4. Avoid using a prosthetic device if skin irritation develops, until examined by a physician.

✎ What are important nursing actions in the care of a patient with an amputation?

1. Provide stump care.
2. Instruct the patient to avoid dangling the stump over the edge of the bed in the immediate postoperative phase to prevent edema.
3. Encourage active ROM exercises of all joints.
4. Instruct the patient to avoid sitting in a chair for prolonged periods of time to prevent development of hip flexion contracture. Lying on his abdomen for 30 minutes several times per day should be encouraged.
5. Consult the physical therapy member of the health care team for exercise and conditioning.
6. Educate the patient regarding stump and prosthesis care.

7. Monitor the patient for complications (hemorrhage, infection) and notify the physician immediately if any develop.
8. Because the patient may experience grief over his lost limb, assist in the grieving process by providing psychological support.

Cancers of the musculoskeletal system

Osteogenic sarcoma

What's osteogenic sarcoma?

An extremely aggressive malignant neoplasm of bone that commonly occurs at the ends (growth plates) of the long bones of the extremities in young people between ages 10 and 25 due to their rapid growth rates

What's the pathophysiologic process of osteogenic sarcoma?

Although the exact cause is unknown, genetics may play a role in the development of this primary bone tumor.

What are the clinical manifestations of osteogenic sarcoma?

Bone pain and swelling, palpation of a mass at the tumor site, and limitation of joint motion (if tumor is near joint)

What's the classic X-ray finding?

"Sunburst" appearance

What complications are associated with osteogenic sarcoma?

Disability, pathologic fractures, adverse reactions to treatments, and death

What's the typical treatment for osteogenic sarcoma?

Surgical resection of the primary lesion or amputation, as well as adjunctive chemotherapy or radiation therapy

What are important nursing actions in the care of a patient with osteogenic sarcoma?

1. Use extreme caution when turning or transferring the patient to prevent pathologic fractures.
2. Encourage the patient to participate in therapeutic activities to prevent complications of prolonged bed rest. Provide frequent rest periods.
3. Administer medications (analgesics, chemotherapeutic agents) as ordered by the physician.
4. Monitor the patient for complications (pathologic fractures) and notify the physician immediately if any develop.

Pharmacology related to the musculoskeletal system

Treatment of muscular disorders

MUSCLE RELAXANTS

How do muscle relaxants work?

Although their exact mechanisms of action vary or may be unclear, their sedative properties are believed to facilitate the relaxation of muscular spasms

What are examples of muscle relaxants?

Baclofen (Lioresal), carisoprodol (Soma), chlorphenesin (Maolate), cyclobenzaprine (Flexeril), diazepam (Valium), metaxalone (Skelaxin), methocarbamol (Robaxin), orphenadrine (Norflex)

✎ What adverse reactions are commonly associated with muscle relaxants?

Central nervous system depression (drowsiness, slurred speech, light-headedness, dizziness), blurred vision, orthostatic hypotension, nausea, vomiting, urinary frequency or retention

⚡ *Physical dependence to muscle relaxants may develop with chronic high-dose therapy.*

✎ What are important nursing actions when administering muscle relaxants?

1. Instruct the patient to take this medication with meals to minimize gastric distress.
2. Instruct the patient to avoid other central nervous system depressants (including alcohol and over-the-counter antihistamines).
3. Instruct the patient to avoid activities that require mental alertness until the effects of muscle relaxants are known.
4. Encourage the patient to change positions slowly due to risk of orthostatic hypotension.
5. Instruct the patient to avoid abrupt discontinuation of baclofen and carisoprodol due to risk of withdrawal symptoms (hallucinations, rebound spasticity).
6. Instruct the patient to avoid concomitant use of cyclobenzaprine and monoamine oxidase inhibitors due to risk of hyperpyretic reaction and seizures.

⚡ *Abrupt discontinuation of baclofen may result in hallucinations, paranoid ideation, and seizures.*

Antigout medications

ANTI-INFLAMMATORY GOUT AGENTS

What's an example of an anti-inflammatory gout agent?	Colchicine
✎ **How does colchicine work?**	Decreases inflammation caused by deposition of urate crystals in acute gouty attacks; unlike many other antigout medications, colchicine does *not* lower the serum uric acid level
✎ **When is colchicine used?**	In the treatment of *acute* gouty arthritis; after the acute phase, it may be taken prophylactically in smaller doses to reduce the frequency and severity of future acute episodes
What adverse reactions are associated with colchicine?	Primarily GI disturbances including nausea, vomiting, abdominal pain, and diarrhea
What life-threatening reactions are associated with long-term colchicine?	Hematologic disturbances including aplastic anemia, thrombocytopenia, and agranulocytosis
What's an advantage of indomethacin over colchicine?	GI adverse effects are far less frequent with indomethacin
✎ **What are important nursing actions when administering colchicine?**	1. Instruct the patient to take this medication with meals to minimize adverse GI effects.
	2. Monitor intake and output. Encourage increased oral fluid intake (6 to 8 glasses of water per day) to maintain adequate urinary output of greater than or equal to 2 L per day.
	3. Instruct the patient to avoid alcohol consumption during therapy (increases urate levels).
	4. Monitor complete blood count periodically throughout therapy.
	5. Monitor for drug toxicity (nausea, vomiting, diarrhea, abdominal pain, fatigue, paresthesia, easy bruising, or bleeding) and notify the physician immediately if any develop.

⚡ *I.V. colchicine use should be limited to 7 days secondary to bone marrow toxicity risks.*

Antigout agents that decrease serum uric acid

How do antigout agents work?

1. *Allopurinol:* decreases uric acid production by inhibiting the enzyme (xanthine oxidase) necessary for the conversion of purines to uric acid
2. *Probenecid and sulfinpyrazone:* increase urinary excretion of uric acid by inhibiting the renal tubular absorption of urate; uricosuric action

What are examples of antigout agents that decrease serum uric acid levels?

Allopurinol (Aloprim, Zyloprim, Purinol), probenecid (Benemid), and sulfinpyrazone (Anturane)

What adverse reactions are commonly associated with antigout agents?

1. *Allopurinol:* headaches, drowsiness, nausea, vomiting, and diarrhea
2. *Probenecid:* headaches, nausea, vomiting, and urinary frequency
3. *Sulfinpyrazone:* nausea and dyspepsia

What life-threatening reactions are associated with antigout agents?

1. *Allopurinol:* exfoliative rash, toxic epidermal necrolysis, hepatitis and hepatic necrosis, renal failure, and hematologic disorders, such as aplastic anemia, agranulocytosis, leukopenia, and thrombocytopenia
2. *Probenecid:* anaphylaxis (sulfa derivative), hepatic necrosis, hemolytic anemia and aplastic anemia; many drug interactions (NSAIDs, salicylates, sulfonylureas)
3. *Sulfinpyrazone:* leukopenia, agranulocytosis, aplastic anemia, and thrombocytopenia

✎ What are important nursing actions when administering antigout agents?

1. Instruct the patient to take antigout agents with meals to minimize adverse GI effects.
2. Monitor intake and output. Encourage increased oral fluid intake (6 to 8 glasses of water per day) to maintain adequate urinary output of greater than or equal to 2 L per day. Neutral or slightly alkaline urine (with sodium bicarbonate or potassium citrate use) is desired to prevent urate stone development.
3. Monitor serum uric acid level periodically during therapy to evaluate response, and monitor complete blood count, hepatic panel, and renal function (blood urea nitrogen and creatinine) periodically during therapy.
4. Inform the patient that peak effects may require up to 6 weeks of therapy to become evident.
5. Instruct the patient to avoid alcohol consumption during therapy (it increases urate level).
6. Inform the patient that drowsiness may result from allopurinol use, and that driving or other activities that

require mental alertness should be avoided until the effects of the drug are known.

7. Instruct the patient to discontinue allopurinol immediately if a rash or fever develops, and to notify the physician.

8. Probenecid and sulfinpyrazone dosages should be reduced in patients with impaired renal function.

9. Instruct the patient to avoid taking NSAIDs (aspirin, indomethacin) during probenecid and sulfinpyrazone therapy due to increased toxicity risk.

Treatment of osteoporosis and metabolic bone diseases

CALCIUM REGULATORS

How do calcium regulators work?	Inhibit bone resorption, decrease mineral release from bone, and increase renal excretion of calcium, phosphate, and sodium
What's an example of a calcium regulator?	Calcitonin (Miacalcin, Osteocalcin, Calcimar, Cibacalcin-human)
What adverse reactions are commonly associated with calcitonin?	Facial flushing, nasal congestion (nasal formulation), nausea, vomiting, urinary frequency, and localized inflammation at injection sites
What life-threatening adverse reaction may occur with the use of calcitonin?	Anaphylactic reaction (salmon or fish sensitivity for nonhuman-derived drugs); skin testing may be performed prior to administration of salmon-derived calcitonin in people with known or suspected allergies

What are important nursing actions when administering calcitonin?

1. Make sure epinephrine is readily available in the event of anaphylactic reaction with first doses.
2. Make sure parenteral calcium is readily available if hypocalcemic tetany occurs with I.V. administration of calcitonin.
3. Perform skin allergy test before using salmon-derived calcitonin.
4. Instruct the patient to take tablets at bedtime to minimize nausea and vomiting, to alternate nostrils daily to prevent nasal irritation (nasal preparations), and to alternate injection sites (parenteral preparations).
5. Monitor the patient for serious adverse reactions, such as hypocalcemic tetany (muscle twitching, spasms, seizures) and anaphylaxis; notify the physician if any develop.
6. Monitor serum calcium and alkaline phosphatase levels.

BISPHOSPHONATES

How do bisphospho-nates work?	Augmentation of bone mass by decreasing rate of bone resorption (suppression of osteoclasts)
What are examples of bisphosphonates?	Alendronate (Fosamax), etidronate (Didronel), risedro-nate (Actonel), and pamidronate (Aredia, only available I.V.)
✎ **What adverse re-actions are commonly associated with bis-phosphonates?**	Primarily GI symptoms, such as diarrhea, constipation, abdominal cramps, nausea, acid reflux, dyspepsia, and gastritis, although musculoskeletal pain and headaches may also occur
✎ **What serious re-action is associated with bisphosphonates?**	Esophagitis

✎ **What are impor-tant nursing actions when administering bisphosphonates?**

1. Instruct the patient to take bisphosphonates 1 hour before breakfast on an empty stomach (improves absorption) and to avoid taking antacids within 2 hours of bisphosphonates.
2. Instruct the patient to take bisphosphonates with a full glass of water and avoid chewing or sucking tablets.
3. Instruct the patient to remain in an upright position for at least 30 minutes after taking this medication to minimize esophagitis.
4. Instruct the patient to wait at least 30 minutes before taking other medications.
5. Monitor serum calcium levels periodically throughout therapy.
6. Inform the patient that improvement may take 3 months or more.

Treatment of rheumatoid arthritis

How do antirheumatic agents work?

1. *COX-2 inhibitors:* block prostaglandin production by cyclooxygenase-2 but not by cyclooxygenase-1
2. *NSAIDs:* inhibit prostaglandin production by blocking both forms of cyclooxygenase (COX-1 and COX-2)
3. *Disease-modifying antirheumatoid agents (DMARDs):* immunomodulatory and anti-inflammatory affects through enzyme inhibition
4. *Antitumor necrosis factor (Anti-TNF) agents:* agents that bind TNF, which minimizes immune response and inflammation

5. *Gold salts:* anti-inflammatory effects by inhibiting activities of lysosomal enzymes; decreases levels of rheumatoid factor and immunoglobulins

What are examples of antirheumatic agents?

1. *DMARDs:* methotrexate, leflunomide (Arava), D-penicillamine (Cuprimine)
2. *Anti-TNF agents:* infliximab (Remicade), etanercept (Enbrel)
3. *Gold salts:* auranofin (Ridaura), aurothioglucose (Solganal)

What adverse reactions are associated with antirheumatic agents?

1. *DMARDs:* elevated liver enzymes (aspartate aminotransferase, alanine aminotransferase), hypertension, diarrhea, rash, alopecia, and respiratory infection
2. *Anti-TNF agents:* headache, fatigue, nausea, abdominal pain, upper respiratory tract infections, and fever, as well as dyspnea, hypotension, hypertension, and chest pain during I.V. use
3. *Gold salts:* nausea, vomiting, abdominal cramps, diarrhea, stomatitis, metallic taste, anemia, dermatitis, pruritus, and chrysiasis (gold deposits result in gray-blue skin discoloration)

What life-threatening reactions are associated with antirheumatic agents?

1. *DMARDs:* hepatic toxicity
2. *Anti-TNF agents:* anaphylactic reactions if preformed mouse antibodies (infliximab is a monoclonal mouse antibody)
3. *Gold salts:* renal failure, interstitial pneumonitis, pulmonary fibrosis, thrombocytopenia, leukopenia, granulocytopenia, seizures, anaphylactic shock (with injection)

✎ What are important nursing actions when administering antirheumatic agents?

1. Monitor the patient for development of infections and lymphomas during anti-TNF therapy.
2. Instruct the patient to avoid live virus vaccines during anti-TNF therapy due to altered immune response.
3. Monitor complete blood count and hepatic function periodically throughout therapy with antirheumatic agents as well as renal (blood urea nitrogen, creatinine, urinalysis) function with gold salt therapy.
4. Inform the female patient taking antirheumatic agents to avoid becoming pregnant during therapy, and to stop the medication and notify the physician immediately if pregnancy is known or suspected.
5. Monitor respiratory status of a patient receiving gold salt therapy due to potential complications, and assess for rash or easy bruising or bleeding (thrombocytopenia). Notify the physician if these conditions develop.

6. Encourage the patient on DMARD and gold salt therapy to avoid exposure to sunlight or ultraviolet light to avoid rash and skin discoloration (gold salts).
7. Instruct the patient to avoid use of cytotoxic agents, immunosuppressive agents (other than low corticosteroid doses), antimalarial agents, and penicillamine during DMARD and gold salt therapy.

Nursing skills

Patient moving and transfers

What's the proper technique for moving a patient up in bed?

1. Place the patient in a supine position and lower the head of the bed so that it's flat.
2. Remove the pillow from under the patient's head.
3. Position one nurse on either side of the bed.
4. Position the bed at a level comfortable for the nurses.
5. Grasp the draw sheet firmly under the patient and with knees and hips flexed, pull the patient up in bed on the count of three while shifting weight to the foot closest to the head of the bed.
6. Replace the pillow under the patient's head and elevate head of bed as tolerated.

What's the proper technique for logrolling a patient?

1. Obtain three people for assistance. One should be positioned at the head of the bed to maintain cervical spine alignment and to ensure adequate airway, while the other two people should be positioned on either side of the patient to maintain alignment of the spine.
2. Place the patient in a supine position. A cervical collar should be worn until the spine is cleared (determined to be uninjured).
3. The person at the head of the bed should grasp either side of the patient's head to maintain cervical-spine alignment, while the two other people grasp the draw sheet on opposite sides of the patient.
4. On the count of three, the two people on the sides lift the draw sheet slowly on the same side so that the patient is rolled over onto the side in one smooth motion, while the person at the head of the bed maintains body alignment.
5. To turn the patient back, the two people on the sides lower the patient back down to the flat position using the draw sheet, while the person at the head maintains body alignment.

What's the proper technique for transferring a patient from a supine to a sitting position on the side of the bed?

1. Elevate the head of the bed to 30 degrees.
2. Turn the patient onto his side.
3. Stand opposite the patient's hips and face the far corner of the foot of the bed.
4. Place feet shoulder length apart with the foot closer to the head of the bed in front of the other foot.
5. Place the arm nearer the head of the bed under the patient's shoulder and place the other arm over the patient's thighs.
6. With one continuous and smooth movement, gently swing the patient by the shoulders and legs so that the legs hang off the side of the bed.

What's the proper technique for transferring a patient from a bed to a wheelchair?

1. Assume a stance with feet shoulder length apart with hips and knees flexed directly in front of the patient.
2. Reach under the patient's axilla and place hands on scapula.
3. Instruct the patient to stand straight up on the count of three.
4. On the count of three, rock the patient up to a standing position while straightening hips and legs using arm and leg muscles to avoid back strain.
5. Assess the patient's stability and ensure that he's strong enough to stand alone.
6. While keeping your hands under the patient's axilla, instruct him to pivot on the foot farther from the chair.
7. Instruct the patient to take small steps back until the chair is felt on the back of his thighs, then instruct him to grab the sides of the chair and flex his knees while lowering himself into the chair. Be sure to flex at the hip and knees while lowering the patient into the chair to avoid back strain.

What's the proper technique for transferring a patient from a bed to a stretcher?

1. Obtain three people for assistance with transfer.
2. Place the patient in a supine position and lower the head of the bed to flat.
3. Position one person on either side of the bed and one at the foot of the bed.
4. Instruct the person on one side of the bed to grasp the draw sheet on the opposite side of the patient and turn the patient towards her, while the person on the other side places a slide board under the draw sheet. Lower the patient back to the supine position.
5. Position the stretcher next to the bed and lock in position.
6. Each person grasps the draw sheet and on the count of three, the person on the same side as the stretcher pulls the patient toward her over the slide board. The person on the opposite side of the bed pushes the

draw sheet toward the stretcher sliding the patient over the slide board, while the nurse at the foot of the bed guides the feet and lower extremities.

7. The slide board is then removed and the side rails are elevated on the sides of the stretcher for safe transfer.

Ambulation

What patient assessments should be made before a patient ambulates?

1. Visual, perceptual, or sensory deficits
2. Environment for potential threats to safety
3. Degree of assistance the patient will require
4. Understanding of type of ambulation to be carried out

What preparations are appropriate to safely ambulate a patient?

1. Demonstrate specific gait technique and decide with the patient how far to ambulate.
2. Place the bed in the lowest position and slowly assist patient to the upright position. Monitor for signs of orthostatic hypotension.
3. Allow the patient (once he's upright) to stand for a few minutes until balance is gained.
4. Assess the patient's strength and balance.

On which side should the nurse stand when a patient ambulates?

On the patient's *stronger* side

On which side should the nurse stand if an assistive device is used?

On the patient's *weaker* side

What's the appropriate action if the patient is weak or unsteady?

Return the patient to bed.

Cane

What are the four different types of canes?

1. *Standard:* provides the least support; used for patients requiring minimal assistance
2. *T-handle:* provides greater stability and is easier to hold; used for patients with hand weakness
3. *Tripod:* provides greater base of support; used for patients with partial or complete leg paralysis
4. *Quad:* provides a bit more stability than a tripod

How should a patient be assisted to ambulate with a cane?

1. Place the cane in the hand *opposite* the affected leg.
2. Place the cane forward 6" (15.2 cm), keeping body weight on both legs.
3. Move the affected leg forward, keeping even with the cane.
4. Advance the unaffected leg forward, keeping even with the affected leg.
5. Repeat.

Crutches

What types of crutches are available?

1. *Axillary:* frequently used by patients on a short-term basis
2. *Lofstrand:* used for paraplegics; the metal bar helps to guide the crutch and allows the patient to free up his hands for opening doors
3. *Platform:* used for those who can't bear weight on the wrists

How should a patient be assisted to ambulate with crutches?

1. Begin in tripod position and place the crutches 6" (15.2 cm) in front and to side of each foot.
2. Instruct the patient to place his weight on the handgrips (not the axillae). Start by moving both crutches forward 6".
3. Next lift and swing his legs to the crutches, letting the crutches support his body weight.
4. Repeat.

Walker

When is a walker indicated?

When a patient is weak or has problems with balance; it's lightweight and easily moveable with a wide base of support for greater security and stability

How is a patient assisted when ambulating with a walker?

1. Instruct the patient to stand in the center of the walker and grasp the handgrips on either side.
2. Instruct the patient to lift the walker and advance it several inches forward, and then set it down.
3. Instruct the patient to take a step forward with either foot and then follow through with the other foot. If one leg is weaker, he should step forward with the weaker leg, support his weight with his arms, and follow through with the uninvolved leg.

Pin care

✎ What's the proper technique for performing pin care?

1. Wash your hands and put on clean gloves.
2. Set up a sterile cup with sterile normal saline.
3. Open a package of sterile cotton-tipped swabs and insert them cotton side down into saline solution.
4. Pick up one applicator from the sterile cup, place the cotton-tipped area next to the pin, and roll it along the skin, away from the insertion site.
5. Dispose of the applicator.
6. Dip a new sterile applicator in normal saline and repeat the process, making sure the tip goes from the insertion site out.

◪ *Never use the same applicator on more than one site due to risk of cross-contamination.*

12

The neurosensory system

Basic concepts of the neurosensory system

What are the four basic functions of the nervous system?

1. Reception of sensory input from internal and external environment
2. Integration of the input
3. Response to the stimuli
4. Rapid maintenance of homeostasis against the endocrine system

✎ What are the two primary cell types that comprise nervous tissue?

1. *Neurons:* functional unit of the nervous system; transmits nerve messages
2. *Glial cells:* provide structural support, oxygen, and nutrients to neurons; astrocytes, oligodendrocytes, microglia, and Schwann cells are specialized types of glial cells

What are ganglia?

Ganglia are collections of neurons in the peripheral nervous system (PNS). Collections of neurons in the central nervous system (CNS) are called nuclei.

✎ What are the three parts of a neuron?

1. *Dendrite:* receives information from another cell and transmits that message to the cell body
2. *Cell body:* contains nucleus, mitochondria, and other organelles
3. *Axon:* conducts messages away from the cell body

✎ What's a myelin sheath?

The fatty insulation surrounding axons that's responsible for the whitish appearance of the white matter of the brain; it serves to increase the speed and efficiency of nerve impulses; conditions that involve demyelination (damage or loss of myelin sheath), such as multiple sclerosis, can produce a disruption of muscle control as well as disturbances of vision and speech

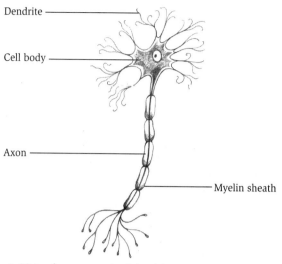

Dendrite

Cell body

Axon

Myelin sheath

What are the three types of neurons?

1. *Motor:* long axon, short dendrites; carry messages from the CNS to muscles or glands
2. *Sensory:* long dendrite, short axon; transmit messages from sensory receptors to the CNS
3. *Interneurons:* connect neuron to neuron; found only in the CNS

What are Schwann cells?

Specialized glial cells that surround nearly all nerve axons in the PNS, forming a protective layer called the myelin sheath; oligodendrocytes are specialized glial cells that insulate nerve axons in the CNS

What's a Node of Ranvier?

The gap that exists between each myelin sheath cell along a nerve axon; an electrical signal jumps from one gap to the next by a process known as saltatory conduction

What's an action potential?

A temporary reversal of the electrical potential (change in polarity) of a membrane, which causes propagation of a nerve impulse along the membrane; reversal of positions of sodium and potassium ions are responsible

What's the refractory period?

A brief period after passage of the action potential in which the membrane can't be stimulated

What's a synapse?

The junction (connection) between two nerve cells; the space between two cells is called the synaptic cleft; neurotransmitters are required for messages to cross the synaptic cleft

What's a neurotransmitter?

Small molecules stored at the axon tip that are released in response to an action potential; they conduct impulses across nerve junctions by binding to receptors on another cell, causing its ion channels to open; neurotransmitters may be excitatory or inhibitory; examples include acetylcholine, norepinephrine, serotonin, and dopamine

What's an afferent pathway?

A sensory pathway that provides input from the body to the CNS

What's an efferent pathway?

A motor pathway that carries signals to muscles and glands

✎ How can the nervous system be divided?

1. *CNS:* consists of brain and spinal cord
2. *PNS:* consists of cranial and spinal nerves as well as the autonomic nervous system; connects the brain and spinal cord with the rest of the body

Central nervous system

What are the three major divisions of the brain?

1. *Forebrain:* largest and most highly developed portion; consists of cerebrum and diencephalons
2. *Midbrain:* uppermost portion of the brain stem; responsible for some reflex actions as well as eye and body movements
3. *Hindbrain:* consists of cerebellum, medulla oblongata, and pons

What's the cerebrum?

The portion of the forebrain responsible for consciousness, intelligence, reasoning, learning, and memory

✎ What are the lobes of the cerebrum?

1. *Frontal:* language, personality, judgment, social behavior, abstract reasoning, language expression, movement (motor)
2. *Temporal:* memory storage and recall, language comprehension, hearing
3. *Occipital:* interpretation of visual stimuli
4. *Parietal:* interpretation and integration of sensations (touch, temperature, pain), interpretation of shapes, sizes, distances

Parietal lobe

Occipital lobe

Temporal lobe

Frontal lobe

What's the corpus callosum?	A mass of nerve fibers that passes from one cerebral hemisphere to the other and permits communication between them
What deep structures lie below the cerebrum?	1. *Limbic system:* lies deep within the temporal lobe, and serves to initiate drives (hunger, sexual arousal, aggression); the hippocampus is one part of the limbic system and is important for learning and memory 2. *Reticular activating system:* a network of hyperexcitable neurons that stimulate wakefulness as well as screen and channel all sensory information to appropriate areas of the brain for interpretation 3. *Basal ganglia:* clusters of neurons that surround the thalamus; responsible for coordination of movement
What's the cerebral cortex?	A layer of gray (nonmyelinated) tissue that coats the surface of the cerebrum; it's the location in which most of the brain's information processing occurs, and it's responsible for thought processes, voluntary movements, language, perception, and reasoning The folds of the brain increase its surface area as well as the amount of "gray matter," which increases the amount of information that can be processed.
What's the diencephalon?	The portion of the forebrain that contains the hypothalamus and thalamus
What's the thalamus?	The portion of the diencephalon that receives sensory information (except smell) and relays the information to the cerebral cortex where the information is processed
What's the hypothalamus?	The portion of the diencephalon that maintains homeostasis by regulating body temperature, appetite, thirst, emotions, pituitary secretions, water balance, and circadian rhythms (sleep/wake cycle); it also connects the nervous and endocrine systems
What's the cerebellum?	The portion of the hindbrain responsible for muscle tone, coordination of muscle, and fine motor movements as well as balance
What's the brain stem?	The portion of the brain responsible for relaying information between the upper and lower nervous system levels; controls some of the most basic life functions, including breathing, heart rate, and blood pressure

What are the components of the brain stem?

1. *Midbrain:* responsible for consciousness and regulation of some eye and body movements; contains cranial nerves (CN) III and IV
2. *Pons:* conveys information about movement from the cerebrum to the cerebellum; contains one of the respiratory centers; contains CN V, VI, and VII
3. *Medulla oblongata:* regulates vasomotor, cardiac, and respiratory functions (blood pressure, heart rate, breathing), as well as reflex centers for vomiting, swallowing, and sneezing; contains CN VIII, IX, X, XI, and XII

What are the meninges?

Three layers of protective tissue that surround the brain and spinal cord

✎ What are the meningeal layers and their spaces?

1. *Epidural space:* a potential space that may exist between the dura mater and the skull
2. *Dura mater:* thick, outermost layer; protects brain from displacement; forms sinuses that carry blood from the brain back to the heart
3. *Subdural space:* a potential space that may exist between the dura mater and arachnoid; contains serous fluid; if bleeding occurs within the cranium, blood may collect here and exert pressure, which can result in brain damage
4. *Arachnoid mater:* impermeable middle membrane that directly covers the brain and spinal cord; contains projections that transfer cerebrospinal fluid (CSF) back into the circulatory system
5. *Subarachnoid space:* space between arachnoid and pia mater that is filled with CSF; all cranial nerves and cerebral arteries and veins pass through this space; site for lumbar puncture ("spinal tap")
6. *Pia mater:* innermost layer that adheres closely to the brain; fuses with lining of ventricles to form the choroid plexus, which is responsible for the production of the CSF

What are the functions of the spinal cord?

1. Receives and processes sensory information from the body
2. Controls muscles through 31 pairs of spinal nerves that branch out to the body

How are the spinal nerves divided?

Cervical (8 pairs), thoracic (12 pairs), lumbar (5 pairs), sacral (5 pairs), and coccygeal (1 pair)

Peripheral nervous system

✎ What are the functions of the 12 pairs of cranial nerves (CN)?

CN I (Olfactory): smell — sensory
CN II (Optic): vision — sensory
CN III (Oculomotor): extraocular eye movement, pupillary constriction, eyelid raising — motor
CN IV (Trochlear): extraocular eye movement — motor
CN V (Trigeminal): innervates head, face, and jaw — motor and sensory
CN VI (Abducens): extraocular eye movement (lateral) — motor
CN VII (Facial): innervates the face — motor and sensory
CN VIII (Acoustic): hearing, sense of balance — sensory
CN IX (Glossopharyngeal): innervates throat, responsible for swallowing and gag reflex — motor and sensory
CN X (Vagus): innervates throat, responsible for swallowing and gag reflex — motor and sensory
CN XI (Spinal accessory): shoulder movement, rotation of head — motor
CN XII (Hypoglossal): innervates the tongue — motor

✎ What's the autonomic nervous system (ANS)?

A portion of the peripheral nervous system (PNS) that consists of motor neurons that control internal organs, such as the heart, lungs, and smooth muscles of the intestine, bladder, and uterus; blood pressure, heart rate, breathing, regional blood flow, cellular metabolism, gastrointestinal motility, secretion of exocrine glands, and body temperature are all regulated by the ANS

◪ *The mind exerts its effects on the functions of the body through the ANS.*

✎ What are the divisions of the ANS?

1. *Sympathetic:* "fight or flight response," norepinephrine, and epinephrine (adrenaline) released; binds to adrenergic receptors; thoracolumbar
2. *Parasympathetic:* "rest and digest," conservation and restoration of energy as well as the reduction of physical and mental stress; acetylcholine released; cholinergic; cranial/sacral

◪ *Both divisions of the ANS innervate the same organs and they act in constant opposition of one another in order to maintain homeostasis.*

✎ What effects do the sympathetic nervous system's release of epinephrine and norepinephrine have on the body?

Increased diaphoresis, decreased digestion, decreased blood flow to abdominal organs, relaxation of bladder smooth muscle, dilation of pupils, and increased energy through the release of glucose stores from the liver (glucagon)

What are the actions of adrenergic receptors?

Alpha 1: peripheral vasoconstriction, mild bronchoconstriction, and stimulation of metabolism
Alpha 2: inhibition of norepinephrine release
Beta 1: increased heart rate
Beta 2: bronchodilation, vasodilation, uterine relaxation
Dopaminergic: dilation of cerebral, renal, and cardiac arteries

◤ *Alpha receptors typically produce excitatory responses of smooth muscle, whereas beta receptors typically produce inhibitory responses of smooth muscle.*

✎ **What effects do the parasympathetic nervous system's release of acetylcholine have on the body?**

Decreased heart rate, increased blood flow to skin and internal organs, intestinal smooth muscle contraction, and constriction of pupils

◤ *The parasympathetic system exerts its affects primarily through the vagus nerve (CN X).*

Sensation and perception

What are the types of sensory receptors?

1. *Mechanoreceptors:* stretching, hearing, and balance
2. *Photoreceptors:* light
3. *Chemoreceptors:* smell and taste
4. *Thermoreceptors:* temperature alterations
5. *Electroreceptors:* electrical currents in surrounding environment

What's an absolute threshold?

The smallest amount of a stimulant that can be perceived

What's adaptation?

The process of becoming less sensitized to a stimulus the more the sensory receptors are exposed to it; the "fading" of perfume throughout the day is a common example

VISION

What are the functions of the various parts of the eye?

1. *Cornea:* clear window of the eye where the majority of focusing occurs
2. *Sclera:* white part of the eye; muscles that move the eyeball connect to the sclera
3. *Anterior chamber or aqueous humor:* front section of the interior of the eye; provides nourishment
4. *Pupil:* point where light enters the eye; changes size in response to amount of light

5. *Iris:* colored membrane that surrounds the pupil and adjusts the amount of light allowed to enter the eye
6. *Lens:* lies behind the pupil and serves as a secondary mechanism of focus
7. *Posterior chamber* or *vitreous humor:* fills the eye to maintain its shape; provides a clear pathway for light to reach the retina from the lens
8. *Retina:* photoreceptor portion of the eye where light is converted into a signal; photoreceptors (rods and cones)
9. *Optic nerve:* pathway for the signals produced by rods and cones to travel from the retina to the brain

What chemical breaks down in response to light, causing a membrane potential that's transmitted to an action potential?

Rhodopsin

What do rods detect?

Differences in light intensity

What do cones detect?

Color

What chemicals bind to cone cells and make them sensitive to a specific wavelength or color?

Opsins; defects in one or more opsin genes can result in color blindness

Different wavelengths produce different colors.

What's the blind spot?

The region of the retina without photoreceptors; any images that fall in this area won't be "seen"

HEARING

What structures are involved with hearing?

1. *Pinna:* cartilaginous outer portion that captures sound waves and reflects them into the auditory canal
2. *Auditory canal:* transmits sound waves from the pinna to the tympanic membrane
3. *Tympanic membrane:* "eardrum"; vibrates in response to sound
4. *Ossicles:* bones of the inner ear that vibrate as the tympanic membrane does; malleus, incus, and stapes
5. *Cochlea:* sensory organ of hearing; contains fluid that vibrates to create wavelike patterns that excite the

cilia in the basilar membrane of the cochlea; also contains organ of Corti

6. *Auditory nerve:* transmits impulses from the ear to the brain

How is sound heard?

Sound waves are collected by the pinna and reflected into the auditory canal, where they cause a vibration of the tympanic membrane. The resulting vibrations of the ossicles are then passed along to the cochlea. The fluid within the cochlea produces a wavelike pattern, which excites the cilia in the basilar membrane. A nerve impulse is generated in the auditory nerve upon excitation of the cilia, and this impulse is then sent to the brain.

✎ What's the function of the vestibular system?

Provides information about movement and the orientation of the body

What's cerumen?

"Ear wax," which acts as a protective barrier for the ear; this sticky wax cleans the the ear canal of dirt and other foreign matter

SMELL (OLFACTION)

What type of receptors are involved with the process of olfaction?

Chemoreceptors, which are located within the olfactory epithelium located in the roof of the two nasal cavities

How does the process of olfaction occur?

Odorants (chemical compounds) from the air come in contact with cilia of the olfactory epithelium in the upper portion of the nasal cavities and bind to receptors on the cilia. This binding induces an enzymatic process, which produces an action potential. This action potential is then conducted along the olfactory nerve to the brain where it's processed.

TASTE (GUSTATION)

What are the sensory organs involved with gustation?

Tongue, palate, pharynx, and epiglottis

What are taste buds?

Specially modified epithelial cells that serve as receptors for chemicals dissolved in saliva

How does the process of gustation occur?

Chemicals in saliva bind to taste receptors, causing them to depolarize. A stimulus is created and is passed along CN VII, IX, or X to the thalamus before it's transmitted to the parietal lobe of the brain, where it's processed

Why do odors frequently elicit memories?

Because of the limbic system's (emotions) involvement in odor processing

⚡ *The senses of smell and taste interact closely with one another.*

What are the four primary tastes?

Sweet, sour, bitter, and salty

TOUCH

How does the sense of touch occur?

Pressure is perceived by mechanoreceptors in the skin. Nerve endings associated with these receptors then transmit the impulses to the brain, where they are processed.

Physical assessment of the neurosensory system

Normal findings

What preparation is necessary for a neurologic evaluation?

1. Provide patient privacy.
2. Obtain a reflex hammer, a penlight, a tongue blade, an ophthalmoscope, an eye chart, a cotton swab, a safety pin, a tuning fork, a dermatome chart, aromatic substances, and a stethoscope.

What categories of function should be included in a complete neurological assessment?

Cognitive function, pupillary response, cranial nerves, motor skills, sensory skills, coordination, and vital signs

⚡ *Level of consciousness is the most effective neurological assessment factor in a conscious patient, and pupillary response is the most effective neurologic assessment factor in an unconscious patient.*

✎ **What factors should be included in a complete cognitive assessment?**

1. *Level of consciousness:* alert, obtunded (confused), stuporous, comatose
2. *Orientation:* person, place, time, purpose
3. *Speech and language:* articulation, rate and rhythm, presence of aphasia

4. *Memory:* short-term (immediate, recent) and long-term
5. *Insight and judgment:* ability to understand and utilize interpretation of behavior and unconscious dynamics; assessment of a patient's ability to function independently at a specific task (signing a consent form, handling finances)
6. *Abstract thinking:* compare and contrast, interpretation of complex concept
7. *Calculations:* counting backwards in specific increments

What's the single most effective factor in assessment of motor function in a conscious patient?

Gait; balance, muscle strength, coordination, and timing can all be assessed by observing a patient's gait.

How is strength assessed?

Ask the patient to perform a specific task (squeeze fingers, flex or extend elbow, knee, ankle) against resistance. Strength is then rated on a scale of 0 to 5, in which 0 is no movement or contraction of the muscle and 5 is normal strength with complete range of motion.

What are the components of a basic sensory assessment?

Light touch and pain sensation in all extremities and assessment of symmetry of sensation by comparing both arms and both legs; more thorough sensory assessments (point localization, response to deep pain and vibration, two-point discrimination) should be performed in people with motor or reflex abnormalities, or skin changes, such as ulcerations or atrophy

How are the reflexes scored?

On a scale of 0 to 4, 0 equals no response and 4 equals hyperactive response with intermittent clonus

What tests may be used to assess coordination?

1. Tapping the index finger against the thumb or a hard surface
2. Touching the finger to the nose and then to the examiner's finger
3. Alternating hands between pronation and supination as quickly as possible
4. Running the heel of one foot up and down along the shin of the other leg
5. Performing a figure-eight movement with the great toe

What are the components of an eye examination?

Inspection of the eyelids, the lacrimal system, the sclera, the cornea, the pupils, pupillary response to light and accommodation, visual field, and acuity

✎ **How is normal pupillary reaction documented?**	PERRLA: **P**upils **E**qual, **R**ound, and **R**eactive to **L**ight and **A**ccommodation. When a light is shined into an eye, the pupil should constrict immediately and then dilate quickly when the light is withdrawn. Accommodation isn't routinely assessed; rather, it's assessed if the pupillary reactions to light are diminished or absent. If accommodation isn't specifically assessed, "PERRL" should be used for accurate documentation.
What's the Rinne test?	A hearing test that uses a vibrating tuning fork placed against the mastoid process to compare the time of bone conduction with air conduction; it's useful in differentiating between conductive and sensorineural hearing loss; normally, air conduction will last longer than bone conduction
What's Weber's test?	A hearing test that uses a vibrating tuning fork against the forehead to identify people with unilateral hearing loss; normally, the sound should be heard equally in both ears
✎ **What's the Whisper test?**	A hearing test in which the patient covers one ear while the examiner whispers two-syllable words into the opposite ear; a soft whisper can normally be heard in each ear

Abnormal findings

What's an altered level of consciousness?	A decreased alertness, awareness, and ability to fully respond to the environment
What's anisocoria?	Unequal size of the pupils; causes are varied, but may include local ophthalmologic conditions (inflammation within anterior chamber, congenital malformation of the iris), dysfunction of CN III, and certain pharmacologic agents (atropine, pilocarpine) 🗲 *Pupils of unequal size can be indicative of increased intracranial pressure (ICP), which causes compression and dysfunction of CN III.*
What's Bell's palsy?	An acute paralysis of CN VII of unknown etiology, which causes unilateral facial paralysis; pain may affect the face and ear: the eye on the affected side tears constantly, the eyelid won't close, and the patient may have difficulty swallowing. There's no definitive treatment; however, prednisone, analgesics, and artificial tears are given for symptom

control. Most cases of Bell's palsy resolve within several months without intervention.

What's trigeminal neuralgia?

Also known as "tic douloureux;" a disorder characterized by severe pain often described as a "lightning bolt" along the path of CN V (trigeminal) with intermittent periods of remission; development of trigeminal neuralgia may occur after trauma or infection, or may be a result of atherosclerosis, tumor, or aneurysm; carbamazepine (Tegretol) is the drug of choice for pain control, although surgery may be necessary to remove the source of pressure along the nerve for intractable pain

What's lethargy?

The state of being sleepy but able to be aroused

What's stupor?

The state of being able to be aroused but with difficulty

What's dysarthria?

Indistinctness in word articulation or enunciation resulting from interference with peripheral speech mechanisms, such as the muscles of the tongue, palate, pharynx, or lips

What's aphasia?

Impairment of language function secondary to damage of the frontal and temporal lobes of the brain; the aphasia may be expressive (impaired ability to speak and write [Broca's aphasia]), receptive (impaired ability to understand written or spoken communication [Wernicke's aphasia]), or global (absence of any intact language skills); it's associated with damage to the left frontal or temporal lobes

What's anomia?

Inability to name objects

What's ataxia?

Lack of coordination in performing a planned, purposeful motion such as walking

What's bradykinesia?

Abnormally slow movement or the inability to initiate movement without difficulty; it's commonly associated with Parkinson's disease; may also be referred to as *hypokinesia*

What's dystonia?

A disorder of hyperkinesis involving sustained, repetitive, or twisting involuntary movements

What's athetosis?

A disorder of hyperkinesis involving spontaneous writhing that results from damage to the extrapyramidal system (basal ganglia), such as occurs with head injuries and strokes; also associated with cerebral palsy and prolonged use of antipsychotics

What's chorea?	Movement similar to athetosis, but on a smaller scale and more abrupt with rapid, arrhythmic motions
✎ **What's tardive dyskinesia?**	A drug-induced disorder of hyperkinesis of slow onset that's characterized by rhythmic tongue movements, "pill-rolling" motions of the fingers, and facial grimacing
✎ **What's the Babinski reflex?**	A superficial plantar reflex involving dorsiflexion of the great toe and fanning of the other toes that is elicited when a stimulus is applied starting at the heel and continues to the great toe; a negative Babinski (downward flexing of the toes) occurs in normal adults, but damage to the corticospinal tracts will cause a positive Babinski reflex
	⚡ *A positive Babinski reflex is considered normal until age 2.*
What's apraxia?	Inability to perform skilled, purposeful movements in the absence of motor, sensory, or coordination losses; has been referred to as "pathological absent-mindedness"
What's paresis?	Weakness
✎ **What's hemiparesis?**	Weakness on one side of the body that commonly occurs after a stroke
What does a hypoactive reflex response indicate?	Lower motor neuron or spinal damage, or a disease involving the muscles or neuromuscular junction
What does a hyperactive reflex response indicate?	Damage of upper motor neuron
✎ **What's a neuropathy?**	A disorder involving a nerve
✎ **What's paresthesia?**	A sensation disturbance characterized by prickling, tingling, or numbness
What's dysesthesia?	An abnormal, unpleasant sensation or pain that results from stimuli that isn't usually painful
✎ **What's tinnitus?**	A sensation of noise in the ear caused by abnormal stimulation of the auditory apparatus; may be described as ringing, buzzing, swishing, roaring, or whistling
What's myopia?	Near-sightedness; parallel rays of light focus in front of the retina as a person looks at a far away object

What's presbyopia?	Loss of lens elasticity leads to the blurring of near objects
What's diplopia?	Double vision
What's nystagmus?	Abnormal eye movements
What's strabismus?	Crossed eyes or abnormal eye alignment, which prohibits focusing simultaneously on a single point; may be congenital or can result from closed head injuries, strokes, or other injuries to the brain or orbit; exercises to strengthen the weakened muscles or glasses are prescribed, but surgical correction may be required to realign the eyes if more conservative therapies are unsuccessful

Major disorders of the sensory system

Eyes

CONJUNCTIVITIS

What's conjunctivitis?	Inflammation of the transparent membrane (conjunctiva) that covers the inner surface of the eyelids; it may be caused by mechanical trauma, infection (viral or bacterial), or allergies; the most common form of conjunctivitis is acute bacterial conjunctivitis ("pinkeye"), which is highly infectious; viral conjunctivitis typically resolves on its own within 1 week
What's the pathophysiologic process of conjunctivitis?	Inflammation of the conjunctiva causes the small blood vessels within the membrane to become more obvious, and the eyes develop a pink or red appearance as a result
What are the clinical manifestations of conjunctivitis?	Reddened eye or eyes, itching of one or both eyes, gritty sensation in the eye or eyes, blurred vision, photosensitivity, and discharge with crusting of the affected eye or eyes
How do bacterial conjunctivitis and viral conjunctivitis differ in their presentations?	Bacterial conjunctivitis typically produces a thick, yellow-green discharge (exudates) and may occur in association with pharyngitis or a respiratory infection, whereas viral conjunctivitis typically produces a watery or mucous discharge; both may be associated with colds
	◤ *Bacterial conjunctival exudates are easily transferred to the uninfected eye, thus leading to a bilateral infection.*
What complications are associated with conjunctivitis?	Temporary blurred vision and possible development of bilateral infections (bacterial)

What's the typical treatment for conjunctivitis?

Warm compresses to clean the eyes and to remove crusty exudate; ophthalmic antibiotic ointment may be prescribed if bacterial etiology is known or suspected

✎ What are important nursing actions when caring for a patient with conjunctivitis?

1. Instruct the patient to keep his hands away from his eyes, and to wash his hands frequently as well as after contact with the affected eye or its discharge.
2. Apply warm compresses to loosen and remove crusty exudates at least daily.
3. Instruct the patient to use a different towel or washcloth each day and to change pillowcases each night.
4. Instruct the patient to avoid sharing towels or handkerchiefs.
5. Instruct the patient to avoid wearing contact lenses and to discard eye cosmetics.
6. Instruct the patient about the proper instillation of ophthalmic ointment (if prescribed).

CORNEAL ABRASION

What's a corneal abrasion?

A superficial injury to the cornea that most commonly results from foreign bodies, such as sand or dust, or from excessive wearing of contact lenses (especially if poorly fitted)

What's the pathophysiologic process of a corneal abrasion?

The corneal surface is denuded or scraped away by external forces

What are the clinical manifestations of a corneal abrasion?

Eye pain, photosensitivity, blurred vision, sensation of foreign object in eye, and watery eyes

What complications are associated with a corneal abrasion?

Serious eye infection can occur if a corneal abrasion is untreated and corneal ulcerations may develop secondary to an infected abrasion

What's the typical treatment for a corneal abrasion?

1. Nonperforating foreign bodies should be removed
2. An antibiotic ointment may be prescribed; however, corneal abrasions typically heal quickly (within 2 days for mild abrasions) without other intervention
3. An eye patch or bandage may be worn for comfort measures

What are important nursing actions when caring for a patient with a corneal abrasion?	1. Administer antibiotic ointment or lubricating eye drops, as ordered by the physician, and apply an eye bandage or a patch, if the patient prefers. 2. Instruct the patient to avoid driving or other potentially hazardous situations until corneal abrasion has healed (2 days). 3. Encourage the use of safety goggles and properly-fitted contact lenses. 4. Determine status of tetanus immunization. If the last immunization was more than 5 years ago, administer a tetanus booster.

CATARACTS

✎ What's a cataract?	Clouding or opacity of the lens that can cause blurred vision and blindness; develops slowly and is painless
What's the pathophysiologic process of a cataract?	Senile cataracts occur as a result of a decrease in protein, increase in sodium, and an accumulation of water. The normal fibers of the lens are disrupted.
What risk factors are associated with cataract development?	Advanced age (over age 60), history of eye trauma, diabetes, prolonged corticosteroid therapy, and excessive exposure to ultraviolet light (more common in those who have worked outdoors or who live in warm, sunny climates)
✎ What are the clinical manifestations of cataracts?	Cloudy white opacity of the pupil, fuzzy or foggy vision, glare sensitivity with lamps or the sun, impaired night vision, halos around lights, and decreased intensity of colors
What complications are associated with cataracts?	Blindness
What's the typical treatment for cataracts?	1. No treatment is necessary for cataracts that aren't bothersome. 2. Surgical removal performed under local anesthesia is the treatment of choice for problematic cataracts, and carries a success rate of 95%. The lens is removed and a lens implant is inserted. Vision can usually be restored to 20/20.
What are the important nursing actions when caring for a patient with cataracts?	1. Instruct the patient to leave the dressing intact until 1 day after surgery. A metal eye shield is worn during sleep for 3 to 4 weeks postoperatively.

2. Instruct the patient to avoid rubbing his eye and sleeping on the operative side for 4 weeks to prevent pressure on the affected eye.
3. Administer medications (stool softeners to prevent constipation, anti-inflammatory drugs, analgesics, antibiotics, ophthalmic drops, and mydriatics to dilate the pupil) as ordered by the physician.
4. Instruct the patient to wear sunglasses when the pupil is dilated.

GLAUCOMA

✎ What's glaucoma?

A group of chronic eye disorders caused by increased intraocular pressure (IOP), resulting in the loss of vision and progression of optic nerve atrophy

What's the patho-physiologic process of glaucoma?

An increase in intraocular pressure is produced when the normal balance of production and drainage of aqueous humor is disrupted. The backup of fluid leads to an increased intraocular pressure, which damages the optic nerve and leads to impaired vision.

What are the clinical manifestations of glaucoma?

Slow loss of vision; progressive loss of peripheral vision, tunnel vision, persistent or acute eye pain, difficulty adjusting to darkness

What complications are associated with glaucoma?

Blindness

What's the typical treatment for glaucoma?

1. Pharmacologic therapy including pilocarpine, timolol (Timoptic), acetazolamide (Diamox), dipivefrin (Propine), and mannitol (Osmitrol) to reduce IOP
2. Surgical intervention (trabeculectomy or laser trabeculoplasty) if pharmacological therapy is ineffective

What are the important nursing actions when caring for a patient with glaucoma?

1. Place a patch over the operative eye.
2. Promote comfort and instruct the patient to lie on his back or nonoperative side.
3. Administer medications (mydriatics, antibiotics, steroids, analgesics) as ordered by the physician.
4. Instruct the patient about the instillation of eye drops.

DIABETIC RETINOPATHY

What's diabetic reti-nopathy?

A complication of vascular disease that results in decreased vision; patients commonly see "floaters" as a result of small hemorrhages within the eye

What's the pathophysiologic process of diabetic retinopathy?

Microaneurysms develop as a result of the thickening of the retinal capillary walls; vision then decreases as retinal veins widen and the vasculature becomes entangled. Small hemorrhages result in scarring, and new vessels grow into the vitreous humor. These new vessels are weak and are prone to rupture.

What are the clinical manifestations of diabetic retinopathy?

Visual disturbances, such as floating specks, dark streaks, or a red film that obscures vision; blurred vision or loss of vision; poor night vision; blind spot in center of visual field; and difficulty adjusting to light

✎ What's the most effective way to prevent diabetic retinopathy?

Maintain optimal glucose control

What complications are associated with diabetic retinopathy?

Abnormal growth of new blood vessels within the eye, which can cause hemorrhage into the vitreous, scar tissue formation with retinal detachment, and development of neovascular glaucoma, which can progress to blindness

What's the typical treatment for diabetic retinopathy?

1. *Photocoagulation:* laser procedure used to create scarring on the peripheral retina, which decreases the ischemia that triggers the formation of new, weak vessels
2. *Vitrectomy:* involves the extraction of the bloody vitreous humor and scar tissue from the posterior chamber; vitreous is replaced with saline or silicone oil

What are important nursing actions in the care of a patient with diabetic retinopathy?

1. Encourage the patient to maintain good blood glucose control.
2. Encourage the patient to maintain normal blood pressure.
3. Promote smoking cessation.
4. Instruct the patient to have annual eye examinations.

DETACHED RETINA

What's a detached retina?

A painless separation of the inner sensory layer of the retina and the outer pigmented layer

What's the patho-physiologic process of a detached retina?

Normally the retina is a multilayered, smooth surface. The retinal layers can separate as a result of trauma, inflammation, or tumor. Degenerative holes or tears in the retina allow the vitreous humor to escape, resulting in detachment. The detachment can have a sudden onset or can occur slowly.

What are the most common causes of retinal detachment?

Bleeding and inflammation related to myopic degeneration and trauma

What are the clinical manifestations of retinal detachment?

Visual disturbances (floating spots, flashes of light, and blurred vision) and loss of vision ("curtain was closed over my eyes")

⚡ *Pain is typically* not *associated with retinal detachment.*

What complications are associated with retinal detachment?

Blindness, if not treated promptly

What's the typical treatment for retinal detachment?

Surgery is the definitive treatment. Retinal tears are typically treated with photocoagulation or cryopexy, in which the portion of the retina surrounding the tear is frozen. Scleral buckling is the most commonly used form of surgery for retinal detachment, and it involves the indentation (buckling) of the sclera by pressing in with a piece of silicone. The buckle is then stitched to the outer portion of the sclera and remains there permanently.

✎ **What are the important nursing considerations post-operatively?**

1. Position the patient with detachment area lowermost (preoperatively, this position prevents further detachment and postoperatively it facilitates approximation of the two retinal layers).
2. Encourage the patient to wear bilateral eye patches to prevent rapid eye movements (can extend the tear).
3. Instruct the patient to avoid bending over with his head below his waist to prevent excessive pressure on fresh surgical site.
4. Administer medications (analgesics) as ordered by the physician and apply cool, moist compresses for comfort.
5. Monitor the patient for complications and notify the physician immediately if any develop. Severe pain is a sign of increased intraocular pressure or hemorrhage.

MACULAR DEGENERATION

What's macular degeneration?

Degenerative changes in the retinal blood vessels that result from the partial breakdown of the retinal pigment epithelium, which typically filters components of blood that are potentially harmful to the retina

What's the pathophysiologic process of macular degeneration?

1. *Neovascular:* fragile new blood vessels appear in the macula and then leak, which leads to scarring and vision loss
2. *Nonneovascular:* more common, atrophy of the choroid and retina occurs as a result of waste products

What are the two types of macular degeneration?

1. *Dry (nonexudative, nonneovascular):* thinning of the retina
2. *Wet (exudative, neovascular):* formation of new blood vessels and leakage of fluid

What are the clinical manifestations of macular degeneration?

1. *Dry:* need for increasingly brighter lights when performing close-up work, washing out or dullness of colors, progressive haziness of vision, and loss of central vision or blind spot in center of visual field (peripheral vision remains intact)
2. *Wet:* distortion of straight lines (appear wavy) and decreased central vision

What complications are associated with macular degeneration?

Loss of ability to read and drive, although complete blindness doesn't occur

What's the typical treatment for macular degeneration?

1. *Dry:* no specific therapy; zinc supplementation may minimize disease progression
2. *Wet:* laser surgery (laser photocoagulation) to coagulate leaking blood vessels, or photodynamic therapy, which involves the chemical destruction of abnormal blood vessels after injection of a light-sensitive medication (Visudyne) through an arm vein and use of a nonthermal laser shone into the eyes

What are important nursing actions in the care of a patient with macular degeneration?

1. Instruct the patient to have annual eye examinations.
2. Encourage the patient to treat other medical conditions, especially high blood pressure.
3. Instruct the patient to wear sunglasses with orange-, yellow-, or amber-tinted lenses to block ultraviolet light (damages retina).
4. Encourage a diet high in antioxidants, such as lutein, zeaxanthin, zinc, and copper (may protect retina).

Ears

EXTERNAL OTITIS

What's external otitis?
An infection (bacterial or fungal) that involves the external ear canal; external otitis is more prevalent in the summer, and is commonly known as "swimmer's ear"

What's the pathophysiologic process of external otitis?
Water becomes trapped in the ear, which facilitates the growth of bacteria and fungi

What are the clinical manifestations of external otitis?
Pain in or around the ear, itching in the ear canal, sensation of fullness in the ear, and drainage from the ear canal (clear or greenish-yellow)

What complications are associated with external otitis?
Temporary hearing loss, chronic external otitis, inflammation and damage to the bones at the base of the skull, and cellulitis

What's the typical treatment for external otitis?
1. Antibiotics (local or systemic) are used to treat external otitis. In the event that the ear canal is swollen shut, a wick can be inserted to allow the antibiotic to enter the ear canal.
2. Analgesics, such as NSAIDs, are used for pain relief.
3. Topical corticosteroids may be used to minimize discomfort and itching.

What are the important nursing actions related to external otitis?
1. Administer medications (antibiotics, analgesics, ear drops) as ordered by the physician. Instruct the patient or his caregiver about the instillation of eardrops.
2. Apply a warm heating pad against the affected ear to minimize discomfort.
3. Instruct the patient to avoid swimming or allowing water to enter the ear canal until the infection has resolved (ear plugs or cotton balls with Vaseline can be used while showering). Once the infection has resolved, encourage the use of earplugs when swimming.

OTITIS MEDIA

What's otitis media?
A nonpurulent bacterial or viral infection of the middle ear that may be mucoid or serous in nature

What's the pathophysiologic process of otitis media?
Swelling and inflammation of the eustachian tubes occurs (usually secondary to an upper respiratory infection), which prevents the tubes from draining fluid completely;

fluid becomes trapped within the ear, which then becomes infected

▧ *Children are more commonly affected by otitis media because they have shorter and narrower eustachian tubes than adults.*

What are the clinical manifestations of otitis media?

Throbbing ear pain, fever, bulging of the tympanic membrane, and drainage from the ear

What complications are associated with otitis media?

Mastoiditis (infection of the mastoid cavity with extension of a middle ear infection) and hearing loss if untreated

What's the typical treatment for otitis media?

1. Broad-spectrum antibiotics for acute infections
2. Surgical intervention (myringotomy) to restore normal middle ear and eustachian tube function may be performed if the infection becomes chronic. A small incision is made in the tympanic membrane, allowing the accumulated fluid to escape. Tubes, which fall out independently at a later time, may be inserted into the incisional area.

What are the important nursing actions when caring for a patient with otitis media?

1. Apply warm compress to the affected ear several times per day to relieve discomfort.
2. Administer medications (antibiotics, analgesics, antipyretics) as ordered by the physician.
3. Instruct the patient to avoid getting water in his ears.

LABYRINTHITIS

What's labyrinthitis?

An inflammatory disorder of the inner ear canals, which causes dizziness or vertigo (pathologic sensation of movement; spinning sensation); it commonly occurs following an ear infection, an upper respiratory infection, head trauma, or ingestion of certain drugs

What's the pathophysiologic process of labyrinthitis?

Although the underlying cause isn't well understood, dysfunction of the vestibular system in the inner ear results in the sensation of dizziness or the perceived instability of one's surroundings

What are the clinical manifestations of labyrinthitis?

Dizziness, vertigo, loss of balance, nausea and vomiting, tinnitus, and hearing loss

What complications are associated with labyrinthitis?	Injury from falls and permanent hearing loss if the condition goes untreated

What's the typical treatment for labyrinthitis?

1. Although it's typically self-limited, symptomatic treatment for acute labyrinthitis may include antihistamines (meclizine [Antivert]), antiemetics (promethazine [Phenergan]), anticholinergics (scopolamine), and benzodiazepines (diazepam [Valium]).
2. Treatment for persistent labyrinthitis may include vestibular rehabilitation, an intensive regimen of home exercises and physical therapy used to strengthen the vestibular, proprioceptive, and visual systems.

What are important nursing actions in the care of a patient with labyrinthitis?

1. Instruct the patient to remain still and to rest during episodes. Potentially hazardous activities, such as driving, should be avoided.
2. Instruct the patient to change position slowly and to gradually resume activity.
3. Instruct the patient to avoid bright lights and reading during episodes.
4. Inform the patient that alcohol should be avoided.
5. Administer medications (antihistamines, antiemetics, anticholinergics, benzodiazepines) as ordered by the physician.

MÉNIÈRE'S DISEASE

What's Ménière's disease?

A syndrome characterized by periods of spinning vertigo, loss of hearing, and tinnitus (ringing in the ears); an attack of Ménière's disease typically lasts several hours; although the underlying cause is unknown, genetics, food allergies, and inner ear injuries are suspected to be contributing factors

What's the pathophysiologic process of Ménière's disease?

The fluid and electrolyte balance is altered when lymph fluids mix, the labyrinth is distended, and volume and pressure increase

What are the clinical manifestations of Ménière's disease?

Vertigo, tinnitus, and hearing loss alternating with sound distortion

What complications are associated with Ménière's disease?

Injuries from falls and permanent hearing loss

What's the typical treatment for Ménière's disease?	1. There's no cure; however, the symptoms are typically treated with sedatives such as diazepam (Valium) and antiemetics such as prochlorperazine (Compazine). 2. Diet therapy may also be effective in minimizing the symptoms. Caffeine, sugar, salt, monosodium glutamate (MSG), and alcohol should be avoided. 3. If symptoms persist and are uncontrolled with medication, surgical removal of the labyrinth may be necessary.
What are important nursing actions in the care of a patient with Ménière's disease?	1. Instruct the patient to lie in a quiet room and close his eyes during acute attacks. 2. Administer medications (sedatives, antiemetics) as ordered by the physician. 3. Instruct the patient to avoid potentially hazardous activities (driving, operating heavy machinery) during attacks or while using antiemetics and sedatives. 4. Instruct the patient to reduce dietary salt.

Major disorders of the neurologic system

Headaches

What's a headache?	Discomfort or pain within the tissues of the cranium that can result from benign muscular or vascular conditions as well as from organic conditions caused by intracranial or extracranial diseases ◆ *A headache is a symptom as well as a disease process.*
What's the pathophysiologic process of a headache?	The pain of headache can be generated by prolonged contraction of skeletal scalp and neck muscles; vascular stretching; or dilatation and inflammation of — or direct pressure on — cranial and cervical contents. It's suspected that serotonin is the neurotransmitter involved in headaches, but the exact pathophysiology is unknown.
How are functional headaches classified?	1. *Tension:* prolonged muscular contraction in the head, neck, and jaws 2. *Migraine:* vasodilatation involving the intracranial and extracranial arteries of the head 3. *Cluster:* vascular origin similar to migraine
◆ **What are the clinical manifestations of a headache?**	1. *Tension:* bilateral pain (commonly in the back of the neck) involving a tight or squeezing sensation; no prodrome or interference with sleep 2. *Migraine:* intense pulsing or throbbing pain (usually unilateral), diaphoresis, nausea, vomiting; may be

preceded by aural phase characterized by weakness, dizziness, and visual defects, such as flashing lights in a quadrant of the visual field

3. *Cluster:* similar to migraine, but occur in "clusters" of weeks to months

▧ *A headache described as the "worst headache of my life" may suggest a subarachnoid hemorrhage.*

What's temporal arteritis?

A unilateral or bilateral headache caused by inflammation of the temporal or occipital arteries that may result in loss of vision

What's the typical treatment for headaches?

1. Nonnarcotic analgesics, such as acetaminophen, NSAIDs, and COX-2 inhibitors are preferred, although analgesic combinations containing butalbital (Fiorinal, Fioricet) or isometheptene (Midrin) may be used as well
2. Muscle relaxants for tension headaches
3. Serotonin agonists, such as ergotamine (Migranal nasal spray), sumatriptan (Imitrex), zolmitriptan (Zomig), and rizatriptan (Maxalt) for migraine and cluster headaches
4. Antiemetics, such as promethazine (Phenergan), for nausea and vomiting
5. Nonpharmacologic therapies, such as massage, relaxation techniques, and biofeedback
6. Prophylactic therapy includes propanolol, verapamil, and tricyclic antidepressants, such as amitriptyline (Elavil) and lithium.

✎ What are important nursing actions for a patient with a headache?

1. Provide a dark, quiet room and minimize other environmental stimuli as much as possible.
2. Administer medications (analgesics, antiemetics, prophylactics) as ordered by the physician.
3. Encourage the patient to keep a headache diary to identify possible triggers. Instruct him to avoid known or suspected triggers.
4. Encourage daily exercise as well as the practice of relaxation techniques and biofeedback.
5. Educate the patient about dietary modifications when appropriate (certain foods may be triggers).

Head injuries

What's a head injury?

Trauma to the scalp, skull, or brain

What's the patho-physiologic process of a head injury?

A blunt or penetrating force is exerted on the skull, which causes the brain to impact the skull

✎ What types of closed head injuries can occur?

1. *Concussion:* transitory change in neurologic function caused by mechanical force; structural changes aren't evident, but cognitive deficits, including brief loss of consciousness and amnesia surrounding the incident, are associated with the injury
2. *Contusion:* a structural alteration leading to a leakage of blood into the brain, similar to a bruise; the contusion can be at the site of the injury (coup) or on the side opposite injury (contrecoup)
3. *Lacerations:* tearing of brain tissue caused by shearing force or a sharp object; more serious as hemorrhage may occur

❧ *A closed head injury results from blunt trauma to the brain, but the skull remains intact.*

✎ What types of hematoma (bleeding) can result from a head injury?

1. *Epidural or extradural:* bleeding (usually arterial) above the dura mater; clot formation compresses the brain, which can quickly progress to herniation and death
2. *Subdural:* bleeding (usually venous) below the dura mater and arachnoid layer, which results in a clot formation; clinical manifestations may be acute, subacute, or chronic
3. *Intracerebral:* bleeding into the brain tissue itself; associated with high mortality rate
4. *Subarachnoid:* an extension of bleeding into the subarachnoid space and cerebrospinal fluid (CSF)

✎ What are the clinical manifestations of a head injury?

Headache, dizziness, nausea, vomiting, amnesia related to the incident, lethargy, change in level of consciousness or behavior, and inability to concentrate; severe head trauma may also result in sensory and motor dysfunction (hemiparesis, hemiplegia, shallow breathing, abnormal size and reaction of pupils) due to cranial nerve injury as well as seizures and coma

✎ What are some of the clinical manifestations of a skull fracture?

Leakage of CSF and blood from nose or ears (presence of glucose indicates CSF), bulging of tympanic membrane by blood or CSF, Battle's sign (ecchymosis behind the ear that develops 24 hours after injury), raccoon's eyes (ecchymosis around eyes), and temporary deafness and loss of consciousness

What complications are associated with a head injury?

Memory loss or difficulty (posttraumatic amnesia), hematoma formation, infection, increased intracranial pressure, cerebral edema, diabetes insipidus, syndrome of inappropriate antidiuretic hormone, posttraumatic epilepsy, coma, brain herniation, and brain death

Increased intracranial pressure (ICP) is the primary cause of death for those who sustain a head injury.

What's the Glasgow Coma Scale?

A scale from 0 to 15 used to assess a patient's level of consciousness, particularly following trauma by assessing the patient's eye-opening, verbal, and motor responses; a score of 13 to 15 indicates a mild head injury, 9 to 12 indicates a moderate head injury, and lower than 8 indicates a severe head injury with coma (absence of ability to follow commands, open eyes, or make verbalizations)

What are the primary goals in the management of a patient with a head injury?

1. Decrease cerebral edema and ICP to prevent cerebral ischemia.
2. Maintain oxygenation.
3. Maintain circulation.
4. Maintain normothermia.
5. Prevent seizures.

What's the typical treatment for a head injury?

1. Bed rest with the head of the bed flat, unless contraindicated by increased ICP
2. Intubation for airway protection
3. Pharmacologic therapy, including osmotic diuretics (mannitol), antibiotics, and anticonvulsants
4. Surgery (craniotomy) may be necessary for evacuation of hematoma or for edema relief

Any patient with a head injury must be presumed to have a spinal cord injury until proven otherwise. A cervical collar should be left in place until imaging studies exclude injury to the spinal cord.

The head of the bed should be elevated to at least 30 degrees if increased ICP is present.

What are the important nursing actions in the care of a patient with a head injury?

1. Immobilize the patient's head and neck until spinal cord injury has been ruled out.
2. Maintain bed rest with the head of the bed flat unless contraindicated by increased ICP.
3. Perform neurologic assessments at intervals determined by the patient's condition.
4. Implement measures to prevent ICP increases. Minimize patient straining or movement, suction only when necessary, and avoid the use of restraints.
5. Administer medications (osmotic diuretics, anticonvulsants) as ordered by the physician.

6. Monitor the patient for complications (behavioral changes, respiratory changes, abnormal size or reaction of pupils), and notify the physician immediately if any develop.
7. Anticipate the need for surgery (craniotomy) if acute subdural or epidural hematoma occurs.

Increased intracranial pressure

What's increased intracranial pressure (ICP)?

A life-threatening pathologic process involving increased pressure within the skull, which compresses the brain structures and blood vessels; increased blood and CSF volumes, as well as swelling of the brain (cerebral edema), can produce an increase in ICP

What's the pathophysiologic process of increased ICP?

Because the cranial vault is rigid and can't expand, a change in volume of any of the components, brain, blood, or cerebrospinal fluid will potentially alter the delicate balance within the skull; the resulting increase in ICP leads to decreased cerebral perfusion, tissue hypoxia, and ischemia, which compromise effective brain functioning

What clinical manifestations are associated with increased ICP?

1. Altered mental status, including decreased level of consciousness (earliest and most sensitive sign), behavioral changes, restlessness, irritability, and confusion
2. Headache
3. Nausea and vomiting
4. Seizures
5. Pupillary changes (asymmetric, fixed and dilated, or nonreactive)
6. Papilledema (edema and hyperemia of the optic disc)
7. Motor weakness and sensory deficits (hemiparesis, hemiplegia)
8. Altered respiratory patterns, including Cheyne-Stokes (rhythmic waxing and waning with apnea), apneustic (prolonged inspiration with a 2- or more second pause), and ataxic (irregular, unpredictable breathing with alternating deep and shallow breaths)
9. Decerebrate posturing: extension of arms and legs with internal rotation; downward pointing toes; backward arching of the head (late)
10. Decorticate posturing: flexion of arms with hyperextension of legs; clenching of fists (late)

Remember that atropine-like medications can cause pupil dilation.

What are the late clinical manifestations associated with increased ICP that comprise the Cushing triad and indicate brain stem involvement?

1. Bradycardia with a full and bounding pulse
2. Hypertension
3. Widening pulse pressure (difference between systolic and diastolic pressures increases)

What complications are associated with increased ICP?

Because the brain is rigidly confined within the skull, any swelling of the brain may lead to compromise of cerebral blood flow, which can progress to brain stem herniation and eventually death.

Cerebral blood perfusion is inversely related to intracranial pressure. Increased ICP diminishes cerebral blood flow.

What methods are used for continuous ICP measurement?

Fiber-optic epidural sensor, subarachnoid bolt or screw, and ventriculostomy catheter

The patient should be in a supine position for an accurate ICP measurement.

What's normal ICP?

Less than 10 mm Hg, although it can vary with activity; coughing and sneezing can raise ICP sharply for brief periods

What are potential causes of acute increased ICP (more than 20 mm Hg)?

Cerebral edema (head injury, encephalitis), subarachnoid hemorrhage, brain tumors, and hepatic encephalopathy

What are typical treatment measures for a patient with increased ICP?

1. Elevate the head of the bed with slight head-up tilt.
2. Use mechanical ventilation to provide hyperventilation in order to reduce $Paco_2$ to 25 to 30 mm Hg (low $Paco_2$ causes vasoconstriction and reduction of ICP).
3. Administer osmotic diuretics (mannitol) and corticosteroids, such as dexamethasone, to decrease edema and thereby increase cerebral blood flow and cerebral oxygen delivery.
4. Sedate the patient with an I.V. anesthetic agent (propofol, thiopental) to reduce metabolic rate, oxygen consumption, and carbon dioxide production.
5. Administer antihypertensives, anticonvulsants, and antipyretics.
6. Drain CSF via ventriculostomy.
7. Administer corticosteroids (Decadron) to decrease edema (primarily with tumors).
8. Remove tumors, hematomas, or abscesses surgically, if necessary.

✎ **What are important nursing interventions for a patient with increased ICP?**

1. Elevate the head of the bed more than 30 degrees at all times.
2. Maintain head-in-midline position.
3. Assess vital signs (especially blood pressure and temperature), neurologic status (Glasgow Coma Scale), and pupils (size, symmetry) at least once an hour. Maintain mean arterial pressure 60 to 160 mm Hg and core body temperature less than 100.4° F (38° C).
4. Minimize patient straining or movement and avoid talking at his bedside.
5. Suction the patient only when needed.
6. Monitor intake and output hourly.
7. Maintain ventilator settings as ordered by the physician.
8. Administer osmotic diuretics (mannitol) as ordered by the physician.
9. Administer I.V. medications (sedatives, paralytic agents, analgesics) as ordered by the physician.

⚡ *Notify the physician immediately if a patient with increased ICP begins posturing or develops seizures, shivering, or pain.*

Epilepsy and seizure disorders

What's a seizure?

An episode of sudden disorganized electrical impulses from neurons in the brain's cerebral cortex; this discharge may trigger a convulsive movement, a decreased level of consciousness, or a combination; can be caused by many factors, including head injury, high fever, metabolic disturbances, toxicities (lead, carbon monoxide), withdrawal from drugs or alcohol, cerebral ischemia, tumor, and infections within the CNS, and certain medications; also called *convulsions*

What's the pathophysiologic process of a seizure?

A hypersensitive group of easily activated neurons fire abnormally

✎ **What are some common types of seizures?**

1. *Petit mal:* a temporary disturbance in brain function produces subtle behavioral changes (blinking, staring into space, pausing in the midst of a conversation) that typically lasts less than 30 seconds; the condition is hereditary and typically occurs in people under the age of 20
2. *Partial:* involves a brief alteration of brain function when a focal point of abnormal electrical activity in

the brain causes symptoms in a particular part of the body; may be simple or complex

3. *Generalized tonic-clonic (grand mal):* muscle rigidity and violent muscle contractions involving the entire body, and loss of consciousness due to abnormal electrical activity at multiple sites in the brain

What's epilepsy?

A condition characterized by recurrent seizures

What are the clinical manifestations of a seizure?

Alteration in mental status (decreased alertness, brief loss of awareness, confusion, behavioral changes), jaw clenching, violent involuntary muscle contractions, incontinence (bowel or bladder), and dyspnea or apnea, which may progress to cyanosis

Manifestations of a seizure vary greatly according to type and, therefore, may be very mild or quite dramatic.

What are common occurrences in the postictal state?

Disorientation, amnesia surrounding the seizure, difficulty speaking, and somnolence

What's an aura?

A sense of awareness of an impending seizure; sensory hallucinations involving sights, tastes, and smells are common

What complications are associated with seizures?

Injury during a seizure, aspiration, development of epilepsy (chronic seizure disorder), respiratory distress, anoxia, and death related to status epilepticus (continuous seizing)

What's the typical treatment for a seizure?

1. Anticonvulsants
2. Identification and treatment of the underlying cause
3. Surgical removal of the seizure focus in the brain (a temporal lobectomy) for intractable, localized seizures, if necessary; a corpus callostomy (severing of connections between brain hemispheres) is occasionally performed to prevent the spread of electrical impulses from one side of the brain to the other, which may decrease the severity and frequency of seizure-related injuries

Never restrain a person experiencing a seizure and don't place anything between the teeth.

What are important nursing actions in the care of a patient with a seizure disorder?

1. Implement seizure precautions (padded side rails).
2. Encourage strict medication compliance with consistent dosing to maintain therapeutic drug levels.
3. Provide safety education, including avoiding driving if uncontrolled seizures are experienced, and avoiding swimming or biking alone.

4. Instruct the patient to maintain a seizure log.
5. Prepare the patient for EEG or other diagnostic studies (magnetic resonance imaging, positron emission tomography scan, magnetic resonance spectroscopy imaging).
6. Encourage the patient to wear medical identification jewelry.
7. During a seizure, protect the patient from harm by clearing the immediate area of furniture and sharp objects, supporting his head with a small pillow, loosening any tight clothing, and turning the patient onto his side if vomiting occurs to prevent aspiration. The physician should be notified of the event as soon as possible, and medications ordered for status epilepticus (anticonvulsants, diazepam, lorazepam) should be administered promptly and as directed. After the seizure has resolved, attempt to reorient the patient, obtain vital signs, and avoid giving anything by mouth until the patient is fully alert. Allow the patient to sleep, if desired.
8. Encourage adequate sleep and discourage the use of alcohol, because it may decrease the effectiveness of anticonvulsants.
9. Monitor plasma drug levels to ensure therapeutic dosing.

Stroke (brain attack)

What's a stroke?	Acute neurologic damage that results from decreased blood flow to the brain; the two major types are ischemic and hemorrhagic
What's the pathophysiologic process of a stroke?	Interruption of the blood supply to the brain deprives it of oxygen and nutrients, resulting in the death of brain tissue
What are the risk factors for a stroke?	Hypertension, hyperlipidemia, coronary artery disease or atherosclerosis, diabetes mellitus, certain cardiac arrhythmias (atrial fibrillation), smoking, obesity, hormonal contraceptive use (rare, but smoking increases risk), cocaine use, heart failure, family history of stroke, and previous transient ischemic attack
What's a transient ischemic attack (TIA)?	A focal ischemic event that causes a brief disturbance in the brain's blood supply, resulting in a temporary neurologic deficit; resolves within 24 hours of symptom onset without residual deficits; also referred to as a "mini stroke" (a stroke is an ischemic event in the brain that lasts longer than 24 hours)

What's a stroke in evolution?	The progression or fluctuation of symptoms for the first 24 to 48 hours after a stroke; a completed stroke is determined by the absence of further deterioration

How can strokes be classified?

1. *Hemorrhagic:* bleeding within the brain due to ruptured or leaking aneurysm, an arteriovenous malformation (AVM), use of anticoagulants, and hypertension; less common than ischemic strokes, but is more commonly fatal
2. *Ischemic (thrombotic, embolic):* due to hypercoagulable states (protein C and S deficiencies), prosthetic heart valves, atrial fibrillation, cancer, and sickle cell disease; most common cause of strokes (80%)

A thrombus is a blood clot. An embolus is a moving blood clot, a piece of plaque, fat, or other material.

Embolic strokes can occur at any time and aren't associated with activity level.

What types of hemorrhagic strokes occur?

1. *Epidural:* bleeding occurs between the skull and meninges
2. *Subdural:* tearing of veins between the dura and brain surface from cranial trauma
3. *Subarachnoid:* refer to bleeding into the subarachnoid; "worst headache of my life"
4. *Intracerebral:* occur as bleeding occurs into the brain tissue itself

Hemorrhagic strokes are named based on the location of the bleed.

What's the most common artery involved in a stroke?

The middle cerebral artery

What are the clinical manifestations of a stroke?

Hemiparesis or hemiplegia, speech or visual disturbances, decreased level of consciousness or loss of consciousness, agnosia (inability to recognize familiar things), abnormal breathing patterns, and unequal pupils (larger on hemorrhage side)

What are the manifestations of right brain damage?

Impaired judgment, impulsive and impatient behavior, short attention span, spatial or perceptual deficits

What are the manifestations of left brain damage?

Speech and language deficits, such as dysarthria and aphasia

What diagnostic tests are used to evaluate for a potential stroke?

Noncontrast computed tomography of the brain to determine if stroke is ischemic or hemorrhagic; an arteriogram may be performed to identify vascular abnormalities (AVM, aneurysm)

What complications are associated with a stroke?

Contractures, muscle spasticity, difficulty swallowing, aspiration, loss of motor or sensory skills in an area of the body, altered communication skills, altered level of consciousness, pressure (decubitus) ulcers, hydrocephalus (from brain bleeding), and death

What's the typical treatment for a stroke?

1. *Pharmacologic therapy:* lorazepam (Ativan), diazepam (Valium), and midazolam (Versed) for extreme agitation; anticonvulsants; antihypertensives; corticosteroids; thrombolytics and anticoagulants for ischemic strokes; analgesics
2. *Surgical intervention (evacuation of hematoma, aneurysm clipping, coil embolization):* for hemorrhagic strokes; a ventriculostomy may be necessary to relieve the pressure from hydrocephalus; a carotid endarterectomy may be performed at a later date to prevent new embolic strokes

◤ *Thrombolytic agents should be initiated within 3 hours of symptom onset.*

◤ *Streptokinase isn't recommended for use with strokes.*

✎ What are important nursing actions in the care of a patient with a stroke?

1. Ensure adequate and effective airway and respirations. Anticipate the need for possible intubation and ventilation.
2. Monitor vital signs and pulse oximetry at frequent intervals. Administer supplemental oxygen if oxygen saturation is less than or equal to 94%.
3. Maintain nothing-by-mouth status and bed rest.
4. Perform neurologic checks at frequent intervals. Evaluate level of consciousness, pupils, assess for facial droop, arm weakness, and speech impairment.
5. Maintain normal ICP and blood pressure. Avoid positions and activities that would increase ICP, and maintain normal body temperature. Elevate the head of the bed slightly and provide stool softeners or laxatives to prevent straining on defecation. Maintain systolic blood pressure less than 220 mm Hg and diastolic pressure less than 120 mm Hg.
6. Monitor intake and output closely and avoid overhydration.
7. Administer medications (thrombolytics, sedatives, antihypertensives) as ordered by the physician.

8. Implement bleeding precautions for at least 24 hours with thrombolytic, antiplatelet, or anticoagulant therapy.
9. Monitor blood test results (prothrombin time or international normalized ratio, partial thromboplastin time).
10. Encourage activities within the patient's physical limitations and participation in physical, occupational, and speech therapy.
11. Assess the need for rehabilitation services beyond discharge and collaborate with social worker and physician.
12. Place frequently used objects on the functional (or unaffected) side and implement safety measures for hemiparesis or hemiplegia.

Multiple sclerosis

What's multiple sclerosis (MS)?

A degenerative neuromuscular disease caused by demyelination of the motor and sensory nerves in the central nervous system; it's thought that the demyelination process is triggered by an autoimmune response or by a virus that causes the loss of Schwann cells, the myelin sheath, and the axon

What's the pathophysiologic process of MS?

Activated T-cells attack the myelin sheath of motor and sensory nerves, causing inflammation. Repeated episodes of inflammation result in destruction of the myelin sheath (demyelination) and scarring (sclerosis), which slows or blocks impulse conduction.

What are the clinical manifestations of MS?

Muscle weakness or spasticity, sensory loss, optic neuritis, tremor, ataxia, fatigue, bladder or bowel dysfunction, visual or speech disturbances, and paresthesia

What complications are associated with MS?

Progressive disability, seizures, and paralysis

What's the typical treatment for MS?

1. Corticosteroids (methylprednisolone, prednisone) to decrease inflammation
2. Muscle relaxants or antispasmodics, such as baclofen, diazepam (Valium), dantrolene (Dantrium), oxybutynin (Ditropan), and tizanidine (Zanaflex), for spasticity
3. Immunosuppressive agents, such as azathioprine (Imuran) and cyclophosphamide (Cytoxan)
4. Pituitary hormones such as corticotropin (ACTH)
5. Interferon beta-1b or glatiramer (Copaxone) for patients with a relapsing or remitting course

6. Physical and occupational therapy to maintain strength and flexibility

✎ What are important nursing actions in the care of a patient with MS?

1. Instruct the patient to avoid factors that can trigger attacks, such as fever, hot baths, stress, and sun exposure.
2. Instruct the patient to take medications consistently.
3. Encourage adequate rest and good nutrition.
4. Encourage regular exercise to maintain muscle tone.
5. Encourage independence with daily activities but provide assistance as appropriate.
6. Administer medications (corticosteroids, interferons, cholinergics) as ordered by the physician.

Guillain-Barré syndrome

✎ What's Guillain-Barré syndrome?

An acute, progressive, ascending paralysis that affects the motor components of the peripheral nervous system (spinal and cranial nerves), particularly the facial nerves; the condition commonly follows a viral illness, such as mononucleosis, herpes simplex, upper respiratory tract infections, and GI tract infections; also referred to as *acute idiopathic polyneuritis*

� *Recovery is possible with Guillain-Barré syndrome because the nerve cell body, axons, and Schwann cells aren't destroyed as they are in multiple sclerosis.*

What's the pathophysiologic process of Guillain-Barré syndrome?

An immune response triggers demyelination of the sheath surrounding the peripheral nerves; transmission of impulses is blocked

What are the clinical manifestations of Guillain-Barré syndrome?

Symmetric and proximal muscle weakness, neuropathy, and paresthesia in a stocking distribution of the legs that ascends to the trunk and arms; difficulty swallowing or breathing and blurred vision may occur, and the cerebrospinal fluid may also contain an increased amount of protein

What complications are associated with Guillain-Barré syndrome?

Impaired mobility, deep vein thrombosis and pulmonary embolism, aspiration, respiratory failure, and paralysis

What's the typical treatment for Guillain-Barré syndrome?

1. Respiratory support is a priority; ventilatory support may be necessary
2. Corticosteroids to reduce inflammation

3. Plasmapheresis to remove antibodies and proteins from the blood
4. High dose immunoglobulin therapy
5. Immunosuppressive therapy with azathioprine (Imuran) and cyclophosphamide (Cytoxan)
6. Anticoagulants, such as heparin, to prevent clot formation from immobility

What are important nursing actions in the care of a patient with Guillain-Barré syndrome?

1. Assess respiratory function including vital capacity measurement. Anticipate the need for intubation and ventilation.
2. Assess muscle strength and swallowing ability.
3. Encourage mobility and assist with transfers or ambulation as needed. Promote self-care.
4. Administer medications (corticosteroids, immunosuppressants) as ordered by the physician.

Myasthenia gravis

What's myasthenia gravis?

A progressive disorder of the neuromuscular junction caused by the destruction of acetylcholine receptors, which results in muscle weakness

What's the pathophysiologic process of myasthenia gravis?

Antibodies are produced that attack acetylcholine receptors, and conduction of nerve impulses across the neuromuscular synapse is impaired; thymus dysfunction is a suspected cause

What are the clinical manifestations of myasthenia gravis?

Generalized muscle weakness that improves with rest, fatigue, visual changes, difficulty chewing or swallowing, decreased cough and gag reflexes, and decreased respiratory rate

What are the complications of myasthenia gravis?

Myasthenic crisis (rapid onset of severe weakness of respiratory muscles), respiratory failure

What's the typical treatment for myasthenia gravis?

1. Anticholinesterases, such as pyridostigmine (Mestinon), to slow the breakdown of acetylcholine, which provides a longer period for it to bind receptors on the postsynaptic membrane
2. Prednisone and other immunosuppressant agents, such as azathioprine (Imuran) and cyclophosphamide (Cytoxan)
3. Thymectomy may be beneficial for young patients with early disease
4. Plasmapheresis
5. I.V. infusion of immune globulin

What are important nursing actions in the care of a patient with myasthenia gravis?

1. Encourage energy conservation and frequent rest periods during activity.
2. Administer medications (anticholinesterases, immunosuppressants) as ordered by the physician.
3. Assess motor strength before and after medication administration.
4. Monitor the patient for complications, such as respiratory difficulty, and notify the physician immediately if any develop.

Parkinson's disease (paralysis agitans)

What's Parkinson's disease?

A chronic, degenerative disorder of the basal ganglia, characterized by hypokinetic movements, such as a resting tremor, and rigidity; Parkinson's disease develops as a primary and idiopathic disease due to insufficient dopamine levels, or it may develop in response to the use of some antipsychotic drugs; it's commonly referred to as *shaking palsy*

What's the pathophysiologic process of Parkinson's disease?

A deficiency of the neurotransmitter dopamine results from the destruction of the substantia nigra in the brain stem. The substantia nigra is a component of the extrapyramidal system, which controls unconscious movements, as well as the initiation, modulation, and completion of movement.

What are the clinical manifestations of Parkinson's disease?

Resting tremor (pill rolling, with rotary motion of thumb and forefinger), cogwheel rigidity (stiff, jerking movements), and bradykinesia (slow movement) are the three cardinal symptoms. Gait disorders (shuffling, stooped posture, decreased arm swing), incoordination, masked facies, drooling, decreased blinking, dementia, and sensory disturbances including hallucinations may occur as secondary symptoms.

What complications are associated with Parkinson's disease?

Progressive disability, dysphagia, and injuries from falls

What are the typical pharmacological agents used in the treatment of Parkinson's disease?

1. Dopamine agonists, such as bromocriptine (Parlodel), pergolide (Permax), pramipexole (Miraplex), and ropinirole (Requip), to stimulate dopamine receptors in the brain
2. Dopamine precursors, such as carbidopa or levodopa (Sinemet), for rigidity, tremor, and bradykinesia
3. Anticholinergics, such as benztropine (Cogentin) and trihexyphenidyl (Artane), for rigidity and tremor

4. Antiviral agents, such as amantadine (Symmetrel), for rigidity, bradykinesia, and dyskinesia
5. Catechol-O-methyltransferase (COMT) inhibitors, such as tolcapone (Tasmar) and entacapone (Comtan), to increase the effectiveness of levodopa
6. MAO-B inhibitors, such as selegiline (Eldepryl), to block the metabolism of dopamine

⚡ *The body converts the medication levodopa into dopamine. Carbidopa is used in conjunction with levodopa to minimize its adverse effects and enhance its actions.*

✎ What are important nursing actions in the care of a patient with Parkinson's disease?

1. Provide supervision and safety through modification of the environment (elimination of clutter to prevent falls, use of door alarms to prevent wandering).
2. Encourage activity and self-sufficiency as much as possible during the early phases of the disease.
3. Establish and maintain routines. Assign the same care provider whenever possible.
4. Provide frequent rest periods to avoid fatigue.
5. Limit environmental stimuli whenever possible (noise, size of groups).
6. Monitor nutritional intake.
7. Administer medications (dopamine agonists, dopamine precursors, anticholinergics, COMT inhibitors, MAO-B inhibitors) as ordered by the physician.
8. Consult social services, physical, and occupational therapy.
9. Provide support and respite care for caregivers.

Alzheimer's disease

✎ What's Alzheimer's disease?

A progressive organic brain disorder that affects the cerebral cortex and causes a loss of cognitive ability as well as behavioral changes; it's a common form of senile dementia and carries a poor prognosis

Genetics and aluminum are suspected factors in the development of Alzheimer's. NSAIDs, vitamin E, and estrogen are believed to offer some protection against development of the disease. A high systolic blood pressure (greater than 160 mm Hg) and an elevated total cholesterol level (greater than 250 mg/dl) has been shown to increase the risk for developing Alzheimer's disease.

What's the patho-physiologic process of Alzheimer's disease?

A loss of cells in the hippocampus, cerebral cortex, and subcortical areas of the cerebrum occurs, which affects memory, cognition, and thought processes; an increased number of neurofibrillary tangles and senile plaques (cellular debris, amyloid or protein deposits, glial cells) are commonly seen in patients with Alzheimer's, although it isn't known whether these findings are a primary cause of the disease process or whether they are a secondary feature

What are the clinical manifestations of Alzheimer's disease?

Forgetfulness, short-term memory loss, repetition of actions or ideas, inability to concentrate, disorientation to time and place, loss of initiative, deterioration in appearance and personal hygiene, inability to verbalize complex thoughts, and poor judgment skills as well as behavioral and personality changes, such as irritability, combativeness, paranoia, and hostility

How is Alzheimer's disease diagnosed?

Other causes of dementia must be excluded based on information obtained through a history and physical examination and laboratory tests. A postmortem brain biopsy provides the only definitive diagnosis.

What complications are associated with Alzheimer's disease?

Progressive disability, incontinence, severe psychosis (delusions, hallucinations), malnutrition, dehydration, aspiration and aspiration pneumonia, injury from patient wandering or violent outbursts, complete loss of short-term and long-term behavior, and death

What's the typical treatment for Alzheimer's disease?

1. Although there's no cure, certain medications may lessen the severity of symptoms. Tacrine may be used to inhibit an enzyme responsible for breakdown of acetylcholine, which temporarily improves memory formation.
2. Other drug therapy may consist of nontricyclic antidepressants such as trazodone, benzodiazepines for anxiety and sleep disturbances, and neuroleptics or antipsychotics such as haloperidol (Haldol) for psychoses and behavioral disturbances.

What are important nursing actions in the care of a patient with Alzheimer's disease?

1. Provide supervision and safety through modification of the environment (eliminate clutter to prevent falls, use door alarms to prevent wandering).
2. Encourage activity and self-sufficiency as much as possible during the early phases of the disease.
3. Establish and maintain routines. Assign the same care provider whenever possible.
4. Provide frequent rest periods to avoid fatigue.
5. Limit environmental stimuli whenever possible (noise, size of groups).

6. Monitor nutritional intake.
7. Administer medications (tacrine, nontricyclic antidepressants, anxiolytics, antipsychotics) as ordered by
   the physician.
8. Consult social services, physical, and occupational
   therapy.
9. Provide support and respite care for caregivers.

Huntington's disease (Progressive hereditary chorea)

✎ What's Hunting-ton's disease?	An autosomal dominant inherited neurological disease that affects the basal ganglia and the extrapyramidal system (like Parkinson's disease); deficiencies of the neurotransmitters acetylcholine and gamma aminobutyric acid (GABA) produce symptoms similar to those of Parkinson's disease
What's the pathophysi-ologic process of Hunt-ington's disease?	An excess of dopamine (opposite of Parkinson's disease) results from a deficiency of the neurotransmitters acetyl-choline and GABA
What clinical manifes-tations are associated with Huntington's disease?	Choreiform movements (abnormal and excessive involun-tary movements), shuffling gait, and a decline in mental capacity
What complications are associated with Huntington's disease?	Dysphagia, aspiration, malnutrition, dramatic intellectual decline, emotional lability, psychosis, and death
What's the typical treatment for Hunting-ton's disease?	Antidepressants, such as amitriptyline (Elavil), imipra-mine (Tofranil), and nortriptyline (Pamelor); antipsy-chotics, such as haloperidol (Haldol) and fluphenazine (Proloxin); and antichorea medications such as reserpine (Serpasil)
What are important nursing actions in the care of a patient with Huntington's disease?	1. Provide supervision and safety through modification of the environment (eliminate clutter to prevent falls, use door alarms to prevent wandering). 2. Encourage activity and self-sufficiency as much as possible during the early phases of the disease. Main-taining physical fitness as much as possible is impor-tant. 3. Establish and maintain routines. Assign the same care provider whenever possible. 4. Provide frequent rest periods to avoid fatigue.

5. Limit environmental stimuli whenever possible (noise, size of groups).
6. Monitor nutritional intake.
7. Administer medications (antidepressants, antipsychotics, antichorea agents) as ordered by the physician.
8. Consult social services, physical, and occupational therapy.
9. Provide support and respite care for caregivers.
10. Recommend genetic counseling.

Meningitis

✎ What's meningitis?

Inflammation of the membranes (meninges) and cerebrospinal fluid (CSF) surrounding the brain and spinal cord that most commonly results from either a bacterial or viral (aseptic) infection; viral meningitis is more common and typically milder than bacterial meningitis, resolving on its own in 1 to 2 weeks; bacterial meningitis is generally more serious and requires prompt hospital-based intervention

What's the pathophysiologic process of meningitis?

Organisms from upper respiratory tract infections, lymphatic drainage of the mastoid or sinuses, or introduction by skull fracture or lumbar puncture, spread to the meninges where they multiply rapidly and become disseminated throughout the CSF.

✎ What are the clinical manifestations of meningitis?

High fever, nausea and vomiting, severe headache, listlessness, irritability, nuchal rigidity (stiff neck; discomfort with neck flexion), photophobia, rash (meningococcal meningitis), seizures, papilledema, positive Kernig test (pain with leg flexion on the abdomen and then straightening), and a positive Brudzinski test (pain, resistance and flexion of the hips and knees with flexion of the neck)

How is meningitis diagnosed?

Lumbar puncture for CSF analysis for bacterial etiology, which is characterized by leukocytosis, decreased glucose, increased protein, and increased spinal fluid pressure

What complications are associated with meningitis?

Hydrocephalus, permanent neurological damage (hearing or vision loss, cognitive deficits), and death

What's the typical treatment for meningitis?	1. *Bacterial:* I.V. antibiotics for 10 to 21 days depending on the organism, analgesics, antiemetics, osmotic diuretics, and anticonvulsants 2. *Viral or aseptic:* symptomatic treatment including analgesics, antipyretics, and hydration

◤ *Meningococcal meningitis is a highly contagious bacterial infection that's spread by droplet secretions from the respiratory tract and the nasopharynx. Isolation precautions should be implemented for at least until 24 hours after antibiotic initiation.*

✎ **What are important nursing actions in the care of a patient with meningitis?**	1. Implement respiratory isolation precautions for meningococcal meningitis. 2. Maintain bed rest and provide quiet environment for the patient. 3. Perform neurologic assessments at frequent intervals. 4. Obtain vital signs at frequent intervals. 5. Implement seizure precautions. 6. Monitor intake and output. 7. Monitor blood tests for fluid and electrolyte imbalances. 8. Administer medications (antibiotics, antipyretics, analgesics, anticonvulsants) as ordered by the physician. Care should be taken to administer antibiotics on time. 9. Monitor for complications, such as hearing impairment (most common), cranial nerve dysfunction, and seizures from increased ICP. 10. Assess the need for immunization with pneumococcal and meningococcal vaccines.

Encephalitis

✎ **What's encephalitis?**	An acute inflammation of the brain tissue that's predominately caused by a viral infection (herpes, West Nile, varicella-zoster), but may also be caused by bacteria, fungi, or protozoa
What's the pathophysiologic process of encephalitis?	The virus crosses the blood-brain barrier and enters neural cells where it disrupts cell functioning and produces an inflammatory response
✎ **What are the clinical manifestations of encephalitis?**	Fever, headache, vomiting, myalgias, seizures, photophobia, nuchal rigidity (stiff neck), visual disturbances (diplopia), and altered mental status (irritability, confusion, drowsiness)

� *Encephalitis and meningitis are clinically two distinct syndromes, but both involve manifestations of meningeal inflammation, including nuchal rigidity, headache, and photophobia.*

What complications are associated with encephalitis?

Seizures, increased ICP, syndrome of inappropriate antidiuretic hormone secretion, coma, and death

What's the typical treatment for encephalitis?

1. I.V. acyclovir if the cause is herpes simplex or varicella-zoster viruses
2. Corticosteroids (dexamethasone) to reduce inflammation
3. Symptomatic care for infection with mosquito and tick-borne viruses (antipyretics, anticonvulsants)

🖎 **What are important nursing actions in the care of a patient with encephalitis?**

1. Maintain bed rest and provide a quiet environment for the patient.
2. Perform neurologic assessments at frequent intervals.
3. Obtain vital signs at frequent intervals.
4. Implement seizure precautions.
5. Monitor intake and output.
6. Monitor blood tests for fluid and electrolyte imbalances.
7. Administer medications (antivirals, antipyretics, analgesics, anticonvulsants) as ordered by the physician.
8. Monitor the patient for complications (increased ICP, seizures, SIADH) and notify the physician if any occur.

Spinal cord trauma and paralysis

🖎 **What's severe spinal cord trauma?**

An injury experienced by the spinal cord, spinal column, or surrounding soft tissues may result in complete or incomplete paralysis. Spinal cord damage affects all neurologic function at and below the level of injury. Most injuries to the spinal cord result from sudden, external trauma.

What's the pathophysiologic process of severe spinal cord trauma?

Trauma to the spinal cord involves both a primary and a secondary injury. Bruising and compression at the site of the injury is the primary injury. The secondary injury involves the body's natural response to trauma, in which edema impairs circulation and ischemia occurs.

🖎 **What two types of spinal cord injury exist?**

1. *Complete:* total loss of sensory and motor function below the level of injury
2. *Incomplete:* some motor and sensory tracts of the cord remain intact with varying degrees of loss

✎ What are the clinical manifestations of a complete spinal cord injury?

Flaccid paralysis; absent spinal reflexes; absent vasomotor tone below the level of injury; and absent sensation to temperature, touch, pressure, and pain

🔋 *Clinical manifestations are dependent upon the level of injury on the spinal cord. The higher the level of injury, the greater the loss of motor and sensory function will be.*

✎ How does the anatomical location of a complete spinal cord injury affect the physical outcome of the patient?

1. *C1-C3:* will require ventilatory support and complete dependence for activities of daily living (ADLs)
2. *C4-C5:* may require ventilatory support; complete dependence for ADLs
3. *C6:* can be independent with a wheelchair and can assist with some ADLs
4. *Thoracic injuries:* intact respiratory function and independence in self-care; orthostatic hypotension is common to patients with an injury above T7
5. *Sacral injuries:* intact ambulation and independence in self-care; bowel and bladder dysfunction

🔋 *The diaphragm is innervated at the C3-C5 level, so a lesion above this level will cause partial or complete paralysis of the diaphragm and will therefore affect the respiratory effort.*

✎ What complications are associated with spinal cord injury?

Spinal shock, autonomic dysreflexia, orthostatic hypotension, respiratory compromise, ileus, skin breakdown, areflexic bowel and bladder, priapism (continuous erection), and depression

🔋 *The parasympathetic nervous system dominates in people with severe spinal cord injury because the sympathetic nervous system can't send impulses beyond a spinal cord lesion.*

✎ What's spinal shock?

An immediate disruption in spinal cord function that begins 30 minutes after the initial injury and produces profound vasomotor failure and promotes vasodilation; hypotension, bradycardia, the inability to perspire below the level of injury, and the equilibration of body temperature with that of the environment, may occur; spinal shock isn't preventable, but it typically resolves in 1 to 6 weeks

✎ What's autonomic dysreflexia?

An exaggerated autonomic nervous system response to noxious stimuli (most commonly a distended bladder or a full bowel) that triggers vasoconstriction due to the release of large amounts of catecholamines; vasodilation occurs above the level of the injury and chilling of the skin (goose bumps) occurs below; hypertension and bradycardia develop; other stimuli include tight clothing, tight shoes, and urinary tract infections; it's most common in people with an injury above T6

What's the typical treatment for a patient with a spinal injury?

1. Corticosteroids, such as dexamethasone, and high-dose methylprednisolone in first 8 hours after injury to minimize the affects of spinal shock
2. Dextran to prevent and treat hypotension and increases capillary blood flow within the spinal cord
3. Atropine to correct bradycardia
4. Dopamine to treat severe hypotension
5. Surgical intervention to relieve spinal cord compression from bone fragments or hematoma (emergent), and spinal fusion and insertion of steel rods (Harrington) for stabilization

✎ What are important nursing actions in the care of a patient with a spinal injury?

1. Maintain spinal column alignment.
2. Assess neurologic function at least every hour for 4 to 6 hours and monitor for any subtle changes in strength and sensation.
3. Ensure effective airway and breathing. Anticipate the need for intubation and mechanical ventilation.
4. Monitor vital signs at frequent intervals. Be alert for bradycardia and hypotension, which can result from loss of vasomotor tone.
5. Turn and reposition the patient every 2 hours (flat bed rest). Use three-person logrolling technique for turning a patient with a spine that's not stabilized. Keep skin dry and use flotation pads, alternating pressure mattresses and pads to prevent pressure ulcers.
6. Administer medications (corticosteroids, vasopressors, atropine) as ordered by the physician.
7. If autonomic dysreflexia occurs, elevate the head of the bed, loosen tight clothing, inspect urinary catheters for kinks, and assess for bladder distention or bowel impaction.
8. Perform passive ROM exercises and utilize devices to prevent footdrop or other contractures for long-term care once the spine is stabilized and edema has resolved.
9. If no indwelling urinary catheter is placed, instruct the patient to empty his bladder at least every 4 hours. Instruct about the use of thigh stroking, pouring warm water over the perineum, and tapping over the bladder area in order to promote bladder contractions. Instruct the patient or his caregiver on bladder training regimen of intermittent catheterizations.

10. Instruct the patient on bowel training program with goal of evacuation every other day with use of suppository or digital stimulation.
11. Encourage adequate fluid intake to prevent constipation.

Brain tumors

What's a brain tumor?

A mass or growth of abnormal cells in the brain tissue that are typically classified as either primary or secondary lesions; primary lesions originate in the brain and may be benign or malignant; secondary brain lesions are malignant and are the result of cancer metastasis from another location in the body; brain tumors are most common in children ages 3 to 12 and in adults ages 40 to 70

What's the pathophysiologic process of a brain tumor?

Abnormal cells arise within the brain tissue, which can exert pressure on the cranial nerves as the tumor enlargers; the underlying cause isn't known

How can brain tumors be classified?

1. Benign or malignant
2. According to location; supratentorial (fold of the dura that surrounds the cerebrum) and infratentorial (in the area of the brain stem structures and cerebellum)
3. According to histologic origin; astrocytoma, glioma, meningioma, glioblastoma, oligodendroglioma

What are the clinical manifestations of a brain tumor?

"Pressure" headaches, usually worse in morning and upon awakening, vomiting (not preceded by nausea), visual changes (decreased visual acuity, diplopia) or loss of visual field, behavioral changes, hemiparesis, hemiplegia, hearing deficits, speech difficulties, and seizures

What complications are associated with brain tumors?

Cranial nerve dysfunction, seizures, temporary or permanent brain damage, increased intracranial pressure (ICP) from hydrocephalus, and death

What's the typical treatment for a brain tumor?

1. Corticosteroids, such as dexamethasone, and osmotic diuretics, such as mannitol, to reduce cerebral edema, anticonvulsants to prevent seizures
2. Surgical procedures including laser destruction of tumor tissue or placement of shunts within the brain to treat hydrocephalus; craniotomy with tumor resection (debulking) when the tumor can be easily accessed and there's a low risk of damage to vital areas
3. Radiation therapy after surgical removal of malignant tumors

4. Chemotherapy administered via various routes, including orally, intravenously, or intrathecally
5. "Gamma knife" therapy, involving specialized, high-dose radiation focused to the tumor that can be performed before or after surgery

◪ *Patients shouldn't be placed on the operative side for at least 8 hours after a craniotomy.*

✎ **What are important nursing actions in the care of a patient with a brain tumor?**

1. Assess neurologic status and report even subtle changes.
2. Implement seizure precautions for patient safety.
3. Assess ICP (if ICP monitor is placed) at frequent intervals and report any sustained elevations to the physician.
4. Assess electrolyte balance.
5. Administer medications as ordered by the physician. Corticosteroids, anticonvulsants, and mild analgesics are typically used because the brain doesn't have pain receptors.

13

The hematologic system

Basic concepts of the hematologic system

✎ What are the components of blood?

1. *Plasma:* fluid portion of blood; protein and salt solution; comprises majority of blood volume
2. *Erythrocytes (red blood cells [RBCs]):* transport oxygen to body tissues by utilizing hemoglobin, and transport carbon dioxide to the lungs
3. *Leukocytes (white blood cells [WBCs]):* participate in inflammatory and immune responses; classified as either granulocytes (neutrophils, basophils, and eosinophils) or mononuclear leukocytes (monocytes and lymphocytes); life span of approximately 24 hours
4. *Thrombocytes (platelets):* control bleeding through hemostasis; formed in and released by megakaryocytes (bone marrow cells); life span of approximately 10 days; spleen serves as a reservoir; adhesion, aggregation, and activation of platelets are all necessary for the clotting process

What are the components of plasma?

Water, proteins (albumin, transferrin, globulins, clotting factors such as fibrinogen), electrolytes (Na^+, Cl^-, K^+, Ca^+), hormones, waste products (nitrogen, creatinine, ammonia, urea), and nutrients (glucose, vitamins, minerals)

What's the difference between plasma and serum?

Plasma is the liquid portion of blood. Serum is the plasma plus clotting factors. Centrifugation, a rapid spinning process, can separate plasma and serum.

✎ What's hematopoiesis?

The formation and development of blood cells from their precursor cells

What's a pluripotent stem cell?

A bone marrow cell that can give rise to five different cell types: neutrophils, monocytes, eosinophils, erythrocytes, and platelets

What's erythropoiesis?

The production of RBCs, which occurs in the red bone marrow found in the vertebrae, sternum, ribs, scapula, skull, pelvis, and proximal long bones (femur, humerus); it's stimulated by hypoxia and by erythropoietin, a hormone produced by the kidneys; when decreased oxygen levels in the blood are detected, the kidney produces more erythropoietin, which stimulates the bone marrow to increase and accelerate the process of erythropoiesis

What other elements and vitamins are needed for RBC production?

Iron, cobalamin (vitamin B_{12}), and folic acid

What are the functions of erythrocytes?

1. Transportation of oxygen to tissues (via attachment to hemoglobin)
2. Transportation of carbon dioxide to the lungs
3. Maintenance of blood pH

What's the average life span of an RBC?

120 days

What's hemoglobin?

An iron-containing protein of the RBC that's responsible for oxygen transportation to tissues; it's composed of a simple protein called *globin* and heme, which contains iron and porphyrin

What's hematocrit?

The percentage of formed elements (RBCs) in the total blood volume; it's an index of the red cell concentration and thus, is indicative of the oxygen-carrying capacity of the blood

Because hematocrit is expressed as a concentration and doesn't reflect the actual number of RBCs, it can fluctuate depending on an individual's hydration status (increased with dehydration and decreased with overhydration).

The hemoglobin level is roughly one-third of the hematocrit level.

How is the RBC eliminated?

By phagocytosis in the reticuloendothelial system utilizing the spleen and liver; the RBC is broken down into heme, which is reused by the liver to produce new hemoglobin; porphyrin is converted into bilirubin and is excreted by the body in feces and urine

What functions do the liver and spleen contribute in the management of RBCs?	The liver and spleen filter out decomposed RBCs. Iron released from the heme is transported by transferrin back to the bone marrow, where it's recycled to make new RBCs. The porphyrin ring of the heme is reduced to bilirubin and eliminated as bile through the intestine.
What's a reticulocyte?	An immature RBC; reticulocytes typically mature into erythrocytes (RBCs) in 1 day
Where's iron stored?	Two-thirds of the body's iron stores are kept in hemoglobin, and one-third is stored in the bone marrow, spleen, and liver.
What's hemolysis?	The destruction of RBC membranes that may be caused by an immune response, sepsis, or mechanical trauma from prosthetic heart valves or vena cava filters

Hemostasis

What's hemostasis?	The balance of coagulation and fibrinolysis, which occur simultaneously as a result of tissue injury; it's the process that terminates bleeding through a complex mechanism that involves vasoconstriction and coagulation
What's the sequence of events involved in hemostasis?	1. Vasoconstriction (due to secretion of serotonin, epinephrine, and lipoprotein upon smooth muscle spasms at site of injury) 2. Platelet aggregation at site of injury and formation of a platelet plug, upon which reactions of the coagulation pathway can occur 3. Activation of the coagulation pathway 4. Formation of a blood clot (fibrin mesh) 5. Clot retraction and clot dissolution (fibrinolysis)
What's coagulation?	A complex process by which the body prevents blood loss through the formation of a blood clot or thrombus
What are the functions of platelets in coagulation?	1. Adherence to collagen fibers at site of injured vessel walls 2. Aggregation into clumps or plugs at the site of injury to the vessel wall 3. Activation of reactions in the coagulation cascade (platelet surface molecules are required for many of the reactions)
What are the two systems of the coagulation pathway?	1. *Extrinsic:* activated after tissue trauma when factor III released from the damaged tissues comes in contact with factor VII (proconvertin) circulating in the blood; initiated by tissue thromboplastin

2. *Intrinsic:* activated after endothelial damage when factor XII (Hageman factor) circulating in the blood comes in contact with collagen; initiated by platelet phospholipids (See flow chart below.)

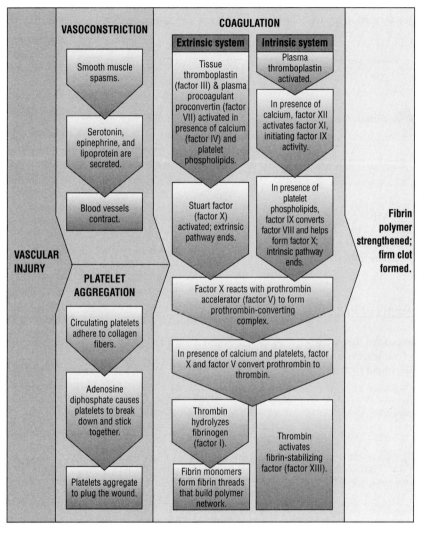

▧ *The goal of the coagulation pathway is the formation of fibrin, which forms a mesh and stabilizes a clot.*

▧ *All of the factors in the coagulation cascade have an inactive and active (denoted by "a") form. Once activated, the factor activates the next factor in the sequence.*

What factors *accelerate* the formation of clots?	Factors V and VIII, because they promote the conversion of prothrombin to thrombin, which then converts fibrinogen to fibrin
What factors *inhibit* the formation of clots?	Proteins C and S and antithrombin III, because they block the actions of various clotting factors

⚡ *Deficiencies of antithrombin III or of proteins C or S can result in hypercoagulable states that may cause strokes. Anticoagulation may be necessary in the management of these deficiencies.*

🔖 **What's fibrinolysis?**	The breakdown of fibrin clots mediated by plasmin, a proteolytic enzyme activated by substances present during coagulation and inflammation (factor XII, thrombin, and lysosomal enzymes); plasmin splits fibrin and fibrinogen into fibrin degradation products, which dissolve the clot
🔖 **What factor is critical in the coagulation pathway as well as in fibrinolysis?**	Thrombin; it converts fibrinogen to fibrin in the coagulation pathway, and it generates the production of plasmin for fibrinolysis to occur

Blood types and compatibilities

What are the two classification systems for blood typing?	ABO system and Rh system
What's the ABO system?	A system in which specific inherited genes determine antigens (A, B, O) on the RBC membrane; blood types are determined by which (if any) antigens are present; type O blood has no antigens on the RBC membrane
🔖 **What blood types are compatible?**	Type O is compatible with only type O. Type A is compatible with type A and type O. Type B is compatible with type B and type O. Type AB is compatible with type AB, A, B, and O.

⚡ *O– is the universal donor and AB+ is the universal recipient.*

What's the result if incompatible blood types are mixed?	A severe hemolytic response, which can be fatal

What's the Rh system?
A complex system of antigens also found on the RBC membrane; an individual is either Rh positive (has the antigen) or Rh negative (doesn't have the antigen); Rh– persons should receive only Rh– blood and Rh+ persons may receive either Rh– or Rh+ blood

◤ *The Rh factor differs from ABO antigens in that it can't cause a hemolytic reaction on* first *exposure to mismatched blood, but is capable of eliciting this response on subsequent exposures. For this reason, women who are pregnant with their second or later child of a different blood type may require an injection of RhoGAM to prevent a hemolytic reaction.*

Physical assessment of the hematologic system

Normal findings

What are important considerations before beginning a physical examination of the hematologic system?
1. Ensure patient privacy and provide warmth.
2. Obtain appropriate supplies and equipment (gown, drapes, ruler, or tape measure).
3. Make sure the examination room is well lit.
4. Instruct the patient to void for comfort.

What factors should be assessed as part of an examination of the hematologic system?
1. *Skin and mucous membranes:* bruises; petechiae; bleeding from wound or I.V. sites; pallor of conjunctivae, lips, or oral mucosa
2. *Neurologic:* dizziness, paresthesia (numbness or tingling), headache, confusion or forgetfulness, ataxia (disturbance in gait), fatigue or weakness
3. *Respiratory:* dyspnea, tachypnea
4. *Cardiovascular:* palpitations, tachycardia, orthostatic hypotension
5. *GI:* gingival bleeding, abdominal pain, hematemesis (bloody, "coffee ground" emesis), hematochezia (black, tarry stools), heme-positive stool
6. *Genitourinary:* hematuria, abnormal menstrual flow

✎ What blood test is most commonly used for general assessment of the hematologic system?
A complete blood count (CBC), which evaluates hemoglobin, hematocrit, red blood cells (RBCs), white blood cells (WBCs) and RBC indices, such as mean corpuscular volume (MCV), mean corpuscular hemoglobin (MCH), and mean corpuscular hemoglobin concentration

What's the importance of the reticulocyte count?
It reflects the blood cell activity rate in the bone marrow in response to erythropoietin. An increased count indicates accelerated RBC production that may occur during

periods of hemolysis, blood loss, hemoglobin S disease (sickle cell anemia), some cancers, and pregnancy as well as after iron replacement for iron deficiency anemia. A decreased reticulocyte count indicates that the bone marrow isn't actively producing RBCs, such as during iron-deficient states, aplastic anemia, chronic infection, chemotherapy, or untreated pernicious anemia.

Abnormal findings

What are the four physiologic disturbances likely to occur in the hematologic system?

1. Decreased number of cells
2. Overproduction of normal or abnormal cells
3. Defects in the clotting mechanism
4. Disorders of the spleen

✎ What laboratory tests may be used to detect bleeding disorders?

1. *Complete blood count with platelet count:* used to monitor hemoglobin, hematocrit, and platelet levels
2. *Prothrombin time (PT):* evaluates clotting factors of the extrinsic pathway (thrombin generation); prolongation of PT may be caused by use of oral anticoagulants (warfarin), hepatic diseases, and deficiencies of fibrinogen, prothrombin, factors V, VII, or X and vitamin K
3. *Partial thromboplastin time (PTT):* evaluates clotting factors of the intrinsic pathway (except VII and XIII); prolongation of PTT may be caused by clotting factor deficiencies (except VII and XIII) or by the use of heparin
4. *Bleeding time or thrombin clotting time:* estimates levels of plasma fibrinogen by measuring the time required for clot formation when thrombin is added to plasma samples from an individual and a normal control; sensitive but not specific; prolongation may be related to heparin therapy, severe hepatic disease, disseminated intravascular coagulation (DIC), and other conditions
5. *Fibrinogen (Factor I):* a protein produced by the liver during coagulation; decreased fibrinogen levels may be associated with liver disease, prostatic cancer, lung disease, bone marrow lesions, a malnourished state, and bleeding disorders caused by fibrinogen abnormalities; low levels may also be seen following large volume blood transfusions (banked blood doesn't contain fibrinogen)
6. *Fibrin degradation (or split) products (FDP):* detects breakdown products of fibrin and fibrinogen caused by plasmin; increased levels result from fibrin or fib-

rinogen destruction, such as occurs with fibrinolysis, DIC, pulmonary embolus (PE), deep vein thrombosis (DVT), MI, and incompatible blood transfusions

7. *Direct Coombs' test:* detects autoantibodies against RBCs; positive results occur in setting of hemolytic diseases

8. *D-dimer:* detects increased levels of fibrin derivatives that are associated with DIC, DVT, PE, and other thromboembolic events

✎ What's thrombocytopenia?

A pathologically low platelet count (less than 50,000/µl), which increases the risk of hemorrhage; it may manifest as petechiae (minute red to purplish flat spots on the skin, especially where clothing constricts circulation, such as the waist), ecchymoses, mild to severe hemorrhage, epistaxis, hematuria or gingival bleeding; spontaneous bleeding may occur if the platelet count is less than or equal to 20,000/µl

✎ What physical findings are suggestive of altered clotting?

Prolonged, excessive, or spontaneous bleeding; easy bruising; petechiae; purpura, tarry stools (melena); bloody stools (hematochezia); hemarthrosis (painful bleeding into a joint); hematuria; and hypotension

What's polycythemia?

A pathologic increase in RBCs in the blood; reddened mucous membranes and plethora (a red, florid complexion) are common physical manifestations

What's porphyria?

A group of inherited disorders that involves an abnormal production of heme pigments, myoglobin, and cytochromes; photosensitivity, and visceral complaints of abdominal pain are common manifestations

Diseases of the hematologic system

Red blood cell disorders

ANEMIA

✎ What's anemia?

An abnormal decrease in red blood cells (RBCs), hemoglobin, or hematocrit, which results in inadequate oxygen supply to body tissues; it results from an imbalance of blood loss (due to bleeding or RBC destruction) and blood production; various types of anemia exist, including iron deficiency anemia, aplastic anemia, megaloblastic anemia (vitamin B_{12} deficiency anemia and pernicious anemia), and acquired hemolytic anemia

✎ What clinical manifestations are suggestive of anemia?

Fatigue, chills, dyspnea on exertion, palpitations, tachycardia, orthostatic hypotension, dizziness, brittle nails, glossitis (sore tongue), beefy red tongue (folic acid deficiencies), tongue lacking papillae (pernicious anemia), jaundice and icterus (hemolytic anemia), pica (unusual food cravings, such as dirt, detergent, or ice associated with iron deficiency), neurosensory disturbances (paresthesia, decreased deep tendon reflexes, confusion, impaired sense of smell, personality changes) due to impaired myelin formation and pallor of nail beds, lips, and oral and conjunctival mucosa

What complications are associated with anemia?

Tissue hypoxia, chronic fatigue, and increased susceptibility to infections

What conditions are usually associated with anemia?

Blood loss, impaired erythrocyte production or increased erythrocyte destruction (hemolysis), or a combination of these factors

How is anemia classified?

Typically, anemia is classified according to cellular morphology of the erythrocyte. Morphologic classification is based upon cell size and hemoglobin content. Cell size (mean corpuscular volume [MCV]) denotes microcytic, normocytic, or macrocytic anemias. The mean corpuscular hemoglobin content (MCHC) denotes normochromic or hypochromic anemias.

✎ What laboratory value is used most often to diagnose anemia?

Hemoglobin (Hb); the severity of anemia can be determined by the serum Hb level; although normal Hb ranges are higher for males than for females, mild anemia is generally defined as a Hb of 10 to 13 g/dl, moderate anemia as a Hb of 6 to 10 g/dl, and severe anemia as a Hb less than 6 g/dl

What laboratory values are most often evaluated to determine anemia classification?

1. *Complete blood count (CBC):* for Hb, MCV, and MCHC
2. *Reticulocyte count:* elevation indicates anemia due to RBC loss or destruction, low level indicates decreased RBC production
3. *Peripheral blood smear:* confirms size and color of RBCs, variation in red cell size (anisocytosis) and shape (poikilocytosis); especially useful in setting of hemolysis
4. *Iron studies:* iron level, percent saturation, total iron binding capacity (TIBC), ferritin, and transferrin

IRON DEFICIENCY ANEMIA: MICROCYTIC OR HYPOCHROMIC

What's iron deficiency anemia?

A decrease in red blood cells (RBCs) that results from insufficient iron caused by inadequate dietary intake, poor iron absorption, or loss of blood

What's the pathophysiologic process of iron deficiency anemia?

Plasma and bone marrow iron stores become depleted, resulting in decreased concentration of serum transferrin. The deficiency results in microcytic, hypochromic cells. Insufficient iron stores lead to a depleted RBC mass with subnormal hemoglobin concentration, and in turn, subnormal oxygen-carrying capacity of the blood.

✎ Who's at risk for developing iron deficiency anemia?

Premenopausal women, pregnant women, infants (particularly premature or low-birth-weight infants), children, and adolescents (especially girls) due to rapid growth

▰ *Iron deficiency anemia progresses gradually, so many patients don't present with overt signs and symptoms.*

What's the typical treatment for iron deficiency anemia?

1. Oral iron preparation, preferably with vitamin C to enhance its absorption
2. Optimization of dietary sources of iron (organ meats, dried beans, spinach, and other green leafy vegetables, raisins, oysters, iron-fortified foods, such as cereal and bread)

✎ What are important nursing actions in the care of a patient with iron deficiency anemia?

1. Monitor vital signs and assess for fatigue, tachycardia, pallor, dyspnea, and signs of GI or other bleeding.
2. Instruct the patient to change positions slowly due to the potential for orthostatic hypotension and falls.
3. Assess the patient for an underlying cause of anemia and possible sources of blood loss.
4. Instruct the patient to increase dietary iron consumption (liver, oysters, lean meats, kidney beans, green leafy vegetables, apricots, raisins).
5. Administer medications (iron supplements such as ferrous sulfate or ferrous gluconate) as ordered by the physician. Instruct the patient to take iron supplements on an empty stomach for better absorption, although they may be taken with food to minimize gastric irritation if necessary. Instruct him to avoid milk and antacids within 2 hours of taking iron supplements. Inform him that vitamin C may enhance iron absorption.
6. Inform the patient that results may not become evident for several weeks to months of supplemental therapy.

7. Inform the patient that I.V. or I.M. injections of iron dextran may be necessary if he can't tolerate oral replacement.

MEGALOBLASTIC ANEMIA

✎ What's mega-loblastic anemia?

A form of anemia in which red blood cells (RBCs) are larger than normal as a result of deficiencies of vitamin B_{12} (cobalamin) or folic acid; these deficiencies may occur secondary to inadequate dietary intake of the vitamin (especially strict vegetarianism), chronic alcoholism, intestinal malabsorption syndromes, or from factors that decrease the production or absorption of intrinsic factor, including gastric or intestinal surgery

✎ What's pernicious anemia?

A decrease in RBCs caused by a deficiency of intrinsic factor, a protein secreted by parietal cells in the stomach, which is necessary for vitamin B_{12} (cobalamin) absorption; deficiency of intrinsic factor may occur as a result of abdominal or intestinal surgery that removes its site of production or absorption

It may also occur secondary to certain GI diseases (Crohn's disease, sprue), certain medications (colchicine, neomycin), and strict vegetarianism (vitamin B_{12} is only obtained through animal sources).

What's the pathophysiologic process of pernicious anemia?

Lack of intrinsic factor in gastric secretions results in inadequate absorption of vitamin B_{12} in the ileum. Vitamin B_{12} deficiency inhibits cell growth, leading to production of few, deformed RBCs with poor oxygen-carrying capacity.

What's a Schilling test?

A urine test used to determine whether the body absorbs vitamin B_{12} normally

What complications are associated with megaloblastic anemia?

Gastric polyps with an increased risk for stomach cancer and permanent neurologic symptoms if not treated within 6 months of presenting symptoms

What's the treatment for megaloblastic anemia?

Vitamin B_{12}; lifelong injections are required for pernicious anemia, whereas oral B_{12} supplementation or short-term injections may be sufficient for dietary inadequacy or until a condition (malabsorption) resolves; concomitant iron and folic acid supplementation is also recommended to prevent the development of iron deficiency anemia; blood transfusions may be necessary for moderate to severe anemia

What are important nursing actions in the care of a patient with megaloblastic anemia?

1. Monitor vital signs and assess for complications of anemia, including neurologic dysfunction (paresthesia, gait disturbances), and GI disease (pernicious anemia).
2. Encourage adequate dietary intake of vitamin B_{12} (animal sources) or discuss need for supplementation.
3. Administer medications (vitamin B_{12}, folate, and iron supplements) as ordered by the physician.
4. Monitor serum B_{12} levels.

APLASTIC ANEMIA

What's aplastic anemia?

A disorder characterized by bone marrow hypoplasia or aplasia resulting in pancytopenia in which insufficient numbers of red blood cells (RBCs), white blood cells, and platelets are produced; although the exact cause is unknown, an autoimmune process is suspected; however, radiation, chemotherapy, and certain drugs, toxins, viral infections, and congenital disorders may also produce aplastic anemia

What's the pathophysiologic process of aplastic anemia?

Damage to or destruction of hematopoietic stem cells occurs via an immune-mediated mechanism, and a decrease in all cell types results (pancytopenia)

What are the clinical manifestations of aplastic anemia?

Pallor, fatigue, exertional dyspnea, tachycardia, and palpitations may occur as a result of decreased RBCs. Easy bruising, nose bleeds, unexplained or prolonged bleeding, petechiae, and ecchymosis may occur secondary to thrombocytopenia. Frequent, recurrent, or severe infections may result from leukopenia.

What complications are associated with aplastic anemia?

Sepsis, hemorrhage, and death

What's the typical treatment for aplastic anemia?

1. Treatment of underlying cause or removal of causative agent
2. Immunosuppressive treatment, which may include anti-thymocyte globulin, a horse serum containing antibodies against human T cells, which permits the bone marrow to resume hematopoiesis (production of blood cells)
3. Blood and platelet transfusions
4. Administration of antibiotics and antifungals
5. Bone marrow stimulating androgens
6. Bone marrow transplantation, which may be indicated for severe cases in which life-threatening conditions arise

What are important nursing actions in the care of a patient with aplastic anemia?	1. Implement infection control measures to minimize the risk of infection (private room, reverse isolation with severe neutropenia). 2. Implement bleeding precautions. Avoid I.M. injections or other invasive procedures. Monitor I.V. sites, wounds, and any broken skin for signs of bleeding. Control bleeding by applying pressure to site. Avoid aspirin and nonsteroidal anti-inflammatory drugs. 3. Monitor platelet count. 4. Administer blood products as ordered by the physician. 5. Avoid exposure to potential toxins (solvents, sprays, paints, pesticides), which may affect bone marrow function.

ACQUIRED HEMOLYTIC ANEMIA

What's acquired hemolytic anemia?	A condition characterized by a decrease in circulating red blood cells (RBCs) due to their premature destruction, which may be caused by some medications or infections as well as autoimmune or inherited disorders; other anemias may develop because the bone marrow can't keep up with the demand of accelerated erythropoiesis due to the active destruction of the RBCs; sickle cell anemia is an example of a hemolytic anemic process
What's the patho-physiologic process of acquired hemolytic anemia?	Premature, accelerated destruction of erythrocytes occurs within blood vessels or in lymphoid tissues that filter blood (spleen and liver) — either episodically or continuously — but the bone marrow is incapable of compensating by increasing the production of new RBCs.
What are the clinical manifestations of acquired hemolytic anemia?	Fatigue, chills, pallor, tachycardia, dyspnea on exertion, and splenomegaly as well as jaundice and dark urine due to elevated bilirubin
What complications are associated with acquired hemolytic anemia?	Hemolytic crisis leading to shock and end organ failure ◥ *Profound anemias can exacerbate preexisting cardiovascular, lung or cerebrovascular disorders.*
What's the typical treatment for acquired hemolytic anemia?	1. Treatment of the underlying disorder or removal of the underlying cause 2. Replacement of fluids and electrolytes 3. Folate and iron supplementation in chronic hemolytic anemia

4. Steroids and other immunosuppressants to treat autoimmune hemolytic anemia
5. Blood transfusions in emergency situations; splenectomy if anemia is severe

What are the important nursing actions in the care of a patient with acquired hemolytic anemia?

1. Monitor vital signs and assess for complications of anemia.
2. Monitor intake and output.
3. Administer medications (blood transfusions, iron and folate supplements, immunosuppressants) as ordered by the physician.
4. Monitor electrolytes, renal function, and complete blood count (hemoglobin level and hematocrit).

THALASSEMIA

✎ What's thalassemia?

A group of inherited blood disorders characterized by defective hemoglobin synthesis that results from insufficient production of globin chains; classification of the disease depends on which globin chain isn't produced (alpha, beta), and whether the defect is inherited homozygously (major) in which both genes responsible for normal hemoglobin production are affected, or heterozygously (minor) in which only one of the genes is affected

Alpha thalassemias are more common in Africa, the Middle East, Southeast Asia, and India; beta thalassemias are more common in persons of Mediterranean descent.

What's the pathophysiologic process of thalassemia?

Polypeptide chains are improperly arranged, which causes a defect in hemoglobin synthesis; extremely thin and fragile erythrocytes with decreased life spans (15 days compared to normal 120 days) are produced as a result, and a gradual and progressive anemia develops that doesn't respond to conventional therapy (iron, folate, or vitamin B_{12} supplementation); the severity of the disease is determined by how the chains have been altered

✎ What are common categories of thalassemia?

1. *Alpha thalassemia major (hydrops fetalis):* complete absence of alpha-chain production, which causes death in utero or shortly after birth due to anoxia, unless the condition was diagnosed before birth and blood transfusions were initiated in utero
2. *Alpha thalassemia minor (trait):* variable clinical manifestations depending on whether genetic defects are on the same chromosome; generally asymptomatic

3. *Beta thalassemia major (Cooley's anemia):* complete absence of beta-chain production; life-threatening anemia develops at age 1 to 2 months; severe hemolysis occurs as the spleen sequesters and destroys the aberrant red cells; lifelong blood transfusions are required (regular transfusions every 2 to 3 weeks), which can cause iron overload; chelation therapy with deferoxamine (Desferal) infusions is necessary to treat iron overload

4. *Beta thalassemia minor (trait):* most common thalassemia; marked by a slight decrease in production of beta chains; normal hemoglobin function; usually asymptomatic, although a mild anemia may result

What are the clinical manifestations of thalassemia?

1. *Minor:* generally produces no symptoms with normal or minimally decreased RBC counts and normal serum iron
2. *Major:* symptoms of anemia (fatigue, dyspnea, jaundice), splenomegaly, neurologic manifestations, such as paresthesias, and bony deformities such as mongoloid-appearing faces

What are the complications of thalassemia?

Severe anemia requiring regular blood transfusions, and cardiac or hepatic complications from iron overload

◤ *Persons with thalassemia should avoid iron supplements and oxidative drugs (sulfonamides) to avoid iron toxicity.*

What's the typical treatment for thalassemia?

1. *Minor:* generally requires no treatment as most patients are asymptomatic
2. *Major:* requires lifelong, routine blood transfusions along with chelating agents, such as deferoxamine (Desferal) to treat iron overload, folate supplementation, and possible splenectomy or bone marrow transplantation

✎ **What are important nursing actions in the care of a patient with thalassemia?**

1. Monitor vital signs and assess for complications.
2. Monitor intake and output.
3. Monitor complete blood count for hemoglobin level and hematocrit.
4. Administer medications (folate, blood transfusions, chelating agents) as ordered by the physician.
5. Instruct the patient to avoid trauma, temperature extremes, and smoking to protect the extremities from injury due to impaired circulation.
6. Instruct the patient to avoid iron supplements, including multivitamins with iron.

SICKLE CELL ANEMIA

✎ What's sickle cell anemia?

An autosomal recessive, chronic disease characterized by red blood cells (RBCs) that contain an abnormal form of hemoglobin (Hb) known as Hb S (S for sickle); periodically, the RBCs become sickled (crescent shaped) and can't pass through small blood vessels; small blood clots form and ischemia results in local tissues, which causes recurrent, painful episodes known as *sickle cell crises*; this particular genetic mutation occurs more commonly in those of African descent, and it's believed to have evolved as a protective mechanism against malaria because people with the sickle cell trait (those who inherited the genetic defect from only one parent) more frequently survived malaria outbreaks

What's the pathophysiologic process of sickle cell anemia?

Abnormal Hb (Hb S) is produced from a genetic mutation in which glutamic acid is switched to valine. Because Hb S is insoluble during hypoxia, RBCs become rigid, rough, and elongated, forming a crescent or sickle shape, and have a shortened life span (less than 60 days). Hemolysis occurs as a result of the sickling. Blood becomes more viscous due to the accumulation of the altered cells in the capillaries and smaller blood vessels. Pain, swelling, and ischemia result from impaired circulation.

What's sickle cell trait?

A condition in which the genetic mutation is inherited from only one parent, and results in normal Hb (Hb A) being produced in larger quantities than Hb S; people with sickle cell trait are simply carriers for the genetic mutation, but are generally healthy and are thought to be immune to malaria

✎ What factors increase the risk of a sickling crisis?

Dehydration, infection, extremes of temperature, stress, and decreased supply of oxygen

✎ What are the clinical manifestations of sickle cell anemia?

Bone or joint pain, fatigue, dyspnea, tachycardia, jaundice, fever, bouts of abdominal pain, increased susceptibility to infections, and delayed growth and puberty; other manifestations may include hematuria, polyuria, polydipsia, and chest pain

Why do infants with sickle cell anemia typically *not* manifest symptoms of the disease before age 6 months?

Fetal Hb (which protects against Hb S) continues to be produced by an infant's bone marrow generally until age 6 months.

What complications are associated with sickle cell anemia?	Bacterial infection or sepsis (due to splenic infarction and damage), hypovolemic shock, sickle cell crisis, growth retardation or delayed puberty, leg ulcers, cholelithiasis (gallstones), retinopathy, blindness, nephropathy, priapism (prolonged, painful erection), stroke, and necrosis of ischemic tissues leading to organ failure and death

✎ What's a sickle cell crisis?

A sudden onset of pain that can last several hours to days and is caused by tissue ischemia from sickled RBCs that form a thrombus

✎ What are the four types of sickle cell crisis?

1. *Hemolytic crisis:* results in breakdown of damaged RBCs
2. *Vaso-occlusive crisis (thrombotic crisis):* most common; results from sickled cells accumulating in the microcirculation eventually causing painful ischemia to local tissues; multiple organ systems may be affected
3. *Aplastic crisis:* results from bone marrow depression and is often associated with viral infections
4. *Splenic sequestration crisis:* rare; affects young children (ages 8 months to 2 years); large amounts of blood become acutely pooled in the liver and spleen

What's the typical treatment for a sickle cell crisis?

1. Hydration, supplemental oxygen, analgesics (acetaminophen, nonsteroidal anti-inflammatory drugs, codeine, morphine), and hydroxyurea (Droxia, Hydrea) to decrease frequency of crises; folic acid supplementation for new RBC production
2. Blood transfusions and possibly RBC exchanges for those with severe complications or refractory pain
3. Bone marrow transplantation can be curative for a select group of patients whose benefits from the procedure outweigh its risks

✎ What are important nursing actions in the care of a patient with sickle cell anemia?

1. Monitor vital signs and assess for complications (infection, hypovolemia, stroke).
2. Monitor intake and output.
3. Administer medications (oxygen, blood products, analgesics, hydroxyurea, folic acid, antibiotics) as ordered by the physician.
4. Assess level of pain to determine effectiveness of therapy.
5. Instruct the patient to avoid factors that may precipitate a crisis. Strenuous exercise, dehydration, alcohol consumption, excessive sun exposure, smoking, infections, emotional stress, and high altitudes should be avoided.
6. Encourage adequate hydration (eight 12-oz glasses of water per day).

7. Encourage administration of preventative vaccines and anti-infectives (pneumococcal vaccine, *Haemophilus influenzae B*, and hepatitis B immunizations can be used for persons of any age; prophylactic penicillin can be used with young children).
8. Encourage genetic counseling.

POLYCYTHEMIA VERA

What's polycythemia vera?

A chronic myeloproliferative disorder of the bone marrow in which there's an overproduction of red blood cells (RBCs; erythrocytosis) primarily, although production of white blood cells (WBCs; leukocytosis) and platelets (thrombocytosis) is increased as well; increased blood volume, viscosity, and hematocrit result, and an increased risk of life-threatening bleeding and clotting accompanies the disorder; polycythemia vera is capable of evolving into a different myeloproliferative disorder or into a leukemia

What's the pathophysiologic process of polycythemia vera?

Although the underlying cause of the disease is unknown, the increased RBC mass produces abnormally viscous blood and impaired blood flow through the microcirculation. Both intravascular thrombosis and hemorrhage result.

What are the clinical manifestations of polycythemia vera?

Headache, tinnitus, blurred vision, ruddy complexion (plethora), reddened mucous membranes, dizziness, vertigo, paresthesia, angina, intermittent claudications, intense pruritus after a warm bath or shower, and early satiety from splenomegaly; bleeding complications, such as epistaxis, gingival bleeding, ecchymosis, and GI bleeding may also be present

What criteria are used to diagnose polycythemia vera?

A red cell mass greater than 36 ml/kg in males and greater than 32 ml/kg in females, arterial oxygen greater than 92%, and splenomegaly are the major diagnostic criteria for the disease. A platelet count greater than 400,000/µl and a WBC greater than 12,000/µl are considered minor diagnostic criteria. The serum erythropoietin level will be decreased.

What complications are associated with polycythemia vera?

Thromboembolic events due to hyperviscosity, such as stroke, myocardial infarction, deep vein thrombosis, portal vein thrombosis (Budd-Chiari syndrome); hypertension; gout from increased uric acid levels; peptic ulcer disease from increased histamine levels; spontaneous hemorrhage; and progression to myelofibrosis or acute leukemia

What's the typical treatment for polycythemia vera?	1. Phlebotomy at intervals determined by complete blood count (CBC) results to maintain hematocrit (HCT) less than 45% is first line of therapy
	2. Myelosuppressive therapy including hydroxyurea (Droxia, Hydrea), interferon alpha, and anagrelide (Agrylin)
	3. Antihistamines such as diphenhydramine (Benadryl) for pruritus
	4. Allopurinol for treatment of hyperuricemia
What's the spent phase of polycythemia vera?	A late phase of the disease in which the bone marrow fails to produce additional cells, resulting in profound anemia for which blood transfusions may be required
✎ What are important nursing actions in the care of a patient with polycythemia vera?	1. Monitor vital signs and assess for complications, such as bleeding or thromboembolism, hypotension, or heart failure.
	2. Administer medications (hydroxyurea, anagrelide, antihistamines, allopurinol, interferon injections) as ordered by the physician.
	3. Monitor CBC (HCT) and phlebotomize to maintain HCT less than 45% for men and less than 42% for women.
	4. Instruct the patient to eat small meals followed by rest periods to avoid early satiety from splenomegaly.
	5. Educate the patient about the risk of thrombosis, and encourage moderate activity.
	6. Advise the patient to avoid hot showers to prevent pruritus.
	7. Teach the patient the proper technique for alpha-interferon injection.
	8. Encourage close follow-up with the hematologist.

Platelet disorders

IDIOPATHIC THROMBOCYTOPENIC PURPURA

✎ What's idiopathic thrombocytopenic purpura (ITP)?	An autoimmune disorder characterized by decreased platelets (thrombocytopenia) in the setting of normal bone marrow; the condition may occur acutely in children following an infection with spontaneous resolution within a few months, or may occur chronically in adults with symptoms persisting for more than 6 months
What's the pathophysiologic process of ITP?	Peripheral destruction of platelets occurs as an autoimmune response induced by antiplatelet antibodies

🔌 **What are the clinical manifestations of ITP?**	Bruising, petechiae (commonly in dependent areas), purpura, epistaxis (nosebleed), hematuria, menorrhagia, gingival bleeding, and spontaneous bleeding if platelet count is less than 20,000/µl
What are risk factors for developing ITP?	Being HIV-positive and using certain medications (sulfonamides, thiazide diuretics, chlorpropamide, quinidine, gold)
What complications are associated with ITP?	Hemorrhage (particularly intracranial) and death

What's the typical treatment for ITP?

1. Administration of glucocorticoids (prednisone) and I.V. immune globulin (IVIG) for platelet count less than 50,000/µl in adults as well as splenectomy if medical therapy fails.
2. Platelet transfusions may become necessary, but they aren't recommended for routine management of ITP.

🔌 **What are important nursing actions in the care of a patient with ITP?**

1. Implement bleeding precautions. Instruct the patient to avoid contact sports and I.M. injections due to the risk of bleeding.
2. Assess for petechiae, purpura, ecchymosis, oozing of blood from venipuncture sites, and other signs of blood loss. Notify the physician immediately if hemorrhage occurs.
3. Administer medications (glucocorticoids, IVIG, platelets) as ordered by the physician.
4. Monitor platelet count.
5. Instruct the patient to avoid aspirin and nonsteroidal anti-inflammatory drugs.
6. Encourage close follow-up with the hematologist.

Hypocoagulable disorders

HEMOPHILIA

🔌 **What's hemophilia?**

An X-linked recessive hematologic disorder characterized by coagulopathy (inability to clot) that results from a deficiency in clotting factor VIII (hemophilia A) or clotting factor IX (hemophilia B or Christmas disease); life-threatening hemorrhage can occur from even a minor injury in persons with these clotting factor deficiencies, although the severity of hemophilia varies greatly and delayed bleeding is more common than immediate hemorrhage

What's the patho-physiologic process of hemophilia?	Abnormal bleeding is caused by a deficiency in clotting factors of the intrinsic coagulation pathway. Platelet plugs may form at a bleeding site, but clotting factor deficiencies impair the formation of stable fibrin clots. Excessive bleeding occurs when clotting factors are reduced by more than 75%.
✎ **What are the clinical manifestations of hemophilia?**	Excessive bleeding or bruising after minor trauma or surgery; pain, swelling, and tenderness due to hemarthrosis (bleeding into joints); hematuria; hematemesis, melena; orthostasis; hypotension; tachycardia; headache; stiff neck; epistaxis, tachypnea, or hemoptysis
What complications are associated with hemophilia?	Intracranial hemorrhage, decreased tissue perfusion, hypovolemic shock, and death

What's the typical treatment for hemophilia?

1. Fresh frozen plasma (FFP) for mild forms of the disease (less commonly used for hemophilia A due to instability of factor VIII in FFP)
2. Administration of recombinant factor VIII concentrate for hemophilia A; administration of recombinant factor IX for hemophilia B
3. Adjunctive therapy to factor VIII such as desmopressin acetate (DDAVP), and antifibrinolytics such as epsilon aminocaproic acid (Amicar) to achieve hemostasis and minimize the need for factor VIII infusions
4. Cold compresses and elevation of bleeding site
5. Analgesics for pain control

✎ **What are important nursing actions in the care of a patient with hemophilia?**

1. Implement bleeding precautions and monitor for acute bleeding. Decrease environmental risk for patient injury by assessing for potential hazards. Avoid I.M. injections due to possible hematoma formation.
2. Administer blood products (FFP, cryoprecipitate, packed red blood cells, clotting factors) during acute bleeding episodes.
3. Instruct the patient to avoid aspirin or aspirin-containing medications due to decreased platelet adherence and possible increased bleeding.
4. Instruct the patient to avoid contact sports due to the risk for bleeding.
5. Provide cold compresses and elevate site of bleeding.
6. Encourage the patient to have hepatitis A and B vaccinations due to the risk of viral transmission in blood products.
7. Inform the patient that prophylactic factor replacement, desmopressin, or aminocaproic acid should be administered prior to invasive procedures, such as tooth extractions and lumbar punctures.

What's von Wille-brand's disease?	An inherited deficiency of von Willebrand factor (vWF), which promotes the clumping of platelets; prolonged bleeding times result; treatment involves the use of desmopressin (DDAVP) to restore clotting functions, or replacement with concentrated vWF or factor VIII

Hypercoagulable disorders

What are hypercoagulable disorders?	A group of disorders of the coagulation pathway that predispose to the formation of blood clots (thromboembolism); a hypercoagulable state may result from genetic defects, prolonged bedrest, dehydration, prolonged sitting or immobility, hormonal contraceptive pills or other sources of estrogen, obesity, recent surgery, trauma, infection or sepsis, pregnancy, and certain types of cancer; may also be referred to as thrombophilia and a prethrombotic state
What are examples of hypercoagulable disorders?	1. *Antithrombin III deficiency:* AT III is a natural anticoagulant; a deficiency of AT III prevents the inactivation of factors IXa, Xa, Xia and thrombin; a hypercoagulable state results, which increases the risk for venous thromboembolisms; may be inherited or acquired 2. *Protein C and S deficiencies:* proteins C and S are naturally occurring vitamin K–dependent anticoagulants; a deficiency in one of these factors predisposes to blood clot formations; may be inherited or acquired 3. *Homocystinemia:* homocysteine is an amino acid that plays an important role in metabolism; increased blood levels of the amino acid are associated with an increased risk of blood clot formation and vascular disease; treatment includes vitamin B supplementation (B_6, B_{12}, and folic acid) to lower the level and anticoagulants may be used to prevent clot formation 4. *Activated protein C resistance (Factor V Leiden):* factor V Leiden is a potent procoagulant that's inactivated by protein C; resistance to protein C predisposes to thrombophilia (clot formation); the condition may be inherited or acquired
What's the pathophysiologic process of hypercoagulable disorders?	Various naturally occurring anticoagulants in the coagulation pathway are inhibited, which produces a hypercoagulable state
What are the clinical manifestations of hypercoagulable disorders?	Hypercoagulable disorders are generally asymptomatic until a complication arises from a thromboembolic event, such as a pulmonary embolus or deep vein thrombosis. Recurrent thromboses, thrombosis at an early age

(younger than age 50) or at an unusual site, and a family history of thromboses may also signify an underlying hypercoagulable disorder.

✎ What complications are associated with hypercoagulable disorders?

Deep vein thrombosis, pulmonary embolism, stroke, and myocardial infarction

What's the typical treatment for hypercoagulable disorders?

1. *Antiplatelet agents:* nonsteroidal anti-inflammatory drugs, ticlopidine (Ticlid), clopidogrel (Plavix), dipyridamole, and aspirin (Aggrenox)
2. *Anticoagulants:* heparin, low molecular weight heparin, such as enoxaparin (Lovenox), and warfarin (Coumadin)
3. *Thrombolytics:* streptokinase, urokinase, tissue plasminogen activator (Alteplase)

✎ What are important nursing actions in the care of a patient with a hypercoagulable disorder?

1. Instruct the patient to avoid smoking and hormonal contraceptive use as well as to maintain normal weight, blood pressure, and cholesterol levels. Encourage regular exercise.
2. Instruct the patient to take anticoagulants consistently (typically at bedtime).
3. Administer medications (aspirin, warfarin, heparin) as ordered by the physician.
4. Monitor PT/INR, PTT and adjust anticoagulants, as indicated in conjunction with the physician's order.
5. Inform the patient that prophylactic heparin should be administered during perioperative periods and inform women of childbearing age that prophylactic heparin should be administered during pregnancy and delivery.
6. Monitor the patient for complications of the disease (thromboembolic events) as well as for adverse reactions to therapy (abnormal bleeding or hemorrhage).

White blood cell (WBC) disorders

✎ What's leukopenia?

A decrease in the total number of white blood cells (WBCs) (granulocytes, lymphocytes, and monocytes) to less than 5,000/µl

What's granulocytopenia?

A decrease in the number of granulocytic cells (neutrophils, eosinophils, and basophils); may be caused by exposure to certain drugs, such as chemotherapeutic agents, phenothiazine derivatives, sulfonamides, and anticonvulsants

What's the pathophysiologic process of granulocytopenia?	May occur in severe prolonged infections where production of granulocytes can't keep up with demand, decreased neutrophil production (hypoplastic or aplastic anemia, leukemia, or drug- or toxin-induced neutropenia), reduced neutrophil survival (autoimmune disorders), and abnormal neutrophil distribution and sequestration

✎ **What's neutropenia?**

A reduction in circulating neutrophils in which the neutrophil count is less than 1,500/µl

What's agranulocytosis?

Severe neutropenia in which the neutrophil count is less than 500/µl; sepsis and death may occur within 3 to 6 days if untreated

✎ **What's the absolute neutrophil count (ANC)?**

The actual number of neutrophils; if the ANC is less than 1,000/µl, the patient is at moderate risk for a bacterial infection; if the ANC is less than 500/µl, the patient is at severe risk for a bacterial infection

What are the clinical manifestations of granulocytopenia?

Fatigue and weakness may result from neutropenia. Fever, chills, and tachycardia may occur if an infection is present.

▉ *The classic signs of infection (erythema, edema, warmth) may not be present in a granulocytopenic patient due to a decreased phagocytic response.*

✎ **What complications are associated with granulocytopenia?**

Infections (primarily bacterial and fungal septicemias or pneumonias) and death

What's the typical treatment for granulocytopenia?

1. Discontinuation of medications associated with bone marrow suppression
2. Implementation of reverse isolation precautions if total granulocytes are less than 1,000/µl
3. Testing of cultures of blood, nose, throat, sputum, and urine
4. Administration of antibiotics if significant infection is evident
5. Administration of granulocyte colony-stimulating factor (G-CSF) if no improvement in granulocyte count

✎ **What are important nursing actions in the care of a patient with granulocytopenia?**

1. Implement reverse isolation precautions with strict hand-washing hygiene by all staff entering the room.
2. Immediately stop the administration of medications causing bone marrow suppression.
3. Monitor laboratory values (CBC with differential).

4. Monitor the patient for signs and symptoms of infection and notify the physician immediately if any develop.
5. Provide frequent oral care; offer lozenges, analgesics, and sedatives as ordered.
6. Reassure the patient and his family that the granulocyte count typically rises to a normal range in 7 to 21 days, once the offending drug or acute illness has stopped.

Cancers of the hematologic system

Leukemias

✎ What's leukemia?

A group of diseases involving the proliferation of immature white blood cells (WBCs); possible causes may include viral infections (Epstein Barr, human lymphotropic virus [HTLV]), environmental factors (radiation, alkylating agents, pesticides, maternal use of tobacco and alcohol), and immunodeficiencies.

What's the pathophysiologic process of leukemia?

In acute leukemia, immature cells accumulate and gradually replace bone marrow. Normal production of red blood cells, WBCs, and platelets is decreased, resulting in anemia, neutropenia, and thrombocytopenia.

✎ What are examples of common leukemias?

1. *Acute lymphocytic leukemia (ALL):* more common in children (especially males) but can affect adults
2. *Chronic lymphocytic leukemia (CLL):* more common in adults older than age 50; most common type of leukemia; involves accumulation of lymphocytes (especially B cells)
3. *Acute myeloid leukemia (AML):* more common in adults, but may affect children younger than age 1
4. *Chronic myeloid leukemia (CML):* more common in adults older than age 60; involves overproduction of granulocytes (neutrophils); associated with Philadelphia chromosome
5. *Hairy cell leukemia:* more common in adult males; abnormal proliferation of B lymphocytes

How do lymphocytic leukemias differ from myeloid leukemias?

Lymphocytic leukemias are malignant forms of lymphoid cells at distinct stages of differentiation (most are B cells); myeloid leukemias involve the infiltration of bone marrow, blood, and other tissues by malignant hematopoietic cells.

✎ What are the clinical manifestations of leukemia?

Lymphadenopathy and hepatosplenomegaly (due to accumulation of immature cells), fatigue, malaise, early satiety, abdominal fullness, weight loss, pallor, easy bruising (petechiae, purpura), abnormal bleeding (epistaxis, heavy menstrual periods), fever, bone or joint pain and tenderness, and night sweats

✎ What complications are associated with leukemia?

Infections, spontaneous or excessive bleeding, disseminated intravascular coagulopathy, hyperuricemia, and relapse

What's the typical treatment for leukemia?

1. *ALL:* chemotherapy (vincristine, prednisone, cyclophosphamide, methotrexate) and bone marrow transplantation; 80% cure rate for children and 30% to 50% for adults
2. *CLL:* chemotherapy (fludarabine, cyclophosphamide, chlorambucil, prednisone), monoclonal antibodies such as alemtuzumab (Campath), radiation, immunoglobulins, interferons
3. *AML:* chemotherapy (cytarabine, daunorubicin, 6-thioguanine), interferons, growth factors (G-CSF, GM-CSF) and bone marrow transplantation; 75% remission rate with 25% cure rate (no evidence of disease after 5 years)
4. *CML:* chemotherapy (cytarabine, imatinib [Gleevec], cyclophosphamide, vincristine), hydroxyurea, interferons (human leukocyte interferon), and bone marrow transplantation (standard of care)
5. *Hairy cell leukemia:* interferon, pentostatin, glucocorticoids (for vasculitis), and splenectomy

✎ What are important nursing actions in the care of a patient with leukemia?

1. Administer medications and blood products (chemotherapy, growth factors, interferons, antibiotics) as ordered by the physician.
2. Monitor the patient for complications from the disease itself (bleeding, infection) and from adverse reactions to therapy (infection).
3. Implement bleeding precautions (soft toothbrush, electric razor).
4. Encourage adequate sleep and rest periods as well as good nutrition with increased proteins and calories.

Lymphomas

HODGKIN'S DISEASE

✎ What's Hodgkin's disease?

A solid hematologic malignancy that originates in the lymphoid system and predominantly involves the lymph nodes and the spleen; an accumulation of dysfunctional, immature lymphoid-derived cells results; characterized by Reed-Sternberg cells; risk factors include immunodeficiency, autoimmune diseases, viral infections (Epstein Barr, HTLV), and exposure to certain chemicals or drugs (chemotherapy, radiation therapy, phenytoin)

What's the patho-physiologic process of Hodgkin's disease?

Lymph node architecture is destroyed locally by monocyte or macrophage hyperplasia, but the disease then spreads to adjacent lymphatics before eventually infiltrating other organs such as the spleen, liver, and lungs.

What are the clinical manifestations of Hodgkin's disease?

Painless and mobile lymphadenopathy localized to single group of nodes (cervical, mediastinal, para-aortic), fever, night sweats, weight loss, abdominal mass, local pain at site of disease with alcohol ingestion, and hepatosplenomegaly

What complications are associated with Hodgkin's disease?

Infections, thromboembolic complications, spinal cord compression, and adverse effects of radiation and chemotherapy (sterility, hypothyroidism, acute leukemia or other secondary malignancies, myelodysplasia)

What's the typical treatment for Hodgkin's disease?

1. Regional radiation therapy for stage I or II disease
2. Chemotherapy, including MOPP regimen (nitrogen mustard, Oncovin, prednisone) or ABVD regimen (Adriamycin, bleomycin, vinblastine, dacarbazine) for disseminated disease
3. Bone marrow transplantation

What are important nursing actions in the care of a patient with Hodgkin's disease?

1. Implement reverse isolation precautions to prevent infection, including strict hand hygiene.
2. Assess the patient for complications of the disease (infection, thromboembolic events) or its therapy.
3. Monitor laboratory values (CBC and platelet count) periodically throughout therapy.
4. Provide comfort measure for adverse effects of chemotherapy and radiation. Administer antiemetics and analgesics to relieve nausea and pain.

Non-Hodgkin's lymphoma

What's non-Hodgkin's lymphoma?

A malignancy of lymphoid tissue arising from T- or B-lymphocytes or their precursors, and is commonly associated with immunosuppressed conditions (transplant recipients, HIV-positive patients), certain viruses (Epstein Barr, HTLV), exposure to herbicides and autoimmune diseases; Burkitt's lymphoma is a form of non-Hodgkin's lymphoma

▙ *The level of differentiation and type of lymphocyte influences course of illness and prognosis.*

What's the pathophysiologic process of non-Hodgkin's lymphoma?

Abnormal white blood cells (lymphocytes) are produced, which grow without regulation and form tumors within the lymphatic system. Occasionally, non-Hodgkin's lymphoma can spread to organs outside of the lymphatic system.

What are the clinical manifestations of non-Hodgkin's lymphoma?

Symptoms will vary according to the involvement of the disease; may include painless enlargement of multiple peripheral lymph nodes, fever, chills, night sweats, weight loss, dyspnea with pulmonary involvement.

What complications are associated with non-Hodgkin's lymphoma?

Infection and death

What's the typical treatment for non-Hodgkin's lymphoma?

1. Chemotherapy, including CHOP regimen (Cyclophosphamide, Hydroxydaunomycin, Oncovin, Prednisone), or BACOP regimen (bleomycin, Adriamycin, cyclophosphamide, Oncovin, prednisone)
2. Radiation therapy (palliative)
3. Bone marrow transplantation

▙ *The prognosis for non-Hodgkin's lymphoma isn't as good as that for Hodgkin's disease.*

What are important nursing actions in the care of a patient with non-Hodgkin's lymphoma?

1. Implement reverse isolation precautions to prevent infection, including strict hand-washing hygiene.
2. Assess the patient for complications of the disease (infections) or its therapy.
3. Monitor laboratory values (CBC and platelet count) periodically throughout therapy.
4. Provide comfort measures for the adverse effects of chemotherapy and radiation. Administer antiemetics and analgesics to relieve nausea and pain.

Multiple myeloma

What's multiple myeloma?

A primary bone malignancy in which bone marrow is predominately replaced by plasma cells; also characterized by abnormal serum immunoglobulins; bones with active marrow such as the long bones, spine, ribs, sternum, skull, and pelvis are the most commonly affected

What's the patho-physiologic process of multiple myeloma?	Plasma cells infiltrate the bone marrow and cause its destruction; also cause the production of osteolytic defects throughout the skeletal system.
What are the clinical manifestations of multiple myeloma?	Back pain, vague bone aches or pain, local swelling or mass, weight loss, periods of immobility, hypercalcemia, and presence of Bence Jones protein in urine
What complications are associated with multiple myeloma?	Anemia (from the destruction of red blood cells), thrombocytopenia, renal failure (due to high protein concentrations), pathologic fractures, and death
What's the typical treatment for multiple myeloma?	1. Management of the neoplasm: usually involves chemotherapy, radiation therapy, steroid therapy, hormone therapy, or a combination of these treatments 2. Management of the symptoms produced by the lesion
✎ **What are important nursing actions in the care of a patient with multiple myeloma?**	1. Use extreme caution when turning or transferring the patient to prevent pathologic fractures. 2. Encourage participation in therapeutic activities to prevent complications of prolonged bed rest. Frequent rest periods should be provided. 3. Administer medications (analgesics, chemotherapeutic agents) as ordered by the physician. 4. Monitor the patient for complications (renal failure, pathologic fractures) and notify the physician immediately if any develop.

Pharmacology related to the hematologic system

Treatment of anemia

IRON SUPPLEMENTATION

How do iron supplements work?	Supply elemental iron, which is essential for hemoglobin formation
What are examples of iron supplements?	Ferrous sulfate, ferrous gluconate, ferrous fumarate, iron dextran (DexFerrum) and polysaccharide iron complex (Niferex, Nu-Iron)
✎ **What adverse reactions are commonly associated with iron supplements?**	GI symptoms, such as nausea, gastric irritation, constipation, abdominal cramps, and dark stools; temporary tooth staining may occur with liquid preparations

What life-threatening reactions are associated with iron supplements?	Overdose (lethargy, nausea, vomiting, abdominal pain, weak and rapid pulse, tarry stools, diffuse vascular congestion, shock, pulmonary edema, seizures); severe hypotension, bradycardia, bronchospasm, and hypersensitivity reactions may occur with I.V. administration of iron

✎ What are important nursing considerations when administering iron supplements?

1. Instruct the patient to take iron supplements on an empty stomach, if tolerable, for better absorption. Taking iron supplements with food may minimize gastric distress, but will decrease absorption. Avoid eggs, milk, cheese, yogurt, tea, and coffee because they further inhibit absorption.
2. If ferrous sulfate isn't tolerated, consider ferrous gluconate or ferrous fumarate. However, avoid interchanging iron salts (gluconate, sulfate, fumarate) because the elemental iron content may vary.
3. Monitor complete blood count (CBC) (hemoglobin, hematocrit) and reticulocyte count during therapy to determine effectiveness.
4. Inform the patient that oral iron may cause darkening of stools.
5. Assess the patient for thalassemia and hemochromatosis prior to initiation of therapy. Iron administration may be lethal in these conditions.
6. Avoid rapid infusion of I.V. iron due to the risk of severe hypotension. Use the Z-track method for I.M. injections.
7. Monitor the patient for complications of drug therapy (gastric distress, constipation, toxicity, hypersensitivity reactions).

▧ *Vitamin C (orange juice) enhances the absorption of iron.*

▧ *Iron-darkened stools may mask melena, and false-positive guaiac tests may occur.*

FOLIC ACID (VITAMIN B$_9$) SUPPLEMENTATION

How do folic acid supplements work?	Stimulate erythropoiesis to correct anemia
What are examples of folic acid supplements?	Folvite

What adverse reactions are associated with folic acid supplementation?	Nausea, bitter taste sensation, confusion, allergic reactions (rash, pruritus, bronchospasm), and discomfort at the injection site
What are important nursing actions when administering folic acid supplements?	1. Avoid use in anemia of unknown origin. Folic acid supplementation may mask pernicious anemia in these patients. 2. Monitor the patient for complications of drug therapy (allergic reactions, confusion). 3. Monitor blood work for CBC and folate level periodically throughout therapy to determine effectiveness.

CYANOCOBALAMIN (VITAMIN B_{12}) SUPPLEMENTATION

How does cyanocobalamin work?	Stimulates hematopoiesis, which aids in the treatment of pernicious anemia or vitamin B_{12} malabsorption
What are examples of cyanocobalamin formulations?	Crystamine, Cyanoject, Rubramin PC, Nascobal (nasal)
What adverse reactions are associated with cyanocobalamin supplements?	Headache, pruritus, transient diarrhea, discomfort at the injection site, and rhinitis or nasal congestion (nasal formulation)
What life-threatening reactions are associated with cyanocobalamin supplements?	Anaphylaxis and heart failure
What are important nursing actions when administering cyanocobalamin?	1. Monitor blood work for vitamin B_{12} levels and CBC periodically throughout therapy to determine effectiveness. 2. Instruct the patient to avoid alcohol during therapy (impairs absorption). 3. Avoid drug exposure to light.

Treatment of sickle cell anemia and polycythemia vera

What are examples of drugs used in the treatment of sickle cell anemia and polycythemia vera and how do they work?	1. *Hydroxyurea (Droxia):* increases production of fetal hemoglobin; used for patients with sickle cell anemia who are older than age 18 and who have had more than three crises per year; decreases need for blood transfusions and frequency of severe pain

2. *Anagrelide (Agrylin):* decreases production of platelets by inhibiting megakaryocyte maturation, thereby reducing the risk of thrombosis

What adverse reactions are associated with agents used in the treatment of sickle cell anemia and polycythemia vera?

1. *Hydroxyurea:* headache, dizziness, anorexia, nausea, vomiting, diarrhea, hyperuricemia, rash, pruritus
2. *Anagrelide:* headaches, confusion, diarrhea, nausea, abdominal pain, gastritis, fluid retention, heart failure, dyspnea, palpitations, rash, purpura

What life-threatening reactions are associated with these agents?

1. *Hydroxyurea:* myelosuppression, leukopenia, thrombocytopenia, seizures
2. *Anagrelide:* thrombocytopenia, arrhythmias, heart failure, stroke

What are important nursing actions when administering hydroxyurea?

1. Monitor blood work for blood urea nitrogen (BUN), creatinine, uric acid, white blood cells, and platelets.
2. Monitor intake and output. Instruct the patient to increase fluid intake to 10 to 12 glasses of fluid per day.
3. Instruct women to avoid becoming pregnant during therapy with hydroxyurea.
4. Monitor the patient for complications of therapy (fever, unusual bleeding or bruising) and notify the physician immediately if any develop.

What are important nursing actions when administering anagrelide?

1. Instruct the patient to take this drug 1 hour before or 2 hours after meals.
2. Monitor blood work for BUN, creatinine, liver function tests, complete blood count, and platelets.
3. Instruct women to avoid becoming pregnant during therapy.
4. Monitor the patient for complications of therapy (abnormal bleeding, bruising, cardiac symptoms, fever) and notify the physician immediately if any develop.

Treatment of hypocoagulable disorders

ANTIFIBRINOLYTICS

How do antifibrinolytics work?

Inhibit fibrinolysis by binding to plasmin, thus preventing the breakdown of clots

What are examples?

Aminocaproic acid (Amicar)

What adverse reactions are associated with antifibrinolytics?

Headache, dizziness, tinnitus, malaise, nausea, diarrhea, abdominal cramps, and myopathy

What life-threatening reactions are associated with antifibrinolytics?	Renal failure, seizures, bradycardia, and arrhythmias
What are important nursing actions when administering antifibrinolytics?	1. Monitor blood work for renal function and hepatic function as well as creatine kinase. 2. Monitor the patient for muscle pain or weakness, hematuria, severe headache, or restlessness, and notify the physician immediately if any develop.

BLOOD DERIVATIVES

How do blood derivatives work?	Replacement of deficient clotting factor
What are examples of blood derivatives?	1. Antihemophilic factor, AHF or factor VIII (Alphanate, Bioclate, Hemofil M, Recombinate, ReFacto) for treatment of hemophilia A 2. Factor IX concentrates (AlphaNine SD), Benefix, Mononine, Proplex T) for treatment of hemophilia B; replaces factors II, VII, IX and X
What adverse reactions are associated with blood derivatives?	1. *AHF:* fever, chills, nausea, chest tightness, wheezing 2. *Factor IX concentrates:* chills, fever, flushing, headache, nausea
What life-threatening reactions are associated with blood derivatives?	1. *AHF:* anaphylaxis, thromboembolic events, thrombocytopenia, small risk of contracting HIV or hepatitis B 2. *Factor IX concentrates:* thromboembolic events, myocardial infarction, disseminated intravascular coagulation, very small risk of contracting HIV or hepatitis B
What are important nursing actions when administering blood derivatives?	1. Administer hepatitis B vaccine before therapy with blood derivatives when possible, particularly for AHF. 2. Refrigerate the product until you're ready to use it and then allow it to warm to room temperature before reconstitution or administration. 3. Obtain baseline pulse before infusions and monitor vital signs closely during infusions. 4. Monitor clotting times, prothrombin time, and partial thromboplastin time periodically to assess response to therapy. 5. Monitor the patient for complications of therapy, such as anaphylactic reactions and thromboembolic events (leg pain and tenderness), and notify the physician immediately if any occur.

Treatment of hypercoagulable disorders

ANTICOAGULANTS

How do anticoagulants work?

1. *Warfarin:* inhibits the effects of vitamin K on various clotting factors (prothrombin and factors VII, IX and X); prolongs prothrombin time (PT) and International Normalized Ratio (INR)
2. *Heparin sodium/calcium:* binds with antithrombin III (AT-III) and inhibits thrombin (factor IIa) as well as factor Xa; prolongs partial thromboplastin time (PTT)
3. *Low molecular weight heparins:* bind with antithrombin III and inhibit factor Xa without affecting thrombin
4. *Danaparoid:* prevents fibrin formation by inhibiting thrombin generation; used for deep vein thrombosis prophylaxis in post-hip replacement patients
5. *Antithrombin III (human):* replaces deficient AT-III to inhibit thromboembolism formation

◤ *INR is a standardized test that accounts for the use of different laboratory reagents.*

What are examples of anticoagulants?

Warfarin (Coumadin); heparin sodium and heparin calcium; low molecular weight heparins, such as enoxaparin (Lovenox), dalteparin (Fragmin), and tinzaparin (Innohep); danaparoid (Organan); and antithrombin III (Thrombate III)

✎ **What adverse reactions are associated with anticoagulants?**

Easy bruising (hematoma at injection sites), increased risk of bleeding, nausea, diarrhea, skin necrosis (warfarin), pruritus, and hematuria

◤ *Protamine is the antidote for heparin.*

◤ *Vitamin K is the antidote for warfarin.*

What life-threatening reactions are associated with anticoagulants?

Hemorrhage, hepatotoxicity, hypersensitivity reactions, and thrombocytopenia (heparin and low molecular weight heparins)

What's the advantage of low molecular weight heparin relative to heparin?

It isn't necessary to monitor the PTT with low molecular weight heparin as it is with heparin sodium, or heparin calcium.

✎ **What are important nursing actions when administering anticoagulants?**

1. Monitor PT, PTT, and INR for proper levels and anticoagulation.
2. Monitor CBC and platelet count as well as hepatic and renal function studies.
3. Monitor the patient for petechiae and excessive bleeding as well as increased bleeding from incisions, I.V. sites, and mucous membranes.
4. Instruct the patient to avoid switching brands of warfarin due to the difference in bioavailability of different brands.
5. When transferring from I.V. heparin therapy to oral warfarin therapy, begin warfarin a minimum of 1 day before stopping heparin therapy.
6. Implement bleeding precautions, such as using soft toothbrushes, careful shaving, and the importance of obtaining regular PT and INR tests for monitoring anticoagulation levels.
7. Administer subcutaneous (S.C.) injections deeply and apply pressure to injection site once the needle is withdrawn, but don't massage the area. Rotate injection sites daily. Avoid I.M. injections of anticoagulants.
8. Instruct the patient to take warfarin at bedtime.
9. Instruct the patient to avoid sudden changes in intake of green leafy vegetables (they contain vitamin K, which alters the effects of warfarin).
10. Instruct the patient to avoid alcohol, which may increase the risk of bleeding.
11. Instruct the patient to refrain from rubbing the injection site after medication administration.
12. Inform the patient that warfarin interacts with many other medications, especially antibiotics.

⚔ *Warfarin takes at least 48 hours to demonstrate a measurable effect on coagulation, so heparin is used as a first-line treatment for hypercoagulable conditions. In addition, initial treatment with warfarin can temporarily* increase *coagulation, which heparin counteracts.*

⚔ *Appropriate injection sites for S.C. anticoagulants include the upper outer portion of the thighs, the area around the navel, and the upper outer portion of the buttocks.*

⚔ *The therapeutic goal of heparin therapy is a PTT of 1 1/2 to 2 1/2 times the control.*

⚔ *The therapeutic goal of warfarin therapy varies according to the indication for its use. An INR of 1 1/2 to 2 is typical for mechanical prosthetic valves or recurrent systemic embolisms. An INR of 2 to 3 is the typical goal for chronic atrial fibrillation.*

ANTI-PLATELET AGENTS

How do anti-platelet agents work?	Prevent platelet aggregation and formation of platelet plug
What are examples of anti-platelet agents?	Aspirin and nonsteroidal anti-inflammatory drugs, ticlopidine (Ticlid), clopidogrel (Plavix), aspirin + dipyridamole (Aggrenox), and glycoprotein (GP) IIB/IIIA inhibitors, such as abciximab (ReoPro), tirofiban (Aggrastat), and eptifibatide (Integrilin)

What adverse reactions are commonly associated with anti-platelet agents?

1. *Ticlopidine:* diarrhea, nausea, vomiting, abdominal pain
2. *Clopidogrel:* headache, dizziness, rash
3. *Aspirin + dipyridamole:* easy bruising, increased risk of bleeding, dizziness, hypotension, headache, nausea, flushing, abdominal discomfort
4. *Glycoprotein IIB/IIIA inhibitors:* hypotension, nausea, dizziness, headache

What life-threatening reactions are associated with anti-platelet agents?

1. *Ticlopidine:* hemorrhage, thrombocytopenia, neutropenia
2. *Clopidogrel:* hemorrhage, thrombocytopenia
3. *Aspirin + dipyridamole:* hemorrhage, thrombocytopenia, renal failure
4. *Glycoprotein IIB/IIIA inhibitors:* hemorrhage, thrombocytopenia, bradycardia

What are important nursing actions when administering anti-platelet agents?

1. Implement bleeding precautions.
2. Monitor blood work for CBC with differential and platelet count as well as renal and hepatic function.
3. Instruct the patient to avoid aspirin and aspirin-containing products during anti-platelet therapy.
4. Inform the patient that bleeding may be prolonged and that direct pressure should be applied to any injuries or trauma.
5. Inform the patient that normal platelet function or aggregation won't return until the drug has been discontinued for at least 5 days. Instruct him to notify all health care providers of anti-platelet therapy before any invasive procedures.
6. Monitor the patient for complications of therapy (abnormal bleeding) and notify the physician immediately if any develop.

THROMBOLYTICS ("CLOT BUSTERS")

How do thrombolytics work?	Break down the fibrin clot after it has formed
What are examples?	Streptokinase (Streptase), urokinase (Abbokinase), tissue plasminogen activator (Alteplase), reteplase (Retavase)
What adverse reactions are commonly associated with thrombolytics?	Transient hypotension and hypertension, headache, dizziness, allergic reactions (especially with streptokinase), and bleeding

🔰 *Aminocaproic acid (Amicar) is the antidote for thrombolytic agents.*

What are the life-threatening effects of thrombolytics?	Hemorrhage, anaphylaxis, and bronchospasm

🔖 **What are important nursing actions when administering a thrombolytic agent?**

1. Assess the patient for conditions that may preclude drug therapy.
2. Monitor the patient for severe bleeding, hemorrhage, and change in status.
3. Monitor ECG, CBC, PT, PTT, liver, and renal function studies.

🔰 *Eligibility for therapy is time limited (3 hours or less from onset of stroke symptoms and 4 hours or less from onset of myocardial infarction).*

Hematologic response modifiers

HUMAN GRANULOCYTE COLONY-STIMULATING FACTOR (G-CSF)

How does human granulocyte colony-stimulating factor (G-CSF) work?	Stimulation of proliferation and differentiation of neutrophils
What's an example?	Filgrastim (Neupogen)
What adverse reactions are associated with G-CSF?	Fatigue, alopecia, nausea, vomiting, diarrhea, mucositis, bone pain, and fever

What life-threatening reactions are associated with G-CSF?	Thrombocytopenia, arrhythmias, and myocardial infarction

What are important nursing actions when administering G-CSF?

1. Store the vial in the refrigerator and allow it to warm to room temperature before use. Avoid shaking the vial and discard a vial that has remained at room temperature for more than 6 hours.
2. Avoid administering within 24 hours of chemotherapy.
3. Instruct the patient about the proper administration of subcutaneous injections as well as the proper disposal of used needles, syringes, and vials.
4. Monitor CBC and platelet count prior to and twice weekly during therapy. Emphasize the importance of keeping follow-up appointments to monitor the response to therapy.
5. Instruct the patient to report fever, chills, severe bone pain, sore throat, and weakness as well as pain or swelling at injection site.
6. Discontinue therapy once neutrophil count is greater than 10,000/µl.

ERYTHROPOIETIN (EPOETIN ALPHA, EPO)

How does erythropoietin work?

Stimulates red blood cell production in the bone marrow

What are examples?

Epogen, Eprex, and Procrit

What are common adverse reactions to erythropoietin?

Headache, arthralgia, fever, fatigue, asthenia, dizziness, edema, nausea, vomiting, diarrhea, rash, cough, shortness of breath, chest pain, hypertension, and increased clotting

What life-threatening reactions are associated with erythropoietin?

Seizures and transient ischemic attacks or stroke

What are important nursing actions when administering erythropoietin?

1. Confirm medical history for anemia associated with renal failure before administration; it isn't intended as a treatment for severe anemia or as a substitute for urgent transfusions.
2. Store the vial in the refrigerator and allow it to warm to room temperature before use. Avoid shaking the vial (may denature the glycoprotein).
3. Instruct the patient about the proper administration of subcutaneous injections as well as the proper disposal of needles, syringes, and vials.

4. Instruct the patient to take supplements (iron, folic acid, vitamin B_{12}) throughout the course of therapy as ordered by the physician.
5. Monitor CBC (especially hematocrit), iron levels, and renal function tests throughout therapy. Determine proper dosage based on hematocrit.
6. Monitor blood pressure during therapy to assess for hypertension.
7. Emphasize the importance of keeping follow-up appointments for blood work before dosing.

Nursing skills

Blood transfusions

✎ **What's the proper technique for administering a blood transfusion?**

1. Confirm the order for blood transfusion, and confirm that the patient has signed a consent form for blood transfusion (a signed consent form is required).
2. Obtain baseline vital signs and inform the patient about the procedure, the blood product to be administered, and the number of units. Determine any previous adverse reactions to blood products. Instruct the patient to immediately report sudden itching, rash, dyspnea, nausea, or chills during transfusion.
3. Ensure patent I.V. access of at least an 18G catheter (large gauge needles prevent damage to red blood cells [RBCs]). Assemble proper tubing (Y-tubing with blood filter) and compatible crystalloid solution (normal saline).
4. Obtain blood from the blood bank and inspect it for color, clots, or excess air. Check the physician order and the blood bag label with the blood bank technician (name of patient, ID number, blood type, Rh group, expiration date).
5. At the bedside, compare the laboratory blood type record with another nurse (name of patient, ID number, blood type, and Rh type, number on blood bag label) and document according to facility policy.
6. Identify the patient by asking him to state his full name and compare it with the name on identification band. Confirm ABO and Rh compatibility by comparing bag labels, bag tag, medical record, or transfusion form.
7. Make sure that the clamps on the Y-set are closed and spike container of normal saline with vented tubing and blood bag with remaining Y-set spike. Hang saline

and blood approximately 36" (90 cm) above the venipuncture site. Open the clamp for the saline tubing, squeeze drip chamber until it's one-third full, and prime the tubing. Connect saline-primed tubing to I.V. needle and open the clamp.

8. Gently invert the blood bag several times to mix cells and plasma. Put on gloves. Expose the injection port on the blood bag and spike it. Open the bloodline clamp and squeeze the drip chamber until it's full with blood. Open the main flow clamp and adjust the drip rate, starting slowly (20 gtt/minute) for the first 15 minutes to monitor for reactions.

9. Observe the patient for at least the first 5 minutes of the infusion (or in accordance with facility policy) and document any adverse reactions. Stop the infusion and notify the physician immediately if any occur.

10. Obtain a second set of vital signs 15 minutes after starting the infusion. If no adverse reactions are noted, the flow rate may be increased. One unit of blood is generally infused in 1½ to 2 hours, depending on the patient's volume status and physician's order. Continue to monitor the patient closely and obtain vital signs every 30 minutes during the transfusion.

11. Once the infusion is complete, put on gloves, clamp the blood tubing, and disconnect it from the primary I.V. line. Flush the primary line with saline solution and discard the blood bag and tubing according to facility policy.

12. Obtain vital signs at completion of infusion.

What are potential complications associated with blood transfusions?

Transfusion reactions, such as acute hemolytic and anaphylactic reactions, generally occur during the initial 50 to 100 ml. Additional transfusion reactions may include allergic, febrile, or septic reactions. Pulmonary edema and heart failure may also result.

What are the clinical manifestations of a transfusion reaction?

Fever, nausea, dyspnea, hypotension, flushing, rash, back or chest pains, and hemoglobinuria

What's the appropriate nursing intervention for a transfusion reaction?

1. Stop the transfusion.
2. Notify the physician immediately.
3. Administer care (oxygen, antihistamines) supportive to the symptoms.

What are important nursing considerations when administering blood products?

1. Observe standard precautions during blood and blood product transfusions because there's a possibility of contact with blood and body fluids.
2. Blood can be stored for 30 minutes at room temperature before infusion, and must be returned to the

blood bank if there's a delay in administration longer than 30 minutes.

3. Completion of the transfusion should occur within 4 hours of its initiation or before expiration of the components (whichever is sooner).

4. Blood products should always be checked at the patient's bedside, and two qualified persons must check each unit to be transfused (one for patient verification and another for blood product verification).

5. Normal saline is the only solution that's acceptable for administration during blood transfusion.

6. No other medications may be administered via the bloodline during the transfusion.

7. Delayed reactions can occur 3 to 10 days after the transfusion.

8. Transfusion of one unit packed RBCs will generally increase the hematocrit by 3%.

9. Common viruses for which blood products are screened include hepatitis (B and C), HIV, human T-cell lymphotrophic virus types I and II (HTLV1 and HTLV2), and syphilis.

14

The endocrine system

Basic concepts of the endocrine system

What's a gland?

A cluster of specialized cells that produce and secrete chemical substances that regulate bodily processes

✎ What's an endocrine gland?

A gland that releases hormones directly into the bloodstream for distribution throughout the body

✎ What's an exocrine gland?

A gland that releases its product into ducts, onto the free surface of the skin, or onto open cavities of the body, such as the digestive, reproductive, or respiratory tracts, for transport to a specific area. Exocrine glands don't release products directly into the blood.

✎ What are the major glands of the endocrine system?

1. *Pituitary:* "master gland" of the body located at the base of the brain; secretes hormones that affect the actions of various other endocrine glands, such as the thyroid, the adrenals, and the ovaries; hypothalamus controls its actions
2. *Pineal:* located at the back of the brain; affects biorhythms, such as daily physiologic cycles, and reproductive development through the production of melatonin
3. *Parathyroids:* four small glands located behind the thyroid gland; <u>maintain calcium levels within normal range; produce a hormone (parathormone) that caus</u>es bones to release calcium into the blood when levels are low
4. *Thyroid:* butterfly-shaped gland located just below the larynx at the base of the neck; <u>regulates body temperature and overall metabolism;</u> plays vital role in development; affects the function of the nervous, immune, reproductive, respiratory, and digestive systems
5. *Thymus:* located below the sternum; produces thymosin and thymopoietin, and produces T-cells for cell-mediated immunity

weight bearing exercise Blood to Bones

6. *Adrenals:* two glands; one gland lies atop each kidney; affect renal function, which helps to maintain blood pressure and salt levels, and to regulate fluid concentrations throughout the body

7. *Islets of Langerhans:* endocrine cells located within the pancreas; regulate blood glucose levels and glucose metabolism, and affect other endocrine cells within the GI tract

8. *Ovaries and testes:* control growth, development, and function of the reproductive system

◤ *The hypothalamus produces various releasing and inhibiting hormones, which regulate the levels of hormones produced by other endocrine glands through their actions on the pituitary gland.*

What system works in conjunction with the endocrine system to exert control on all physiologic processes?

The nervous system

◤ **What's a hormone?**

A chemical produced and secreted by specialized cells within an organ or tissue that enters the bloodstream and is carried throughout the body to exert its actions on target cells; once the hormone binds to its target cell, a cascade of events within the cell affects its function

◤ *The physiologic effect of a hormone is primarily determined by its concentration in the blood and extracellular fluid.*

What must target cells have in order to respond to a specific hormone?

A receptor specific for the hormone; these receptors may be located on the cell's surface or within the cell, depending on the type of hormone; once a hormone binds its receptor, unique physiologic changes occur that are dependent upon the hormone's target site and its particular action at that site

◤ *A hormone may produce different effects at different target sites.*

What are the three types of hormonal action?

1. *Endocrine:* hormone exerts its action by binding to distant target sites

2. *Paracrine:* hormone acts locally; diffuses from its source to affect nearby target cells

3. *Autocrine:* hormone exerts its effects on the same cell that produced it

✎ How is hormonal production primarily controlled?

By feedback loops, which serve to prevent hormonal over- or under-secretion — negative feedback loops (output of a pathway inhibits input into the pathway) are more common; control of the secretion of thyroid hormones is an example of a negative feedback loop; increased blood levels of triiodothyronine (T_3) and thyroxine (T_4) inhibit the secretion of thyroid-releasing hormone (TRH), which in turn inhibits the secretion of thyroid-stimulating hormone (TSH) so that thyroid hormone secretion is reduced

✎ What hormones does the anterior pituitary produce?

1. *Growth hormone (GH) or somatotropin:* promotes growth indirectly through stimulation of insulin-like growth factor (IGF-1) production by the liver; regulates metabolism of proteins, lipids, and carbohydrates; stimulates protein synthesis and growth; main target sites include liver and adipose tissue (adipocytes)
2. *TSH or thyrotropin:* produced in response to signal (TRH) from hypothalamus; stimulates production and secretion of thyroid hormones, T_4 and T_3; main target site is the thyroid gland
3. *Corticotropin:* stimulates secretion of glucocorticoids (cortisol) from the adrenal cortex; released from the anterior pituitary in response to corticotropin-releasing hormone (CRH), which is produced in response to various forms of stress; main target site of corticotropin is the adrenal cortex
4. *Prolactin:* promotes development of glandular tissue in the female breast during pregnancy and stimulates the production of milk after birth; primary source is anterior pituitary, but is also secreted from other cells, including lymphocytes; the hypothalamus inhibits prolactin secretion from the pituitary, and dopamine is the primary inhibiting factor; main target sites include the mammary glands
5. *Gonadotropic hormones, such as follicle-stimulating hormone (FSH) and luteinizing hormone (LH):* regulate reproductive function; secretion is regulated by gonadotropin-releasing hormone (GnRH); main target sites are ovaries and testes

What effect do GH and IGF-1 have on metabolism?

1. *Protein:* anabolic effect due to increased amino acid uptake and protein synthesis as well as decreased protein oxidation
2. *Fat:* stimulates breakdown and oxidation of triglycerides, which enhances the utilization of fat
3. *Carbohydrate:* helps maintain normal range of blood glucose along with other hormones; anti-insulin activity; inhibits insulin's ability to stimulate peripheral tissue uptake of glucose

What hormones control the production of GH?

1. *Growth hormone–releasing hormone (GH-RH):* stimulates production and secretion of GH; is a hypothalamic hormone
2. *Somatostatin (SS):* inhibits secretion of GH; is a hypothalamic hormone
3. *Ghrelin:* stimulates GH secretion; is secreted from the stomach

Production and secretion of GH occurs in a pulsatile pattern due to the combination of multiple factors, including nutrition, sleep, exercise, and stress as well as levels of GH-RH, SS, and GH itself.

What are the effects of LH?

In males, it stimulates the production and secretion of testosterone. In females, a surge of LH induces ovulation, and it stimulates the formation of the corpus luteum and its production of progesterone.

What are the effects of FSH?

It stimulates the maturation of ovarian follicles and their production of estrogen in females, and it's necessary for spermatogenesis in males.

What hormones are produced by the posterior pituitary?

1. *Oxytocin:* stimulates uterine contractions and milk ejection; primary stimulus for oxytocin; may play role in initiation of labor; main target sites include uterus and mammary tissue
2. *Antidiuretic hormone (ADH) or vasopressin:* promotes conservation of body water by decreasing urine output; promotes reabsorption of water by binding to receptors on the distal or collecting tubules; high concentrations can increase arterial pressure by constricting arterioles; main target site is the kidney

3 ways to conserve H2O.
vassopressin

What factor is the most important regulator of ADH secretion?

Plasma osmolarity, or solute concentration in blood; increased plasma osmolarity causes ADH to be secreted; plasma osmolarity is decreased while urine osmolarity is increased

ADH secretion is also affected by blood pressure and volume; decreases in blood pressure and volume activate stretch receptors in the heart and large arteries, and ADH secretion is stimulated.

What hormones are produced by the thyroid gland?

1. T_4 and T_3: help regulate body temperature, metabolism, heart rate, and protein production; T_4 is the most abundant form produced by the thyroid gland, but it's converted to T_3 by tissues in the body; T_3 is the metabolically active form of the hormone; amount of thyroid hormones produced is determined by the amount of T_3 and T_4 in the blood; high blood levels of

thyroid hormones inhibit their production via a negative feedback loop

2. *Calcitonin:* decreases serum calcium levels by inhibiting the activity of osteoclasts (suppresses resorption of bone)

> ◥ *Thyroid hormone production is dependent on an adequate iodine supply. To produce thyroid hormone, 100 to 200 mcg of dietary iodine is required.*

✎ What hormone is produced by the parathyroid glands?

Parathyroid hormone (PTH) or parathormone, which helps maintain the calcium and phosphorus balance in the body; PTH increases serum calcium levels by causing its release from bones (through activation of osteoclasts), causing the kidneys to increase calcium absorption from the blood and causing the intestine to increase its absorption of dietary calcium; the parathyroid glands increase PTH secretion in response to low calcium levels in the blood, and it decreases PTH production when blood calcium levels are high

> ◥ *PTH is the most important regulator of blood calcium levels.*

What are the two parts of the adrenal glands?

The medulla (inner portion) and the cortex (outer portion); medullary activity is regulated by hypothalamic nerve impulses and cortical activity is controlled by the negative feedback loop that exists between the hypothalamus and corticotropin; the medulla can be removed without life-threatening effects, but the cortex is essential to life

✎ What hormones are produced by the adrenal cortex?

1. Mineralocorticoids, such as aldosterone, cause renal conservation of sodium and water.
2. Glucocorticoids, such as cortisol, increase blood glucose levels by stimulating gluconeogenesis (conversion of fat and protein into glucose) in the liver during stress; produce anti-inflammatory effects by suppressing the immune response.
3. Gonadocorticoids or sex hormones, such as androgens (testosterone), become important only if excessive production occurs.

> ◥ *All cortical hormones are steroid hormones chemically.*

What hormone stimulates the adrenal cortex?

Corticotropin

✎ What hormones are produced by the adrenal medulla?

Epinephrine (adrenalin), norepinephrine (noradrenalin), and dopamine

✎ What are catecholamines?

The hormones epinephrine, norepinephrine, and dopamine are collectively referred to as *catecholamines*. These hormones are secreted in response to stress, such as trauma, exercise, and hypoglycemia. Catecholamines prepare the body for the "fight or flight" response by increasing the heart, respiratory, and metabolic rates, increasing blood glucose levels, dilating pupils and bronchi, and shunting blood from the skin and viscera, such as the digestive organs, to the brain, coronary arteries, and skeletal muscles. Corticotropin secretion from the anterior pituitary is also increased.

▜ *Catecholamines bind to adrenergic receptors on their target cells, producing a response that mimics that of direct sympathetic nervous stimulation.*

What types of adrenergic receptors exist?

1. *Alpha:* stimulated by epinephrine, norepinephrine, and phenylephrine; blocked by phentolamine. Alpha$_1$-receptors are located primarily in smooth muscles of gut, skin, arterioles, veins, and eye; cause smooth muscle contraction; alpha$_2$-receptors are located at the pre-synaptic terminals of adrenergic nerves
2. *Beta:* stimulated by isoproterenol (strongest stimulus), epinephrine, and norepinephrine; blocked by propranolol; beta$_1$-receptors are located in cardiac muscle and the kidneys; increase heart rate and cardiac contractility and promotes rennin release from the kidneys; beta$_2$-receptors are located in metabolic tissues and smooth muscles that relax with stimulation; decreases motility of GI system, produces bronchodilation, vasodilation within cardiac and skeletal muscles, and promotes glycogenolysis within the liver

✎ What hormones are produced by the islets of Langerhans in the pancreas?

1. *Insulin:* secreted by beta cells in response to high blood glucose levels; decreases blood glucose levels by facilitating its entry into cells; stimulates glycogen and fat synthesis; increases protein synthesis
2. *Glucagon:* secreted by alpha cells in response to low blood glucose levels; stimulates glycogen breakdown (hydrolysis) and gluconeogenesis
3. *Somatostatin:* secreted by delta cells; inhibits the release of insulin and glucagon; inhibits gastrin secretion

▜ *The pancreas serves both endocrine and exocrine functions.*

✎ What does insulin do? | Insulin promotes glucose uptake by the cells, which decreases serum glucose levels; stimulates the conversion of glucose to glycogen (storage form), lipids to fats, and amino acids to proteins

What hormones oppose the action of insulin? | Glucagon, cortisol, catecholamines, and GH
need fuel

✎ What hormones do the ovaries produce? |
1. *Estrogen:* secreted by developing follicles; influences maturation of reproductive organs, development of secondary sex characteristics, and endometrial growth during menses
2. *Progesterone:* secreted by corpus luteum; causes endometrial thickening in preparation for pregnancy

✎ What hormone does the testes produce? | Testosterone (an androgen), which is produced by Leydig's cells within the testes; testosterone affects the development of the reproductive organs and secondary sex characteristics

What are examples of other organs that produce hormones? |
1. *Kidneys:* produce and secrete erythropoietin and renin
2. *Stomach:* produces and secretes gastrin (stimulates histamine release, which then acts on parietal cells to produce hydrochloric acid) and pepsin production necessary for digestion
3. *Liver:* produces various growth factors (IGF, epidermal growth factor, platelet-derived growth factor) and binding proteins necessary for normal hormonal function
4. *Small intestine:* secretes secretin (neutralizes stomach acid through production of bicarbonate ions by the pancreas) and cholecystokinin (stimulates gall bladder contraction to release bile and stimulates secretion of digestive enzymes and bicarbonate from the pancreas)
5. *Heart:* upper chambers produce atrial natriuretic factor (ANF), which maintains cardiovascular homeostasis

✎ What hormones are responsible for breast development? |
1. *Estrogen:* stimulates ductal tissue growth and fat depositions
2. *Progesterone:* stimulates glandular development

Where is the majority of glandular tissue located in the female breast? | In the upper outer quadrant of the breast, also known as the *tail of Spence*

▉ *The glandular tissue of the breast is a potential site for malignancy. Because the largest portion of this tissue lies in the upper outer quadrants, most malignancies of the female breast occur in this area.*

> ◩ *Males have a small amount of glandular tissue beneath the nipples, but women have glandular tissue more widely distributed throughout the breasts.*

Physical assessment of the endocrine system

Normal findings

What are important nursing actions prior to beginning a physical examination of the endocrine system?

1. Ensure patient privacy and that the room is a comfortable temperature and well lit.
2. Obtain the necessary equipment (tape measure, stethoscope, watch with a second hand, glass of water with a straw).

✎ What general items should be assessed during an endocrine examination?

Vital signs, height, weight, proportionality of body parts, fat distribution, apparent age relative to chronological age, and mental and emotional status

What physical assessments should be made of the endocrine system?

1. Inspection of general body development; skin pigmentation; amount, distribution, and texture of hair; nail growth and condition; shape and symmetry of facial features; neck symmetry and midline positioning of trachea; symmetry; shape of breast and development of external genitalia; appearance of extremities (no muscle atrophy); condition of skin on feet and between toes
2. Palpation of thyroid gland
3. Auscultation of thyroid if abnormalities are found on palpation

What are the only endocrine glands accessible to palpation?

Thyroid and testes

Where is the thyroid gland located?

In the front of the neck, just below the larynx

✎ How is the thyroid examined?

1. Stand behind the patient and, using both hands, place your fingers on either side of his trachea, just beneath the cricoid cartilage.
2. Instruct the patient to swallow as the thyroid is gently palpated. One lobe should be palpated at a time, and the patient should be instructed to lower his chin and flex his neck slightly to the side being assessed.
3. To assess the right lobe, use your left hand to displace the patient's trachea to the right. Palpate right lobe with fingers of your right hand.

4. To palpate the right lateral border of the right lobe, hold the sternocleidomastoid muscle with your right hand while placing your middle fingers deep into and in front of it.
5. To assess the left lobe, use your right hand to displace the trachea slightly to the left and use your left hand to palpate.

▌ *Although the thyroid generally can't be palpated unless the patient has a very thin neck, the isthmus (center portion that connects the two lobes) may be palpated.*

If an enlarged thyroid gland is palpated, what's the next step in the examination?

Auscultation of the thyroid with the bell of the stethoscope to assess for systolic bruits while the patient holds his breath. The presence of a bruit indicates increased blood flow through the thyroid, which may indicate hyperthyroidism.

Abnormal findings

What subjective findings are commonly associated with endocrine disorders?

Fatigue, mental status changes (lethargy, memory problems), altered sleep habits (increased sleep requirements, insomnia, frequent awakenings), heat or cold intolerance, and unintentional weight loss or gain

What are examples of some abnormalities that should be noted on a physical examination of the endocrine system?

1. *Inspection:* pigmentation abnormalities of the skin; abnormal distribution or amount of hair; thickness, cracking, brittleness of nails or separation of nail bed; protrusion of the eyeballs (exophthalmos) or incomplete eyelid closure; asymmetry or enlargement of the neck; asymmetry of the shape or size of the breasts (some slight variations are normal, especially during puberty); nipple discharge not associated with pregnancy or lactation; gynecomastia; muscle wasting of upper extremities
2. *Palpation:* knot or swelling in front of neck; firm, fixed nodules in front of neck
3. *Auscultation:* bruits

Polyuria and polydipsia may be indicative of what endocrine disorders?

Diabetes mellitus or diabetes insipidus

Polyphagia may be indicative of what endocrine disorders?

Diabetes mellitus or hyperthyroidism

✎ **Heat intolerance might be indicative of what endocrine disorder?**	Hyperthyroidism
✎ **Cold intolerance might be indicative of what endocrine disorder?**	Hypothyroidism
✎ **Thick, dry skin may be indicative of what endocrine disorder?**	Hypothyroidism
✎ **Purple striae of the breasts and abdomen and ecchymosis may be indicative of what endocrine disorder?**	Cushing's syndrome
✎ **Widening of the bones of the hands and feet may be indicative of what endocrine disorder?**	Acromegaly
✎ **A protrusion of the eyeballs and a gritty sensation of the eyes may be indicative of what endocrine disorder?**	Graves' disease
✎ **Hypertension may be associated with what endocrine disorders?**	Pheochromocytoma, hyperthyroidism, and Cushing's syndrome
Hypotension may be associated with what endocrine disorder?	Hypothyroidism
✎ **Tachycardia (more than 100 beats/ minute) may be associated with what endocrine disorders?**	Hyperthyroidism and thyroid tumors

✎ Bradycardia (less than 60 beats/minute) may be associated with what endocrine disorders?

Myxedema and hypopituitarism

✎ Hyperpigmentation of sun-exposed body areas as well as joints, genitals, palmar creases, and recent scars may be indicative of what endocrine disorder?

Addison's disease

✎ What's gynecomastia?

Overdevelopment of breast tissue that usually results from hormonal alterations — idiopathic systemic disorders, such as endocrine disorders, disease of the liver, pituitary adenoma; drugs such as cimetidine, phenytoin, reserpine, nifedipine, theophylline, diuretics; neoplasms such as testicular tumors; and in association with lung cancer; occurs most commonly in adolescents and men older than age 50

✎ What's hirsutism?

Excessive hair growth on the face or body that results from increased sensitivity to (or abnormally elevated levels of) androgens (male sex hormones such as testosterone); can result from androgen-secreting tumors, polycystic ovary disease, or even certain medications, including hormonal contraceptives and anabolic steroids

Major disorders of the endocrine system

Disorders of insulin regulation

DIABETES MELLITUS

✎ What's diabetes mellitus?

A syndrome of disordered metabolism with inappropriate hyperglycemia due to either an absolute deficiency of insulin secretion or production, or a reduction in the sensitivity of cells to insulin

What's the pathophysiologic process of diabetes mellitus?

Cells can't take up glucose from the bloodstream so that blood glucose levels increase. Because glucose is a hyperosmolar substance, hyperglycemia produces hyperosmolarity and excessive amounts of fluid are drawn out of cells as a result. Glucose then overflows into the urine where it's excreted along with fluid (responsible for polyuria). As a result, glucose passes out of the body unused, causing cells to be starved of energy (responsible for polyphagia, or increased appetite) and also to become dehydrated (responsible for polydipsia, or increased thirst).

✎ What are the three types of diabetes mellitus?

1. *Type 1:* juvenile onset (typically before age 30); rapid onset; decreased insulin production; lean body build; autoimmune process in which antibodies destroy beta cells of the pancreas so that little or no insulin is produced; genetic association
2. *Type 2:* typically of adult onset (older than age 40); slow onset; usually begins with insulin resistance in which cells can't use insulin effectively and insulin production eventually decreases; commonly associated with obesity and sedentary lifestyle in combination with hypertension and hyperlipidemia; represents majority (90%) of total diabetics; more common in African Americans, Native Americans, Asian and Pacific Islanders, and Hispanic populations
3. *Gestational diabetes:* occurs during pregnancy and disappears after birth of baby; mother is at increased risk for development of type 2 diabetes later

✎ What are the clinical manifestations of diabetes mellitus?

Polyuria, polydipsia, polyphagia, fatigue, weight loss, blurred vision, frequent infections (type 2), chronic non-healing wounds (type 2)

How is the diagnosis of diabetes mellitus made?

Random glucose level greater than 200 mg/dl in association with symptoms of diabetes, a fasting glucose level greater than 126 mg/dl, or a glucose level greater than 200 mg/dl 2 hours following an oral glucose tolerance test (OGTT) in which 75 g of glucose is dissolved in water and drunk

✎ What's a hemoglobin A_{1c}?

Also referred to as *glycosylated hemoglobin*; it's a blood test that reflects average blood glucose over the previous 3 months. Maintenance of a hemoglobin A_{1c} level less than 6% is ideal, because it significantly decreases the rate of complications from diabetes.

▶ *Blood glucose increases 30 mg/dl for every 1% increase in hemoglobin A_{1c}, and the risk of complications increases accordingly.*

What's an insulin C-peptide?

Connecting peptide, or C-peptide, is a subunit of insulin with no known function. However, C-peptide levels reflect insulin production (for every one C-peptide molecule in the blood, there's one insulin molecule) and are therefore useful in differentiating between endogenous (produced by the body) and exogenous (from injection into the body) insulin production in type 2 diabetics.

✎ What complications are associated with diabetes mellitus?

Hypoglycemic and hyperglycemic episodes, gastroparesis, acute metabolic disturbances (diabetic ketoacidosis [DKA], hyperglycemic hyperosmolar nonketotic syndrome [HHNS], acidosis from excess ketone body production), cardiac and vascular disorders (peripheral vascular disease, painless myocardial infarction, diabetic foot or leg ulcerations, chronic wounds, retinopathy, nephropathy, neuropathy, cataracts), and increased susceptibility to infections

⚡ *Patients with blood glucose levels greater than 350 mg/dl are at risk for progression to DKA or HHNS.*

⚡ *ACE inhibitors are commonly used to prevent or delay renal failure in diabetics.*

✎ What's the typical treatment for diabetes mellitus?

1. *Type 1:* insulin (via injections or an insulin pump) and diet (less than 30 g carbohydrates per meal); pancreas or islet cell transplantation
2. *Type 2:* diet, exercise, medications including oral hypoglycemic agents, such as sulfonylureas (Glucotrol), metformin (Glucophage) and rosiglitazone (Avandia), and insulin

What are the benefits of exercise for a patient who has, or is at risk for developing, type 2 diabetes?

Exercise stimulates glucose uptake by active muscle cells and can increase tissue sensitivity to insulin, so that less insulin is required. Exercise also facilitates weight loss, which can prevent or delay the onset of diabetes.

What are the two primary causes of hypoglycemia (blood glucose less than 70 mg/dl)?

Underproduction of glucose (hormonal deficiencies, liver disease) or an overproduction of insulin (insulinoma)

✎ What are the clinical manifestations of hypoglycemia?

Shaking, diaphoresis, weakness, fatigue, dizziness, confusion, headache, anxiety, hunger, tachycardia, impaired or blurred vision, irritability

✎ What's the standard treatment for hypoglycemia in an alert person?

Replacement of glucose with approximately 15 g of carbohydrates; examples include $^1/_2$ cup of fruit juice or regular soda, 1 cup of milk, 6 pieces of hard candy, or 2 teaspoons of sugar or honey; if blood glucose remains below 70 mg/dl 15 minutes later, then another 15 g of carbohydrates should be consumed

✎ What's the typical treatment for hypoglycemia in an unconscious person?

Administration of 25 g of dextrose 50% (D_{50}) followed typically by I.V. fluids such as dextrose 5% in normal saline (D_5NS)

⚡ *It's important to determine the timing of the last dose of hypoglycemic medications in order to determine if and when another hypoglycemic episode might occur.*

What's the Somogyi effect?

Also known as the *rebound effect,* it's the tendency of the body to overcompensate for hypoglycemia so that hyperglycemia occurs. Counter-regulatory hormones, such as glucagon, are released from the liver during untreated hypoglycemia so that glycogen is converted into glucose, which raises blood glucose levels. Nightmares, elevated blood glucose levels upon awakening, and a morning headache are common manifestations.

What's the "dawn phenomenon"?

A condition in which blood glucose levels are fairly stable overnight but increase near dawn due to the circadian rhythmic release of growth hormone (GH); it doesn't occur secondary to an insulin reaction, as does the Somogyi effect

⚡ *Insulin resistance occurs naturally in nondiabetics in response to GH secretion that typically occurs from 4 a.m. to 9 a.m.*

✎ What are examples of appropriate snacks for a diabetic patient?

Those containing protein and starch, such as a cup of milk with crackers, or crackers with peanut butter or cheese

✎ What are the clinical manifestations of hyperglycemia?

Extreme thirst, frequent urination, blurred vision, drowsiness

✎ How is a blood glucose greater than 400 mg/dl typically treated?

Infusion of I.V. insulin and aggressive fluid resuscitation; insulin is discontinued when the blood glucose is approximately 250 mg/dl, and a hypertonic I.V. fluid containing dextrose, such as $D_5\frac{1}{2}NS$, is used to minimize the risk of hypoglycemia, hypokalemia from rapid or overcorrection of hyperglycemia, and cerebral edema from hyponatremia

⚡ *Because insulin causes cellular uptake of glucose and potassium, serum potassium levels may decrease rapidly following insulin administration.*

✎ What are important nursing actions in the care of a patient with diabetes mellitus?

1. Educate the patient about appropriate dietary management, including the consumption of high-complex carbohydrates and high-fiber foods. Fasting, skipping meals, and ingestion of simple sugars should be avoided. Meals should be taken at consistent times each day for type 1 diabetes, and carbohydrate intake should be spread out evenly throughout the day.
2. Instruct the patient on proper blood glucose monitoring.
3. Educate the patient about proper insulin administration, including rotating injection sites (prevents lipodystrophy). Teach the patient to draw up regular insulin into the syringe first if two types of insulin are being combined. Instruct the patient to take regular and longer-acting insulin 30 minutes before meals, and rapid-acting insulin immediately before meals. Emphasize the importance of coordinating the timing of insulin injections with meals.
4. Encourage physical activity, especially for patients with type 2 diabetes. Exercise is best performed after a meal when blood glucose levels are rising, but it should be avoided during peak insulin action times.
5. Administer medications (oral hypoglycemic agents, insulin) as ordered by the physician.
6. Monitor the patient for complications of diabetes (infections, cardiovascular problems) and its treatment (hypoglycemic episodes).
7. Educate the patient about symptoms, prevention, and treatment of hypoglycemia and hyperglycemia, DKA, or HHNS. Patients with diabetes should be prepared for hypoglycemic episodes by carrying hard candy or other rapid-acting glucose sources with them at all times.
8. Instruct the patient to examine his feet daily for sores or ulcerations.
9. Encourage routine ophthalmologic examination as well as close follow-up with diabetes specialists, including an endocrinologist, diabetes educator, and dietitian.

DIABETIC KETOACIDOSIS

✎ What's diabetic ketoacidosis (DKA)?

An acute metabolic disorder characterized by a persistent state of hyperglycemia that occurs primarily with severe insulin deficiency in type 1 diabetics; it can result from noncompliance with insulin regimen, or as a result of an acute illness, trauma, infection, surgery, pancreatitis, or extreme emotional stress; massive ketone formation and osmotic diuresis occur

What's the pathophysiologic process of DKA?	Cells are deprived of glucose during acute hyperglycemia because endogenous insulin isn't available to facilitate glucose entry into the cells. As a result, alternative fuel sources, such as stored glycogen, protein, and fat, are used in an attempt to provide glucose to the cells
	However, the persistent lack of insulin also prevents this additional glucose from entering the cells, which results in a worsening of the hyperglycemia. In addition, ketones are formed from the breakdown of fat, which lower the serum pH and produce metabolic acidosis.
Why do type 2 diabetics generally *not* develop DKA?	Type 2 diabetics typically produce some amount of endogenous insulin, whereas type 1 diabetics don't.
✎ **What are the clinical manifestations of DKA?**	Mental status changes (drowsiness, stupor, and unresponsiveness if left untreated), dry mucous membranes, extreme thirst, fruity odor of the breath (acetone), nausea and vomiting, tachycardia, hypotension, high urine output initially followed by decreased output, and Kussmaul's respirations (rapid, deep respirations) as a result of metabolic acidosis
	◥ *Increased urinary output is indicative of hyperglycemia while decreased urinary output is indicative of dehydration and hypovolemia.*
	◥ *Diabetics typically spill glucose into their urine until blood glucose levels are greater than 300 mg/dl, while nondiabetics tend to spill glucose into their urine when blood glucose levels are less than 180 mg/dl.*
What clinical indicators are used to diagnose DKA?	Hyperglycemia (300 to 800 mg/dl), ketones present in blood and urine, serum osmolarity greater than 350 mOsm/L, and presence of metabolic acidosis (pH less than 7.35) with resultant hyperventilation (to blow off carbon dioxide)
What complications are associated with DKA?	Dehydration, hemoconcentration, metabolic disturbances, shock, and death (10% or less mortality)
What's the typical treatment for DKA?	Insulin infusion and aggressive I.V. hydration; once the blood glucose level reaches 250 mg/dl an I.V. solution with 5% to 10% glucose, such as D_5NS, is used in combination with I.V. or S.C. insulin to reduce the risk of hypoglycemia and hypokalemia that can result from treatment

✎ What are important nursing actions in the care of a patient with DKA?

1. Administer insulin and I.V. fluids as ordered by the physician.
2. Monitor intake and output at least once per hour during the acute phase.
3. Assess vital signs at least once per hour during the acute phase, particularly respiratory rate, oxygen saturation, and lung sounds.
4. Monitor blood glucose levels hourly during the acute phase.
5. Perform neurologic assessments at least every 4 hours or more often, as the patient's condition dictates.
6. Assess urine for glucose and ketone levels at regular intervals.
7. Monitor the patient for complications of hyperglycemia (neurologic impairment) and treatment (fluid overload, hypoglycemia, hypokalemia). Ensure 50% dextrose for I.V. administration is readily available to treat hypoglycemia secondary to aggressive insulin therapy.

HYPEROSMOLAR HYPERGLYCEMIC NONKETOTIC SYNDROME

✎ What's hyperosmolar hyperglycemic nonketotic syndrome (HHNS)?

A life-threatening state of chronic hyperglycemia that occurs in people with uncontrolled type 2 diabetes due to the inhibition of insulin action or as a result of noncompliance with hypoglycemic agents; intracellular and extracellular dehydration eventually occur

Precipitating factors may include infection, renal failure, surgery, trauma, pancreatitis, heart failure, myocardial infarction, or the use of total parenteral nutrition, glucocorticoids, diuretics, or beta-adrenergic blockers.

◤ *Hyperglycemia associated with HHNS tends to be more severe and to progress at a more rapid rate than hyperglycemia associated with DKA.*

What's the pathophysiologic process of HHNS?

Insulin is produced in adequate amounts to prevent DKA, but the amount is insufficient to prevent severe hyperglycemia, osmotic diuresis, and depletion of extracellular fluid.

✎ What are the clinical manifestations of HHNS?

Polyuria, mental status changes (lethargy, confusion, mental obtundation), and possibly fever

◤ *Unlike DKA, pH and ventilation are normal in HHNS.*

What are the diagnostic criteria for HHNS?

Hyperglycemia (greater than 600 mg/dl), serum osmolarity greater than 350 mOsm/L, and arterial pH greater than 7.35

What complications are associated with HHNS?	Seizures, coma, and death
How is HHNS typically treated?	Aggressive fluid and electrolyte (potassium) replacement, administration of insulin, and treatment of precipitating factors

> ⚡ *The treatment of both DKA and HHNS is similar, although patients with HHNS typically require greater fluid replacement.*

✎ **What are the important nursing actions for a patient with HHNS?**	1. Administer insulin and I.V. fluids as ordered by the physician.
	2. Monitor intake and output at least once per hour during the acute phase.
	3. Assess vital signs at least once per hour during the acute phase, particularly respiratory rate, oxygen saturation, and lung sounds.
	4. Monitor blood glucose levels hourly during the acute phase.
	5. Perform neurologic assessments at least every 4 hours or more often, as the patient's condition dictates.
	6. Assess urine for glucose and ketone levels at regular intervals.
	7. Monitor the patient for complications of hyperglycemia (neurologic impairment) and treatment (fluid overload, hypoglycemia, hypokalemia). Make sure 50% dextrose for I.V. administration is readily available to treat hypoglycemia secondary to aggressive insulin therapy.

Disorders of the pituitary gland

HYPOPITUITARISM

✎ **What's hypopituitarism?**	A rare endocrine disorder in which underactivity of the anterior pituitary gland results in the deficiency of various critical hormones, including growth hormone (GH), thyroid-stimulating hormone (TSH), corticotropin, antidiuretic hormone (ADH), luteinizing hormone (LH), follicle-stimulating hormone (FSH), prolactin, and oxytocin; causes may include hypothalamic or pituitary tumors, surgical removal of the pituitary, infections of the brain, head trauma, radiation treatment of the brain, or certain metabolic disorders such as hemochromatosis

What's the pathophysiologic process of hypopituitarism?	Because the pituitary is responsible for the production of hormones that affect the function of other glands throughout the body, its underactivity can result in the deficiency of one or more pituitary hormones and loss of function of the specific gland or organ that it regulates.

What's dwarfism?

A condition of growth retardation caused by a deficiency in GH or receptor defects

Manifestations of abnormal GH production are dependent upon the age of onset of the disorder.

What are the clinical manifestations of hypopituitarism?

Symptoms of TSH deficiency or hypothyroidism (fatigue, weight gain, cold intolerance, impaired memory, constipation), symptoms of GH deficiency (growth retardation and delayed sexual maturation in children, delayed wound healing, decreased exercise intolerance and weakness in adults), symptoms of corticotropin deficiency (weight loss, abdominal pain, altered mental status, decreased axillary and pubic hair, myalgias, arthralgias, adrenal crisis), symptoms of ADH deficiency (polydipsia, polyuria, diabetes insipidus), symptoms of gonadotropin (FSH, LH) deficiency (hypogonadism, decreased libido, erectile dysfunction, altered menstrual cycles, lack of sexual development in children), symptoms of prolactin deficiency (inability to produce milk after childbirth), and symptoms of oxytocin deficiency (decreased milk ejection during lactation)

Manifestations of hypopituitarism vary according to which hormone isn't being produced, and the manifestations of that deficiency may occur over years or may develop suddenly and dramatically.

What's the typical treatment for hypopituitarism?

1. Surgical resection or radiation therapy of any pituitary tumor
2. Lifelong hormonal therapy to replace deficient hormones, including corticosteroids, thyroid hormones, GH, and estrogen or testosterone

What complications are associated with hypopituitarism?

Adrenal crisis (corticotropin deficiency) and infertility

What are important nursing actions in the care of a patient with hypopituitarism?

1. Emphasize the importance of taking medications consistently.
2. Administer medications (hormones) as ordered by the physician.
3. Monitor the patient for complications such as adrenal crisis.

4. Encourage routine medical follow-up.
5. Encourage the patient to wear medical identification jewelry and to notify health care providers of his condition.
6. Tell the patient that increased doses of corticosteroids may be needed during periods of increased physical stress (surgery, trauma, major infections).

DIABETES INSIPIDUS

What's diabetes insipidus (DI)?

A disorder of water metabolism caused by decreased or ineffective secretion of antidiuretic hormone ([ADH]; vasopressin) by the posterior pituitary; central DI involves decreased ADH secretion, which may be caused by head trauma, neurosurgery, or pituitary tumors; nephrogenic DI involves an inability of the kidneys to respond to ADH, which may be the result of long-standing renal disease and some medications

What's the pathophysiologic process of DI?

A deficiency of ADH prevents renal reabsorption of water, resulting in the excretion of large volumes of urine; dehydration causes increased thirst

What are the clinical manifestations of DI?

Marked polyuria (5 to 10 L of very dilute urine/24 hours), polydipsia (due to dehydration), and hypernatremia

What test is used to differentiate central from nephrogenic DI?

A water deprivation test, in which hourly samples are analyzed for plasma and urine osmolality following I.V. administration of ADH (vasopressin)

Prolonged withholding of water from a patient with DI can be dangerous and should be avoided, as these patients typically produce many liters of water per day.

What complications are associated with DI?

Severe dehydration and hypovolemic shock

What's the typical treatment for DI?

1. *Central:* administration of exogenous ADH, such as desmopressin (Pitressin) or desmopressin (DDAVP), via injection or nasal spray, and removal of pituitary tumor, if present
2. *Nephrogenic:* discontinuation of any causative drug being taken and treatment with a thiazide diuretic

✎ What are important nursing actions in the care of a patient with DI?

1. Administer I.V. fluids and medications (vasopressin, desmopressin) as ordered by the physician.
2. Monitor intake and output carefully. Encourage increased oral intake of fluids.
3. Assess vital signs at frequent intervals.
4. Obtain daily weight.
5. Monitor serum and urine osmolality and serum electrolyte levels (particularly sodium).
6. Assess the patient for complications, such as dehydration and hypovolemic shock, and notify the physician immediately if any develop.

HYPERPITUITARISM

✎ What's acromegaly?

A chronic endocrine condition in adults that results from excessive growth hormone (GH) production and is characterized by progressive, marked enlargement and elongation of the bones of the face, jaw, hands, and feet; metabolic abnormalities, including glucose intolerance, may also result; a pituitary tumor is the most common cause of acromegaly

What's the pathophysiologic process of acromegaly?

GH is produced in excessive amounts after completion of normal skeletal growth; changes in appearance occur secondary to overgrowth of bone and connective tissue

✎ What's giantism?

A condition in which excessive amounts of GH are produced in children or adolescents

✎ What are the clinical manifestations of acromegaly?

Enlargement of hands and feet, protruding jaw (prognathism), enlargement of facial bones and tongue, increased spacing between teeth, hoarseness, widening of fingers and toes, broad and bulbous nose, slanting forehead, thickened and oily skin, frontal bossing (horns), arthralgias, diaphoresis, hirsutism (abnormal hair growth) and amenorrhea in females, hypogonadism, and glycosuria

✎ What complications are associated with acromegaly?

Cardiovascular disease, diabetes mellitus, hypertension, hypopituitarism (insufficient amounts of other pituitary hormones may be secreted), arthritis, carpal tunnel syndrome, and limited mobility or disability from arthralgias

What's the typical treatment for acromegaly?

Surgical removal of the tumor or the pituitary gland (transsphenoidal hypophysectomy) is the treatment of choice. Radiation of the pituitary gland and pharmacologic therapy (octreotide, Pegvisomant) may be used to decrease the secretion of GH or to block its effects in some people.

✎ What are important considerations for a patient who has undergone a transsphenoidal hypophysectomy?

1. Elevate the head of the bed 30 degrees during the postoperative period (prevents headaches).
2. Avoid persistent coughing, sneezing, or straining on defecation in immediate postoperative period (prevents cerebrospinal fluid [CSF] from leaking from surgical site). Stool softeners and laxatives should be used.
3. Test any clear nasal drainage for glucose (drainage is CSF if glucose is present).
4. Avoid bending or Valsalva's maneuver for first 2 postoperative weeks (prevents disruption of surgical site by pressure).

What are important nursing actions in the care of a patient with acromegaly?

1. Encourage routine follow-up of pituitary function.
2. Monitor the patient for disease complications, including compromised cardiovascular functioning and the development of diabetes.

SYNDROME OF INAPPROPRIATE ANTIDIURETIC HORMONE

✎ What's syndrome of inappropriate antidiuretic hormone (SIADH)?

An endocrine disorder of the posterior pituitary characterized by hyponatremia and hypoosmolality that are caused by the continued (and inappropriate) secretion of ADH/vasopressin despite opposing regulatory signals, such as euvolemia; the cause may be idiopathic, due to tumors (lung cancer) that secrete ADH, trauma, pulmonary disease, and certain medications (oxytocin, vincristine, thiazide diuretics, carbamazepine)

What's the pathophysiologic process of SIADH?

The inability to suppress vasopressin secretion results in water retention and volume expansion. Weight gain and natriuresis (excretion of sodium in the urine) occur as a result.

✎ What are the clinical manifestations of SIADH?

GI symptoms (anorexia, nausea, vomiting, abdominal pain), neuropsychiatric alterations (headache, confusion, blurred vision, personality changes, lethargy, stupor), muscle weakness and cramps, and weight gain due to fluid retention

From what do most manifestations of SIADH stem?

Hyponatremia

What laboratory findings are indicative of SIADH?

1. Urinary sodium greater than 20 mEq/L coupled with increased urinary osmolality (greater than 100 mOsm/kg)

2. Hyponatremia (less than 125 mEq/L) and hypoosmolality (less than 280 mOsm/kg water)
3. Low or normal albumin levels and normal renal, thyroid, and adrenal function

What complications are associated with SIADH?

Complications secondary to volume overload (hypertension, heart failure, pulmonary edema, anasarca) and hyponatremia (cerebral edema, seizures, coma, irreversible brain damage)

What's the typical treatment for SIADH?

1. Fluid restriction of 500 ml or less per 24 hours for asymptomatic patients; patients with central nervous system manifestations of hyponatremia are treated with administration of hypertonic sodium chloride solution and loop diuretics, such as furosemide (Lasix) to promote the removal of excess water, and osmotic diuretics
2. Surgery to correct a vasopressin-secreting tumor
3. ADH antagonists, including lithium and demeclocycline (Declomycin), for chronic SIADH

▶ *Fluid restriction is the foundation of treatment for SIADH.*

▶ *Thiazide diuretics, such as metolazone (Zaroxolyn), can exacerbate hyponatremia associated with SIADH and should be avoided.*

What condition is commonly associated with rapid correction of hyponatremia?

Central pontine myelinosis, which can result in permanent brain damage

✎ What are important nursing actions in the care of a patient with SIADH?

1. Monitor intake and output carefully. Ensure strict adherence to fluid restrictions. Obtain and record daily weight.
2. Obtain vital signs, especially blood pressure, at regular intervals.
3. Implement safety precautions for disoriented or weak patients.
4. Administer medications (hypertonic sodium solution, furosemide, sodium and potassium replacements) as ordered by the physician.
5. Monitor the patient for complications of SIADH or its treatment, such as volume overload or too rapid correction of electrolyte abnormalities, and notify the physician immediately if any develop.

Disorders of the thyroid gland

HYPERTHYROIDISM

What's hyper-thyroidism?

A condition involving the excess production of thyroxine (T_3), which may be caused by Graves' disease (most common), goiter, thyroid adenoma, thyroiditis, toxic multinodular goiter, and ingestion of excessive thyroid hormone; it typically occurs in young and middle-aged adults, and women are affected more frequently than men; a familial tendency exists

What's the patho-physiologic process of hyperthyroidism?

Overactivity of the thyroid gland causes increased thyroid hormone synthesis and increased metabolic rate

What are the clinical manifestations of hyperthyroidism?

Rapid weight loss (due to increased metabolic rate) despite adequate dietary intake, tachycardia, irregular heart rate, palpitations, emotional lability (anxiety, irritability), heat intolerance, diaphoresis, sleep disturbances, menstrual irregularities, exophthalmos (proptosis), visual disturbances (diplopia), increased frequency of bowel patterns, resting tremor of extremities, hyperactive reflexes; proximal muscle weakness, thin and brittle nails, fine and thinly distributed hair, and diffuse, nontender and symmetric thyroid enlargement (goiter)

What laboratory results are diagnostic of hyperthyroidism?

Increased T_3 and triiodothyronine (T_4) levels, but low or undetectable thyroid-stimulating hormone (TSH) levels

What's Graves' disease?

An autoimmune condition in which antibodies stimulate the thyroid to produce excess T_3; typical onset occurs between ages 20 and 40, and women are affected more commonly than men

What are the clinical manifestations of Graves' disease?

Reddened or swollen eyes, photosensitivity, myopia or diplopia, goiter, exophthalmos (protrusion of eyeball, which causes excessive tearing in response to drying of eye), and dermopathy

What's Graves' dermopathy?

A complication of Graves' disease involving localized myxedema in which subcutaneous swelling develops on the anterior portion of the legs with indurated and edematous skin

What's a toxic multinodular goiter?

A form of hyperthyroidism in which adenomas (benign or malignant) of the thyroid produce excessive amounts of thyroxine; manifestations develop more slowly and tend to be less severe than those of Graves' disease

✎ **What complications are associated with hyperthyroidism?**	Cardiac complications (atrial fibrillation, heart failure), osteoporosis (if untreated), and hyperthyroid crises (thyrotoxicosis, thyroid storm)
✎ **What's thyrotoxicosis?**	The clinical syndrome that results when tissues are exposed to high levels of unbound thyroid hormone, irrespective of whether the primary source is the thyroid gland
✎ **What's thyroid storm?**	A life-threatening condition manifested by marked increase in manifestations of hyperthyroidism, high fever, and altered mental status (irritability, delirium); death can occur in 48 hours if the condition is untreated; infection, trauma, diabetic ketoacidosis, radiation, and thyroiditis are factors that may precipitate a thyroid storm
In what diseases is thyroid storm most likely to occur?	Graves' disease and toxic multinodular goiter; trauma to the neck can precipitate thyroid storm in patients with Graves' disease

What's the typical treatment for hyperthyroidism?

1. *Anti-thyroid agents:* use of thioamides, such as propylthiouracil (PTU) or methimazole, to inhibit production of thyroid hormone, or use of glucocorticoids such as hydrocortisone to block its action (treatment of thyroid storm)
2. *Beta-adrenergic blockers:* propranolol (Inderal) to alleviate symptoms of hyperthyroidism, including palpitations, tremor, and heat intolerance
3. *Radioactive iodine (^{131}I) therapy:* oral administration slows the production of thyroid hormones by ablating the thyroid gland; followed by lifelong need for thyroid hormone replacement (due to resultant hypothyroidism)
4. *Surgery:* such as a subtotal thyroidectomy, followed by lifelong need for thyroid hormone replacement

⚡ *Adrenergic agents and sympathomimetic agents such as pseudoephedrine should be avoided in patients with hyperthyroidism. Symptoms of thyrotoxicosis mimic those of adrenergic excess, and sympathomimetic agents can exacerbate thyrotoxic symptoms.*

✎ **What are important nursing considerations for a patient who has undergone a thyroidectomy?**

1. Place the patient in a semi-Fowler's position. Avoid flexion of the neck and tension on suture line.
2. Assess the patient every 2 hours for 24 hours for complications, including hemorrhage (assess surgical site dressings and behind the neck), thyroid storm (from manipulation of thyroid during surgery), tracheal compression, excessive neck swelling, and respiratory difficulties such as laryngeal stridor from tracheal ede-

ma. A tracheostomy tube should be kept at the bedside throughout the postoperative period.

3. Monitor the patient for tetany, which can occur secondary to accidental removal of or trauma to the parathyroid glands (hypocalcemia results). I.V. calcium should be administered if tetany occurs.

4. Inform the patient that hoarseness is normal for several days following surgery secondary to edema.

5. Provide analgesics (meperidine, morphine) for pain control as ordered by the physician.

6. Inform the patient that caloric intake should be decreased to prevent weight gain after recovery from thyroidectomy.

What are important nursing actions in the care of a patient with hyperthyroidism?

1. Maintain a cool and quiet environment conducive to sleep.

2. Administer medications (anti-thyroid agents, beta-adrenergic blockers, radioactive iodine) as ordered by the physician.

3. Emphasize the importance of strict medication compliance.

4. Inform the patient about the potential for weight gain after correction of hyperthyroidism. Although a high-calorie diet is necessary before thyroid function is restored to normal, the patient should be instructed to decrease dietary intake and to engage in an exercise regimen after the condition is corrected through surgery or medications.

5. Monitor the patient for complications, such as thyrotoxicosis and hypothyroidism, and notify the physician immediately if any develop.

6. Encourage routine follow-up to monitor thyroid function. Surgically or radioiodine-treated patients should have their thyroid function tested annually.

HYPOTHYROIDISM

What's hypothyroidism?

A condition involving a deficiency in T_4 production despite adequate or high levels of TSH; causes may include an inability of the thyroid to produce adequate quantities of T_4 (primary cause), insufficient release of TSH from the pituitary gland (secondary cause), or from an error within the hypothalamus (tertiary cause), which regulates the endocrine system; specifically, removal of the thyroid gland, radiation to the head and neck, treatment with radioactive iodine, use of certain medications (lithium), iodine deficiency and some autoimmune processes (Hashimoto's or chronic thyroiditis) can cause hypothyroidism; the condition more commonly affects women over age 40 and the obese

What's the patho-physiologic process of hypothyroidism?

Damage to or loss of thyroid tissue results in decreased production of thyroid hormones

✎ **What's cretinism?**

An endocrine disorder involving the thyroid gland in which insufficient thyroid hormone is secreted in an infant; impaired physical development and mental retardation result

✎ **What are the clinical manifestations of hypothyroidism?**

Fatigue, weakness, increased cold sensitivity, constipation, unexplained weight gain (primarily fluid; myxedema, or mucinous edema), puffy face, pale and dry skin, thinning hair or hair loss, brittle nails, impaired memory or slowed mental functioning, decreased hearing, depression, lack of facial expression, hoarseness, arthralgias or myalgias, decreased libido, abnormal menses, hypercholesterolemia (primarily low-density lipoprotein [LDL]), and bradycardia

✎ **What complications are associated with hypothyroidism?**

Goiter, myxedema coma, cardiomyopathy or heart disease (due to high LDL cholesterol); higher rate of infertility, miscarriage and birth defects in children born to women with thyroid disease

✎ **What's a goiter?**

Enlargement of the thyroid gland that results from its constant stimulation to release more hormones; Hashimoto's thyroiditis (underactive thyroid gland results from its chronic inflammation), Graves' disease (overactive thyroid gland), inflammation, pregnancy, and thyroid cancer are all potential causes of goiters; the condition is generally painless, but may become uncomfortable or interfere with breathing or swallowing if the goiter is large

Conservative treatment includes the use of thyroid hormone replacement therapy, potassium iodine solutions (Lugol's) for iodine deficiency or radioactive iodine to shrink the thyroid gland. A thyroidectomy may be necessary for symptomatic cases refractory to conservative treatments.

✎ **What's myxedema coma?**

An advanced, life-threatening form of hypothyroidism that results from being undiagnosed or undertreated; physical stress, including infections, illnesses, exposure to cold and the use of sedatives, may initiate the condition

Symptoms of myxedema may include severe drowsiness, marked cold intolerance, subnormal temperature, hypotension, hypoventilation, profound lethargy, loss of consciousness, and coma. I.V. thyroid replacement and steroids are the primary treatment measures.

What's the typical treatment for hypothyroidism?

Lifelong thyroid hormone replacement with a synthetic form, such as levothyroxine (Synthroid, Levothroid); dosages are adjusted based on TSH levels

What are important nursing actions in the care of a patient with hypothyroidism?

1. Obtain routine vital signs and weight daily.
2. Monitor intake and output and assess for edema.
3. Maintain warm environment (cold insensitivity).
4. Implement preventative measures for skin breakdown.
5. Administer medications (levothyroxine) as ordered by the physician. Sedatives should be avoided in altered or impaired mental status. Emphasize the importance of consistent use of thyroid replacement medications. Advise the patient not to skip medications, even if he starts to feel better.
6. Monitor the patient for complications of hypothyroidism or its treatment. Use stool softeners, increased dietary bulk, and exercise to treat constipation.
7. Instruct the patient to notify the physician if a change of brands occurs (dosage may need to be altered).
8. Educate the patient about symptoms of hypothyroidism or hyperthyroidism (can result from overtreatment) and instruct the patient to notify the physician immediately if any develop.

Disorders of the parathyroid glands

HYPERPARATHYROIDISM

What's hyperparathyroidism?

A condition in which the parathyroid glands produce excessive amounts of parathyroid hormone (PTH), resulting in hypercalcemia; primary causes include adenomas (benign growths) and hyperplasia (enlargement) of the parathyroid glands, and secondary causes (the result of another medical condition) include renal failure, rickets (chronic vitamin D deficiency), and chronic hypocalcemia; women are affected twice as often as men, and the risk for development of hyperparathyroidism increases with age

What's the pathophysiologic process of hyperparathyroidism?

The relationship between serum calcium levels and PTH secretion is interrupted, and PTH is produced in excess

✎ What are the clinical manifestations of hyperparathyroidism?	Mild conditions may produce no symptoms, or may produce muscle weakness, fatigue, and vague aches and pains (back pains), as well as hypercalcemia and hypophosphatemia. More significant symptoms may develop over time, including polyuria and polydipsia (due to hypercalciuria), and confusion or memory difficulties. GI symptoms include nausea, vomiting, anorexia, and dyspepsia, and gastroesophageal reflux disease (excess calcium stimulates acid production in the stomach).
How is hyperparathyroidism diagnosed?	Based on increased serum calcium levels and increased PTH levels
✎ What complications are associated with hyperparathyroidism?	Nephrolithiasis (renal calculi), urinary tract infections, kidney damage, osteoporosis, and pathologic bone changes (fractures, compression fractures of the vertebrae, kyphosis) from chronic calcium loss from the bones, peptic ulcer disease due to excess stomach acid production (induced by hypercalcemia), pancreatitis, hypertension, and cardiac arrhythmias
What's the typical treatment for hyperparathyroidism?	1. *Primary:* no treatment necessary for mild hyperparathyroidism, although periodic blood studies to monitor serum calcium levels and renal function and bone studies (DEXA scan) should be performed routinely; surgery (parathyroidectomy) may be necessary for moderate to severe disease with complications; minimally invasive radio guided parathyroidectomy (MIRP) is a less invasive procedure involving the use of radioisotopes to locate the abnormal gland before surgery 2. *Secondary:* restoration of normal calcium level, administration of hormone replacement therapy with calcitonin, and treatment of the underlying disorder
What complications can occur following a parathyroidectomy?	Nerve damage involving the vocal cords and chronic hypocalcemia
✎ What are important nursing actions for a patient with hyperparathyroidism?	1. Promote increase fluid intake to prevent the formation of renal calculi. 2. Administer medications (vitamin D supplements, such as calcitonin) as ordered by the physician. 3. Instruct the patient to restrict dietary calcium intake. 4. Monitor the patient for complications of hypercalcemia, including nephrolithiasis, hypertension, and pancreatitis. 5. Prevent immobility. Encourage weight-bearing and strengthening exercises and smoking cessation to prevent bone loss.

6. Consider hormone replacement therapy for post-menopausal women at risk for osteoporosis.
7. Encourage routine blood studies (serum calcium levels, renal function) and bone density scans.

HYPOPARATHYROIDISM

What's hypoparathyroidism?

An endocrine disorder in which the production of parathyroid hormone (PTH) is either decreased or ineffective, resulting in hypocalcemia and hyperphosphatemia; may be either hereditary (absent at birth or fail to develop afterwards) or acquired (surgical removal of parathyroids)

▶ *PTH, vitamin D, and calcitonin work in conjunction with one another to regulate serum calcium levels.*

What's the pathophysiologic process of hypoparathyroidism?

Normal serum calcium levels aren't maintained due to a deficiency of PTH; serum phosphate levels rise concomitantly

What's the most common cause of hypoparathyroidism?

Damage to the parathyroids during thyroid surgery

What are the clinical manifestations of hypoparathyroidism?

Hyperreflexia, paresthesia, and muscle cramps or spasms (tetany) from neuromuscular irritability

▶ *Manifestations of hypoparathyroidism are similar to those of hypocalcemia.*

What complications are associated with hypoparathyroidism?

Clonic-tonic seizures, stridor and wheezing from laryngeal spasm, and severe respiratory compromise; inadequate tooth development and mental retardation may occur in children

What's the typical treatment for hypoparathyroidism?

1. *Acute:* administration of I.V. calcium salts to treat tetany
2. *Chronic:* lifelong administration of calcium, active vitamin D supplements (calcitriol), and oral phosphate binders; diuretics may be prescribed to prevent excessive urinary excretion of calcium

▶ *I.V. push calcium salts should be administered slowly due to risk for hypotension and cardiac arrest.*

🖎 **What are important nursing actions in the care of a patient with hypoparathyroidism?**	1. Encourage a diet high in calcium (dark green vegetables, dairy products, soy beans) and low in phosphorus (no dairy products or egg yolks). 2. Administer medications (calcium and vitamin D supplements; oral phosphate binders) as ordered by the physician. Calcium supplements should be taken 2 hours after meals. 3. Monitor the patient for complications, such as tetany and paresthesia, and notify the physician immediately if any develop. 4. Encourage routine follow-up for assessment of serum calcium and phosphorus levels.

Disorders of the adrenal glands

ADRENAL INSUFFICIENCY (ADDISON'S DISEASE)

🖎 **What's Addison's disease?**	An endocrine disorder of adrenal insufficiency in which cortisol and aldosterone secretion are decreased; the condition can be caused by an autoimmune response, certain infections (tuberculosis, human immunodeficiency virus, fungal), a tumor of the adrenal glands, or an inherited defect in the corticotropin receptor on adrenal cells; Addison's disease is life-threatening, and lifelong treatment with replacement hormones is required
What's the pathophysiologic process of Addison's disease?	Hyposecretion of glucocorticoids and mineralocorticoids occurs secondary to destruction or dysfunction of the adrenal cortex
🖎 **What are the clinical manifestations of Addison's disease?**	Progressive fatigue, weakness, and weight loss; hyperpigmentation or bronzing of sun-exposed skin and mucous membranes (increased melanin production secondary to stimulation from excess corticotropin) with or without areas of vitiligo (due to autoimmune damage to melanocytes); vague GI manifestations, including pain, anorexia, diarrhea, nausea, vomiting, and constipation; dehydration from increased urinary losses of sodium, chloride, and water (potassium is retained); manifestations of postural hypotension, such as dizziness, syncopal or near syncopal episodes; enhanced olfactory, auditory, and taste sensations; abnormal craving for salt; increased insulin sensitivity (decreased insulin requirements); decreased libido and impotence in males; decreased pubic or axillary hair as well as amenorrhea in women
What complications are associated with Addison's disease?	Electrolyte imbalances (hyponatremia, hyperkalemia), hypoglycemia, and addisonian crisis

✎ What's an addisonian crisis?

Also known as an *adrenal crisis*, it's an acute and potentially fatal condition involving extreme manifestations of adrenal insufficiency.

Manifestations may include nausea, vomiting, high fever, confusion, cyanosis, and shock due to vascular collapse. Precipitating factors include physical stress, such as persistent vomiting or diarrhea, infection, surgery, trauma, or noncompliance with replacement steroids. Treatment involves the administration of hydrocortisone (I.V. or I.M.), volume resuscitation with an I.V. isotonic sodium solution, and correction of the precipitating factor. Glucose supplementation may also be required.

What's the typical treatment for Addison's disease?

Replacement of glucocorticoids (prednisone, dexamethasone); mineralocorticoid replacement (fludrocortisone) may be necessary for primary adrenal insufficiency

▧ *Glucocorticoid dosing is designed to mimic diurnal production of endogenous glucocorticoids, and because they stimulate the central nervous system, they shouldn't be taken at bedtime.*

✎ What are important nursing actions in the care of a patient with Addison's disease?

1. Maintain a calm, quiet environment to minimize physical stress. Noise, light, and environmental temperature extremes should be avoided.
2. Obtain vital signs (particularly blood pressure) at frequent intervals.
3. Monitor intake and output carefully.
4. Obtain daily weight.
5. Monitor serum electrolyte levels.
6. Administer medications (I.V. or I.M. hydrocortisone, prednisone, fludrocortisone) as ordered by the physician.
7. Emphasize the importance of taking medications consistently and inform the patient of the danger of abrupt discontinuation of glucocorticoids.
8. Monitor the patient for complications, such as electrolyte imbalances and addisonian crisis.
9. Instruct the patient to increase his salt intake during hot weather.
10. Encourage the patient to wear medical identification jewelry and to inform emergency personnel and other health care providers of addisonian condition. Instruct the patient and caregiver that hydrocortisone should be administered (or prednisone dose increased) in the event of surgery or a major procedure, trauma, or other stressful event.

Hyperadrenal disorders

CUSHING'S SYNDROME

✎ What's Cushing's syndrome?

An endocrine disorder in which excessive levels of adrenal hormones (particularly cortisol) are produced; causes may include overproduction of corticotropin by the anterior pituitary, overproduction of adrenal hormones, or long-term glucocorticoid (steroid) therapy for a separate disorder (most common cause), such as prednisone used to treat rheumatoid arthritis or other inflammatory conditions, and steroid inhalers used to treat asthma

▌ *Cushing's syndrome is essentially the opposite of Addison's disease.*

What's Cushing's disease?

The term used for Cushing's syndrome when the cause is a pituitary tumor; Cushing's disease is a common cause of Cushing's syndrome

What's the pathophysiologic process of Cushing's syndrome?

Adrenal hyperfunction causes the overproduction of the stress hormone, cortisol

✎ What are the clinical manifestations of Cushing's syndrome?

Weight gain: fat deposition described as truncal obesity (obese trunk and abdomen with thin extremities due to muscle wasting), "moon face," and "buffalo hump"; hypertension; facial flushing or hirsutism; glucose intolerance; skin changes (acne; thin and atrophic skin; hyperpigmentation or acanthosis of hair and skin; purple striae or stretch marks); easy bruising; muscle weakness (particularly in upper extremities); polydipsia and polyuria; metabolic disturbances (hyperglycemia, hypokalemia, metabolic alkalosis); mood swings; depression; and impotence in males or irregular menses in females

What tests may be used to confirm a high cortisol level?

1. *24-hour urine cortisol level test:* increased levels are indicative of Cushing's syndrome
2. *Dexamethasone suppression test:* administration of synthetic steroid similar to cortisol suppresses corticotropin secretion (and therefore decreases cortisol levels) in normal individuals
3. *Repeat serum cortisol levels:* typical diurnal variations aren't apparent in persons with Cushing's syndrome

✎ What complications are associated with Cushing's syndrome?

Osteoporosis, increased susceptibility to infections, diabetes, stroke, and death (if not treated promptly)

What's the typical treatment for Cushing's syndrome?	1. Treatment of underlying cause (gradual discontinuation of corticosteroids)
	2. Surgical removal of pituitary tumor (transsphenoidal resection or removal of entire pituitary gland); adrenalectomy is used to treat adrenal tumors; radiation therapy is commonly used in combination with surgery; cortisol production usually resumes within the first year following surgery, however, lifelong replacement therapy may be necessary in some instances
✎ **What are important nursing actions in the care of a patient with Cushing's syndrome?**	1. Obtain vital signs (particularly blood pressure) at frequent intervals.
	2. Obtain daily weight and assess for edema.
	3. Monitor serum electrolyte levels.
	4. Monitor the patient for complications, including serious infections and diabetes, and notify the physician immediately if any develop.
	5. Encourage the patient to wear medical identification jewelry and to notify emergency health care providers of his condition.

HYPERALDOSTERONISM

What's hyperaldosteronism?	An endocrine disorder that results from excessive aldosterone production by the adrenal gland; primary hyperaldosteronism is caused by adrenal hyperplasia or an adrenal tumor (usually benign) that produces aldosterone (referred to as Conn's syndrome if a single adrenal tumor); secondary hyperaldosteronism is caused by factors outside of the adrenal glands that cause excessive production of aldosterone or renin
What's the pathophysiologic process of hyperaldosteronism?	Because aldosterone regulates sodium and potassium levels, its overproduction results in salt retention and potassium loss, which causes hypertension
✎ **What are the clinical manifestations of hyperaldosteronism?**	Moderate hypertension, orthostatic hypotension, constipation, muscle weakness with intermittent paralysis, polyuria, polydipsia, headache, and personality changes
What complications are associated with hyperaldosteronism?	Hypertensive complications, including renal failure, stroke, and myocardial infarction
What's the typical treatment for hyperaldosteronism?	1. Surgical removal of the adrenal tumor
	2. Pharmacologic agents including calcium channel blockers and diuretics, such as spironolactone (Aldactone) and amiloride (Midamor), which block effects of aldosterone

| **What are important nursing actions in the care of a patient with hyperaldosteronism?** | 1. Monitor vital signs, particularly blood pressure.
2. Administer medications (diuretics, calcium channel blockers) as ordered by the physician.
3. Instruct the patient to restrict dietary sodium (if secondary hyperaldosteronism).
4. Monitor the patient for complications, such as renal failure and MI, and notify the physician immediately if any develop. |

PHEOCHROMOCYTOMA

✎ **What's a pheochromocytoma?**	A highly vascular tumor of the adrenal medulla that produces excessive amounts of catecholamines (epinephrine, norepinephrine) at inappropriate times; manifestations may be triggered by allergic reactions, physical exertion, extreme emotional distress, or may occur without identifiable stimulus.
What's the pathophysiologic process of pheochromocytoma?	Because a pheochromocytoma isn't innervated like healthy adrenal medulla tissue, secretion of catecholamines isn't induced by neural stimulation. As a result, excessive amounts of catecholamines are secreted inappropriately.
✎ **What are the clinical manifestations of pheochromocytoma?**	Hypertension (intermittent or persistent) with postural hypotension (due to volume contraction), tachycardia, palpitations, diaphoresis, tremor, hyperglycemia, polyuria, severe headache, café au lait spots, pallor, anxiety, irritability, nausea, epigastric pain, constipation, weight loss, and neurofibromas
✎ **What complications are associated with pheochromocytoma?**	Hypertensive crisis, stroke, cardiac arrhythmias, and metastasis (10% of pheochromocytomas are malignant) ▸ *Pheochromocytoma is commonly referred to as "the ten percent tumor": 10% are malignant, 10% are found in both adrenal glands, 10% occur in children, 10% are diagnosed after a patient presents with a stroke, and 10% will recur in five to ten years.*
What are common precipitating events for a hypertensive crisis?	Use of certain medications (anesthesia, opiates, cold medications, tricyclic antidepressants, dopamine antagonists, cocaine), use of radiographic contrast media, and childbirth
How is the diagnosis made for pheochromocytoma?	Analysis of a 24-hour urine collection for creatinine, total catecholamines, metanephrines (epinephrine and norepinephrine metabolites), and vanillylmandelic acid; a cloni-

dine suppression test may be used to differentiate between essential hypertension and pheochromocytoma

> ◤ *Clonidine inhibits the release of catecholamines from nerve endings, but it doesn't affect their release from tumor cells.*

What's the typical treatment for a pheochromocytoma?

Tumor resection (laparoscopic adrenalectomy) is the preferred treatment. Due to the risk of an intraoperative hypertensive crisis, alpha- and beta-adrenergic blockers, such as phenoxybenzamine (Dibenzyline) and propranolol (Labetalol), are prescribed preoperatively to inhibit catecholamine effects on blood pressure. Additional alpha and beta blockers, such as phentolamine (Regitine), may be used intraoperatively.

What are important nursing actions in the care of a patient with pheochromocytoma?

1. Provide a calm, quiet environment. Minimize environmental stimulation.
2. Monitor vital signs (especially blood pressure) at frequent intervals.
3. Administer medications (alpha- and beta-adrenergic blockers preoperatively) as ordered by the physician. Inform the patient of the need to change positions slowly to prevent orthostatic hypotension during treatment with alpha- and beta-blockers.
4. Monitor the patient for complications, such as a hypertensive crisis, stroke, or cardiac arrhythmias.

Pharmacology related to the endocrine system

Diabetes management

ORAL HYPOGLYCEMIC AGENTS

How do oral hypoglycemic agents work?

1. *Sulfonylureas and meglitinides:* stimulate insulin production from pancreatic beta cells
2. *Biguanides:* decrease glucose production in the liver and increases the body's sensitivity to insulin
3. *Alpha glucosidase inhibitors:* decrease the absorption of starches or carbohydrates through its affect on the stomach and small intestine, resulting in a smaller increase in postprandial blood glucose levels
4. *Thiazolidinediones:* increase sensitivity of insulin receptors in muscles, the liver, and adipose tissues

What are examples of oral hypoglycemic agents?

1. *Sulfonylureas:* glipizide (Glucotrol, Glucotrol XL), glyburide (Micronase), glimepiride (Amaryl), chlorpropamide (Diabinese)
2. *Biguanides:* metformin (Glucophage, Glucophage XR)
3. *Alpha glucosidase inhibitors:* miglitol (Glyset), acarbose (Precose)
4. *Thiazolidinediones:* rosiglitazone (Avandia), pioglitazone (Actos)
5. *Meglitinides:* repaglinide (Prandin), nateglinide (Starlix)
6. *Combination agents:* glyburide + metformin = Glucovance

What adverse reactions are commonly associated with oral hypoglycemic agents?

1. *Sulfonylureas:* nausea, constipation, jaundice, headache, dizziness, drowsiness, rash, photosensitivity, renal insufficiency, and arthralgias and myalgias (glyburide)
2. *Biguanides:* nausea, vomiting, bloating, abdominal cramping, diarrhea, altered taste sensations (metallic), renal insufficiency
3. *Alpha glucosidase inhibitors:* abdominal pain, bloating, nausea, diarrhea
4. *Thiazolidinediones:* headache, diarrhea, fatigue, edema, myalgias, toothaches, upper respiratory infection
5. *Meglitinides:* nausea, vomiting, diarrhea, myalgias, arthralgias, back pain, flulike symptoms, headache, upper respiratory infection
6. *Combination agents:* diarrhea, abdominal pain, nausea, headache, dizziness, upper respiratory tract infection

What life-threatening reactions are associated with oral hypoglycemic agents?

1. *Sulfonylureas:* anaphylaxis (sulfa allergy), hypoglycemia, hematologic disorders (leukopenia, thrombocytopenia, aplastic anemia), hepatitis (glyburide), and disulfiram-like (Atabuse) reactions (chlorpropamide)
2. *Biguanides:* lactic acidosis
3. *Thiazolidinediones:* hepatic injury
4. *Meglitinides:* hypoglycemia

What are important nursing actions when administering an oral hypoglycemic agent?

1. Instruct the patient to take oral hypoglycemic agents with meals (extended-release forms are generally taken at least 30 minutes before meals).
2. Instruct the patient to monitor blood glucose levels as directed to assess response and about the need for dosage adjustments.
3. Encourage adherence to diet, exercise, and weight loss regimens.
4. Instruct the patient not to change the dosage without first consulting a physician.

5. Monitor hemoglobin A_{1c} every 3 months to assess long-term glycemic control.
6. Assess the patient for sulfa allergy before initiation of sulfonylurea agent.
7. Monitor the patient for complications, such as hypoglycemia, and signs of impending renal insufficiency.
8. Monitor complete blood count and platelet count as well as renal and hepatic function periodically throughout therapy.
9. Instruct the patient to avoid alcohol (chlorpropamide).

INSULIN

How does insulin work?

It promotes cellular uptake of glucose and stimulates the conversion of glucose to glycogen (storage form), lipids to fats, and amino acids to proteins.

By what methods can insulin be administered?

Through subcutaneous injections with a syringe or an insulin pen or by an insulin pump; nasal inhalation therapy is being studied as an alternative route of administration, but isn't yet approved for general use

What are examples of insulin?

1. *Quick-acting:* lispro (Humalog); onset of action 15 minutes; peak effect at 1 to 3 hours; duration of action 3 to 5 hours
2. *Short-acting:* regular (Humulin R, Novolin R); onset of action 30 to 60 minutes; peak effect at 2 to 3 hours; duration of action 6 to 8 hours
3. *Intermediate-acting:* NPH (Humulin N, Novolin N) or lente (Humulin L, Lente L); onset of action 1 to $2^{1}/_{2}$ hours; peak effect at 4 to 12 hours (NPH) and 7 to 15 hours (Lente); duration of action 24 hours
4. *Long-acting:* ultralente (Humulin U Ultralente); onset of action 4 to 8 hours; peak effect at 10 to 30 hours; duration of action 36 hours
5. *Steady state:* glargine (Lantus); duration of action 24 hours
6. *Combination agents:* 70/30 (70% NPH and 30% Regular); onset of action 30 minutes; peak effect at 4 to 8 hours; duration of action 12 to 24 hours

Lantus insulin (glargine) can't be combined with any medications, including other forms of insulin.

What adverse reactions are commonly associated with insulin?

Local reaction at injection site (edema, erythema, pruritus), hypoglycemia, and rash

What life-threatening reactions are associated with insulin?	Anaphylaxis (pork allergies) and profound hypoglycemia
✎ **What are appropriate body sites for subcutaneous insulin injections?**	The abdomen, thighs, and upper arms are sites commonly used **⚡** *Injection sites should be rotated to prevent the development of lipodystrophy.*
Why is insulin not available in an oral form?	It's a protein and would be degraded by digestive enzymes before it could exert its effects.
What type of insulin is used in conjunction with a sliding scale?	Regular insulin
✎ **What are important nursing actions when administering insulin?**	1. Monitor serum glucose levels, as ordered, to assess response and to ensure appropriate dosage. Anticipate the need for dosage adjustments during times of trauma, infection, or extreme stress, or in relation to activities and diet. 2. Ensure that the proper dosage is drawn up into syringe by having another nurse check it (especially for pediatric patients). 3. Educate the patient about proper administration (technique, rotation of sites). Instruct him to roll the vial between his hands to disperse the insulin suspension uniformly, but to avoid vigorous shaking. 4. Instruct the patient to store insulin in a cool place protected from direct sunlight (refrigerator). Inform him that prefilled syringes are stable for 1 week if refrigerated. 5. Encourage the patient to wear medical identification jewelry and to notify emergency personnel of his diabetic status. **⚡** *If two forms of insulin are to be mixed, the regular insulin should be drawn up first.*

Treatment of thyroid disorders

THYROID HORMONES

How do thyroid replacement agents work?	Increases metabolic rate in all body tissues

What are examples of thyroid replacement agents?	Levothyroxine (Synthroid, Levoxyl, Levoxine, Levothroid), liothyronine (Cytomel, Triostat), and liotrix (Thyrolar)

> ⚡ *These medications aren't bioequivalent, and therefore aren't interchangeable with one another. Dosage adjustments are typically required if one form is switched to another.*

What adverse reactions are commonly associated with thyroid replacement agents?	Tachycardia, palpitations, nervousness, tremor, insomnia, diaphoresis, diarrhea, and menstrual irregularities

> ⚡ *Adverse reactions to thyroid replacement agents are similar to the clinical manifestations of hyperthyroidism.*

What life-threatening reactions are associated with thyroid replacement agents?	Arrhythmias

✎ What are important nursing actions when administering a thyroid replacement agent?

1. Instruct the patient to take thyroid replacements consistently at the same time each day and to avoid skipping doses or to abruptly stop taking this drug. Breakfast is an ideal time to take this medication because it minimizes insomnia.
2. Educate the patient about adverse reactions, and instruct him to notify the physician immediately if chest pains or palpitations occur.
3. Inform the patient that the medication will be started at the lowest dose but will be adjusted according to clinical symptoms and laboratory results of thyroid function (TSH levels).
4. Instruct the patient to inform the physician if a change in the type of thyroid replacement hormone occurs because the need for dosage adjustments is likely.
5. Emphasize the importance of routine medical follow-up for evaluation of thyroid function and medication dosage adjustments.
6. Encourage the patient to wear medical identification jewelry and to inform emergency health care workers of the need for this medication.

THYROID ANTAGONISTS

How do thyroid antagonists work?	Block formation of thyroid hormones, or limit their secretion through the destruction of thyroid tissue (^{131}I)

| **What are examples of thyroid antagonists?** | Methimazole (Tapazole), potassium iodide saturated solution (SSKI), strong iodine solution (Lugol's solution), propylthiouracil (PTU), and radioactive iodine (^{131}I) |

What are common adverse reactions of thyroid antagonists?

1. *Methimazole and PTU:* rash, headaches, drowsiness, paresthesia, neuritis, nephritis, nausea, vomiting, diarrhea, arthralgias, myalgias, hair loss, unusual bruising, or bleeding
2. *Potassium iodide:* metallic taste, inflammation of salivary glands, rash, burning mouth and throat, sore teeth and gums, diarrhea
3. *^{131}I:* neck fullness, sore throat, temporary hair thinning, rash, tachycardia

What life-threatening reactions are associated with thyroid antagonists?

1. *Methimazole and PTU:* hepatotoxicity, hematologic disorders (leukopenia, thrombocytopenia, aplastic anemia)
2. *Potassium iodide:* potassium toxicity, anaphylaxis (iodine allergy)
3. *^{131}I:* hematologic disorders (anemia, leukopenia, thrombocytopenia)

✎ **What are important nursing actions when administering a thyroid antagonist?**

1. Implement radiation precautions during ^{131}I therapy (avoid exposure to pregnant women; follow guidelines for the proper disposal of emesis, urine, sputum production).
2. Instruct the patient to take thyroid antagonists with food to minimize adverse GI reactions.
3. Instruct the patient to use a straw when taking liquid iodides to prevent tooth discoloration.
4. Discourage the use of iodized salt and the consumption of shellfish because they may alter the effectiveness of thyroid antagonists.
5. Monitor laboratory results routinely for thyroid function, CBC, platelet count, and hepatic function.
6. Educate the patient about symptoms of hypothyroidism and serious adverse medication reactions, and instruct the patient to notify the physician immediately if any develop.

Treatment of parathyroid disorders

PARATHYROID-LIKE AGENTS

How do parathyroid-like agents work?

1. *Calcitonin:* inhibits activity of osteoclasts, which prevents bone breakdown
2. *Calcitriol:* analogue of vitamin D that increases calcium absorption from the GI tract and facilitates calcium movement from bone to blood

What are examples of parathyroid-like agents?	Calcitonin (Miacalcin, Cibacalcin) and calcitriol/1,25-dihydroxycholecalciferol (Rocaltrol, Calcijex)
What are common adverse reactions associated with parathyroid-like agents?	1. *Calcitonin:* nasal congestion, rhinitis, increased urination, facial flushing, headache, nausea, pedal edema 2. *Calcitriol:* none reported
What life-threatening reactions are associated with parathyroid-like agents?	Calcitonin: anaphylaxis (if salmon derivative)
✎ **What are important nursing actions when administering a parathyroid-like agent?**	1. Instruct the patient to take calcitonin at bedtime to reduce nausea and vomiting. 2. Monitor serum calcium levels periodically during therapy. 3. Monitor the patient for signs of hypocalcemia or hypercalcemia as well as symptoms of vitamin D toxicity (calcitriol), and notify the physician immediately if any develop.

Treatment of pituitary disorders

PITUITARY HORMONES

How do pituitary hormones work?	1. *Desmopressin and vasopressin:* promote water reabsorption by increasing permeability of renal tubules 2. *Corticotropin:* stimulates hormonal secretion by the adrenal cortex
What are examples of pituitary hormones?	Desmopressin (DDAVP), vasopressin (Pitressin), and corticotropin (ACTH)
What are common adverse reactions to pituitary hormones?	1. *Desmopressin:* headache, flushing, nausea, abdominal cramps, fluid retention, mild hypertension 2. *Vasopressin:* water intoxication, diaphoresis, tremor, abdominal cramps 3. *Corticotropin:* retention of sodium and fluid, hypertension, headaches, insomnia, mood swings, hyperglycemia, cushingoid features, thin and fragile skin
What life-threatening reactions are associated with pituitary hormones?	1. *Vasopressin:* hypersensitivity reactions, arrhythmias, and cardiac arrest 2. *Corticotropin:* increased intracranial pressure, seizures, shock, bronchospasm, and pancreatitis

What are important nursing actions when administering a pituitary hormone?	1. Instruct the patient about a low-sodium diet to minimize edema.
	2. Monitor weight changes.
	3. Instruct the patient to avoid abrupt discontinuation of the drug (corticotropin).
	4. Instruct the patient to avoid using nonsteroidal anti-inflammatory drugs and alcohol due to increased risk of ulcers (corticotropin).
	5. Instruct the patient to drink only enough water to satisfy thirst, but to avoid additional fluid intake due to risk for water intoxication (desmopressin and vasopressin).
	6. Monitor the patient for complications from therapy and notify the physician immediately if any develop.
	7. Instruct the patient to rotate injection sites (vasopressin).

Treatment of adrenal disorders

CORTICOSTEROIDS

How do corticosteroids work?	By various methods, including suppression of the inflammatory and immune responses, stimulation of bone marrow, and effects on the metabolism of carbohydrates, fats, and proteins
What are examples of corticosteroids?	Prednisone (Deltasone), prednisolone (Prelone, Delta-Cortef, Pediapred), methylprednisolone (Medrol, Solu-Medrol, Depo-Medrol), cortisone, hydrocortisone (Hydrocortone, Cortef, Solu-Cortef), dexamethasone (Decadron), betamethasone (Celestone), triamcinolone (Azmacort, Trilone, Aristocort), and fludrocortisone (Florinef)
✎ What are common adverse reactions to corticosteroids?	Cushingoid features ("moon face"), increased susceptibility to infections, impaired wound healing, osteoporosis, insomnia, emotional lability, hypertension, edema, cataracts and glaucoma (long-term use), GI irritation, peptic ulcerations, striae, thin and fragile skin, hyperglycemia, and hypercholesterolemia
✎ What life-threatening reactions are associated with corticosteroids?	Adrenal crisis (if discontinued abruptly), seizures, and pancreatitis

✎ **What are important nursing actions when administering corticosteroids?**

1. Instruct the patient to take corticosteroids with food or milk to minimize GI distress. Ulcer preventative agents may be necessary.
2. Instruct the patient to take medication consistently in the morning (mimics normal circadian rhythms and maintains stable production of basal cortisol) and to avoid skipping doses and abrupt discontinuation (risk of adrenal crisis).
3. Monitor glucose levels, blood pressure, and weight periodically during therapy.
4. Inform the patient of the need for an increased dose of steroids during stressful situations, such as infections, trauma, surgery, and major procedures.
5. Encourage close medical follow-up, and inform the patient of the need for regular ophthalmic examinations and DEXA scans for patients on maintenance steroids.

▌ *Abrupt discontinuation of glucocorticoids should be avoided due to the risk of precipitating an adrenal crisis.*

▌ *Patients with diabetes may require increased insulin during corticosteroid therapy.*

Nursing skills

Blood glucose monitoring

What supplies are needed in order to perform blood glucose monitoring?

Disposable gloves, alcohol wipes, glucometer with appropriate test strips, lancets, and gauze

How often should finger sticks be performed?

The frequency is usually determined by the onset, peak, and duration of the type of insulin used.

✎ **What's the proper technique for performing blood glucose monitoring?**

1. Instruct the patient to wash his hands in warm water (warm water cleans skin and brings blood to surface) and dry thoroughly.
2. Select a finger and wipe the tip with an alcohol swab.
3. Put on disposable gloves and grasp the joint closest to the tip of the finger, squeezing for several seconds.
4. While squeezing fingertip, use a lancet to prick the skin. If no blood appears, hold the hand downward to increase blood flow.

5. Apply a large drop of blood to the test strip area and insert the test strip into the glucometer for analysis.
6. Cover the lanced finger with gauze until bleeding stops.
7. Obtain the glucose reading from the glucometer and record.
8. Dispose of sharps and blood-contaminated supplies in an appropriate container.
9. Discard gloves and wash hands.

Adrenocorticotropic stimulation test (cortrosyn or cosyntropin)

What's an adreno-corticotropic (ACTH) stimulation test?

A series of blood tests performed over a 1-hour time period to determine the functionality of the adrenal cortex; specifically, its ability to synthesize cortisol in response to ACTH

⧉ *Normal cortisol levels vary over a 24-hour period, and these fluctuations are referred to as diurnal variations.*

⬧ When are cortisol levels highest in a normal individual?

Early morning hours (6 a.m. to 8 a.m.)

⬧ When are cortisol levels lowest in a normal individual?

Around midnight

How is an ACTH stimulation test performed?

1. Obtain a blood sample before administration of cortrosyn for determination of the baseline cortisol level.
2. Administer cortrosyn (synthetic ACTH) either I.V. or I.M.
3. Obtain blood samples at 30 minutes and 60 minutes following cortrosyn administration.

⧉ *Results are considered normal if the baseline cortisol level is doubled, or if one of the cortisol values is greater than 20.*

15

The respiratory system

Basic concepts of the respiratory system

What structures comprise the respiratory system?

The upper and lower airways and the thoracic cage (ribs, sternum, vertebrae)

What structures comprise the upper respiratory system?

1. *Nose:* contains rolling projections (turbinates), which increase the surface area and warm and moisten the air; protective function by filtering air for passage into remainder of respiratory tract
2. *Nasopharynx:* contains adenoids
3. *Oropharynx:* contains tonsils
4. *Epiglottis:* small flap at the base of the tongue, which closes off the trachea and prevents the food entry
5. *Larynx:* contains vocal cords
6. *Trachea:* cylindrical tube supported by U-shaped cartilage; divides into left and right branches at the manubriosternal junction (carina, or Angle of Louis)

What structures comprise the lower respiratory system?

1. *Bronchi:* tubes that allow air passage from the trachea to the lungs; two branches, each leading to a lung
2. *Lungs:* a pair of elastic, spongy organs used for breathing and gas exchange; oxygen is extracted from inhaled air and carbon dioxide is expelled in exhaled air; the left lung is smaller than the right (2 lobes versus 3) to accommodate the heart
3. *Bronchioles:* encircled by smooth muscles that constrict and dilate in response to different stimuli; site of some gas exchange
4. *Alveoli:* small compartments that are the functional units of the lung; primary site of gas exchange; connected to one another by pores of Kohn

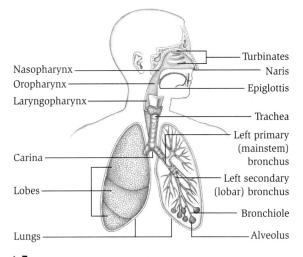

Nasopharynx — Oropharynx — Laryngopharynx —

Turbinates — Naris — Epiglottis — Trachea — Left primary (mainstem) bronchus

Carina —

Lobes —

Lungs —

Left secondary (lobar) bronchus — Bronchiole — Alveolus

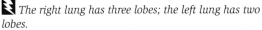 *The right lung has three lobes; the left lung has two lobes.*

✎ What two gases are exchanged in the bronchioles and alveoli?

Oxygen and carbon dioxide

Which lung is more likely to be affected if a foreign object is aspirated?

The right lung; the right bronchus is shorter, wider, and straighter than the left bronchus

What's surfactant?

A phospholipid secreted from cells of the alveolar surface that decreases the surface tension in the alveoli, preventing their collapse

What's the pleura?

A serous membrane that covers the surface of both lungs and the walls of the thorax and diaphragm; the thoracic cavity is divided into two distinct pleural cavities that are separated by the mediastinum

What role does the diaphragm play in respiration?

It's the primary muscle involved in respiration; it descends to expand the chest cavity during inspiration and its elevation is responsible for expiration.

What's ventilation?

The act of breathing; movement of air into and out of the lungs

What's respiration?

The process of gas exchange that occurs with ventilation

✎ **What two processes are involved with ventilation?**

1. *Inspiration:* movement of air into the lungs as a result of a change in intrathoracic pressure (pressure in lungs less than atmospheric pressure); air rushes in, diaphragm flattens; active process
2. *Expiration:* movement of air out of the lungs as the diaphragm relaxes; recoil of chest wall and lungs; passive process

⚡ *The intrapleural pressure (that around the lungs) is always negative, unless there's an opening in the chest cavity.*

How is blood supplied to the lungs?

The pulmonary arteries receive deoxygenated blood from the right ventricle. Gaseous exchange between oxygen and carbon dioxide occurs within the lungs, and the pulmonary veins carry the oxygen-rich blood back to the heart.

⚡ *In the pulmonary circulatory system, arteries carry deoxygenated blood and veins carry oxygen-rich blood, which is opposite of the arteries and veins of the systemic circulation.*

Physical assessment of the respiratory system

Normal findings

What equipment should be obtained before performing an examination of the respiratory system?

A stethoscope, a centimeter ruler, a marking pen, and an alcohol swab

What types of information should be obtained during history-taking for a respiratory examination?

Smoking history, family history of respiratory problems, environmental exposure, presence of allergies, exercise tolerance, use of medications to aid breathing, presence of a cough (wet, dry, productive, barking, whooping), amount and color of sputum produced, presence of dyspnea, history of respiratory illnesses

⚡ *Pack-year history is determined by multiplying the number of packs smoked per day by the total number of years smoked.*

How should the patient be positioned when performing the physical examination?

Seated on the side of the bed or at the end of the examination table with his arms either on an over-bed table or crossed on his chest to spread the scapula; if the patient is bedridden, raise the head of the bed to at least 45 degrees to examine the anterior chest, then turn the patient onto his side to examine the posterior chest

What should be the sequence of examination techniques?

Inspection, palpation, percussion, and auscultation; perform the entire examination on the anterior chest and then the posterior chest, or vice versa; compare one side to the other

✎ What's the usual ratio of inspiration to expiration?

1:3; expiration typically lasts three times longer than inspiration

What conditions can affect this ratio?

Exertional dyspnea could decrease the ratio to 1:1 because breaths may be shallow and fast; conditions that cause air trapping (chronic obstructive pulmonary disease) can prolong the expiratory phase

What factors should be assessed during inspection of the respiratory system?

1. Skin color and presence of clubbing of the fingers
2. Shape and configuration of the chest wall
3. Respiratory pattern: rate, rhythm, depth, effort
4. Signs of labored breathing: nasal flaring, intercostal retractions, or use of accessory muscles

▌ *The normal respiratory rate for adults is 12 to 20 breaths/minute at rest.*

✎ What's the normal shape of the chest?

The anterior-to-posterior diameter (anteroposterior, or front to back) compared to lateral (side to side) is a 1:2 ratio; the chest is twice as wide side to side as front to back

How should the nose be examined?

1. Assess the alignment of the septum.
2. Assess patency of the nostrils by holding the back of the hand several inches from the nares to feel for airflow as the patient blocks one nare at a time and breathes in and out deeply.
3. Use a light and inspect the nasal mucosa for color, moistness, and presence of polyps.

How are the sinuses palpated?

Facing the patient, use the thumbs to press up into the bony brow on either side of the nose to assess the frontal sinuses. Then use the thumbs to press underneath the zygomatic processes (cheekbone) to assess the maxillary sinuses. Note if either area is tender.

✎ What factors should be assessed with palpation of the anterior and posterior chest?

1. *Respiratory excursion:* palpation technique used to assess for symmetry of chest expansion with inspiration; thumbs are placed at the 10th ribs bilaterally on the posterior chest wall and the patient is instructed to inhale deeply while thumb movement is assessed for

symmetry; asymmetry can occur with a pneumothorax

2. *Tactile (vocal) fremitus:* detection of vibrations by holding the ball of the hand against the chest of a person who is speaking (repeating "ninety-nine" or "blue moon") in a normal voice; the further one moves from the main stem bronchi, the less vibration is felt; increased tactile fremitus can occur in the setting of a fluid-filled lung or consolidation of the underlying lung tissue, as occurs in pneumonia; decreased fremitus indicates obstruction of sound transmission, as occurs if the lung is hyperinflated (chronic obstructive pulmonary disease); it may be absent if the lung is incompletely expanded, as occurs with a pneumothorax or atelectasis

✎ **What factors should be assessed during percussion of the anterior and posterior chest?**

1. Sound over lung fields
2. Diaphragmatic excursion — percussion technique used to determine the depth of diaphragmatic movement between inspiration and expiration

How is assessment of diaphragmatic excursion performed?

Locate the level of diaphragmatic dullness on both sides by percussing posteriorly downward from an area of resonance to dullness where the lung tissue ends. Note the level where the sound changed. Instruct the patient to take a deep breath in and hold it, while percussion is performed from the initial site of dullness inferiorly until dullness is reached again.

The distance from one area of dullness to the other is measured. Each side of the diaphragm should have moved 1″ to 2″ (2.5 to 5 cm), although abnormal findings can occur in the setting of a pneumothorax or emphysema, which can impede the movement of the diaphragm.

▶ *The diaphragm is normally higher on the right side because of the liver.*

▶ *Percussion is used to determine the relative amounts of air, fluid or solid material within the underlying lung tissue.*

✎ **What types of sounds may be noted over the lung fields on percussion?**

1. *Flat:* short, high-pitched sound; occurs over large amounts of fluid such as occurs with a large pleural effusion
2. *Dull:* sound of medium pitch and duration with a "thudlike" quality; occurs with fluid (pneumonia), consolidation, or tumors

3. *Resonant:* loud, low-pitched sound of long duration; occurs with normal lung tissue and with bronchitis
4. *Hyperresonant:* very loud, low-pitched sound of long duration; occurs with increased amounts of air, such as in emphysema or pneumothorax
5. *Tympany:* loud, high-pitched sound; occurs with large pneumothorax

✎ What's the proper technique for percussion of the chest?

1. Hyperextend the middle finger of one hand and place the distal interphalangeal joint firmly against the patient's chest.
2. Using the tip (not the pad) of the opposite middle finger, use a quick flick of the wrist to strike the first finger, followed by a quick removal of the striking finger. Two to three strikes should be performed in each examination area.
3. Percuss from side to side and from top to bottom, omitting the areas over the scapulae. Compare findings from one side to the other, noting any asymmetry. Note the location and quality of the percussion sounds heard.
4. Locate the level of diaphragmatic dullness on both the right and left sides.

What factors should be assessed during auscultation of the anterior and posterior chest?

Presence of normal breath sounds, presence of abnormal breath sounds, and presence of voice sounds

✎ What are the three types of normal breath sounds?

1. *Bronchial (tracheal):* harsh and discontinuous high-pitched sounds heard over the trachea and on the posterior chest; result from air passage over the walls of the trachea; prolonged on expiration (1:2 inspiration to expiration ratio)
2. *Bronchovesicular:* continuous, soft, breezy, and lower-pitched sounds than bronchial; heard anteriorly over the mainstem bronchi in the 1st and 2nd intercostal space, and posteriorly between the scapulae; result from transitional airflow moving through the branches of the smaller bronchi and bronchioles; are equally audible during inspiration and expiration (have a nearly equal inspiratory-expiratory ratio)
3. *Vesicular:* soft, breezy lower-pitched sounds than bronchovesicular; heard throughout most of lung, but best at lung periphery; inaudible over the scapulae; result from laminar airflow moving through the alveolar ducts and alveoli at low flow rates; prolonged on inspiration and almost silent on expiration (inspiratory-expiratory ratio of 3:1)

◤ *In the upright position, breath sounds are symmetrical and louder in intensity in the lung bases than in the apices.*

◤ What's the proper technique for ausculta tion of the chest?

1. Warm the stethoscope by placing it between your hands.
2. Instruct the patient to take deep breaths through his mouth, and place the diaphragm of the stethoscope directly on his skin (not on clothing).
3. In a systematic manner, assess the anterior and lateral thorax for normal breath sounds, noting any areas of abnormalities. Start at the upper lobes and move from side to side and downward (as for percussion). A point on one side of the chest should be auscultated followed by auscultation at the same site on the opposite side of the chest for comparison.
4. Auscultate the right 4th to 6th intercostal spaces to assess the right middle lung.
5. Auscultate at least one complete respiratory cycle at each site.

◤ *An intercostal space is named for the rib that lies above it.*

Where's the xiphoid process?

At the bottom of the sternum

Where's the supra-sternal notch located?

At the top of the sternum

◤ What's the costal angle?

The area located between the two lower borders of the ribcage near the xiphoid process

What's the angle of Louis located?

The angle between the manubrium and the body of the sternum; it's the location where the trachea bifurcates into the left and right bronchi; may be referred to as the carina

Abnormal findings

◤ What's tracheal deviation

A non-midline trachea with a palpable space between the sternocleidomastoid and trachea; may indicate tension pneumothorax, a mass, or thyroid enlargement

◤ *With tension pneumothorax, a shift of the mediastinum can occur with displacement of the trachea to the side opposite of the collapse.*

✎ **What unusual chest shapes might be noted on inspection of the chest?**

1. *Barrel chest:* increased anteroposterior chest diameter due to increased functional residual capacity and air trapping from alveolar collapse; anteroposterior ratio is close to 1:1; commonly occurs with chronic obstructive pulmonary disease

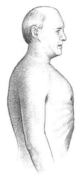

2. *Pectus excavatum:* "funnel chest;" sternum is depressed and seems to nearly touch the vertebrae

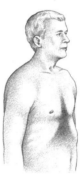

3. *Pectus carinatum:* "pigeon chest;" sternum protrudes from the chest

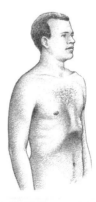

What are examples of adventitious (extra) breath sounds that might be noted on auscultation of the chest?

1. *Crackles:* short, discontinuous sounds heard during inspiration (and usually in the lung bases); classified as fine or coarse; caused by the passage of air over airway secretions; associated with restrictive diseases, such as pulmonary fibrosis and heart failure; rales are coarse crackles

2. *Wheezes or rhonchi:* continuous musical sound of high or low pitch that is best heard on exhalation; rhonchi are longer and lower-pitched wheezes with a "snoring" or "gurgling" quality; sibilant rhonchi have a shrill or squeaking quality and are caused by narrowing of the airway, as occurs with an asthmatic attack; sonorous rhonchi are lower-pitched with a snoring quality and are caused by secretions in large airways, as occurs with bronchitis

3. *Pleural friction rub:* creaking, grating, or leather-like sound usually heard both on inspiration and expiration; caused by rubbing together of inflamed pleura

To differentiate a pleural friction rub from a pericardial friction rub, instruct the patient to hold his breath briefly. A pericardial friction rub continues with each heartbeat, while a pleural friction rub is absent when the breath is held.

What's stridor?

A continuous high-pitched, harsh sound that occurs as a result of partial obstruction of the larynx or trachea, as occurs with laryngeal edema or choking; a sign of respiratory distress that requires immediate attention

What features of adventitious breath sounds should be noted?

Inspiratory or expiratory, continuous or discontinuous, and high- or low-pitch

When might breath sounds be decreased or absent?

In conditions in which there is an increased filtration of sound (pleural thickening, pleural effusion), or a decreased movement of air (severe asthma, emphysema, pneumothorax)

What are voice sounds (or voice resonance)?

The spoken voice transmits through the pulmonary tree and may be heard during auscultation. Voice sounds should be assessed if chest inspection, palpation, percussion, or auscultation reveal any abnormalities. Voice sounds may be heard with atelectasis, pleural effusion, or consolidation of tissue, which resonates the voice and transmits it more loudly.

If there's distance between the spoken voice then the voice sounds would be diminished, such as chronic obstructive pulmonary disease or pneumothorax, and the nurse would record "voice sounds decreased or absent."

▶ *Voice sounds are vibrations through lung fields on auscultation; tactile fremitus is sound vibration through lung fields on palpation.*

▶ *Voice resonance is typically only assessed when abnormal breath sounds are noted on auscultation.*

What types of voice sounds may be heard?

1. *Egophony:* patient states the letter "E" continuously, but it sounds like "A," or the spoken syllable has a particular nasal quality; caused by compression of the lung by fluid, as occurs with pleural effusions
2. *Whispered pectoriloquy:* whispered word ("ninety-nine") is distinctly heard in an area of the lung; normally, absent or faint sounds only are heard
3. *Bronchophony:* spoken word ("ninety-nine") is heard loud and clear and seems close to the ear; sounds are normally muffled or indistinct

What are accessory muscles?

Muscles other than the diaphragm and intercostals that are used for abnormal, labored breathing (forced inspiration and active expiration); the pectoral, scalenus, sternocleidomastoid, trapezius, and abdominal rectus muscles are commonly used as accessory muscles for respiration

What are intercostal retractions?

The visible use of the muscles located between the ribs to assist with breathing; occur with labored breathing, such as with acute exertional dyspnea, respiratory distress, or chronic obstructive pulmonary disease

What's bradypnea?

A respiratory rate that's less than normal for the age-group (adult or pediatric); less than 10 breaths/minute for an adult

What's tachypnea?

A persistent, rapid and shallow type of breathing; more than 20 breaths/minute for an adult

What's dyspnea?

A sense of shortness of breath or inability to catch one's breath

What's orthopnea?

Dyspnea that occurs in the recumbent position; "two pillow orthopnea" indicates a need to use two pillows to avoid lying flat and experiencing shortness of breath

What's hemoptysis?

Presence of blood in sputum

What's hyperpnea?

Deep or labored respirations; hyperpnea is a normal response to exercise or physical exertion, but may occur abnormally with fever, pain, or metabolic acidosis

What's hypercapnia?

The condition characterized by increased arterial levels of carbon dioxide; commonly occurs in chronic obstructive pulmonary disease.

What's hyperventilation?

An abnormal rate of ventilation that's more rapid that the rate metabolically necessary for respiratory gas exchange; results in excessive oxygen intake along with a loss of carbon dioxide; may occur with acid-base imbalances or secondary to anxiety

What's hypoventilation?

An abnormally decreased rate and depth of respiration that results in an inadequate volume of air within the alveoli for gas exchange and retention of carbon dioxide; may occur with opioid overdose, neurologic impairment, or secondary to postoperative pain

What's apnea?

The absence of respirations

What's sleep apnea?

A disorder characterized by temporary airflow obstruction of the pharynx by the tongue and soft palate that occurs during sleep; excessive daytime sleepiness, frequent awakenings at night, loud snoring, morning headaches (from retention of carbon dioxide), and irritability from fragmented sleep are common manifestations; commonly associated with obesity

Treatment measures include weight loss, avoidance of supine position during sleep, avoidance of alcohol, avoidance of sedatives, use of continuous positive airway pressure or bilevel positive airway pressure, or use of surgical procedures, such as uvulopalatopharyngoplasty, which removes obstructing tissues.

What are apneustic respirations?

A breathing pattern with long inspiration and short expiration

What's Cheyne-Stokes respirations?

An abnormal breathing pattern consisting of periods of apnea followed by respirations of increasing depth and frequency; commonly occurs in the final stages of life or with drug-induced respiratory depression

What are Kussmaul's respirations?

Very deep respirations similar to gasping that commonly occurs with metabolic acidosis, such as in severe diabetic ketoacidosis and coma

What's atactic breathing?

Respiratory pattern characterized by unpredictable irregularity

What's hypoxemia?

A condition characterized by a blood oxygen level lower than normal (less than 80 mm Hg) that occurs secondary to reduced alveolar oxygen tension or hypoventilation; may exhibit symptoms of a deficiency in tissue oxygenation, depending on the degree of hypoxemia

What's hypoxia?

A deficiency in tissue oxygenation associated with manifestations of inadequate oxygen delivery to vital organs, such as the brain and heart

What's cyanosis?

A bluish or purplish discoloration of the skin and mucous membranes caused by decreased arterial levels of oxygen; reflects hemoglobin unsaturated with oxygen; manifestations of central cyanosis may include a bluish tinge under the tongue and on the mucous membranes, face, or lips; peripheral cyanosis may be noted on the nails, nose, and ears and only implies vasoconstriction, which may appear when one is chilled

Cyanosis is a late sign of hypoxia.

What's clubbing?

An abnormal enlargement of the distal phalanges that occurs secondary to chronic hypoxemia; flattening of the angle between skin and nail base occurs

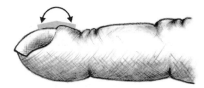

What's atelectasis?

A condition characterized by collapsed, airless alveoli that result from exudates or retained secretions that obstruct the bronchioles, causing alveolar collapse distal to the obstruction; breath sounds may be decreased or absent over affected areas

Postoperative and immobile patients are at the highest risk and usually presents as dyspnea, cough, and a fever 24 to 48 hours following surgery. Early ambulation and deep breathing and coughing exercises should be used to prevent the development of atelectasis.

What's bronchiectasis?

A condition characterized by the irreversible dilatation of one or more large bronchi that occurs secondary to damage of the elastic and muscular structures of the bronchial walls; bacterial infections and obstructive processes (tumors of the lungs or thoracic cavity, thick secretions from chronic bronchitis) are common causes; manifestations include a paroxysmal cough productive of mucopurulent sputum that worsens with position changes, hemoptysis, exertional dyspnea, weight loss, fetid breath, and recurrent episodes of pneumonia; antibiotics, bronchodilators, mucolytic agents, and expectorants may be used in the treatment of bronchiectasis, and deep breathing exercises should be encouraged

What's a pleural effusion?

Fluid accumulation in the pleural space that occurs secondary to blocked lymphatic drainage or a change in colloid osmotic pressure; worsening dyspnea and pleuritic pain may result; small effusions may be observed without the need for any invasive treatment, but a thoracentesis (removal of pleural fluid with a needle) may be performed for large effusions

What are the causes of pleural effusion and how are they classified?

1. *Transudative:* protein content of the fluid is low; occurs with noninflammatory conditions, such as heart failure (increased hydrostatic pressure) or chronic liver or renal disease (decreased oncotic pressure from low serum albumin)
2. *Exudative:* protein content of the fluid is high; occurs with inflammatory processes where capillaries are more permeable, such as pulmonary cancers, infections, emboli, and GI disease

What's pleurisy (also called pleuritis)?

Inflammation of the pleura that can cause pain with breathing; a pleural effusion may develop from pleurisy, and a pleural friction rub may be noted over the affected area; most common cause is tuberculosis, pneumonia, neoplasms, chest trauma, and pulmonary embolisms or infarctions

Although the condition can be self-limited, analgesics should be given for moderate to severe pain, and fluid may need to be drained from around the lungs (thoracentesis). Adhesions (scar tissue) may form within the pleura as a result of the inflammation.

What's pleuritic pain?

Pain that worsens with breathing and coughing and is very localized; patients tend to compensate for the pain by breathing rapidly and shallowly

What's an empyema?

An infected fluid collection within the pleural space; clinical manifestations include fever, night sweats, weight loss, and cough; drainage of the infected fluid via thoracentesis or insertion of a closed thoracotomy tube or a chest tube may be performed; antibiotics are administered

What's an area of consolidation?	An area in the lung characterized by a dense mass that occurs secondary to solidification of fluid or an infection; air in the lungs is replaced with fluid or a mass
What's nasal flaring?	Periodic outward movements of the nostrils that occurs with inspirations, indicating an increased effort to breathe
✎ **What's allergic rhinitis?**	An inflammatory reaction (immunoglobulin E antibody) of the nasal mucosa to an allergen; also known as hay fever; common manifestations include nasal congestion, tearing, itchy eyes, and pale, boggy, and edematous nasal turbinates with increased mucous secretion; antihistamines and decongestants are commonly used in treatment
✎ **What's sinusitis?**	Inflammation of the sinus cavities, which typically occurs secondary to a viral upper respiratory infection, but may also be associated with rhinitis, a tooth abscess, and nasal surgery; severe pain located over the affected sinuses, headaches, fever, malaise, and decreased transillumination of the sinuses (from fluid accumulation) are common manifestations
✎ **What's epistaxis?**	A nosebleed, which can occur as a result of internal or external nose trauma, hypertension, inflammation, or tumor growth; direct pressure should be applied to the bleeding nostril and a seated position should be assumed by the patient; the use of cool compresses and ice may be used to slow the bleeding; nasal packing with petroleum jelly or ribbon gauze may be necessary in some instances

Major disease processes of the respiratory system

Infectious diseases

PNEUMONIA

What's pneumonia?	An infectious process that causes inflammation within the alveolar spaces and the interstitial tissue of the lungs; the pathogen may be bacterial, viral (influenza, respiratory syncytial virus, rhinovirus, adenovirus), or fungal; typical pathogens include *S. pneumonia* (pneumococcus), *Haemophilus*, and *Staphylococcus* species, and atypical organisms include *Mycoplasma*, *Chlamydia*, and *Legionella* species; immunocompromised individuals (very old, very young, persons with chronic diseases) are at the greatest risk for development of pneumonia; the condi-

tion may be classified as community acquired (occurs within first 2 days of hospitalization), or health care facility acquired (occurs 72 hours or longer after admission)

What's the patho-physiologic process of pneumonia?

Pathogens enter the lungs by inhalation, aspiration, or via circulation. Within the lungs these organisms infect alveolar cells, multiply, and then are spread from alveolus to alveolus, producing inflammation and consolidation; all pneumonias result in decreased ventilation, low ventilation-perfusion ratio in the diseased area, and hypoxemia

What's aspiration pneumonia?

Pneumonia that typically occurs in individuals with altered consciousness and an impaired gag reflex who aspirate food or other substances; can be minimized by proper positioning of patients with head of bed elevated to at least 30 degrees

What's opportunistic pneumonia?

Pneumonia that occurs in individuals with severely depressed immune systems (chemotherapy, acquired immunodeficiency syndrome, organ transplant recipients); common organisms are *Pneumocystis carinii* pneumonia and cytomegalovirus

What are the clinical manifestations of pneumonia?

1. *Bacterial:* sudden onset of fever and shaking chills, productive cough with purulent (yellow-green, gray, or rust-colored) or bloody sputum, pleuritic chest pain, exertional dyspnea, tachypnea, myalgias, pulmonary consolidation on chest X-ray, decreased or bronchial breath sounds, dullness to percussion over affected area, crackles in affected lobe, positive voice sounds; pleural friction rub, and altered mental status
2. *Viral:* low-grade fever, malaise, mild dyspnea, and nonproductive cough (initially)
3. *Mycoplasma:* slower onset of milder symptoms (malaise, headache, fever, prolonged, paroxysmal cough); common cause of "walking pneumonia" because affected individuals aren't usually bedridden by the infection

What complications are associated with pneumonia?

Pleurisy (inflammation of the pleura), pleural effusion, atelectasis, empyema, pulmonary abscess, pericarditis or endocarditis, bacteremia and sepsis, respiratory failure, acute respiratory distress syndrome, and death

What's the typical treatment for pneumonia?

1. *Bacterial:* antibiotics, such as macrolides (azithromycin, erythromycin), although the class of antibiotics used will depend on the causative organism; administration of oxygen, analgesics (for pleuritic pain), and antipyretics; hydration with I.V. fluids

2. *Viral:* hydration, administration of oxygen for dyspnea or hypoxemia; antiviral agents (acyclovir, ganciclovir); antibiotics may be used because many viral pneumonias occur in the setting of a coexisting bacterial pneumonia

3. *Mycoplasmal:* antibiotics (used for bacteriostatic actions in this setting); commonly self-limited with resolution in 2 to 4 weeks without treatment in otherwise healthy individuals

✎ What are important nursing actions in the care of a patient with pneumonia?

1. Implement respiratory isolation precautions for patients with viral or mycoplasmal pneumonia.
2. Administer supplemental oxygen as ordered by the physician.
3. Assess the patient's respiratory status and breath sounds. Obtain pulse oximetry at frequent intervals. Notify the physician of oxygen saturation less than 92%, or according to the physician's order or facility policy.
4. Maintain a patent airway with coughing, deep breathing, and high Fowler's or semi-Fowler's positioning. Provide bronchial hygiene (suctioning, chest physiotherapy, positioning) to prevent atelectasis, if ordered by the physician. Maintain the head of bed at 30-degree angle to prevent aspiration pneumonia.
5. Hydrate with 3 L of fluids/day I.V. or orally, unless contraindicated. Monitor intake and output.
6. Obtain vital signs at least every 4 hours (more often if indicated or ordered by the physician).
7. Administer medications (antibiotics, analgesics, antipyretics, cough suppressants) as ordered by the physician.
8. Encourage adequate intake of high-calorie foods.
9. Monitor for complications, including respiratory distress or sepsis, and notify the physician immediately if any develop.
10. Emphasize the importance of completing the entire antibiotic course upon discharge.
11. Encourage smoking cessation and vaccinations.

How can viral influenza pneumonia be prevented?

By receiving an annual influenza vaccination

How can some forms of bacterial pneumonia be prevented?

By receiving the pneumococcal vaccine; all persons older than age 65 and persons with diabetes mellitus, alcoholism, asplenia, or chronic cardiac, pulmonary, or liver disease should receive the vaccination

TUBERCULOSIS

✎ What's tuberculosis (TB)?

A bacterial infection caused by *Mycobacterium tuberculosis* that primarily affects the lungs (pulmonary TB), although it can affect other organs and body structures; it's transmitted through respiratory droplets; the disease may be an active process or it may remain dormant for a lifetime; immunocompromised persons (HIV-positive, malnourished, alcoholics) are at the highest risk for development of TB; Asians, Pacific Islanders, and Mexicans have the highest rates of infection

What's the pathophysiologic process of TB?

The *Mycobacterium tuberculosis* bacilli are inhaled and then become deposited within the lungs where they may be killed by the host's immune system, may become dormant without causing symptoms, or may produce primary TB by reproducing. It's possible for the bacilli to proliferate after a period of dormancy, causing reactivation of TB. Cavitations may be produced within the lung tissue.

⚡ *Contraction of TB typically requires close, repeated contact over a long period of time.*

✎ How is the diagnosis made?

The Mantoux test (commonly known as the purified protein derivative [PPD] or skin test) is the gold standard for screening. Skin tests should be read 48 to 72 hours after PPD administration. A positive test is determined by the size of the area of induration (hardened and raised area).

An induration of 15 mm or greater is considered positive for persons without risk factors; 10 mm or greater is considered positive for persons with low risk factors (staff at health care facilities, residents of long-term care facilities, foreign-borne persons, I.V. drug users who are HIV-negative); and 5 mm or greater is considered positive for persons with high risk factors (HIV-positive, close contact with a person with infectious TB, I.V. drug user with unknown HIV status). A chest X-ray is performed for persons with positive skin tests and for persons with symptoms suggestive of pulmonary TB.

⚡ *The presence of erythema isn't used to determine if a TB skin test is positive; only the size of the induration (hard, raised area) is diagnostic.*

✎ Is a positive PPD indicative of active TB?

Not necessarily; in addition to active TB, it may also mean that an individual has been exposed to someone with TB; that person now is infected with the bacillus and has latent disease instead of active disease

✎ What are the clinical manifestations of pulmonary TB?

1. *Latent disease:* usually produces no symptoms
2. *Active disease:* fever, productive cough, night sweats, unintentional weight loss, chest pain, increase fatigue, malaise, and hemoptysis

What complications are associated with pulmonary TB?

Dissemination throughout body (miliary TB), such as the bones, joints, bone marrow, and central nervous system; pleural effusion; TB pneumonia; and multidrug-resistant TB

What's multi-drug resistant TB?

A form of TB that's resistant to at least two of the standard medications used to treat TB; usually results from under treatment or noncompliance with drug regimen

✎ What's the typical treatment for TB?

1. *Prophylactic treatment:* isoniazid (INH) daily for 6 to 12 months
2. *Active disease:* usually a combination of INH, rifampin, ethambutol, and pyrazinamide for 6 to 12 months; combination drugs, such as Rifater (isoniazid, rifampin, pyrazinamide), and new formulations of medicines requiring once a week dosing, such as rifapentine (Priftin), may improve medication compliance

⚡ *Rifampin should be avoided in persons taking protease inhibitors (commonly used for HIV management) because the effectiveness of both drugs is reduced when they're used concomitantly.*

✎ What are important nursing actions in the care of a patient with active TB?

1. Implement appropriate isolation precautions by placing the patient in a room with negative pressure. Make sure you wear a respirator mask when entering the patient's room, and instruct all visitors to do the same. Instruct the patient to cough into tissues and to wear a mask when leaving the hospital room.
2. Monitor the patient's respiratory status, including breath sounds and oxygen saturation.
3. Administer medications (isoniazid, rifampin, ethambutol, pyrazinamide) as ordered by the physician.
4. Encourage consumption of high-protein and high-carbohydrate foods to enhance nutritional status.
5. Monitor for complications from the disease process or its treatment (evidence of hepatotoxicity) and notify the physician immediately if any develop.
6. Monitor laboratory results periodically during therapy, particularly hepatic and renal function.
7. Educate the patient about the importance of strict compliance with medications for the entire duration prescribed. Inform him about adverse effects of anti-tuberculosis medications, including reddish orange discoloration of body fluids (tears, sweat, urine) with

rifampin. Educate him about hepatotoxicity associated with some antituberculosis drugs, and instruct him to notify the physician immediately if jaundice occurs.

8. Encourage close medical follow-up.

Restrictive lung diseases

PNEUMOTHORAX

What's pneumothorax?

A condition characterized by air collecting within the intrapleural space, which results in the total or partial collapse of the affected lung; mediastinal structures can be displaced and cardiopulmonary function can be compromised

Pneumothoraces may be associated with medical or surgical procedures (mechanical ventilation, lung biopsy, thoracentesis, cardiopulmonary resuscitation, invasive procedures involving the subclavian vein), or trauma resulting in fractured ribs as well as smoking and chronic obstructive pulmonary disease in which a bleb on the lung ruptures. Spontaneous pneumothoraces occur more commonly in males ages 20 to 40, especially those who are tall and thin (particularly prevalent in Marfan syndrome).

What's the pathophysiologic process of pneumothorax?

Positive pressure in the intrapleural space causes partial or total lung collapse, and as the pneumothorax enlarges, the affected lung becomes smaller. Hypoxia and decreased cardiac output result.

✎ What are the clinical manifestations of pneumothorax?

Dyspnea, air hunger, tachypnea, tachycardia, chest pain, absent or decreased breath sounds over affected area, and mental status changes may be seen initially; hypotension, cyanosis, and tracheal deviation are late findings

▧ *Displacement of the trachea occurs to the unaffected side with pneumothorax.*

What complications are associated with pneumothorax?

Empyema, pulmonary edema (after lung re-expansion), tension pneumothorax (may result from kinking or obstruction of the chest tube), hemopneumothorax, respiratory arrest, and cardiac arrest

✎ What's the typical treatment for pneumothorax?

1. *Small pneumothorax (less than 15%):* observation, if the patient is asymptomatic; aspiration of the air with a large bore needle, if the patient is symptomatic
2. *Large pneumothorax:* administration of oxygen; commonly a chest tube is placed via a thoracostomy and is connected to water seal drainage; a Heimlich valve

(rubber, one-way flutter valve) may be used for the outpatient management of a pneumothorax; pleurodesis (sclerosis) may be performed after re-inflation of the lung to prevent pneumothorax recurrence

◆ What are important nursing actions in the care of a patient with pneumothorax?

1. Administer supplemental oxygen as ordered by the physician and assess oxygenation status (arterial blood gas values and pulse oximetry).
2. Monitor respiratory status, breath sounds, and vital signs at frequent intervals. Encourage deep-breathing exercises.
3. Evaluate for proper functioning of chest tubes and drainage systems. Ensure patency of tubing and maintain drainage system in an upright position below the level of the heart. Assess the integrity of the occlusive dressing at the insertion site and change them daily, or more often as indicated. Assess for the presence of air leaks by instructing the patient to take a deep breath and cough (bubbling in the water seal is indicative of an air leak). Observe the amount and type of fluid drainage. Evaluate for the presence of subcutaneous emphysema at the insertion site.
4. Make sure emergency equipment is readily available (petroleum jelly impregnated gauze, padded clamps, sterile saline, tape).
5. Reposition the patient every 2 hours.
6. Assess the patient's anxiety and comfort level.
7. Administer medications (analgesics) as ordered by the physician.
8. Monitor for complications, such as problems with the chest tube or its drainage system, bleeding from the drain insertion site, development of tension pneumothorax, or respiratory distress.
9. Encourage smoking cessation to minimize recurrence of pneumothorax.

Vascular disorders of the respiratory system

PULMONARY EDEMA

◆ What's pulmonary edema?

Abnormal accumulation of fluid in the alveolar and interstitial spaces of the lungs; commonly develops suddenly and is a medical emergency; associated with cardiac disorders, such as coronary artery disease or valvular diseases, but it can also occur as a result of other conditions, such as pneumonia, severe allergic reactions, and smoke inhalation

What's the patho-physiologic process of pulmonary edema?

Fluid fills the alveoli due to altered capillary permeability, increased pulmonary capillary pressure, decreased oncotic pressure, or failure of the heart to maintain adequate blood circulation, as occurs in heart failure; gas exchange is impaired as a result

✎ What are the clinical manifestations of pulmonary edema?

Dyspnea, anxiety, restlessness, hypoxemia, orthopnea, wheezing or crackles, tachypnea, tachycardia, hypertension, jugular vein distension, decreased air exchange on auscultation, peripheral edema, weight gain, and use of accessory muscles of respiration; cyanosis and pink-tinged and frothy sputum are late findings, and are highly suggestive of heart failure

What complications are associated with pulmonary edema?

Electrolyte disturbances (from diuretic therapy), arrhythmias, acute myocardial infarction, and respiratory distress

What's the typical treatment for pulmonary edema?

1. *Oxygen therapy:* via face mask or nasal cannula
2. *Pharmacologic agents:* diuretics such as furosemide (Lasix); nitrates such as nitroprusside or nitroglycerin; and analgesics (morphine) to decrease anxiety

✎ What are important nursing actions in the care of a patient with pulmonary edema?

1. Administer supplemental oxygen as ordered by the physician.
2. Elevate the head of the bed to high Fowler's position to aid breathing and to reduce venous return.
3. Assess respiratory status (breath sounds, oxygen saturation). Assess for presence of crackles in the bases and determine if it's worsening (if the crackles are ascending).
4. Monitor intake and output. Place an indwelling urinary catheter.
5. Obtain daily weight.
6. Restrict fluids and sodium as ordered by the physician.
7. Monitor vital signs at frequent intervals.
8. Administer medications (nitrates, diuretics) as ordered by the physician.
9. Provide a calm environment, and administer I.V. morphine to relieve anxiety.
10. Anticipate the need for continuous positive airway pressure, bilevel positive airway pressure or, possibly, intubation with mechanical ventilation.
11. Monitor electrolytes periodically throughout diuretic therapy.

PULMONARY EMBOLUS AND INFARCTION

✎ What's a pulmonary embolus (PE)?

An obstruction within the pulmonary circulatory system caused by a clot; blood clots that originate from the deep veins of the legs are the most common cause, however fat, air, and tumor emboli may also occur

Risk factors for the development of a PE include prolonged immobility, venous disease of lower extremities, atrial fibrillation, cancer (produces hypercoagulable state), heart failure, surgery or trauma involving the pelvic area or lower extremities, pregnancy, hormonal contraceptive use, previous history of deep vein thrombosis, and obesity.

What's the pathophysiologic process of PE?

A clot forms within the deep veins of the lower extremities as a result of venous stasis, injury to the intima of the vein, or a hypercoagulable state; the clot breaks away from its site of formation, is carried through the circulatory system, and becomes lodged in the pulmonary vascular system; the obstruction produces varying degrees of respiratory distress

▧ *A thrombus is a blood clot that forms within a blood vessel, and an embolus is a thrombus that has become dislodged and is carried through the blood stream before becoming lodged in a small vessel.*

▧ *Virchow's triad, which are three factors that enhance thrombosis, consists of the processes of venous stasis, injury to the intima of the vein, and hypercoagulability.*

✎ What are the clinical manifestations of a PE?

Sudden dyspnea, feeling of impending doom, anxiety, pleuritic chest pain, cough, tachycardia, tachypnea, hemoptysis, altered mental status, low-grade fever, accentuation of pulmonic heart sound, and crackles on inspiration

What complications are associated with a PE?

Pulmonary infarction (death of lung tissue), pulmonary hypertension, respiratory failure, and death

What are the typical treatment measures?

1. *Supplemental oxygen:* via nasal cannula or face mask
2. *Thrombolytic agents (streptokinase, urokinase):* to dissolve blood clots; must be given within 48 hours of embolic event
3. *Surgery:* pulmonary embolectomy may be performed urgently for severe pulmonary arterial obstruction that doesn't respond to conservative treatment; placement

of Greenfield filter may be performed in persons with recurrent emboli despite anticoagulation

4. *Anticoagulants:* to prevent recurrent emboli; I.V. heparin, low molecular weight heparin (Enoxaparin), and warfarin (Coumadin) with international normalized ratio goal of 2.0 to 3.0

✎ What are important nursing actions in the care of a patient with a PE?

1. Administer 100% oxygen via face mask.
2. Place the patient in semi-Fowler's or high Fowler's position.
3. Establish I.V. access for possible crystalloid solutions and vasopressors to treat hypotension and heparin for anticoagulation.
4. Monitor vital signs and respiratory status (breath sounds, oxygen saturation level, arterial blood gas levels) at least every 15 minutes until stable.
5. Administer medication (analgesics, heparin bolus, and thrombolytic agents, such as streptokinase, urokinase, tissue plasminogen activator) as ordered by the physician.
6. Monitor for complications from the condition (severe respiratory distress) or from its treatment (excessive bruising, hemorrhaging), and notify the physician if any occur.
7. Educate the patient about prevention of PE and deep vein thrombosis. Encourage ambulation at least every hour while on long car or plane rides.
8. Educate the patient about the use of Coumadin, including avoiding foods high in vitamin K, and about avoiding the use of straightedge razors, stiff toothbrushes, and rectal thermometers.

Obstructive lung diseases

CHRONIC OBSTRUCTIVE PULMONARY DISEASE

✎ What's chronic obstructive pulmonary disease (COPD)?

A term used to identify pulmonary disorders characterized by airflow obstruction; the classic triad of COPD includes chronic bronchitis (predominately) with overlapping features of emphysema and possibly asthma

Smoking is the most common cause (90% of cases), but other factors may include exposure to air pollution and occupational dusts and chemicals, hyperreactive airways, a genetic predisposition (alpha$_1$-antitrypsin deficiency), and childhood infections (severe respiratory, viral). Forced expiratory volume (FEV_1), an index of airflow obstruction, is reduced on pulmonary function tests.

What's the patho-physiologic process of COPD?

In general, progressive airflow obstruction occurs secondary to the chronic inflammatory response of the lungs to noxious particles or gases

✎ What's emphysema?

A pulmonary disorder characterized by irreversible destruction of the airways distal to the terminal bronchioles

Because elastin and collagen in the lungs are destroyed in emphysema, the elastic recoil of the lungs is lost, further limiting airflow and predisposing the bronchioles to collapse (particularly on expiration). Air trapping occurs within the distal alveoli, and their resultant hyperinflation is responsible for the characteristic "barrel chest" (increased anteroposterior diameter of the chest) of emphysema; blebs (large air spaces within the visceral pleura) and bullae (large air spaces within the lung tissue) form as progressive destruction and coalescence of the alveoli occur. Persons with emphysema compensate for the loss of surface area available for the exchange of oxygen within the alveoli by hyperventilating

▚ *Persons with emphysema are referred to as "pink puffers" because hyperventilation prevents the development of cyanosis.*

▚ *Air enters the lungs easily in persons with emphysema but it becomes trapped in the lungs because they can only partially deflate on expiration.*

✎ What's chronic bronchitis?

A condition characterized by the presence of a productive cough for 3 months, during each of 2 consecutive years in association with excessive mucus production; the smooth muscle of the airways becomes inflamed, the bronchial walls thicken, mucous plugs form, and the airways become narrow with limitation of airflow; because the bronchioles become clogged with mucus, a physical barrier to ventilation is created

Persons with chronic bronchitis have a diminished respiratory drive, and hypoventilation and retention of carbon dioxide occur. Hypoxemia and polycythemia develop from the ventilation-perfusion mismatch. The pathologic changes that occur are somewhat more reversible than those that occur with emphysema.

▚ *Persons with chronic bronchitis are referred to as "blue bloaters" due to the ensuing hypoxemia and cyanosis that occur.*

▚ *Acute bronchitis is a condition characterized by inflammation of the tracheobronchial tree that's usually caused by an infectious agent (typically in winter months following an upper respiratory illness), but may also be the result of exposure to an allergen, pollutant, or irritant.*

✎ What are the clinical manifestations of COPD?

1. *Emphysema:* progressive dyspnea, tachypnea, and possibly wheezing (especially on exertion); thin and underweight or cachectic from protein-calorie malnutrition; barrel chest (due to hyperinflation from air trapping); prolonged expiration with use of pursed lips and accessory muscles; decreased breath sounds diffusely with hyperresonance on percussion; late onset of cough that's typically worse in the mornings and produces colorless sputum; and peripheral edema and finger clubbing in advanced disease
2. *Chronic bronchitis:* malaise, fever, myalgia, sore throat, normal weight or heavyset, purulent cough, frequent pulmonary infections, and rhonchi may be noted; edema and cyanosis if right sided heart failure occurs

What are the general arterial blood gas analysis findings in persons with COPD?

Early stages: normal or slightly decreased level of Pao_2 with normal $Paco_2$

Later stages: decreased Pao_2, elevated $Paco_2$, decreased pH, and increased bicarbonate level

What complications are associated with COPD?

1. *Emphysema:* acute exacerbations, frequent pulmonary infections (pneumonia), protein-calorie malnutrition (loss of lean muscle mass and subcutaneous fat), pneumothorax from bullae (bleb) formation, cyanosis, cor pulmonale (enlargement of right side of the heart from pulmonary hypertension) and possibly right heart failure (peripheral edema, jugular vein distension); increased incidence of peptic ulcer disease and esophageal reflux
2. *Chronic bronchitis:* frequent pulmonary infections (pneumonia), polycythemia with hemoglobin typically 20 g/dl or more (from increased production of red blood cells in response to chronic hypoxemia), cor pulmonale and possibly right heart failure, and increased incidence of peptic ulcer disease and esophageal reflux

✎ What's the typical treatment for COPD?

1. *Avoiding or eliminating the underlying cause:* smoking cessation should be strongly encouraged; nicotine patches or gum and the use of bupropion (Zyban) may be helpful
2. *Using inhaled bronchodilators:* decrease muscle tone in small airways and increase ventilation; albuterol (Proventil, Ventolin), pirbuterol (Maxair), metaproterenol (Alupent), salmeterol (Serevent), and ipra-

tropium (Atrovent); corticosteroid inhalants, such as fluticasone (Flovent) and budesonide (Pulmicort) may be used to decrease the frequency of exacerbations; a spacer may be used to enhance aerosol delivery

3. *Using oral pharmacologic agents:* theophylline (Theo-Dur, Slo-bid), leukotriene modifiers (such as montelukast [Singulair] and zafirlukast [Accolate]), corticosteroids (prednisone) to treat exacerbations and using antibiotics to treat bacterial infections because chronic infections and colonization of the lower airways is common in persons with COPD; antitussives and expectorants, such as guaifenesin and dextromethorphan (Humibid Dm, Robitussin DM) and guaifenesin and codeine (Robitussin A-C) may be used; magnesium and mucolytic agents such as N-acetylcysteine (to reduce sputum viscosity and improve clearance of secretions) may also be of some benefit

4. *Prescribing long-term oxygen therapy:* if Pao_2 is 59 mm Hg or less or if Sao_2 is 90% or less

5. *Intervening with surgery:* including bullectomy for large bullae, lung volume reduction surgery to remove diseased portions of the lung (allows the remaining, healthier lung to function more effectively), or lung transplantation

6. *Intervening with pulmonary rehabilitation:* including education, medications, exercise training, breathing retraining techniques (pursed lip breathing to prevent alveolar collapse and air trapping, diaphragmatic breathing for maximum inhalation, and slowed respiratory rate), and chest physiotherapy with percussion (cupped hands create an air pocket between examiner's hand and patient's chest), vibration (rhythmic massage with palm of hand during prolonged exhalation), and postural drainage (bronchial drainage via gravity)

▰ *Inhaled beta$_2$ agonists are the initial treatment of choice for acute exacerbations of COPD.*

▰ *Hypoxemia is the primary respiratory stimulant for persons with COPD due to the chronic elevation of carbon dioxide; the administration of excessive oxygen can depress the respiratory drive, causing breathing to slow or stop altogether.*

What are symptoms of an acute exacerbation of COPD?

Classic symptoms include worsening dyspnea, increased sputum purulence, and increased sputum production; may also have upper respiratory infection, wheezing, fever, increased cough, and increased heart and respiratory rate; COPD is generally treated with inhaled bronchodilators, such as terbutaline (Brethaire), albuterol (Proventil), theophylline (Theo-Dur), ipratropium (Atrovent), a combination of ipratropium and albuterol (Combivent) and, possibly, systemic corticosteroids; antibiotics may be prescribed if an infectious process is suspected; ventilatory support may be necessary in severe cases

◥ *Beta-adrenergic blockers should be avoided in persons with COPD.*

✎ What are important nursing actions in the care of a patient with COPD?

1. Place the patient in high Fowler's position to facilitate breathing.
2. Administer oxygen, if ordered by the physician.
3. Monitor respiratory status (respiratory effort, oxygen saturation level) at regular intervals.
4. Instruct the patient to increase fluid intake to 3 L/day to thin secretions, unless contraindicated.
5. Provide frequent rest periods and teach energy conservation methods.
6. Administer medications (bronchodilators, oxygen, antibiotics) as ordered by the physician.
7. Monitor blood studies for complete blood count (polycythemia), electrolyte levels (potassium, magnesium, and calcium may be lowered as a result of therapy), and theophylline levels periodically during therapy.
8. Monitor the patient for complications, such as worsening respiratory status or infections, and notify the physician immediately if any develop.
9. Educate the patient about long-term care of COPD. Instruct him on the use of a metered dose inhaler or other device. Demonstrate how to clean inhalers and how to determine if they are empty.
10. Educate the patient about the use of oxygen, if appropriate. Also, educate him about prevention and treatment of acute exacerbation of COPD, pulmonary hygiene, such as coughing and deep breathing, pursed lip breathing, diaphragmatic breathing, and medications.
11. Encourage adequate nutrition such as five or six small, high-calorie, high-protein meals per day (to prevent early satiety and malnutrition). Instruct the patient to consume high-calorie foods first and encourage the use of butter, mayonnaise, and sauces for additional calories. Avoid gas-forming foods (impede diaphragmatic movement) and foods that require a lot of chewing.
12. Strongly encourage smoking cessation. Discuss options of nicotine replacement therapies (patches, gum) and cessation programs. Encourage the patient to set a stop date.

13. Encourage exercise 3 to 5 times per week, particularly aerobic, strengthening, and flexibility. Remind the patient that walking is great exercise.
14. Promote stress reduction and teach relaxation exercises.
15. Encourage flu vaccine yearly and pneumococcal pneumonia vaccine every 8 to 10 years.

ASTHMA

✎ What's asthma?

A condition characterized by hyperactive airways with episodes of bronchospasms that are typically initiated by respiratory infections (most common), allergic reactions, inhalation of irritants, exercise, or stress; a prolonged expiratory phase results from airway narrowing

What's the patho-physiologic process of asthma?

Hyperresponsiveness of the airways to an initiating stimulus (allergen or nonallergen) causes mast cells to release a variety of mediators (histamine, leukotrienes), which produce an inflammatory reaction in which the airway diameter is reduced and airway resistance is increased

✎ What are the clinical manifestations of asthma?

Dyspnea, wheezing, cough, and chest tightness, which usually worsens with exercise or on exposure to allergens and pollutants

✎ What complications are associated with asthma?

Pneumonia, atelectasis, pneumothorax, status asthmaticus (a life-threatening asthma attack of prolonged duration) with possible respiratory arrest and death

What's the typical treatment for asthma?

Bronchodilators such as beta$_2$ agonists by metered dose inhaler (MDI) or handheld nebulizer is the mainstay of therapy. Severe respiratory distress may require administration of corticosteroids, oxygen, and intubation with mechanical ventilation. Treatment is typically guided by peak expiratory flow rate, pulse oximetry, and arterial blood gas results.

▨ *Short-acting beta$_2$ agonists, such as albuterol, are used as rescue medications as they provide quick relief of bronchospasm: up to three treatments of 2 to 4 puffs at 20-minute intervals or a single nebulized treatment.*

What medications should be avoided in persons with asthma?

Non-selective beta-adrenergic blockers such as propranolol

✎ **What are important nursing actions in the care of a patient with asthma?**

1. Place the patient in high Fowler's position during exacerbations to facilitate breathing.
2. Administer medications (bronchodilators, corticosteroids, oxygen) as ordered by the physician.
3. Monitor respiratory status, including breath sounds, oxygenation status, respiratory rate, and use of accessory muscles.
4. Encourage breathing in through the nose and slow expiration through pursed lips.
5. Encourage effective diaphragmatic coughing.
6. Monitor the patient for complications, including worsening respiratory distress or pulmonary infections.
7. Educate the patient about long-term management of asthma. Desensitization (allergy shots) may be indicated. Instruct him on the use peak flow meters, inhalers, and MDIs as well as on the importance of regular mouthpiece cleaning to prevent infections (candida).
8. Instruct the patient to avoid asthma triggers by cleaning the house regularly to minimize dust and pet dander; using synthetic bedding materials; washing linens and mattress pads weekly in hot water; controlling house mites by encasing pillows, mattresses, and box springs in allergen-impermeable covers; removing stuffed toys, upholstered furniture, and carpets from the bedroom; closing windows during pollen season; and maintaining a low humidity environment (40% to 50%) with a dehumidifier.
9. Develop an Asthma Action Plan, which defines peak flow zones (green, yellow, and red). It should also address what the patient should do in case of worsening symptoms at 50% to 80% (yellow zone) of personal best peak flow. Instruct the patient to seek urgent medical care if rescue therapy doesn't work and peak flow is less than 50% of personal best (red zone).

CYSTIC FIBROSIS

What's cystic fibrosis (CF)?

An autosomal recessive disease in which abnormal function of the exocrine glands of the lungs, pancreas, and sweat (apocrine) glands produce copious amounts of abnormally thick secretions

What's the pathophysiologic process of CF?

The exocrine glands' ducts become obstructed by the thick secretions produced; this obstructive process eventually causes fibrosis of the distal glands.

✎ What are the clinical manifestations of CF?

Delayed growth in childhood, a chronic cough with production of mucus, tachypnea, clubbing, steatorrhea (fatty bowel movements), high sodium and chloride concentrations in sweat (due to sweat duct's inability to reabsorb chloride)

✎ What complications are associated with CF?

Malabsorption of fats, protein and fat-soluble vitamins; recurrent pulmonary infections (bronchitis, pneumonia); hemoptysis; pneumothorax (due to bleb rupture); diabetes mellitus (if fibrosis affects islets of Langerhans); biliary cirrhosis (if liver involved); cor pulmonale; and death

What's the typical treatment of CF?

1. Aerosol and nebulization treatments with N-acetylcysteine (Mucomyst) and bronchodilators (beta$_2$ agonists, theophylline)
2. Chest physiotherapy (percussion, vibration, postural drainage)
3. Pancreatic enzyme replacements, such as Creon and Pancrease
4. Fat-soluble vitamin supplements (A, D, E, and K)
5. Antibiotics, if bacterial infection is known or suspected

✎ What are important nursing actions in the care of a patient with CF?

1. Provide frequent rest periods throughout the day.
2. Encourage aerobic exercise as tolerated for airway clearance.
3. Encourage adequate intake of high-calorie foods.
4. Encourage adequate fluid intake to thin secretions and encourage replacement of salt losses, especially during hot weather and excessive sweating.
5. Provide chest physiotherapy.
6. Administer medications (bronchodilators, pancreatic enzymes, fat-soluble vitamins) as ordered by the physician.
7. Monitor the patient for complications (pulmonary infections, hemoptysis, pneumothorax), and notify the physician immediately if any develop.

Cancers of the respiratory system

LARYNGEAL CANCER

What's laryngeal cancer?

A condition characterized by malignant cells within the tissues of the larynx. Tumors can develop in any of the three regions of the larynx: the glottis, supraglottis, or subglottis; prolonged use of tobacco, prolonged consumption of alcohol, and prolonged exposure to some noxious fumes and chemicals are risk factors; a genetic predisposition and viral etiology are suspected

What's the pathophysiologic process of laryngeal cancer?

Cells within the tissues of the larynx exhibit abnormal cellular growth and differentiation, resulting in tumor formation

What are the clinical manifestations of laryngeal cancer?

Sore throat, painful swallowing, referred ear pain, hoarseness or change in voice quality (if vocal cords affected), a sensation of a lump in the throat, dyspnea, a palpable neck mass, tracheal deviation, stridor, and lymphadenopathy in the neck

What complications are associated with laryngeal cancer?

Malnutrition (from swallowing difficulty), respiratory distress, metastatic disease, and death

What's the typical treatment for laryngeal cancer?

1. Radiation and chemotherapy
2. Surgery — removal of part of the vocal cords (cordectomy) or hemi-laryngectomies (partial laryngectomy) for early vocal cord lesions; total laryngectomy with modified or radical neck dissection (removal of cancerous lymph nodes and other structures in the head and neck to minimize metastasis) with skin grafting is used for advanced lesions; chemotherapy may be used after surgical interventions

What complications are associated with surgical procedures performed for head and neck cancer?

A cordectomy or hemi-laryngectomy may result in hoarseness, and a total laryngectomy results in no natural voice (permanent tracheostomy is required). A radical neck dissection can result in stooped shoulders, limitation of head and neck rotation, and restricted arm movements due to damage to nerves, muscles, and veins in the neck.

✎ What are important nursing actions in the care of a patient with laryngeal cancer?

1. Place the patient in semi-Fowler's position to minimize edema and tension on suture line during the postoperative period.
2. Obtain vital signs at frequent intervals, especially temperature and blood pressure (risk of infection and hemorrhage) during the postoperative period.
3. Monitor viability of the skin graft (if used with the neck dissection) per facility protocol.
4. Provide tracheostomy care, if tracheostomy was performed. Keep extra laryngectomy and tracheostomy tubes with obturator at the patient's bedside at all times.
5. Establish an alternate method of communication, such as a writing pad, for the patient to use during the postoperative period.

6. Provide the patient meticulous mouth care during the preoperative period. Encourage saline gargles, sucking on ice, topical viscous lidocaine or mouthwashes or oral anesthetic sprays for sore throat. Provide increased fluid intake and the use of humidifiers, artificial saliva, chewing gum or hard candy to minimize dry mouth (salivary glands may be affected). Provide frequent mouth suction postoperatively (patient can't swallow).

7. Monitor the patient for complications of the condition (malnutrition) or its treatment (wound infection, hemorrhage), and notify the physician if any develop.

8. Monitor the patient's nutritional status. Postoperatively, a feeding tube will likely be in place for nutritional support while the wound is healing. After the tube is removed, the patient is at risk for aspiration and should be monitored closely.

9. Educate the patient about stoma care. The site around the stoma should be cleaned daily and the laryngectomy tube should be cleaned every 4 to 5 days. Instruct the patient to cover the stoma with his hand or a tissue when coughing, avoid swimming, wear plastic or rubber collar when in shower, and increase fluid intake, especially during hot weather.

10. Inform the patient of the need to perform Valsalva's maneuver to swallow after surgery (compensates for loss of epiglottis).

11. Instruct the patient to avoid sun exposure to the neck area.

12. Consult speech pathologist so that esophageal speech where air is "burped" can be taught. Mechanical devices, which are placed against the neck or cheek, may also be used.

13. Encourage smoking cessation and avoiding alcohol and chewing tobacco.

LUNG CANCER

What's lung cancer?

A condition characterized by abnormal cell growth and differentiation within the lung tissue or parenchyma; smoking accounts for approximately 85% of the cases, although exposure to secondhand smoke, asbestos, or radon gas also increases the risk

What's the pathophysiologic process of lung cancer?

Bronchogenic carcinoma arises from the bronchial mucosa as a result of chronic injury or damage to the mucosa, most commonly from cigarette smoke or environmental toxins. Chronic damage to the bronchial mucosa results in excessive proliferation of the bronchial cell, chronic inflammation, and DNA damage—all of which promote the development of cancer.

How is lung cancer categorized?

1. *Small-cell:* aggressive metastasis; occurs predominantly in smokers
2. *Non-small-cell:* more common; further divided into squamous cell, adenocarcinoma, and large cell carcinoma

What are the clinical manifestations of lung cancer?

Although lung cancer typically produces no symptoms in the initial phase, a chronic cough, hemoptysis, chest pain, dyspnea, fatigue, anorexia, and weight loss typically develop later in the course of the disease. Headaches, bone pain, and lymphadenopathy can occur secondary to metastatic disease.

What complications are associated with lung cancer?

Pneumonia, metastatic disease, and death

What's the typical treatment for lung cancer?

1. Surgical resection (wedge resection, lobectomy, pneumonectomy) if tumor is confined.
2. Chemotherapy (with or without radiation treatment), depending on size and staging of tumor

What are important nursing actions in the care of a patient with lung cancer?

1. Encourage smoking cessation. Discuss options of nicotine patches or chewing gum and the use of antidepressants, such as bupropion (Wellbutrin, Zyban), to facilitate smoking cessation.
2. Provide skin care for patients receiving radiation treatment. Avoid removing any radiation markings.
3. Encourage adequate intake of high-calorie foods.
4. Administer medications (oxygen, opioid analgesics) as ordered by the physician.
5. Provide frequent rest periods to minimize fatigue.
6. Monitor the patient for complications of the disease process (respiratory distress, hypercalcemia) or its treatment (leukopenia, increased risk of infections).
7. Encourage close medical follow-up.

Pharmacology related to the respiratory system

Treatment of allergies

ANTIHISTAMINES

✎ How do antihistamines work?

Selectively blocks or antagonizes H_1-receptors in the periphery and prevents histamine release

What are examples of antihistamines?

Cetirizine (Zyrtec), desloratidine (Clarinex), diphenhydramine (Benadryl), chlorpheniramine (Chlor-Trimeton), clemastine (Tavist), fexofenadine (Allegra), loratadine (Claritin), cetirizine/pseudoephedrine (Zyrtec-D), fexofenadine/pseudoephedrine (Allegra-D), loratadine/pseudoephedrine (Claritin-D)

✎ What are the most common adverse reactions of antihistamines?

Dry mouth, sedation (especially diphenhydramine), fatigue, paradoxical excitement (restlessness, nervousness), hypertension, tachycardia, palpitations, and thickened bronchial secretions

What life-threatening reactions are associated with antihistamines?

Seizures, hematologic abnormalities (such as thrombocytopenia), and anaphylactic shock (particularly with diphenhydramine)

⚡ *Avoid antihistamines in persons with cardiovascular disease, narrow angle glaucoma, bladder neck obstruction, or benign prostatic hyperplasia.*

✎ What are important nursing actions when administering an antihistamine?

1. Assess for hypertension, cardiovascular disease, prostatic hyperplasia, and increased intraocular pressure before administration of antihistamine.
2. Monitor for changes in cardiovascular system, such as palpitations, tachycardia, and blood pressure alterations.
3. Monitor for excessive sedation.
4. Inform the patient of hazards in driving or other activities that could be dangerous if the antihistamine causes drowsiness. Instruct him to avoid alcohol (increases central nervous system depression).
5. Encourage the use of hard candy, sugarless gum, or ice chips to treat dry mouth.
6. Instruct the patient to monitor his heart rate and blood pressure at home for long-term antihistamine use and to report any significant elevations.
7. Encourage the use of sun block to protect from photosensitivity reactions (diphenhydramine, loratadine).

DECONGESTANTS

How do decongestants work?	Stimulate vasoconstriction in mucous membranes within nasal passages, which increases the patency of the airway and improves ventilation
What's an example of a decongestant?	Pseudoephedrine (Drixoral, Sudafed, Afrin)
🖋 **What are the common adverse reactions with a decongestant?**	Dry mouth, restlessness, nervousness, tremor, tachycardia, palpitations, and difficulty urinating
What life-threatening reactions are associated with decongestants?	Arrhythmias

🖋 **What are important nursing actions when administering a decongestant?**

1. Assess the patient for hypertension, cardiovascular disease, diabetes, glaucoma, hyperthyroidism, and prostatic hyperplasia, before administration of a decongestant.
2. Assess vital signs for blood pressure and heart rate.
3. Monitor the patient for palpitations, tachycardia, and arrhythmias.
4. Inform the patient that decongestants shouldn't be taken within 2 hours of bedtime (risk of insomnia).
5. Instruct the patient to monitor his blood pressure and heart rate periodically and to report significant elevations to the physician.

Treatment of asthma and COPD

BRONCHODILATORS

How do bronchodilators work?

1. *Beta$_2$ agonists:* stimulate relaxation of bronchial smooth muscle
2. *Anticholinergics:* inhibit bronchoconstrictive effects of acetylcholine within the large airways
3. *Xanthines:* produce relaxation of smooth muscles of bronchial airways and pulmonary vasculature by inhibiting phosphodiesterase; chemically related to caffeine

> 🔖 *Because beta$_2$ agonists exert their effects rapidly, they're typically only used for rescue therapy.*

What are examples of bronchodilators?

1. *Beta₂ agonists:* albuterol (Proventil, Ventolin), salmeterol (Serevent), metaproterenol (Alupent), pirbuterol (Maxair), and isoproterenol (Isuprel)
2. *Anticholinergics:* ipratropium (Atrovent)
3. *Xanthines:* theophylline (Theo-Dur, Uniphyl, Slo-Phyllin)

✎ What adverse reactions are associated with bronchodilators?

1. *Beta₂ agonists:* tachycardia, hyperactivity, anxiety, restlessness, tremor, palpitations
2. *Anticholinergics:* headache, nervousness, dizziness, bad taste in mouth
3. *Xanthines:* similar to caffeine (tachycardia, anxiety, diuresis, tremor, insomnia) and many drug interactions

⚡ *Regular and frequent use of beta₂ agonists can actually worsen asthma.*

What life-threatening reactions are associated with bronchodilators?

Bronchospasms (beta₂ agonists), tachyarrhythmia, and seizures

✎ What's a therapeutic range for theophylline levels?

10 to 20 mcg/ml

What clinical manifestations are associated with theophylline toxicity?

Nausea, vomiting, tachycardia, arrhythmias, and seizures

✎ What are important nursing actions when administering bronchodilators?

1. Assess the patient for cardiovascular disease, hypertension, hyperthyroidism, and diabetes mellitus before administration of beta₂ agonists.
2. Monitor for complications of therapy, including bronchospasms (beta₂ agonists).
3. Educate the patient about the proper use of metered dose inhalers, dried powder inhaler, or nebulizer, including how to tell if the canister is empty. Instruct him to wait 2 minutes between inhalations.
4. Instruct the patient to use beta₂ agonists (albuterol) for rescue therapy when wheezing, shortness of breath, chest tightness, and cough occur. Instruct him to use this medication just before exercise or exposure to known triggers. Reinforce that salmeterol (Serevent), inhaled corticosteroids (triamcinolone, beclomethasone, fluticasone), theophylline, and anticholinergics (Ipratropium) shouldn't be used for rescue therapy.
5. Monitor theophylline levels periodically during therapy (if used); goal is 10 to 20 mcg/ml.

6. Inform the patient of the potential for many drug interactions with theophylline. Encourage him to contact his physician before takir g any new medications, including over-the-counter preparations.

INHALED CORTICOSTEROIDS

How do inhaled corticosteroids work?

By anti-inflammatory actions that minimize mucosal edema, coughing, wheezing and dyspnea

What are examples of inhaled corticosteroids?

Triamcinolone (Azmacort), beclomethasone (Beclovent, Vanceril), fluticasone (Flovent), budesonide (Pulmicort), and flunisolide (AeroBid)

What adverse reactions are associated with inhaled corticosteroids?

Oral candidiasis (thrush), hoarseness, and sore throat

What life-threatening reactions are associated with inhaled corticosteroids?

Bronchospasm and angioedema

What are important nursing actions when administering inhaled corticosteroids?

1. Instruct the patient to rinse his mouth and gargle after each inhaler use.
2. Instruct the patient to clean the inhaler periodically with soap and warm water.
3. Inform the patient that inhaled corticosteroids aren't to be used as rescue therapy.
4. Assess oral mucosa for evidence of fungal infection (white, flaky patches).
5. Instruct the patient to wait 1 to 2 minutes between inhalations.

MAST CELL STABILIZERS

How do mast cell stabilizers work?

By preventing histamine release

What's an example of a mast cell stabilizer?

Cromolyn (Intal)

What adverse reactions are associated with mast cell stabilizers?

Throat and tracheal irritation, sneezing, bad taste in mouth, cough, urinary frequency

What life-threatening reactions are associated with mast cell stabilizers?	Angioedema and bronchospasm

What are important nursing actions when administering a mast cell stabilizer?

1. Inform the patient that corticosteroid inhalers shouldn't be used as a rescue medication, due to their delayed response.
2. Inform the patient that complete effects of drug therapy may take 4 weeks.

LEUKOTRIENE MODIFIERS

How do leukotriene modifiers work?

By inhibiting leukotriene production, thereby preventing bronchoconstriction, reducing edema, and decreasing production of mucus

What are examples of leukotriene modifiers?

Montelukast (Singulair) and zafirlukast (Accolate)

What adverse reactions are associated with leukotriene modifiers?

Dry mouth, drowsiness, and headache

What life-threatening reactions are associated with leukotriene modifiers?

Hepatotoxicity

What are important nursing actions when administering leukotriene modifiers?

1. Instruct the patient to take zafirlukast 1 hour before or 2 hours after meals.
2. Emphasize the importance of daily use.
3. Inform the patient that leukotriene modifiers aren't effective as rescue medications.

Treatment of coughs

ANTITUSSIVES

How do antitussives work?

Suppress coughs by acting on the cough center in the medulla

What are examples of antitussives?

1. *Nonopioids:* dextromethorphan (Robitussin DM), benzonatate (Tessalon, Tessalon Perles)
2. *Opioids:* codeine and hydrocodone

What adverse reactions are associated with antitussives?	1. *Opioid:* sedation, abuse potential, respiratory depression, nausea, constipation 2. *Nonopioid:* occasional drowsiness, dizziness
✎ **What life-threatening reactions are associated with antitussives?**	Respiratory depression with opioid combinations
What are important nursing actions when administering an antitussive?	1. Assess frequency and nature of cough as well as the type and amount of sputum produced. Auscultate breath sounds. 2. Advise the patient to seek medical attention if cough lasts for more than 1 week or is accompanied by a fever, chest pain, persistent headache, or increased productive sputum. 3. Instruct the patient to avoid hazardous activities (driving) until response to drug is known (with opioid use). 4. Instruct the patient to avoid other irritants such as smoking. 5. Encourage the patient to maintain adequate hydration to thin secretions.

EXPECTORANTS

How do expectorants work?	Facilitate production of secretions from respiratory tract
What are examples of expectorants?	Guaifenesin (Robitussin, Humibid L.A.) and dornase alpha (Pulmozyme)
What are the most common adverse reactions to expectorants?	Occasional nausea, dizziness, headache, and drowsiness
What are important nursing actions when administering an expectorant?	1. Assess lung sounds, frequency and type of cough, and character of secretions. 2. Maintain adequate hydration of 2 L/day to thin secretions. 3. Instruct the patient to inform the physician or other health care professional if cough lasts more than 1 week.

Nursing skills

Chest physiotherapy and postural drainage

What activities comprise chest physiotherapy (PT)?

Chest percussion, vibration, and postural drainage

What's the purpose of chest PT and postural drainage?

Mobilization and drainage of areas of the lung to prevent atelectasis and pneumonia; commonly used in the management of cystic fibrosis, bronchiectasis, and chronic obstructive pulmonary disease; may also be used postoperatively

What's the proper technique for chest PT and postural drainage?

1. Administer bronchodilators before treatment and assess breath sounds.
2. Use breath sounds, chest X-ray, and physical therapy or physician referral to determine which lobes are to be drained and the best position in which to drain.
3. Perform chest PT in the correct sequence: postural drainage (usually starting with the most dependent lobes first), percussion, and vibration.
4. Correctly position the patient to facilitate drainage.
5. Position yourself so that you can see the patient's face while you're percussing.
6. If possible, have the patient assume positions that allow for drainage of the affected lung areas for 5 to 15 minutes each before starting percussion.
7. Instruct the patient to breathe in through his nose slowly and out through pursed lips.
8. While the patient is in position to facilitate drainage, percuss 1 to 2 minutes over the lung area with cupped hands. Avoid percussing over uncovered skin, breast, spine, sternum, and kidneys.

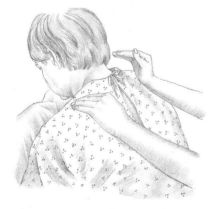

9. For vibration, firmly press your fingers and palms of your hands over the area that was percussed. With arms straight, lean into the patient. Using an isometric action or vibration, apply moderate pressure during the patient's expiratory phase. Repeat for about 3 breaths.

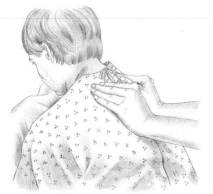

10. Encourage diaphragmatic coughing after each exhalation.
11. Assess breath sounds.

When are the best times to perform chest PT and postural drainage?

Upon arising and before bedtime or as ordered by the physician

When should chest PT and postural drainage be avoided?

For 1½ to 2 hours after meals

What are potential complications associated with chest PT and postural drainage?

Hypoxemia, dyspnea, and vomiting (especially if performed after eating)

Immediately place the patient in an upright position in the event of hypoxemia or dyspnea during chest PT.

Pulse oximetry

What's the purpose of pulse oximetry?

To monitor the patient's oxygen saturation either intermittently or continuously

How does a pulse oximeter work?

A beam of light passes through tissue and measures the absorption of light by the oxyhemoglobin. Blood that's well oxygenated (red) absorbs light differently than blood that is deoxygenated (blue). The machine provides a digital reading of pulse and oxygen saturation.

What's the proper technique for obtaining a pulse oximetry reading?

1. Assess for any factors that may give inaccurate (low) readings, such as fingernail polish and cold hands.
2. Apply the probe (may be similar to a pinch type clothespin) to a finger, earlobe, bridge of the nose, or forehead.
3. Note the reading displayed and document it in the patient's chart. Notify the physician if the reading is less than 91%, or as orders or facility policy mandate.

Aside from decreased oxygen saturation in the blood, what other factors might cause low readings?

Fingernail polish or acrylic nails, cold hands, and poor perfusion, and dark skin color

What's a normal reading?

Oxygen saturation greater than 91%

◤ *Results less than 86% should be reported to the physician immediately.*

Arterial blood gas analysis

What's an arterial blood gas (ABG) analysis?

A blood test used to determine the levels of various gases in the arterial blood, primarily oxygen and carbon dioxide; an ABG analysis is useful in the assessment of a patient's oxygenation and acid-base statuses

What are the indications for obtaining an ABG analysis?

Assess acid-base balance, assess ventilation status and need for or adjustment of oxygen therapy, evaluate the patient's response to treatments or therapy, and a change in ventilator setting or response to weaning of a ventilator

✎ What are the primary components of an ABG analysis?

1. *pH:* indicates normal, acidotic or alkalotic state
2. *Pao_2:* partial pressure of oxygen dissolved in the blood; indicative of tissue oxygenation
3. *$Paco_2$:* partial pressure of carbon dioxide in the blood; representative of the respiratory component of acid-base regulation
4. *Bicarbonate (HCO_3^-):* amount of HCO_3^- in the blood; representative of the renal or metabolic component of acid-base regulation
5. *Sao_2:* the percentage of oxygen carried by the hemoglobin relative to the amount it can carry

✎ **What are typical ABG values?**

1. *pH:* 7.35 to 7.45
2. *Pao$_2$:* 85 to 100 mm Hg
3. *Paco$_2$:* 35 to 45 mm Hg
4. *HCO$_3$$^-$:* 22 to 26 mEq/L
5. *Sao$_2$:* 94% to 98%

✎ **What are key points to remember when interpreting ABG results?**

1. *Acidosis:* increased hydrogen ions; decreased pH (less than 7.35)
2. *Alkalosis:* decreased hydrogen ions; increased pH (greater than 7.45)
3. *Respiratory disturbance:* change in Paco$_2$ matches the change in the pH
4. *Metabolic disturbance:* change in HCO$_3$$^-$ matches the change in the pH
5. *Compensation:* unaffected system attempts to restore acid-base balance

What's the nurse's role in assisting with ABG analysis?

1. Indicate the percentage of oxygen or liter flow that the patient is receiving. Avoid changing the level of oxygen or performing interventions that would likely change the patient's oxygen level 20 minutes before ABG levels are obtained (suctioning, exercising).
2. Obtain a cup of ice.
3. Assist with positioning of the arm (for radial blood draw).
4. Make sure blood is obtained in a heparinized syringe.
5. Immediately place the blood-filled syringe in the cup of ice.
6. Apply firmly pressure to the puncture site for at least 5 minutes, longer for a patient taking anticoagulants.
7. Apply a pressure bandage (if indicated) at the puncture site.

Sputum studies

What's the purpose of sputum studies?

Identify an infecting organism via culture and determine the sensitivity to various antibiotics; may also be performed to identify the presence of malignant cells

What are the indications for a sputum study?

Development of purulent secretions or to aid in the diagnosis of lung cancer

By what methods can a sputum sample be obtained?

Expectoration, endotracheal suctioning, and bronchoscopy

What's the proper technique for obtaining a sputum sample by expectoration?

1. Obtain the proper sterile collection container.
2. Perform mouth care for the patient.
3. Instruct the patient in diaphragmatic breathing and coughing to facilitate expectoration.
4. Collect a specimen in the appropriate container, and make sure the specimen is mucoidlike and not saliva.
5. Label the specimen and send to the laboratory promptly.

⚡ *Sputum for cytology must be collected in the early morning and usually requires a container with a special preservative.*

Peak flow meters

✎ **What's a peak flow meter and what does it measure?**

A handheld device that provides an objective measure of the relative degree of airway obstruction; it requires the patient take a maximal inspiration (preferably in a standing position) and quickly and forcefully blow into the device to attain the peak expiratory flow

New readings are compared to the patient's current "personal best" reading. Less than 80% may indicate a need for additional therapy and less than 50% indicates an emergency situation.

How are peak flow measurements obtained?

1. Connect the mouthpiece to the peak flow meter and set the marker to the bottom of the scale.
2. Instruct the patient to take a deep breath, place his lips tightly around the mouthpiece, and exhale as hard and fast as possible.
3. Note the position of the marker on the numeric scale after complete exhalation.
4. Repeat the process two more times and report the highest reading of the three.

16

The cardiovascular system

Basic concepts of the cardiovascular system

The heart

What are the layers of the heart?

1. *Epicardium:* the outer protective layer of the heart that consists of connective tissue covered by epithelium; contains blood and lymph capillaries as well as nerve fibers
2. *Myocardium:* the relatively thick middle layer that consists primarily of cardiac muscle tissue, which is responsible for the pumping action of the heart
3. *Endocardium:* inner layer that lines all of the heart chambers and covers heart valves; contains many elastic and collagenous fibers; is continuous with the intima of the blood vessels

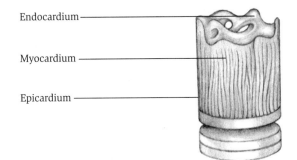

Endocardium

Myocardium

Epicardium

What's the pericardial sac?

A fibrous sac of double walls that contains a lubricating fluid between the layers

What are the four chambers of the heart?

1. *Right atrium:* site where blood enters heart through the vena cava
2. *Right ventricle:* pumps blood into the lungs via the pulmonary artery for gas exchange within the pulmo-

nary vasculature before the pulmonary veins carry the blood into the left atrium

3. *Left atrium:* pumps blood through the mitral valve into the left ventricle

4. *Left ventricle:* forcefully pumps blood into the systemic circulation through the aortic valve and into the aorta

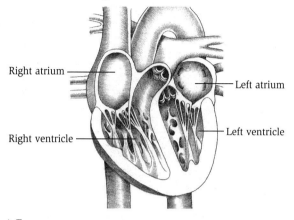

Right atrium

Left atrium

Right ventricle

Left ventricle

▧ *Although the same events occur on the right and left sides of the heart, pressures are lower on the right.*

▧ *The ventricles are the more muscular chambers of the heart, which contract with a twisting motion, squeezing blood into arteries.*

✎ **What are the valves of the heart?**

1. *Tricuspid valve:* separates the right atrium from the right ventricle
2. *Mitral:* separates the left atrium and left ventricle
3. *Pulmonic:* separates the right ventricle and pulmonary artery
4. *Aortic:* separates the left ventricle and the aorta

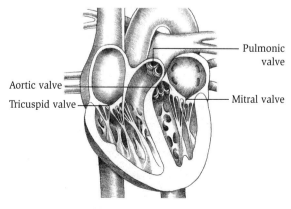

Aortic valve

Tricuspid valve

Pulmonic valve

Mitral valve

▶ *The sympathetic and parasympathetic nervous systems are in constant opposition with one another in order to regulate the heart rate.*

What's the cardiac cycle?

The series of electromechanical events consisting of two phases (systole and diastole) that occur during an individual heartbeat; each cardiac cycle lasts approximately 0.8 seconds and covers the period from the end of one cardiac contraction to the end of the subsequent cardiac contraction

▶ *Although the atria and ventricles act simultaneously, they function as separate units because they enter systole and diastole at different times: when the atria are in systole, the ventricles are in diastole.*

▶ *Blood tends to flow from an area of high pressure to one of lower pressure.*

What's systole?

The period of ventricular contraction

What's diastole?

The period of ventricular relaxation; usually lasts longer than systole

▶ *Seventy-five percent of ventricular filling occurs during diastole.*

▶ *Contraction and relaxation of the heart muscle produces sequential pressure changes within the chambers of the heart and the blood vessels, which results in the orderly passage of blood.*

What's the sinoatrial (SA) node?

A group of specialized conduction cells located in the superior aspect of the right atrium that trigger a heart beat about once every 0.8 seconds; commonly known as the pacemaker of the heart for its ability to spontaneously generate an action potential; depolarization of the SA node marks the beginning of the cardiac cycle; the SA node regulates the heart rate at 60 to 100 beats/minute

What's the atrioventricular (AV) node?

A group of specialized conduction cells in the inferior aspect of the right atrium that serves as a bridge between the atria and ventricles; in the AV node, a delay (0.1 second) in the transmission of the electrical impulse from the atria to the ventricles occurs so that blood has time to empty out of the atria before the ventricles contract

What are the bundle branches?

Nerve fibers that carry electrical impulses from the AV node; divided into left and right bundle branches

What's the bundle of His?

Conduction fibers that transmit the electrical impulse at a rapid rate throughout the ventricular myocardium

What are Purkinje fibers?

Very large, specialized conduction fibers that transmit the electrical impulse from the AV node throughout the walls of both ventricles simultaneously; conduct action potential at six times the velocity of normal cardiac muscle

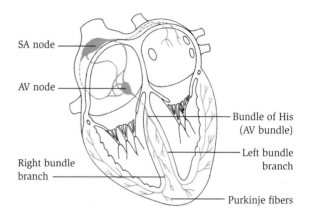

What are the coronary arteries?

The arteries that supply the cardiac muscle with oxygen-rich blood; any coronary artery disorder that reduces blood flow to the heart can result in myocardial infarction and, possibly, death

What are the two main coronary arteries?

The right coronary artery (RCA) and the left coronary artery (LCA)

What are the branches of the two main coronary arteries?

The RCA branches into the right posterior descending artery and a marginal branch, which provide blood to the ventricles, right atrium, and SA node; the LCA branches into the left anterior descending artery (LAD) and the circumflex branch, which supply blood to the front of the heart and the back of the heart, respectively; smaller divisions of the coronary arteries include the acute marginal, posterior descending, obtuse marginal, and diagonals

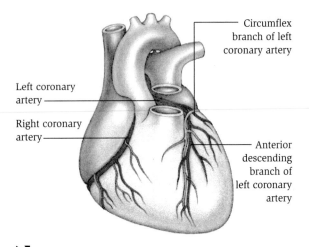

Left coronary artery

Right coronary artery

Circumflex branch of left coronary artery

Anterior descending branch of left coronary artery

The LAD is commonly referred to as the "widow maker" because it supplies blood to 75% of the left ventricle, and a sudden occlusion within this artery is usually fatal.

What's stroke volume?	The volume of blood ejected from each ventricle in a single beat at systole
What's cardiac output (CO)?	Stroke volume (SV) × heart rate (HR); CO is an important indicator of cardiac function; normal CO is 4 to 6 L/minute
What's cardiac index (CI)?	CO divided by body surface area; a normal CI is 2.5 to 4.0 L/minute/m²
Why is CI a better indicator of left ventricular function than CO?	CO varies according to body size, whereas CI does not.
What's preload?	Ventricular volume at the end of diastole, or the amount of stretch on the ventricular myocardium prior to its contraction; an increase in preload produces an increase in stroke volume; it's primarily dependent on venous blood return from the body
What's afterload?	The resistance to ventricular ejection, which is caused by the systemic vascular resistance (resistance to flow in the systemic circulation); stroke volume decreases as afterload increases
What's contractility?	The myocardium's ability to contract and empty the ventricle in the absence of a change in preload or afterload;

the sympathetic nervous system is the most critical influence on contractility

What's the ejection fraction (EF)?

An index of the contractile status of the heart; a normal EF is greater than 50% and can be measured by an echocardiogram or cardiac catheterization

What produces the characteristic "lub-dup" heart sounds?

Vibrations caused by closure of the heart valves in various parts of the cardiac cycle; the "lub" sound occurs at the beginning of systole and is due to the closure of the mitral and tricuspid valves; the "dup" sound marks the beginning of diastole and is due to the closure of the aortic and pulmonary valves

In a healthy heart, the only detectable heart sounds are those of closure of the valves.

What's an S_1?

The first heart sound, which is produced by closure of the mitral and tricuspid valves

The closure of the mitral and tricuspid valves occurs so closely together that they're commonly perceived as a single sound.

What's an S_2?

The second heart sound, which is produced by closure of the aortic and pulmonic valves; the interval between the closure of the two valves widens with inhalation

What's a pulse?

The rhythmic arterial expansion that's produced by the ejection of blood from the left ventricle

What's blood pressure?

The force exerted on the walls of arteries as blood is pumped through the body; a product of the cardiac output and total peripheral resistance (TPR) (blood pressure = cardiac output × TPR); blood pressure is measured with a sphygmomanometer and is described as systolic pressure over diastolic pressure

What's systolic blood pressure?

The point at which arterial blood pressure is at its highest level

What's diastolic blood pressure?

The point at which arterial blood pressure is at its lowest level

An increase in cardiac output usually produces an increase in systolic pressure. An increase in peripheral resistance (vasoconstriction) usually produces an increase in diastolic pressure.

⚡ *Because of the relationship between heart rate and cardiac output (heart rate × stroke volume = cardiac output), any factor that increases the heart rate will also increase the blood pressure, and any factor that increases the blood pressure will also increase the heart rate.*

What's the pulse pressure?

An important component of blood pressure; the difference between the systolic and diastolic blood pressures; reflective of the pulsatile nature of the arterial blood flow — typically about 40 mm Hg

✎ What are the two basic mechanisms for blood pressure regulation?

1. *Short-term:* regulation of blood vessel diameter, heart rate, and contractility
2. *Long-term:* regulation of blood volume, primarily via the conservation of body fluids through renal mechanisms and stimulation of water intake; involves renin-angiotensin-aldosterone mechanism and release of anti-diuretic hormone

What factors are involved in the short-term regulation of *rising* blood pressure?

Rising blood pressure stretches the arterial walls, stimulating baroreceptors, which send impulses to the brain. Parasympathetic activity is then increased and the sympathetic activity is decreased, which in turn decreases the heart rate, relaxes the vascular smooth muscle, and increases the arterial diameter. Blood pressure is lowered as a result.

What factors are involved in the short-term regulation of *decreasing* blood pressure?

Baroreceptors are inhibited by decreasing blood pressure, parasympathetic activity is decreased, and sympathetic activity is increased due to decreased impulses to the brain; heart rate, contractility, and vasoconstriction are increased due to release of epinephrine and norepinephrine by the adrenal glands; blood pressure is raised as a result.

✎ What factors are involved in the long-term regulation of low blood pressure?

Renin is released by the kidney juxtaglomerular cells in response to a drop in blood pressure. Renin binds to angiotensinogen, an inactive plasma protein, as it travels through the circulatory system. This binding process activates angiotensinogen to angiotensin I. Angiotensin I is converted to angiotensin II as it passes through the lung, and angiotensin II travels to the adrenal glands where it stimulates the release of aldosterone. Aldosterone then increases sodium reabsorption from the distal convoluted tubules; water follows the movement of sodium into the bloodstream, and blood volume and blood pressure are increased as a result. In addition, antidiuretic hormone (ADH) is released by the posterior pituitary in response to increased osmolarity (dehydration). ADH promotes water reabsorption in the kidney and stimulates the thirst center, which decrease the osmolarity of the blood volume and increases blood pressure.

The vascular system

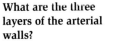 **What types of blood vessels comprise the vascular system?**

1. *Arteries:* carry oxygenated blood away from the heart; thick walls of three layers
2. *Capillaries:* are the site of exchange of water, macromolecules, metabolites, and waste products between blood and tissue; highly branched vessels of thin (single layer) walls
3. *Veins:* carry deoxygenated blood from the capillary bed towards the heart; contain valves to prevent backflow of blood; contain 70% of circulating blood volume

The pulmonary artery and pulmonary veins are the exception to the rule regarding arteries carrying oxygenated blood and veins carrying deoxygenated blood: the pulmonary artery carries deoxygenated blood to the pulmonary vasculature for gas exchange, the pulmonary veins carry oxygenated blood back to the heart from the pulmonary vasculature.

What are the three layers of the arterial walls?

Tunica adventitia, tunica media, and tunica intima

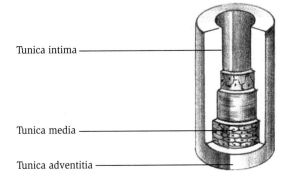

Tunica intima

Tunica media

Tunica adventitia

Physical assessment of the cardiovascular system

Normal findings

✎ At what sites are arterial pulses typically palpated?

Carotid, brachial, radial, femoral, popliteal, dorsalis pedis, and posterior tibial areas

How are arterial pulses palpated?

Via gentle palpation with the index and middle fingers over the location of the artery to be palpated; a systematic progression from head to toe should be used

⚡ *Light palpation is necessary so as not to obliterate the pulse.*

What features of the arterial pulse should be assessed?

Rate, rhythm, symmetry, contour, and strength at each arterial site

✎ What are the four primary cardiac auscultation sites?

1. *Aortic area:* second intercostal space along the right sternal border
2. *Pulmonic area:* second intercostal space at the left sternal border
3. *Tricuspid area:* fourth intercostal space along the left sternal border
4. *Mitral area:* fifth intercostal space near the midclavicular line

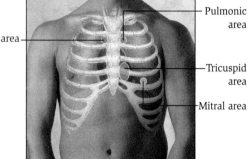

⚡ *Auscultation is the most important assessment technique for the cardiovascular system.*

In what positions should a patient be placed for cardiac auscultation?	1. Forward leaning best detects high-pitched sounds from aortic and pulmonic valves 2. Left lateral recumbent best detects low-pitched sounds from the mitral valve or extra heart sounds
 **What's the point of maximum impulse (PMI)?**	Located at the site at the midclavicular line in the fifth intercostal space, it's the location in which pulsations are best detected.

Abnormal findings

If an abnormal heart sound is detected on auscultation, what general physical assessments should be made?	Distension of jugular veins, abnormal respiratory sounds, and cyanosis
How is jugular vein distention (JVD) assessed?	1. Place the patient in semi-Fowler's position and expose the neck and thoracic areas. Jugular veins should *not* be prominent in this position if the right heart is functioning properly. Bilateral distention of the jugular veins in the semi-Fowler position is typically associated with advanced cardiopulmonary disease, while unilateral distention is more commonly associated with local obstruction. 2. Identify the highest visible point of distention of the internal jugular vein; measure from the sternal angle to this highest point to determine its vertical height. 3. Repeat this process on the other side of the patient's neck.
What's a murmur?	A blowing, whooshing, or rumbling sound that lasts longer than a heart sound and is the result of abnormal blood flow patterns; may be pathologic or benign and is generally associated with turbulent blood flow through the heart valves Conditions that can produce a murmur in adults include mitral insufficiency, mitral stenosis, aortic insufficiency, aortic stenosis, tricuspid insufficiency, tricuspid stenosis, pulmonic insufficiency, and pulmonic stenosis. Atrial and ventricular septal defects and patent ductus arteriosus are conditions that commonly cause murmurs in children.
How are murmurs classified?	1. *Intensity:* grade, volume, presence, or absence of a thrill 2. *Timing:* systolic or diastolic 3. *Shape:* crescendo, decrescendo, or holosystolic

> ◪ *Diastolic murmurs, such as mitral stenosis and aortic insufficiency, are usually pathologic; systolic murmurs aren't.*

✎ How is the intensity of a murmur graded?

On a scale of I to VI over VI; for example, I/VI would indicate a murmur that's barely detectable to the examiner, while a VI/VI would indicate a murmur that can still be heard when the stethoscope is completely off the chest

What's an ejection murmur?

An abnormal heart sound that results from the opening of the aortic and pulmonic valves during rapid ejection of blood out of the ventricles; an ejection murmur may be indicative of valve disease or intracardiac shunts

What's a split S_2?

The heart sound produced when the right and left ventricles contract at slightly different times; may be a normal variant in some persons, but it may also indicate left ventricular hypertrophy; an echocardiogram may be performed for further evaluation

✎ What's a gallop?

An abnormal heart rhythm marked by a low-pitched extra sound during diastole; usually referred to as S_3 or S_4

✎ What's an S_3?

The low-pitched third heart sound that results from the rapid ventricular filling during diastole; also referred to as a ventricular gallop; may be normal in children, but is usually associated with heart failure in adults

A left ventricular S_3 is best detected using the bell of the stethoscope during expiration with the patient in the left lateral decubitus position, whereas a right ventricular S_3 is best auscultated with the bell of the stethoscope over the left sternal border during inspiration.

✎ What's an S_4?

The low-pitched fourth heart sound that occurs secondary to atrial contraction against a noncompliant left ventricle; a presystolic heart sound best detected with the bell of the stethoscope; S_4 is commonly associated with systemic hypertension, aortic stenosis, hypertrophic cardiomyopathy, and ischemic heart disease; also referred to as an *atrial gallop*

What's a click?

A high-pitched abnormal heart sound auscultated at the apex during mid- to late systole; commonly precedes a late systolic murmur

✎ What are palpitations?

Sensation of skipped heart beats or of pounding or racing of the heart

✎ What's a pericardial friction rub?

A harsh scraping or creaking sound auscultated over the left third intercostal space; may occur during systole, diastole, or both

What's pulsus paradoxus?	An exaggerated inspiratory decrease in systolic blood pressure greater than 10 mm Hg (normal inspiratory drop is less than 10 mm Hg); occurs in association with cardiac tamponade
What's bradycardia?	A slow heart rate, generally less than 60 beats/minute
What's tachycardia?	A rapid heart rate; generally greater than 100 beats/minute
What's fibrillation?	An erratic, quivering of the myocardium that prevents the heart from effectively pumping blood
What's flutter?	A disorder characterized by extremely rapid yet regular contractions of the atria or ventricles; may produce no symptoms
What's ischemia?	Inadequate blood flow to tissues, resulting in oxygen deprivation; usually caused by a constriction or obstruction of an artery
What's an infarction?	An area of dead tissue caused by the obstruction of blood flow
What's valvular stenosis?	The inability of a valve to open to its normal position
What's valvular regurgitation or insufficiency?	The inability of a valve to effectively close and prevent the backward flow of blood
What's mitral valve prolapse?	A mild abnormality of the mitral valve in which the valve leaflets flap backwards as the heart contracts
What's Valsalva's maneuver?	A type of movement involving forcible exhalation while the mouth and nose remain closed (bearing down, as if having a bowel movement), which causes an increase in intrathoracic pressure and a slowing of the heart rate; can be used to diagnose certain cardiac abnormalities and to correct certain rapid heart beats; usually taught to persons with multiple sclerosis to aid in fully emptying the bladder

Valsalva's maneuver should be avoided in patient's with severe coronary artery disease, a recent history of myocardial infarction, or a significant reduction in blood volume.

What's arteriosclerosis?

The loss of vessel elasticity; commonly known as hardening of the arteries

What's atherosclerosis?

A form of arteriosclerosis characterized by the gradual accumulation of plaque or an atheroma, which causes the arteries to narrow and become less elastic; as a result, blood flow through the arteries is obstructed; a diet high in fat and cholesterol, smoking, diabetes, and hypertension accelerate the process of plaque formation and are risk factors for atherosclerosis; coronary artery disease is a form of atherosclerosis

What's an atheroma?

Atherosclerotic plaque consisting of deposits of fats, cholesterol, cellular debris, calcium, and fibrin

What's a bruit?

An abnormal, murmurlike heart sound associated with turbulent blood flow through a major vessel

What's a thrill?

A vibrating sensation similar to a cat purring that frequently accompanies a bruit and is also indicative of turbulent blood flow

What's a thrombus?

A blood clot consisting of platelets, fibrin, and possibly, other blood components that develop inside a blood vessel or within a cavity of the heart

What's an embolus?

A clot that moves through the circulatory system until it becomes lodged in a narrowed blood vessel where it blocks blood flow, producing ischemia beyond the site of obstruction; most emboli arise from thrombi, although fat, air bubbles, and plaque can also be considered emboli

What's an aneurysm?

A bulging, ballooning, or abnormal enlargement of an artery that results from damage to or weakness of the blood vessel wall; most occur in the abdomen (abdominal aortic aneurysm) or brain (cerebral aneurysm)

What's vasculitis?

A condition characterized by an inflammation of blood vessels, commonly the arteries; thickening, weakening, or scarring of the blood vessel wall can result; blood clots may develop

What are varicose veins?

Veins that are swollen, torturous, and bulging above the skin surface as a result of congestion within the vein due to weakness of its valve; may be dark blue or purple and are found most commonly on the lower extremities; genetics, hormones, pregnancy, obesity, and prolonged standing are contributing factors to the development of varicose veins

Major disorders of the heart

Hypercholesterolemia

What's hypercholesterolemia?

A condition characterized by elevated serum cholesterol levels (240 mg/dl or greater) that's associated with an increased risk for coronary heart disease and other atherosclerotic diseases such as thrombotic strokes

Hypercholesterolemia occurs in association with a genetic predisposition and excessive intake of saturated fat, trans fatty acid, and cholesterol (believed to decrease low density lipoprotein receptors in the liver). Long-term use of glucocorticoids, anabolic steroids, and progestins may also adversely affect cholesterol levels.

What's the pathophysiologic process of hypercholesterolemia?

Elevated serum cholesterol levels occur secondary to increased production of low-density lipoprotein (LDL) or decreased catabolism of LDL; the excess lipids then promote atherogenesis by attaching to a site of vessel injury and attracting clusters of monocytes, which contribute to the formation of fatty streaks

What are clinical manifestations of hypercholesterolemia?

Usually produces no symptoms and is typically found at the time of routine screening; xanthomas (slightly raised and yellow skin lesions that frequently are located on the eyelids) may indicate extreme hypertriglyceridemia

What's a normal total cholesterol level?

Below 200 mg/dl

A full lipid panel should be performed after the patient has fasted for 9 to 12 hours.

What are lipoproteins?

Fat-carrying proteins that encapsulate lipids for transportation in the blood; core contains cholesterol esters and triglycerides

Lipoproteins are classified according to the type and ratio of proteins to fats they contain. The size and density of lipoproteins are also determined by their protein and fat content.

What are the classes of lipoproteins?

1. *Chylomicrons:* formed in the intestine; transport fats from intestine to liver and adipose tissue
2. *Very low-density lipoproteins (VLDL):* produced by the liver; carry largest amounts of lipids (triglycerides); can be converted to low-density lipoproteins
3. *Low-density lipoproteins (LDL):* primary carriers of cholesterol, and as a result, are reflective of serum

cholesterol level; "bad cholesterol;" normal levels are considered to be below 160 mg/dl

4. *High-density lipoproteins (HDL):* cholesterol scavengers that remove excess cholesterol from peripheral tissues and carry it back to the liver for catabolism and excretion; HDL level above 40 mg/dl is considered a risk factor for coronary artery disease

◥ *VLDL and LDL lipoproteins are atherogenic.*

What complications are associated with hypercholesterolemia?

Increased risk for coronary artery disease and thrombotic strokes

What's the typical treatment for hypercholesterolemia?

1. *Dietary modifications:* fat intake less than 30% of calories, saturated fat less than 7% of calories, polyunsaturated fat 10% or less of calories, monounsaturated fat 10% to 15% of calories, carbohydrates 50% to 60% of calories, and cholesterol less than 200 mg/dl; include plant sterol and plant stanol esters, such as certain margarine substitutes (Benecol), omega-3 fatty acids, eicosapentaenoic acid (EPA) and docosahexaenoic acid (DHA)

2. *Pharmacologic agents:* statins, or HMG-CoA reductase inhibitors, such as atorvastatin (Lipitor), pravastatin (Pravachol), simvastatin (Zocor), fluvastatin (Lescol), and lovastatin (Mevacor); fibrates, such as fenofibrate (Tricor) and gemfibrozil (Lopid); bile acid sequestrants or resins, such as cholestyramine (Questran), colestipol (Colestid), and colesevelam (Welchol); niacin such as SR niacin (Niaspan, Niacor, Slo-Niacin); and cholesterol absorption inhibitors such as ezetimibe (Zetia)

◥ *Liver function tests should be obtained before initiation of statin therapy, at 6 and 12 weeks after initiation of therapy, and every 6 months thereafter. Statin drugs should be discontinued for elevation of transaminases (aspartate aminotransferase, alanine aminotransferase) that are more than three times higher than the upper limit of the normal range.*

✎ **What are important nursing actions in the care of a patient with hypercholesterolemia?**

1. Instruct the patient to consume foods low in cholesterol and saturated fat. High-fiber foods and complex carbohydrates should be encouraged as well as plant sterol and plant stanol esters such as certain margarine substitutes.

2. Encourage aerobic exercise (improves HDL and triglyceride levels).

3. Instruct the patient to take medications consistently as prescribed for optimal results.

4. Administer medications (statins, fibrates, niacin, bile acid sequestrants, and cholesterol absorption inhibitors) as ordered by the physician.
5. Monitor liver function tests periodically during statin therapy. Obtain baseline liver function tests prior to initiation of therapy, at 6 and 12 weeks after initiation, and every 6 months thereafter for 1 year.
6. Encourage routine medical follow-up.
7. Encourage smoking cessation to decrease risk of coronary artery disease.

Hypertension

What's hypertension?

A condition characterized by a chronic blood pressure that exceeds 140/90 mm Hg; primary or essential hypertension defines high blood pressure without an identifiable cause; secondary hypertension has a specific cause, such as another medical condition (typically renal disease) or a medication

Although the cause of hypertension is commonly multifactorial, the potential consequences are the same: end organ damage as a result of blood vessel damage, primarily involving the kidneys, heart, and brain.

What's the pathophysiologic process of hypertension?

Blood pressure is ultimately determined by the balance between cardiac output and vascular resistance. An uncompensated rise in one variable will produce an increase in the mean blood pressure. Untreated hypertension can damage the intima of blood vessels, predisposing them to atherosclerotic plaque deposition.

What are the risk factors for hypertension?

Positive family history, increased age, black race, obesity, sedentary lifestyle, high-salt diet, heavy alcohol consumption, and use of hormonal contraceptives; smoking, high cholesterol levels, diabetes, and left ventricular enlargement

How is hypertension classified?

1. *Prehypertension:* systolic blood pressure 120 to 139 or diastolic blood pressure 80 to 89 mm Hg
2. *Stage 1 hypertension:* systolic blood pressure 140 to 159 or diastolic blood pressure 90 to 99 mm Hg
3. *Stage 2 hypertension:* systolic blood pressure 160 or greater or diastolic blood pressure 100 mm Hg or greater

What are the clinical manifestations of hypertension?

Headaches, dizziness, and a pounding sensation of the heart as well as vision disturbances, nausea, vomiting, and chest pain in severe hypertension

✎ What complications are associated with hypertension?

Heart disease, myocardial infarction, heart failure, renal failure, peripheral vascular disease, retinopathy, or stroke

▰ *Untreated hypertension can damage the intima of blood vessels, which facilitates the accumulation of fats and calcium and the formation of an atherosclerotic plaque.*

▰ *The higher the blood pressure, the higher the risk of myocardial infarction, heart failure, renal disease, and stroke.*

What's the typical treatment for hypertension?

1. *Prehypertension:* although no antihypertensives are indicated, lifestyle modifications (sodium restriction, weight loss if obese, and stress reduction) should be encouraged
2. *Stage 1 hypertension:* diuretic therapy (usually thiazide) should be initiated with consideration of other agents (angiotensin-converting enzyme (ACE) inhibitors, angiotensin receptor blockers, beta-adrenergic blockers, and calcium channel blockers); lifestyle modifications should also be emphasized
3. *Stage 2 hypertension:* combination of two drugs (typically thiazide diuretic along with ACE inhibitor, angiotensin receptor blocker, beta-adrenergic blocker, or calcium channel blocker); lifestyle modifications should also be emphasized

✎ What are important nursing actions in the care of a patient with hypertension?

1. Instruct the patient to consume a low-salt, low-fat, and low-cholesterol diet. The consumption of omega-3 fatty acids (fish oil) should be encouraged.
2. Encourage healthy lifestyle modifications, such as weight loss if the paient is obese, and yoga, biofeedback, guided imagery, or meditation for stress reduction.
3. Encourage good diabetes control (insulin resistance and the resultant increase in blood insulin levels can cause sodium retention, which increases blood pressure). Instruct the patient to consume consistent amounts of carbohydrates.
4. Instruct the patient to take medications consistently.
5. Monitor for complications, such as myocardial infarction, renal dysfunction or failure, and stoke, and notify the physician immediately if any occur.
6. Educate the patient about the importance of close medical follow-up and routine blood pressure screenings.
7. Consider potassium, calcium, and magnesium supplementation.

Coronary artery disease

What's coronary artery disease (CAD)?

A form of atherosclerosis in which the coronary arteries (those that supply blood and oxygen to the heart muscle itself) become severely narrowed by plaques or atheromas

What's the pathophysiologic process of CAD?

A lipid-containing fatty streak becomes deposited in the intima of arteries, and macrophages are attracted to this area. Over time this area can become calcified, causing a decrease in the vessel's elasticity, or hardening of the arteries. Increased resistance to blood flow results, which causes an increase in blood pressure.

The lumen of a coronary artery must typically be reduced by 75% or more to significantly affect perfusion.

What are nonmodifiable risk factors for CAD?

Male gender, advanced age, positive family history of CAD, postmenopausal women, and black race

What are modifiable risk factors for CAD?

Cholesterol levels (particularly high low-density lipoproteins and low high-density lipoproteins), smoking, excessive alcohol use, uncontrolled hypertension, uncontrolled diabetes, sedentary lifestyle, obesity (more than 20% above ideal body weight), elevated homocysteine levels, elevated C-reactive protein, and uncontrolled stress or anger (type A personality)

Homocysteine is an amino acid; increased levels have been proven to cause premature development of cardiovascular disease and are associated with low levels of B vitamins and renal disease.

What are the clinical manifestations of CAD?

Usually produces no symptoms, but angina (especially with exertion), dyspnea, and claudication may occur

What complications are associated with CAD?

Angina, myocardial infarction, transient ischemic attack, or stroke

What's the typical treatment for CAD?

1. *Pharmacologic agents:* antilipemics (gemfibrozil, atorvastatin, simvastatin), inhibitors of platelet aggregation (aspirin, ticlopidine, clopidogrel), and anticoagulants (warfarin)
2. *Angioplasty:* invasive procedure in which a catheter with a small balloon tip is used to open blocked arteries by compressing the plaque against the arterial wall

and stretching open the artery in order to improve blood flow to the heart

3. *Stent placement with potential brachytherapy:* small, stainless steel mesh tube that's used to hold an artery open; if stenosis of the stent occurs, radiation may be administered via a ribbon of radioactive isotopes at the site of narrowing

4. *Rotablation:* rapidly spinning catheter tip is used to grind away plaque

5. *Atherectomy:* special catheter is used to shave off plaque

6. *Surgery:* an endarterectomy (surgical removal of plaques) or coronary artery bypass grafting (CABG) in which a blood vessel (commonly the internal mammary artery or saphenous vein) is removed or redirected from one area of the body around the area of narrowing in order to bypass it and re-establish normal blood flow to the myocardium; heart transplantation may be a treatment option for some patients with CAD who have failed other methods or have developed cardiomyopathy

7. *Left ventricular assist device (LVAD):* a type of mechanical heart placed inside the chest to pump oxygen-rich blood throughout the body; used to rest the heart as a bridge to heart transplantation

✎ What are important nursing actions in the care of a patient with CAD?

1. Promote smoking cessation and achievement or maintenance of ideal body weight.

2. Encourage a low-cholesterol (less than 300 mg/day), low-fat, and low-salt diet. Total fat grams should be limited, avoiding or minimizing saturated fats and emphasizing monounsaturated fats. Encourage foods rich in B vitamins (fruits and green, leafy vegetables) and a folic acid supplement to help lower homocysteine levels.

3. Encourage regular aerobic exercises, such as walking or jogging, if approved by the physician. Instruct the patient to avoid exercising in temperature extremes, to stop exercising if chest pain, dizziness, light-headedness, or dyspnea occur and to avoid sudden bursts of energy.

4. Encourage restriction of alcohol consumption to no more than one drink per day for women and two drinks per day for men.

5. Instruct the patient to take medicines exactly as prescribed to ensure good blood pressure and blood glucose control.

6. Administer medications (antilipemics, antihypertensives, hypoglycemic agents) as ordered by the physician.

7. Monitor for complications, such as angina, myocardial infarction, transient ischemic attack, or stroke, and notify the physician immediately if any develop.

Ischemic heart disease

ANGINA PECTORIS

What's angina?

Chest discomfort or pain that occurs secondary to decreased oxygen delivery to the myocardium, typically due to a blockage within the coronary arteries; indicative of underlying coronary artery disease

Stable angina occurs during periods of increased myocardial oxygen demand, such as during physical exertion, temperature extremes, heavy meals, cigarette smoking, or intense emotions. Unstable angina commonly occurs as a result of a thrombus formation in a coronary artery at the site of ruptured plaque and is typically of longer duration than stable angina. Unstable angina occurs without any precipitating factors (little to no exertion) and may be less responsive to medications than stable angina. Prinzmetal's (variant) angina is a rare form of unstable angina that involves coronary artery spasm.

Stable angina is a symptom of myocardial ischemia, but differs from myocardial infarction (MI) in that the symptoms of angina are of shorter duration and are commonly relieved by rest or sublingual nitroglycerin (usually within 15 minutes). Stable angina rarely results in permanent damage to the myocardium unless it remains untreated. It causes ST-segment depression on the electrocardiogram.

Unstable angina is a medical emergency because it's an acute coronary syndrome that can progress to MI. It causes ST-segment depression or ST-segment elevation on the electrocardiogram.

What's the pathophysiologic process of angina?

An imbalance between myocardial blood flow and the metabolic demand of the myocardium occurs when the coronary arteries can't provide an adequate amount of oxygenated blood to the heart; the chest pressure, pain, or discomfort that results occurs secondary to the ischemic process

What are clinical manifestations of angina?

Substernal pressure, squeezing, or pain sensation that may radiate to the left shoulder, left arm, jaw, abdomen, or back that typically lasts less than 15 minutes and is relieved by rest and nitroglycerin; indigestion; dyspnea; palpitations; rapid, bounding heart beat; light-headedness or dizziness; and nausea, vomiting, and diaphoresis

What complications are associated with angina?

1. *Stable angina:* may progress to unstable angina, MI, or sudden death due to lethal arrhythmias (ventricular fibrillation, ventricular tachycardia)
2. *Unstable angina:* progression to MI or sudden death due to lethal arrhythmias

◥ *The duration of the ischemia determines the extent of the damage done to the myocardium; the longer the period of ischemia, the more extensive the damage.*

What's the typical treatment for angina pectoris?

1. *Pharmacologic agents:* nitrates (nitroglycerin) to temporarily dilate the coronary arteries and veins throughout the body, increasing oxygen delivery to myocardium and decreasing the cardiac workload; beta-adrenergic blockers to decrease the heart rate and reduce the force of the myocardial contraction; calcium channel blockers to prevent coronary artery spasms; and antiplatelet medications (aspirin, clopidogrel) to prevent platelet aggregation in unstable angina
2. *Angioplasty, percutaneous transluminal coronary angioplasty (PTCA), or balloon dilatation:* a nonsurgical procedure that involves inserting a small balloon catheter into an artery in the groin or arm that's then advanced to the narrowed coronary artery; the balloon is inflated at the site of the narrowing to enlarge the diameter of the artery; this will improve oxygen delivery to the heart
3. *Surgery:* such as coronary artery bypass grafting (CABG)
4. *Transmyocardial revascularization:* (laser transmyocardial revascularization or percutaneous transluminal myocardial revascularization) small holes are drilled into the myocardium, which allow blood and oxygen to enter
5. *Enhanced external counterpulsation:* application of gentle, yet firm pressure on the veins in the lower extremities is used to increase blood flow to the heart, which may stimulate the formation of collateral vessels (small branches of blood vessels) that form a natural bypass around narrowed arteries; treatment lasts 1 to 2 hours per day, 5 days per week for a total of 7 weeks

◥ *One sublingual nitroglycerin should be taken every 5 minutes to a maximum of three doses for the relief of anginal pain. Chest pain or heaviness that persists beyond* three doses of nitroglycerin (and 15 minutes) may indicate unstable angina or MI, and medical care should be sought immediately.

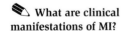

What are important nursing actions in the care of a patient with angina?

1. Instruct the patient to carry nitroglycerin at all times, and replace it every 6 months to ensure its effectiveness.
2. Encourage smoking cessation and maintenance of healthy weight.
3. Educate the patient about the importance of modifying risk factors, including controlling blood pressure, diabetes, and cholesterol level.
4. Administer medications (nitroglycerine, antiplatelet agents, beta-adrenergic blockers) as ordered by the physician.
5. Monitor for complications, including MI and arrhythmias.

Myocardial infarction

What's myocardial infarction (MI)?

A condition in which an area of the myocardium dies or is irreversibly damaged as a result of insufficient oxygen delivery to the area relative to its myocardial demand; commonly caused by a plaque rupture with subsequent spasm and thrombus formation within a coronary vessel, which obstructs blood and oxygen flow to the cardiac muscle; also known as a *heart attack*

What's the pathophysiologic process of MI?

An acute reduction of blood flow to the myocardium of more than 4 to 6 hours duration that produces irreversible myocardial damage and necrosis (cell death); necrotic tissue is replaced by scar tissue, which inhibits cardiac contractility and the remainder of the heart muscle is left to compensate for the loss

The greater the area affected by the ischemia, the greater the loss of overall contractility.

Reperfusion to the ischemic area within 4 to 6 hours of the inciting event can salvage the myocardium and decrease the associated morbidity and mortality.

What are clinical manifestations of MI?

Chest discomfort, pain, or pressure that occurs across the anterior precordium and isn't relieved by rest or nitroglycerin (commonly described as a tight band around chest, or an elephant sitting on chest); radiation of pain into jaw, neck, or arms (particularly left arm); feeling of indigestion, dyspnea, and nausea; vomiting; diaphoresis, light-headedness, syncope, and anxiety (sense of impending doom)

⚡ *A silent heart attack occurs without symptoms and is more common in patients with diabetes.*

How are angina and MI differentiated symptomatically?

Symptoms of MI last 30 minutes or longer and aren't relieved by rest or sublingual nitroglycerin

✎ What laboratory tests are typically performed to diagnose MI?

1. *Troponin (I and T):* highly specific for myocardial injury (particularly troponin I, which is released only when necrosis of myocardium occurs); increase 3 to 6 hours following MI and may remain elevated for several days or as much as 2 weeks (troponin T)
2. *Creatine kinase (CK, CK-MB):* most CK is located in skeletal muscle; three isoenzymes exist, with the CK-MB being more specific for cardiac muscle than either total CK or any of the other isoenzymes; good marker for myocardial injury; rises within 4 hours following myocardial injury, peaks at approximately 18 to 24 hours, and begins to decrease and finally dissipate in 1 to 3 days; less specific for myocardial injury than troponin, but serial sampling (multiple blood draws over time to follow the trend) increases sensitivity of test; upper limit of normal values is 3% to 6% of total CK
3. *Myoglobin:* highly sensitive indicator of muscle injury, but not specific for cardiac muscle; extent of rise can help determine the infarction size; rises even before CK-MB

indicator only for muscle damage, just muscle damage.

⚡ *Cardiac enzymes are released into the circulation when the myocardium is damaged.*

What's the cardiac index?

A ratio of total CK to CK-MB; a good indicator of early MI

✎ What electrocardiogram findings may be indicative of MI?

ST-segment elevation, new Q-waves, and T-wave inversions

⚡ *ST-segment depression is more commonly associated with ischemia, while ST-segment elevation is more commonly associated with infarction.*

What's a transmural MI?

An MI that involves the entire thickness of the left ventricular wall (endocardium to epicardium)

✎ What complications are associated with an MI?

Bradyarrhythmias (second-degree heart blocks) or tachyarrhythmias (sinus tachycardia, premature ventricular contractions), cardiogenic shock, heart failure (jugular vein distention, crackles, presence of an S_3), extension of the infarction, re-infarction, mural thrombosis, pericarditis, formation of ventricular aneurysms, myocardial wall rupture (with possible tamponade), and sudden death

✎ What's cardio-genic shock?

A condition in which the pumping action of the heart is reduced, systolic blood pressure decreases, and inadequate tissue perfusion occurs; the overall result is an increased cardiac workload in an attempt to maintain coronary and cerebral perfusion; caused by any factor that can reduce myocardial function (most commonly MI), and is associated with a high mortality rate (80% for hospitalized patients) due to complications, such as cardiopulmonary arrest, multiple organ dysfunction syndrome, and thromboembolic events

What's the typical treatment for an MI?

1. *Oxygen therapy:* reduces the workload of the heart, even if blood oxygen levels are normal
2. *Pharmacologic agents:* such as analgesics (morphine), sublingual or I.V. nitroglycerin, anxiolytics, thrombolytic agents (streptokinase or tissue plasminogen activator) if within 6 hours of onset of chest pain, antiplatelet agents, anticoagulants (heparin for 48 to 72 hours followed by warfarin therapy), and beta-adrenergic blockers to decrease heart rate and myocardial oxygen demand
3. *Percutaneous transluminal angioplasty (PTCA):* for those with no response to thrombolytics; may involve stenting
4. *Surgery:* coronary artery bypass grafting (CABG) may be necessary once stabilized; infarct exclusion surgery (infarcted area of myocardial tissue or aneurysm that occurs following MI is removed, which returns the heart to a more normal shape and function)
5. *Implantable left ventricular assist device (LVAD):* a mechanical pump that's surgically placed beneath the ribs; allows weakened heart to rest by aiding it in pumping blood throughout the body; commonly used for cardiomyopathy and heart failure

▰ *The primary goals of therapy are to increase the myocardial oxygen supply and decrease the myocardial oxygen demand.*

✎ What are important nursing actions in the care of a patient experiencing MI?

1. Administer supplemental oxygen at 4 L/minute via nasal cannula and place the patient in an upright position. Maintain oxygen saturation above 90%.
2. Administer medications, such as morphine (2 to 4 mg I.V. push), nitroglycerin (sublingual or I.V.), and aspirin as ordered by the physician.

3. Establish two large bore I.V. accesses for administration of fluids and medications (heparin and thrombolytic agents).
4. Monitor vital signs and respiratory status (oxygen saturation level) at least every 15 minutes until stable, and place on continuous cardiac monitor if available.
5. Ensure that the code cart is readily available.
6. Maintain nothing-by-mouth status.
7. Promote bed rest and provide the patient with a bedside toilet.
8. Prevent performance of Valsalva's maneuver (administer stool softeners to prevent straining with defecation).
9. Educate the patient about modification of risk factors upon stabilization (weight loss, low cholesterol diet, smoking cessation, and control of hypertension).

↑main risk factor - hypertension (sodium)

Heart failure

What's heart failure?

A condition characterized by a weakening of the heart's pumping ability, which causes blood to circulate more slowly throughout the heart and body as well as an increase in the pressure within the heart; the kidneys respond by causing the retention of fluid and sodium, which results in edema and vascular congestion

MI is the most common cause of left-sided heart failure, but hypertension, cardiomyopathy, and aortic insufficiency are also contributing factors. Right-sided heart failure can be caused by left-sided heart failure, obstructive lung disease, and congenital heart defects.

Factors affecting one side of the heart will eventually affect both sides.

What's the pathophysiologic process of heart failure?

As a result of biventricular failure, the heart can't pump sufficient amounts of blood to meet the tissue metabolic demands

What are clinical manifestations of heart failure?

1. *Left-sided:* pulmonary congestion and decreased systemic blood pressure
2. *Right-sided:* systemic venous congestion (hepatomegaly, splenomegaly, peripheral edema) and decreased output to the lungs, which in turn produces signs of left heart failure

What complications are associated with heart failure?

Pulmonary edema, pleural effusions, left ventricular thrombosis, and decompensated heart failure

What's the typical treatment for heart failure?

1. *Pharmacologic agents:* diuretics, angiotensin-converting enzyme (ACE) inhibitors, beta-adrenergic blockers, digoxin, and anticoagulants for deep vein thrombosis (DVT) prophylaxis
2. *Surgery:* CABG, valve repair or replacement, infarct exclusion surgery, and heart transplantation
3. *Implantable left ventricular assist device (LVAD):* allows heart to rest by aiding it in pumping blood throughout the body

✎ **What are important nursing actions in the care of a patient with heart failure?**

1. Elevate the head of the bed during acute episodes.
2. Monitor respiratory status and oxygen saturation.
3. Implement fluid and sodium restrictions.
4. Obtain daily weight.
5. Provide rest periods for the patient throughout the day and plan activities accordingly.
6. Encourage regular exercise, if approved by the physician.
7. Promote smoking cessation and discourage the use of alcohol.
8. Encourage weight loss if the patient is overweight.
9. Instruct the patient to take all medications (diuretics, digoxin, anticoagulants) regularly and as prescribed.
10. Monitor for complications, including pulmonary edema and DVT, and notify the physician immediately if any develop.
11. Encourage vaccinations against the flu and pneumonia in order to prevent respiratory infections.

no fluid overload to heart b/c add stress to heart muscle.

CARDIOMYOPATHY

✎ **What's cardiomyopathy?**

A progressive disease involving the heart muscle (myocardium) characterized by an abnormal enlargement, thickening, or stiffening, which reduces the contractility of the heart; heart failure and congestion of blood in the lungs or other areas of the body, and arrhythmias can result

What are the three types of cardiomyopathy?

1. *Dilated cardiomyopathy:* characterized by enlargement and stiffening of the left ventricle, which reduces the ejection fraction; severe coronary artery disease, chronic alcoholism, diabetes, viral infections of the heart, cardiac valve abnormalities, drug toxicity affecting the heart, thyroid disease, and genetics are potential causes; idiopathic dilated cardiomyopathy is the term used when a cause can't be identified
2. *Hypertrophic cardiomyopathy:* characterized by an asymmetric increase in the muscle mass of the ventri-

cles due to an abnormal growth of muscle fibers; the heart's pumping action is impaired due to the abnormal thickening of the cardiac muscle, and blood flow out of the heart is obstructed secondary to abnormal functioning of the cardiac valves; may be caused by hypertension, increasing age, or a genetic predisposition

3. *Restrictive cardiomyopathy:* rare; characterized by abnormal rigidity and inability of the ventricles to expand with the filling of blood; the cause is often unknown, but amyloidosis (accumulation of fats and proteins within the myocardium), hemochromatosis (excessive iron deposits in the heart), radiation exposure of the chest, various connective tissue diseases, and scar tissue formation following MI are potential contributing factors

What are clinical manifestations of cardiomyopathy?

Chest pain or pressure (commonly occurs with physical activity or exercise), dyspnea, fatigue, lower extremity edema, weight gain, light-headedness or dizziness, palpitations, and syncope from abnormal heart rhythms

What complications are associated with cardiomyopathy?

Heart failure, arrhythmias, syncope, and sudden cardiac death (severe cases)

What's the typical treatment for dilated cardiomyopathy?

1. Pharmacologic agents, including beta-adrenergic blockers, ACE inhibitors, and diuretics; anti-arrhythmics may be necessary to regulate the heart rate; dobutamine or milrinone "training"; continuous I.V. therapy
2. Biventricular pacemaker involving the pacing of right and left ventricles to improve symptoms
3. Implantable cardioverter-defibrillator (ICD): used for persons at risk for life-threatening arrhythmias or sudden cardiac death; detects abnormal heart rhythms and delivers energy to the myocardium causing it to beat in a normal rhythm
4. Surgery to repair the left ventricle or heart transplantation
5. Left ventricular assist device (LVAD)

What are important nursing actions in the care of a patient with dilated cardiomyopathy?

1. Encourage sodium restriction (2 to 3 g/day).
2. Encourage noncompetitive aerobic exercise, if cleared by the physician, and avoidance of heavy weight-lifting.
3. Instruct the patient to avoid alcohol.
4. Encourage weight loss if the patient is overweight.

5. Administer medications (diuretics, vasodilators, digoxin, calcium channel blockers, beta-adrenergic blockers) as ordered by the physician.
6. Monitor for complications, including heart failure and arrhythmias, and notify the physician immediately if any develop.

What's the typical treatment for hypertrophic cardiomyopathy?

1. Lifestyle modifications, including less physical exertion (if significant blood flow or electrical abnormalities)
2. Pharmacologic agents, including beta-adrenergic blockers, anti-arrhythmics, and calcium channel blockers
3. Surgery, including implantation of pacemaker or ICD, ethanol ablation (injection of alcohol into an enlarged septal wall during cardiac catheterization), or septal myectomy (small amount of enlarged septal wall is removed)

What are important nursing actions in the care of a patient with hypertrophic cardiomyopathy?

1. Encourage sodium restriction (2 to 3 g/day).
2. Encourage noncompetitive aerobic exercise, if cleared by the physician, and avoidance of heavy weight-lifting.
3. Instruct the patient to avoid alcohol.
4. Encourage weight loss if the patient is overweight.
5. Administer medications (diuretics, vasodilators, digoxin, calcium channel blockers, beta-adrenergic blockers) as ordered by the physician.
6. Monitor for complications, including heart failure and arrhythmias, and notify the physician immediately if any develop.
7. Educate the patient about increased risk for endocarditis and increased need for prophylactic antibiotics prior to surgical or dental procedures.

What's the typical treatment for restrictive cardiomyopathy?

Treatment of the underlying cause (if known), the use of pharmacologic agents (beta-adrenergic blockers, ACE inhibitors, diuretics) to treat heart failure, surgery to improve myocardial blood flow, and possibly, heart transplantation

What are important nursing actions in the care of a patient with restrictive cardiomyopathy?

1. Encourage sodium restriction (2 to 3 g/day).
2. Encourage noncompetitive aerobic exercise, if cleared by the physician and avoidance of heavy weight-lifting.

Arrhythmias

✎ What's an arrhythmia?

An irregular heart rate or rhythm that's caused by a disturbance in the electrical conduction system of the heart; persons with coronary artery disease, valvular disorders, or electrolyte abnormalities are at an increased risk for arrhythmias and their complications

What's an ectopic focus?

An area of myocardial tissue that overtakes the pacemaker function of the sinoatrial node, producing rapid and spontaneous electrical discharges; any foci that isn't sinus node is ectopic

✎ What are examples of types of arrhythmias?

1. *Atrial flutter:* rapid, but regular heart rhythm; symptoms may include light-headedness, pounding heart rate, and dyspnea
2. *Atrial fibrillation (A fib):* rapid, irregular rhythm that originates from multiple sites within the atria, producing more rapid, irregular, and incomplete contractions of the ventricles; palpitations, tachycardia, chest discomfort, light-headedness, and dyspnea may result
3. *Premature atrial contractions (PACs):* benign, early extra beats of the heart that originate in the atria
4. *Premature ventricular contractions (PVCs):* skipped heart beats; may be caused by stress, caffeine, nicotine, or excessive exercise
5. *Heart block:* delay or total block of the electrical impulse from the sinus node to the ventricles; heart may beat irregularly
6. *Ventricular tachycardia (VT):* rapid heart rate caused by abnormal impulses originating from a single area of the heart that overtake the pacemaking function of the sinoatrial (SA) node; V tach is usually regular in appearance; light-headedness, syncope, blind spots, unconsciousness, and may result in cardiac arrest
7. *Ventricular fibrillation (V fib):* rapid and irregular heart rate caused by abnormal impulses from multiple areas of the heart that overtake the pacemaking function of the SA node; blood is ineffectively pumped to the brain and body tissues, resulting in unconsciousness, cardiac arrest, or death

▧ *The inability of the atria to contract properly increases the risk of a blood clot formation (thrombus), which can travel to distant sites and become lodged. Anticoagulation therapy is usually necessary for thrombus prophylaxis in persons with atrial fibrillation.*

✎ What are the common manifestations of arrhythmias?

Palpitations, dizziness or light-headedness, pallor, syncope or near syncopal episodes, chest pain, dyspnea, or pulse abnormalities

What complications are associated with arrhythmias?

Angina, MI, heart failure, stroke, or sudden cardiac death

What's sudden cardiac death?

Unexpected death caused by loss of heart function that results from a sudden irregularity of the electrical system

What's the typical treatment for arrhythmias?

1. *Pharmacologic agents:* anti-arrhythmics, anticoagulants, and antiplatelets
2. *Cardioversion or defibrillation:* use of electrical impulses to disrupt arrhythmia
3. *Implantation of a temporary pacemaker:* disrupts the arrhythmia; most commonly used for bradyarrhythmias, but also used for heart failure and hypertrophic cardiomyopathy
4. *Insertion of implantable cardioverter-defibrillator (ICD):* identifies arrhythmias and uses electrical impulses to correct them
5. *Radiofrequency catheter ablation:* for treatment of atrial flutter or atrial fibrillation

✎ What are important nursing actions in the care of a patient with an arrhythmia?

1. Instruct the patient to limit or stop caffeine intake.
2. Instruct the patient to avoid stimulants, such as those found in over-the-counter cough and cold medications.
3. Emphasize the importance of compliance with medications (antiarrhythmics, anticoagulants).
4. Monitor for complications, including MI or stroke, and notify the physician immediately if any develop.

Inflammatory disorders of the heart

Infective endocarditis

✎ What's infective endocarditis?

An infectious process involving the endocardium (inner lining), cardiac valves or leaflets that may be caused by bacteria (*Streptococcus viridans*), virus, fungi, or other pathogens; the condition may develop acutely or slowly (subacute); normal alignment of the cusps is prevented, which can result in incomplete closure of the valves or regurgitation, and cardiac murmurs

What's the pathophysiologic process of infective endocarditis?	Pathogens (usually bacteria) in the bloodstream become lodged on abnormal heart valves or damaged cardiac tissue. Infectious growths (vegetations) can become dislodged, sending clots to the lungs, brain, kidneys, or spleen.
What are clinical manifestations of infective endocarditis?	Fever, chills, fatigue, malaise, headache, diaphoresis or night sweats, weight loss, hematuria, splenomegaly, petechiae, splinter hemorrhages beneath the fingernails, anemia, Osler's nodes (painful, red nodes in the pads of the fingers and toes), edema, and dyspnea
What complications are associated with infective endocarditis?	Arrhythmias, heart failure, thromboembolisms (stroke, brain abscess), glomerulonephritis, and severe valve damage
What's the typical treatment for infective endocarditis?	Long-term, high-dose I.V. antimicrobial therapy, including antibiotics

Prophylactic antibiotics should be administered before surgical or dental procedures in persons at risk for developing endocarditis, such as those with prosthetic heart valves or artificial joints, a prior history of endocarditis, congenital heart or valve defects (murmurs, mitral valve prolapse), valvular damage or scarring from rheumatic fever, and hypertrophic cardiomyopathy.

What are important nursing actions in the care of a patient with infective endocarditis?	1. Educate the patient about the need for prophylactic antibiotics before dental or surgical procedures.
	2. Administer medications (antibiotics) as ordered by the physician.
	3. Monitor for complications, including arrhythmias, heart failure, and stroke, and notify the physician immediately if any develop.

Pericarditis

What's pericarditis?	An inflammation of the pericardial sac, which causes an increase in the fluid between the two layers of the pericardium; compliance of the pericardial membrane is reduced due to the thickening or fibrotic changes that occur, and ventricular filling is restricted as a result; causes include open heart surgery, viral or bacterial infections, MI, or trauma; commonly associated with rheumatoid arthritis, lupus, and renal failure
What's the pathophysiologic process of pericarditis?	Excessive fluid accumulation within the pericardial sac causes an increase in the pericardial pressure. This increased pressure results in a reduction of cardiac output

and hypotension. Fibrosis and scarring can occur if the inflammation is chronic.

✎ What are the clinical manifestations of pericarditis?

Pericardial friction rub; sharp chest pain located behind the sternum that worsens with deep inhalation; fever, malaise, and tachycardia

What complications are associated with pericarditis?

Constrictive pericarditis (layers of the pericardium become rigid and stick together), pericardial effusions, and cardiac tamponade

What's the typical treatment for pericarditis?

Activity restrictions, analgesics or anti-inflammatories (nonsteroidal anti-inflammatory drugs [NSAIDs], morphine), antibiotics (if bacterial source), and removal of fluid with needle (pericardiocentesis)

What are important nursing actions in the care of a patient with pericarditis?

1. Place the patient in a comfortable position (usually upright).
2. Administer medications (NSAIDs, morphine, antibiotics) as ordered by the physician.
3. Restrict activity until condition improves.
4. Monitor for complications, such as arrhythmias, and notify the physician if any develop.

Myocarditis

✎ What's myocarditis?

An inflammation of the myocardium that results from viral (commonly coxsackievirus), bacterial or fungal infections, or radiation- or chemical-induced damage

What's the pathophysiologic process of myocarditis?

An immunologic response results in an inflammatory process that causes edema and damage to the myocardial cells; pinpoint hemorrhages may occur as a result

What are clinical manifestations of myocarditis?

Initially produces no symptoms; fever, chills, malaise, fatigue, dyspnea, and palpitations occur later

What complications are associated with myocarditis?

Heart failure, pericarditis, and cardiomyopathy

What's the typical treatment for myocarditis?

Decreased activity level, antibiotics, diuretics, low-salt diet, and steroids may be used to manage myocarditis. If arrhythmias are present, anti-arrhythmics may be used as well as pacemaker or defibrillator insertion.

What are important nursing actions in the care of a patient with myocarditis?	1. Place the patient in a comfortable position (usually upright). 2. Restrict activity until condition improves. 3. Administer medications (diuretics, antibiotics) as ordered by the physician. 4. Monitor for complications, including heart failure, and notify the physician if any develop.

Valvular heart disease

What are types of valvular heart disease?	Mitral stenosis, mitral insufficiency, aortic stenosis, aortic insufficiency, tricuspid stenosis, tricuspid insufficiency, pulmonic insufficiency, and pulmonic stenosis 🔋 *Stenosis is the impedance of forward flow through an open valve; insufficiency is the backward leaking of blood through a closed valve.*
What's mitral stenosis?	A valvular disorder in which thickening, scarring and, possibly, fusing of the mitral valve leaflets occurs, thereby impairing blood flow from the left atrium to the left ventricle; as a result, blood backs up within the pulmonary vasculature and symptoms of pulmonary congestion occur; mitral stenosis is a common complication of rheumatic fever
What's mitral insufficiency?	A valvular disorder in which the valve leaflets fail to close properly during systole, and blood is allowed to flow back through the mitral valve into the left atrium; left ventricular hypertrophy occurs as a result of the increased blood volume; rheumatic fever is the most common cause of this condition, but it can also occur secondary to age-related deterioration, endocarditis, chest trauma, or left ventricular hypertrophy from a prior MI 🔋 *Mitral insufficiency is best detected with auscultation at the cardiac apex.*
What's mitral valve prolapse?	Usually produces no symptoms, but may manifest as a systolic murmur, palpitations, chest pain, dizziness, dyspnea, or light-headedness that typically worsens with stress
What's aortic stenosis?	A condition involving a stiffening of the aortic valve with narrowing of the opening; a heart murmur is best heard at the aortic area with radiation to the neck; the left ventricle must work harder to create a higher pressure so that

normal blood flow is maintained; causes include rheumatic valvular disease, a bicuspid aortic valve, and calcifications of the aortic valve with increasing age

✎ What's aortic insufficiency?

A condition in which the aortic valve permits the backflow of blood into the left ventricle from the aorta; consequently, the left ventricle must pump more blood than usual so that normal blood flow is delivered throughout the body; causes include chronic hypertension, rheumatic valvular disease, endocarditis, some congenital defects, and autoimmune diseases (lupus, rheumatoid arthritis)

✎ What's tricuspid stenosis?

A condition involving excessive tightness of the tricuspid valve that occurs secondary to rheumatic valvular disease

✎ What's tricuspid insufficiency?

A condition characterized by leaking of the tricuspid valve, which allows the backward flow of blood from the right ventricle to the right atrium

✎ What's pulmonic insufficiency?

A condition in which the pulmonic valve permits the backflow of blood into the right ventricle from the pulmonary artery

✎ What's pulmonic stenosis?

A condition characterized by narrowing of the pulmonic valve

✎ What are the common manifestations of valvular disorders?

Palpitations, dyspnea, light-headedness, dizziness, chest pressure, and edema of lower extremities

What's the typical treatment of valvular disorders?

1. *Pharmacologic agents:* ACE inhibitors, anticoagulation, diuretics, and digoxin (if ventricular contractility is decreased)
2. *Surgery:* repair (valvuloplasty) or replacement of diseased valves

✎ What are important nursing actions in the care of a patient with a valvular disorder?

1. Educate the patient about the need for prophylactic antibiotics before dental or surgical procedures with certain valvular disorders (aortic valve disorders).
2. Administer medications (anticoagulants, ACE inhibitors, diuretics, digoxin, and antibiotics) as ordered by the physician.
3. Monitor for complications, including heart failure, and notify the physician if any develop.
4. Monitor clotting times periodically during anticoagulant therapy.

Major vascular disorders

Aortic disorders

ABDOMINAL AORTIC ANEURYSM

What's an abdominal aortic aneurysm?	A ballooning of the lower portion of the aorta that extends into the abdominal area; causes may include weakening of the arterial walls by atherosclerosis, hypertension, blunt trauma, or other disease processes, including diabetes, congenital defects, or Marfan's syndrome
What's the pathophysiologic process of abdominal aortic aneurysm?	The media (middle layer) of the aorta degenerates secondary to atherosclerotic changes. Widening of the vessel lumen and a decrease in its structural integrity result.
✎ **What are clinical manifestations of an abdominal aortic aneurysm?**	Pulsating and possibly tender mass in the midline of the abdomen, or pain in the back, abdomen, or groin (commonly mistaken for nephrolithiasis or a ruptured disc)

⚑ *Most aneurysms develop slowly over many years and produce no symptoms until the aneurysm suddenly expands or ruptures, or an aortic dissection occurs.*

What complications are associated with an abdominal aortic aneurysm?	Rupture of the aneurysm with life-threatening internal bleeding, infection, thromboembolisms (aneurysms may contain small blood clots that can break loose), compression of local structures (nerves), and aortic dissection
What's aortic dissection?	A condition in which a tearing of the arterial lining occurs with leakage of blood into the arterial wall; causes may include atherosclerosis, hypertension, congenital weakness of the aorta, pregnancy, and valvular disorders of the heart
	Manifestations may include sudden, sharp, stabbing, or tearing chest pain that may radiate to the shoulder, neck, jaw, arm, abdomen or hips; mental status changes (confusion, disorientation); pallor; tachycardia; diaphoresis; anxiety; light-headedness; dizziness; dyspnea; clammy skin; a weak or absent pulse; and a blowing murmur over the aorta.

⚑ *The location of the pain may change as the aortic dissection progresses.*

What's the typical treatment for an abdominal aortic aneurysm?	Antihypertensives (beta-adrenergic blockers), routine monitoring of the aneurysm size with ultrasound or other imaging studies, and surgical repair for large aneurysms (larger than 5 cm)

What are important nursing actions in the care of a patient with an abdominal aortic aneurysm?	1. Educate the patient about lifestyle modifications (diet, exercise) to reduce risks for atherosclerotic disease. 2. Administer medications (antihypertensives) as ordered by the physician. 3. Anticipate a consultation with a vascular surgeon if the aneurysm is larger than 3 cm. 4. Encourage close medical follow-up for serial ultrasounds to monitor size of aneurysm. 5. Monitor for complications, including rupture of the aneurysm, infections, and thromboembolisms, and notify the physician immediately if any occur.

Vasculitis

BUERGER'S DISEASE (THROMBOANGIITIS OBLITERANS)

✎ What's Buerger's disease?	An inflammatory condition involving the arteries, veins, and nerves; the exact cause is unknown, however an autoimmune or genetic process is suspected; most commonly occurs in middle-aged men who are heavy smokers
What's the pathophysiologic process of Buerger's disease?	The inflammatory process produces a thickening of the blood vessel walls due to infiltration of white blood cells
✎ What are clinical manifestations of Buerger's disease?	Bluish, whitish, or reddish discoloration of fingers or toes upon exposure to cold; sensation of coldness in affected extremity, sweaty feet (due to overactive sympathetic nerves), and intermittent claudication as blood vessels become progressively blocked
What complications are associated with Buerger's disease?	Ischemic skin ulcerations and gangrene, possibly requiring amputation
What's the typical treatment for Buerger's disease?	Smoking cessation generally produces marked improvement; sympathectomy may be necessary if pain persists
What are important nursing actions in the care of a patient with Buerger's disease?	1. Encourage smoking cessation. 2. Instruct the patient to avoid exposure to cold weather. 3. Monitor for complications, including skin ulcerations and possibly infections, and notify the physician if any develop.

RAYNAUD'S PHENOMENON (ARTERIOSPASTIC DISEASE)

✎ **What's Raynaud's phenomenon?**	A condition involving arterial spasms in the fingers and toes, which produces ischemia of the affected extremities; exposure to cold temperatures, smoking and, possibly, emotional factors can exacerbate this disorder
What's the pathophysiologic process of Raynaud's phenomenon?	Spastic constriction of blood vessels of the fingers and toes causes ischemia of the affected extremities
✎ **What are clinical manifestations of Raynaud's phenomenon?**	Bluish discoloration and pain in the digits (usually occurs bilaterally), numbness, paresthesias, and cold affected digits
What complications are associated with Raynaud's phenomenon?	May progress to ischemic ulcerations and gangrenous infections (rare)
What's the typical treatment for Raynaud's phenomenon?	Pharmacologic agents, such as calcium channel blockers and phenoxybenzamine, may be used
What are important nursing actions in the care of a patient with Raynaud's phenomenon?	1. Instruct the patient to avoid exposure to cold weather. Encourage the patient to wear thick gloves and socks. 2. Encourage smoking cessation. 3. Monitor for complications, including ulcerations (rare), and notify the physician immediately if any develop.

Vein disorders

Thrombophlebitis

✎ **What's thrombophlebitis?**	A condition in which a blood clot and inflammation occur in one or more veins, most commonly involves the lower extremities; prolonged inactivity is a common cause
What's the pathophysiologic process of thrombophlebitis?	Blood clot formation in a vein causes irritation or injury to the vein

✎ What are clinical manifestations of thrombophlebitis?	Erythema, edema, warmth, and tenderness of the affected area; low-grade fever
What complications are associated with thrombophlebitis?	Pulmonary embolism with deep vein clots, formation of varicose veins, and venous insufficiency with stasis pigmentation and skin ulcerations
What's the typical treatment for thrombophlebitis?	Application of heat, elevation of the affected extremity, and administration of a nonsteroidal anti-inflammatory drug (NSAID) if the clot is superficial; deep vein clots will require anticoagulation therapy
✎ What are important nursing actions in the care of a patient with thrombophlebitis?	1. Apply heat to the affected area and elevate the extremity. 2. Administer medications (NSAIDs, possibly anticoagulants) as ordered by the physician. 3. Encourage periodic ambulation during long car or plane rides, flexing ankles, using support stockings, and taking aspirin before long trips to prevent clot formation.

Deep venous thrombosis

What's deep venous thrombosis (DVT)?	A blood clot in a deep vein (usually occurs in lower leg, thigh, or pelvis)
✎ What are common causes of a DVT?	Recent major surgery (50% of cases occur within 24 hours of surgery), immobilization, fracture or trauma, malignancy, thrombophlebitis, obesity, smoking, and estrogen therapy
✎ What are the clinical manifestations of a DVT?	Pain isolated to one leg, unilateral edema, warmth and erythema of the affected area, pain on calf flexion (Homans' sign), palpable cord and, possibly, a low-grade fever
What diagnostic tests should be anticipated in the event of a suspected DVT?	Venous duplex Doppler or contrast venogram; other diagnostic tests include the cuff pain test of Löwenberg (lower threshold for pain occurs when blood pressure cuff inflated around affected extremity) and impedance plethysmography (based on electrical conduction of the blood); baseline coagulation studies should also be obtained before administration of antithrombotic agents
✎ What complications may be prevented with early intervention?	Pulmonary embolus (breaking off of a clot) that becomes lodged in the lungs or chronic leg swelling and pain

✎ **What are important nursing interventions for a patient with a DVT?**	1. Elevate the affected extremity above the level of the heart. 2. Avoid any unnecessary activity involving the affected extremity. 3. Administer anticoagulants (heparin initially) as ordered to maintain partial thromboplastin time between $1\frac{1}{2}$ to $2\frac{1}{2}$ times the control. 4. Monitor vital signs at frequent intervals and assess for signs of pulmonary embolus. 5. Monitor intake and output and ensure adequate hydration. 6. Prepare the patient for possible radiologic studies and thrombolytic therapy.

Pharmacology related to the cardiovascular system

Management of hypercholesterolemia

ANTILIPEMICS

How do antilipemic agents work?	1. *Statins:* inhibit cholesterol synthesis within the liver by inhibiting an enzyme (HMG-CoA reductase) required for its production; decrease low-density-lipoprotein (LDL) and triglycerides, and slightly increase high-density-lipoprotein (HDL) ("good" cholesterol) 2. *Nicotinic acid:* decreases LDL and triglyceride levels and increases HDL levels 3. *Bile acid resins:* deplete body's supply of cholesterol by binding bile in the intestines and preventing it from being absorbed into the bloodstream (bile is primarily made from cholesterol) 4. *Fibric acid derivatives:* decrease triglyceride production and increase HDL levels 5. *Cholesterol absorption inhibitors:* inhibit intestinal absorption of cholesterol
What are examples of antilipemic agents?	1. *Statins:* atorvastatin (Lipitor), pravastatin (Pravachol), lovastatin (Mevacor), fluvastatin (Lescol), simvastatin (Zocor) 2. *Nicotinic acid:* niacin (Niaspan, Nicolar) 3. *Bile acid resins:* cholestyramine (Questran), colestipol (Colestid), colesevelam (Welchol) 4. *Fibric acid derivatives:* gemfibrozil (Lopid), clofibrate (Atromid-S), fenofibrate (Tricor) 5. *Cholesterol absorption inhibitors:* ezetimibe (Zetia)

✎ What adverse reactions are associated with antilipemic agents?

1. *Statins:* intestinal problems, muscle tenderness (myopathy, rhabdomyolysis), elevated liver enzymes (aspartate aminotransferase (AST), alanine aminotransferase (ALT)
2. *Nicotinic acid:* facial flushing, headache, pruritus
3. *Bile acid resins:* constipation; inhibits absorption of many other drugs; increased risk for bleeding tendencies (due to decreased vitamin K absorption in the intestines)
4. *Fibric acid derivatives:* rhabdomyolysis and myoglobinuria when used in conjunction with statins

✎ What are important nursing actions when administering an antilipemic agent?

1. Instruct the patient to follow a low-cholesterol, low-fat (especially saturated fat and trans fatty acids) diet in addition to taking antilipemics.
2. Instruct the patient to avoid drinking grapefruit juice.
3. Monitor liver function tests, particularly transaminases (AST, ALT) throughout statin therapy. Obtain baseline liver function tests before initiation of statin therapy, at 6 and 12 weeks after initiation, and every 6 months thereafter (may be stopped or decreased in frequency if normal after 1 year on a stable dose). Discontinue statin if transaminases become three times higher than the upper limit of normal.
4. Assess for muscle weakness or tenderness routinely throughout therapy. Instruct the patient to contact the physician immediately if muscle aches or weakness occur. Discontinue statin if symptoms of myopathy or rhabdomyolysis occur, or if creatine kinase levels become elevated.
5. Instruct the patient to avoid alcohol during therapy.
6. Instruct the patient to prepare powdered cholestyramine in a glass of water, milk, or juice.
7. Monitor blood pressure regularly.

Management of hypertension

BETA-ADRENERGIC BLOCKERS

How do beta-adrenergic blockers work?

Decrease heart rate and cardiac output, which in turn lower blood pressure

▪ *In addition to hypertension, angina and heart failure, beta-adrenergic blockers are also prescribed for migraine headaches and glaucoma.*

What are examples of beta-adrenergic blockers?	Metoprolol (Lopressor, Toprol XL), propranolol (Inderal), labetalol (Normodyne), atenolol (Tenormin), nadolol (Corgard), carvedilol (Coreg), acebutolol (Sectral), esmolol (Brevibloc)

🔼 *Beta-adrenergic blockers should be used cautiously in persons with asthma, emphysema, diabetes, hypercholesterolemia, and depression.*

🖎 **What adverse effects are associated with beta-adrenergic blockers?**	Bradycardia, confusion, nightmares, decreases in HDL, erectile dysfunction, hyperglycemia, and asthma exacerbations

🖎 **What are important nursing actions when administering a beta-adrenergic blocker?**

1. Assess the patient for asthma or emphysema before administration of a beta-adrenergic blocker.
2. Instruct the patient to take this medication with meals or shortly after meals.
3. Assess pulse rate before administration of a beta-adrenergic blocker. If pulse is less than 60 beats/minute don't administer the drug and be sure to document this action in the patient's chart.
4. Inform the patient that beta-adrenergic blockers may increase blood glucose levels.
5. Instruct the patient to change positions slowly to prevent orthostatic hypotension.
6. Monitor blood pressure regularly and instruct the patient to do the same at home.
7. Inform the patient that results may take weeks to become evident.
8. Inform the patient that abrupt discontinuation should be avoided. Gradual withdrawal of drug over 2 weeks should be performed to minimize serious reactions.

🔼 *Beta-adrenergic blockers should be withheld if the patient's pulse is less than 60 beats/minute.*

ANGIOTENSIN-CONVERTING ENZYME INHIBITORS

How do angiotensin-converting enzyme (ACE) inhibitors work?	By blocking an enzyme necessary for the formation of a substance that causes vasoconstriction; vasodilation is the result, which facilitates the flow of blood through the blood vessels, which decreases blood pressure; ACE inhibitors also increase water and sodium excretion in the urine, which also results in the lowering of blood pressure

> ⚡ *ACE inhibitors don't affect blood glucose levels as do beta-adrenergic blockers; ACE inhibitors may protect against the development of renal failure in diabetics.*

What are examples of ACE inhibitors?

Captopril (Capoten), enalapril (Vasotec), lisinopril (Prinivil), fosinopril (Monopril, Zestril), quinapril (Accupril), benazepril (Lotensin), ramipril (Altace), and moexipril (Univasc)

What adverse reactions are associated with ACE inhibitors?

Nonproductive cough, rash, pruritus, tachycardia, and hypotension

What life-threatening reactions are associated with ACE inhibitors?

Angioedema and hyperkalemia (particularly in the presence of renal disease)

What are important nursing actions when administering an ACE inhibitor?

1. Instruct the patient to take this medication on an empty stomach, preferably 1 hour before meals.
2. Monitor blood pressure regularly and instruct the patient to do the same at home.
3. Monitor renal function and potassium levels periodically during therapy.
4. Encourage consumption of low-potassium foods (ACE inhibitors cause potassium retention). Instruct the patient to avoid salt substitutes because they contain potassium in place of sodium.
5. Instruct the patient to change positions slowly to prevent orthostatic hypotension.

CALCIUM CHANNEL BLOCKERS

How do calcium channel blockers work?

Inhibit vasoconstriction by preventing the movement of calcium into myocardial cells and blood vessels; increases myocardial supply of blood and oxygen, and reduces cardiac workload

What are examples of calcium channel blockers?

Diltiazem (Cardizem, Cardizem CD, Cardizem SR, Dilacor XR, Tiazac), amlodipine (Norvasc), felodipine (Plendil), isradipine (DynaCirc), nifedipine (Procardia XL, Adalat), verapamil (Calan, Calan SR, Covera, Isoptin, Verelan), and nisoldipine (Sular)

What adverse reactions are associated with calcium channel blockers?

Dizziness, headache, flushing, peripheral edema, bradycardia or tachycardia, drowsiness, increased appetite, constipation, hypotension, and syncope

What life-threatening reactions are associated with calcium channel blockers?	Arrhythmias, heart failure and, possibly, MI ◪ *Calcium channel blockers should be used cautiously in patients with arrhythmias or heart failure.*
What are important nursing actions when administering a calcium channel blocker?	1. Instruct the patient to take this medication with food or milk and to avoid grapefruits and grapefruit juice during therapy. 2. Monitor blood pressure and pulse before administration. If the systolic pressure is less than 90 mm Hg or if the pulse is more than 60 beats/minute, withhold the medication and notify the physician. 3. Instruct the patient to avoid alcohol. 4. Monitor for signs and symptoms of heart failure, and notify the physician if any occur.

ANGIOTENSIN II RECEPTOR BLOCKERS

How do angiotensin II receptor blockers work?	By inhibiting the action of a hormone that causes vasoconstriction and increasing the urinary excretion of water and sodium; commonly substituted for an ACE inhibitor if the patient develops a cough from the medication
What are examples of angiotensin II receptor blockers?	Losartan (Cozaar, Hyzaar), irbesartan (Avapro), candesartan (Atacand), and valsartan (Diovan)
What adverse reactions are associated with angiotensin II receptor blockers?	Dizziness, headache, diarrhea, dyspepsia, myalgias, and upper respiratory tract infections
What are important nursing actions when administering an angiotensin II receptor blocker?	1. Monitor blood pressure regularly and instruct the patient to do the same at home. 2. Monitor renal function (blood urea nitrogen, creatinine) periodically during therapy. 3. Encourage the patient to change positions slowly to prevent orthostatic hypotension. 4. Instruct women of childbearing age to notify the physician immediately if pregnancy is known or suspected. 5. Instruct the patient to avoid salt substitutes due to the risk of hyperkalemia. 6. Inform the patient that results may take several weeks to become evident.

VASODILATORS

How do vasodilators work?

Decrease peripheral vascular resistance by causing vasodilation

What are examples of vasodilators?

Clonidine (Catapres, Catapres-TTS), terazosin (Hytrin), prazosin (Minipress), methyldopa (Aldomet), minoxidil (Loniten), isosorbide (Isordil, Iso-Bid, Isorbid, IMDUR), and apresoline (Hydralazine)

What adverse reactions are associated with vasodilators?

Dizziness, syncope, tachycardia, palpitations, headache, edema, hypotension, drowsiness, fatigue, dry mouth, erectile dysfunction, hair growth (minoxidil), peripheral edema, and paresthesia of fingers and toes

⚡ *Rebound hypertension can occur if these medications are stopped abruptly.*

What are important nursing actions when administering a vasodilator?

1. Instruct the patient to take medications with meals.
2. Monitor blood pressure regularly and instruct the patient to do the same at home.
3. Inform the patient that abrupt discontinuation of these medications should be avoided due to risk of rebound hypertension. Gradual withdrawal is necessary to prevent this complication.
4. Inform the patient that this medication may cause drowsiness during initial use (typically resolves over a short period).
5. Instruct the patient to change positions slowly to prevent orthostatic hypotension.

INOTROPICS

How do inotropics work?

Strengthen the contraction of the heart by facilitating the movement of calcium from the extracellular to the intracellular space

What are examples of inotropics?

Digoxin (Lanoxin, Lanoxicaps), milrinone (Primacor), and inamrinone (Inocor)

What adverse reactions are associated with inotropics?

Drowsiness, anorexia, nausea, vomiting, headache, confusion, palpitations, bradycardia, and visual changes, including yellow or green haze, and seeing halos around objects

What life-threatening reactions are associated with inotropics?

Arrhythmias

What are important nursing actions when administering inotropics?

1. Instruct the patient to take apical pulse for 1 minute before each administration of digoxin. Withhold dose if heart rate is less than 60 beats/minute.
2. Inform the patient that digoxin may cause drowsiness.
3. Monitor digoxin levels periodically during therapy; therapeutic levels are 0.5 to 2 ng/ml.
4. Assess for signs of toxicity (bradycardia, halos around objects, yellow or green hazes).
5. Instruct the patient to avoid alcohol (increases adverse reactions).
6. Monitor potassium levels periodically during therapy (may cause hypokalemia).

⚡ *The apical pulse should be taken for 1 full minute before the administration of inotropic agents such as digoxin; the medication should be withheld if the apical pulse is less than 60 beats/minute.*

Management of arrhythmias

ANTIARRHYTHMICS

How do antiarrhythmics work?

By a variety of mechanisms, including slowing conduction through the atrioventricular node, and via selective actions that affect heart rate and contractility

What are examples of antiarrhythmics?

Amiodarone (Cordarone), procainamide (Procanbid), flecainide (Tambocor), and sotalol (Betapace)

What adverse reactions are associated with antiarrhythmics?

Syncope, blurred vision, dyspnea, peripheral edema, bradycardia or tachycardia, dizziness, altered taste sensations (bitter or metallic taste), anorexia, cough, photosensitivity, diarrhea or constipation, and increased liver function tests

What life-threatening reactions are associated with antiarrhythmics?

Worsening arrhythmias, allergic reactions, and chest pain

What are important nursing actions when administering an antiarrhythmic?

1. Instruct the patient to take antiarrhythmics exactly as prescribed.
2. Monitor blood pressure and heart rate regularly and instruct the patient to do the same at home.

3. Evaluate hepatic function and potassium levels periodically throughout therapy.
4. Monitor for complications, including worsening arrhythmias.

Management of ischemic heart disease

ANTIANGINALS

How do antianginals work?

Decreases preload (left ventricular end-diastolic pressure) and afterload (systemic vascular resistance), and increases blood flow through collateral coronary vessels

What are examples of antianginals?

Nitroglycerin (Nitro-Bid, Nitro-Dur, Transderm-Nitro) and amyl nitrite

What adverse reactions are associated with antianginals?

Headache, dizziness, hypotension, palpitations, tachycardia, flushing, nausea, and rash (transdermal preparations)

What are important nursing actions when administering an antianginal?

1. Instruct the patient to have antianginal medications readily available and that the medication should be stored in a cool, dark place.
2. Inform the patient that nitroglycerin should be taken promptly at the onset of angina, and that sitting down and resting is important. Tablets should be placed under the tongue and allowed to dissolve. Dosage may be repeated every 5 minutes up to a total of three doses over 15 minutes if the discomfort persists. Medical care should be sought immediately if the discomfort persists despite three doses of nitroglycerin.
3. Instruct the patient to avoid abrupt discontinuation of nitroglycerin due to risk of coronary vasospasm. Dosage should be tapered gradually.
4. Encourage the patient to change positions slowly to prevent orthostatic hypotension.
5. Inform the patient that transdermal doses should be applied to a hairless part of the body and shouldn't be rubbed into the skin. Excess paste should be removed by wiping the skin clean before another dose is applied. Avoid getting ointment on fingers or hands.
6. Instruct the patient to monitor blood pressure regularly during therapy.

17

The gastrointestinal system

Basic concepts of the GI system

What structures comprise the upper GI system?

1. *Mouth:* composed of lips and oral (buccal) cavity; teeth, tongue, and salivary glands located in oral cavity; responsible for speech (lips and hard and soft palate), chewing (teeth), taste (tongue), and swallowing; initial site of digestion (breakdown of starches)
2. *Esophagus:* hollow and muscular tube that uses peristalsis to propel food toward the stomach and secretes mucus
3. *Stomach:* alkaline environment; stores and mixes food to produce chemical changes; minimal digestion of starches and fats; absorbs small quantities of water, glucose, electrolytes, and alcohol
4. *Liver:* largest internal organ; responsible for various metabolic functions as well as the production of bile and the storage of glucose (in form of glycogen), fat-soluble vitamins, and some minerals (iron and copper); filters blood of bacteria and old red blood cells, and converts hemoglobin to bilirubin and biliverdin
5. *Pancreas:* long gland located behind the stomach; divided into the head, body, and tail; has both endocrine and exocrine functions; secretes pancreatic enzymes, insulin, and glucagon
6. *Gallbladder:* sac located beneath the liver; responsible for storage and concentration of bile for fat emulsification

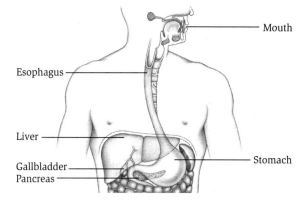

Mouth

Esophagus

Liver

Gallbladder

Pancreas

Stomach

What structures comprise the lower GI system?

1. *Small intestine:* responsible for digestion and absorption of digestive end products; separated from the pylorus of the stomach by the pyloric sphincter
2. *Large intestine:* responsible for water and electrolyte absorption and formation of feces; intestinal bacteria responsible for synthesis of vitamin K and deamination of some amino acids (which are then converted to urea in liver); secretion of mucus to lubricate and protect the mucosa; separated from the ileum of the small intestine by the ileocecal valve

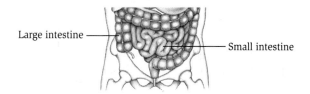

Large intestine

Small intestine

What processes are involved with the function of the GI system?

1. *Ingestion and propulsion:* intake and movement of food
2. *Digestion:* chemical and physical breakdown of food into absorbable substances, such as nutrients, electrolytes, and water; waste products are produced
3. *Absorption:* transfer of digested food products across the intestinal wall and into the circulatory system for cellular use; primarily occurs in the duodenum and jejunum of the small intestine, the stomach absorbs alcohol and the large intestine absorbs water
4. *Elimination:* excretion of waste products that result from digestion

What are the four layers that comprise the GI tract?

Mucosa (innermost lining), submucosa, muscularis (three layers), and serosa (outer most lining)

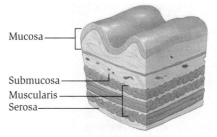

Mucosa

Submucosa
Muscularis
Serosa

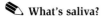 *The GI tract is innervated by both the parasympathetic (primarily excitatory) and the sympathetic (primarily inhibitory) nervous systems.*

Where's the appetite center located?

In the hypothalamus; it's stimulated directly or indirectly by various factors, including an empty stomach, hypoglycemia, decreased body temperature, and the sight, smell, and taste of food; inhibitory factors include stomach distension, hyperglycemia, nausea, vomiting, febrile illness, and some medications such as amphetamines

What's saliva?

A substance consisting of water, protein, mucin, inorganic salts, and salivary amylase (ptyalin) that's produced by the salivary glands in the oral cavity in response to chewing, or the sight, smell, taste, and thought of food; serves to lubricate and soften the food mass and is responsible for the breakdown of starches to maltose

Digestion begins in the oral cavity with the breakdown of starches by saliva.

What's peristalsis?

Wave-like contractions that move food through the GI tract

What are the three portions of the stomach?

1. *Fundus:* uppermost portion; contains chief cells and parietal cells
2. *Body:* central portion
3. *Antrum:* lower portion

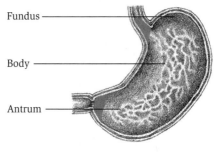

Fundus

Body

Antrum

What's the pylorus?

A small portion of the antrum that's located just prior to the beginning of the duodenum

✎ What's the function of the chief cells?

Secretion of pepsinogen (converted to pepsin in presence of hydrochloric acid), which aids in the breakdown of proteins

✎ What's the function of the parietal cells?

Secretion of hydrochloric acid and intrinsic factor

✎ What's the function of intrinsic factor?

It promotes the absorption of vitamin B_{12} in the small intestine

⬛ *Gastric emptying time is typically 3 to 4 hours.*

✎ What hormone does the stomach produce?

Gastrin, which stimulates the gastric mucosa to secrete hydrochloric acid; gastrin release is stimulated by presence of peptides and amino acids in the stomach

✎ What are villi?

The functional units and sites of absorption of the small intestine, villi are finger-like projections in the mucous membrane that increase the surface area for absorption; contain absorptive cells and goblet cells (secrete mucus)

✎ What are the different segments of the small intestine?

1. *Duodenum:* first portion of the small intestine; responsible for completion of carbohydrate, fat, and protein digestion
2. *Jejunum:* middle portion of the small intestine; responsible for the majority of nutrient absorption
3. *Ileum:* lower portion of the small intestine; opens into the large intestine

Duodenum

Jejunum

Ileum

✎ What digestive processes occur within the small intestine?

1. Conversion of carbohydrates to monosaccharides
2. Conversion of fats to glycerol and fatty acids
3. Conversion of proteins to amino acids

What's chyme?

A mixture of food and gastric secretions in the stomach

✎ What are the predominant hormones involved with digestion?

1. *Gastrin:* stimulates the gastric mucosa to secrete hydrochloric acid
2. *Secretin:* stimulates the pancreas to secrete sodium bicarbonate, which neutralizes the acidic content of

chyme; increases rate of bile secretion from gallbladder

3. *Cholecystokinin:* produced in the duodenum; responsible for stimulating gallbladder contraction and relaxation of the sphincter of Oddi, which allow bile flow from the common bile duct into the duodenum; also stimulates release of pancreatic enzymes responsible for the breakdown of carbohydrates, fats, and proteins

The absorption of what nutritional factors occurs in the small intestine?

Simple sugars, fatty acids, amino acids, water, electrolytes, and vitamins

What are the divisions of the large intestine?

1. *Cecum:* blind pouch-like section that comprises the first 2″ to 3″ (5 to 7.5 cm) of large intestine from which the appendix extends
2. *Ascending colon:* located along right border of the abdomen vertically; begins in right lower quadrant of the abdomen and ends at the transverse colon in the right upper quadrant of the abdomen
3. *Transverse colon:* located across the abdomen horizontally above the small intestine
4. *Descending colon:* located along the left border of the abdomen vertically
5. *Sigmoid colon:* S-shaped portion that curves downward and joins the rectum
6. *Rectum:* last 7″ to 8″ (17.5 to 20 cm)
7. *Anus:* opening at the end of the GI tract through which feces is expelled

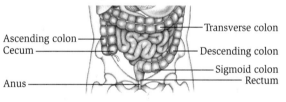

Ascending colon
Cecum
Anus
Transverse colon
Descending colon
Sigmoid colon
Rectum

What are some of the metabolic functions of the liver?

1. *Carbohydrate metabolism:* glycogenesis (conversion of glucose to storage form, glycogen), glycogenolysis (breakdown of glycogen to glucose), and gluconeogenesis (production of glucose from fatty acids and amino acids)
2. *Protein metabolism:* synthesizes plasma proteins, clotting factors, and nonessential amino acids, and forms urea from ammonia
3. *Fat metabolism:* produces lipoproteins, ketone bodies, and fatty acids; synthesizes and breaks down choles-

terol; breaks down triglycerides into glycerol and fatty acids

4. *Steroid metabolism:* conjugates and excretes adrenal and sex steroids

5. *Detoxification:* inactivates drugs and other harmful substances; excretion of their end products

What's bile?

A substance produced by the liver that consists of bile salts, bile pigments (primarily bilirubin), and cholesterol; important for the emulsification of fats prior to their digestion; serves as a means of excreting cholesterol and bile pigments

What digestive enzymes does the pancreas secrete?

1. *Trypsinogen:* aids in protein digestion
2. *Chymotrypsin:* aids in protein digestion
3. *Amylase:* converts starches to disaccharides
4. *Lipase:* aids in fat digestion

What hormones are produced by the pancreas that affect metabolism?

1. *Insulin:* affects carbohydrate metabolism primarily (decreases blood glucose), but also has a role in protein and fat metabolism
2. *Glucagon:* primarily increases glycogenolysis, thereby raises blood glucose levels
3. *Somatostatin:* hinders the release of insulin and glucagon

What's deglutination?

The process of swallowing

What's mastication?

The process of chewing

What's defecation?

Commonly referred to as a bowel movement, it's a reflexive action involving the expulsion of feces from the rectum; both voluntary and involuntary reflexes are involved.

What's feces?

Also known as *stool;* a substance that consists of undigested solid materials, water, mucus, sloughed cells of the intestinal lining, ions, and bacteria that's expelled through the anus during the process of defecation

What's Valsalva's maneuver?

An action in which the intra-abdominal pressure is increased as a result of the contraction of the chest muscles on a closed glottis with simultaneous contraction of the abdominal muscles; facilitates defecation

Valsalva's maneuver should be avoided in patients with head injuries, certain cardiac disorders, and those who have had recent eye surgery.

Physical assessment of the GI system

Normal findings

What are important considerations before beginning an examination of the GI system?

1. Ensure patient privacy in a well-lit room.
2. Place the patient in a supine position with his knees flexed with pillows placed underneath and the head of the bed elevated (relaxes the abdominal muscles).
3. Encourage the patient to empty his bladder to prevent obscured bowel sounds.

What inspections should be made of the oral cavity?

Color and symmetry of lips; condition of tongue (white coating on top and smooth underneath); condition of teeth and gums; presence of distinctive breath odor; midline location of uvula and soft palpate

▧ *Any suspicious areas within the oral cavity should be palpated.*

✎ What's the correct order of an abdominal examination?

Auscultation should precede percussion and palpation because they can alter intestinal activity and bowel sounds; always examine any painful quadrant last

✎ What are two common methods for identifying abdominal landmarks?

1. *Quadrant method:* right upper, right lower, left upper and left lower quadrants
2. *Nine regions method:* right hypochondriac, right lumbar, right inguinal, epigastric, umbilical, suprapubic or hypogastric, left hypochondriac, left lumbar and left inguinal regions

What organs or structures are located in the right upper quadrant?

Liver, gallbladder, pyloric sphincter, duodenum, head of the pancreas, right adrenal gland, portion of the right kidney, hepatic flexure of the colon, and portions of the ascending and transverse colon

What organs or structures are located in the right lower quadrant?

Lower pole of the right kidney, cecum, appendix, portion of the ascending colon, right ovary and fallopian tube, right spermatic cord, and right ureter

What organs or structures are located in the left upper quadrant?

Left lobe of the liver, spleen, stomach, body of the pancreas, left adrenal gland, portion of the left kidney, splenic flexure of the colon, and portions of the transverse and descending colon

What organs or structures are located in the left lower quadrant?

Lower pole of the left kidney, sigmoid colon, portion of the descending colon, left ovary and fallopian tube, left spermatic cord, and left ureter

✎ What's the proper technique for auscultation of the abdomen?

1. Place the patient in a supine position with his knees flexed and his head slightly elevated.
2. Warm the stethoscope by placing it between your hands.
3. Using the diaphragm of the stethoscope, listen for bowel sounds in the epigastrium and in all four abdominal quadrants; auscultation should be performed for at least 5 minutes in each quadrant before the abscence of bowel sounds can be declared.
4. Auscultate for presence of aortic bruits (swooshing or roaring sound heard over turbulent blood flow in a vessel).

◪ *The diaphragm of the stethoscope is used to detect high-pitched sounds (bowel sounds), and the bell of the stethoscope is used to detect lower-pitched sounds.*

✎ What's the proper technique for percussion of the abdomen?

1. Place the patient in a supine position with his knees flexed and his head slightly elevated.
2. Begin by percussing below the umbilicus in the right midclavicular line; percussion should be performed until dullness is detected, which defines the lower border of the liver.
3. Percussion should begin again at the nipple line in the right midclavicular line in a downward direction until dullness is again detected, which defines the upper border of the liver; measure the distance between the two areas of dullness to determine the liver size (normally $2^{1}/_{2}''$ to 5″ [6 to 12.5 cm] in the right midclavicular line).

◪ *Percussion of the abdomen is performed to detect the presence of fluid, distention, or masses based on the sound produced.*

✎ What's the proper technique for palpation of the abdomen?

1. Instruct the patient to get in a supine position, flex his knees and elevate his head slightly. Perform light palpation by using the pads of fingertips to gently depress the abdominal wall (about $^{1}/_{2}''$ [1 cm]) in a smooth and systematic manner. Note any areas of tenderness, muscular resistance, or masses.
2. Perform deep palpation by using the palmar surfaces of the fingers to press more deeply in order to delineate abdominal organs and any masses.
3. Palpate the liver by using the left hand to support the patient's right 11th and 12th ribs and placing the right hand on the patient's right abdomen with the fingertips placed just below the lower border of liver dullness. Press fingertips gently inwards and upwards and instruct the patient to take a deep breath (allows the

liver to drop). Assess for the liver edge, which should be smooth, firm, and sharp.

4. Palpate the spleen by performing a similar technique just below the left costal margin. The spleen normally isn't palpable.

◤ *If the spleen is palpable, discontinue the manual compression so that the enlarged spleen doesn't rupture.*

◤ **What constitutes normal bowel sounds?**	Soft, gurgling sounds in an irregular pattern occurring every 5 to 15 seconds
What's the predominant abdominal percussion sound?	Tympany; dullness is usually detected over solid objects and tympany is usually detected over air
◤ **What are contraindications to percussion or palpation?**	Suspected abdominal aortic aneurysm (pulsating midline mass); percussion and palpation should be performed cautiously when appendicitis is suspected

Abnormal findings

◤ **What constitutes hypoactive bowel sounds?**	Three to five bowel sounds per minute; indicates decreased bowel motility, possibly from complete obstruction, peritonitis, or paralytic ileus
◤ **What constitutes absent bowel sounds?**	No bowel sounds auscultated in any of the four quadrants after 5 minutes; may indicate an immobile bowel possibly from peritonitis, complete obstruction, or paralytic ileus
◤ **What constitutes hyperactive bowel sounds?**	Greater than 34 bowel sounds per minute; may indicate anxiety, infectious diarrhea, or irritation of the intestinal mucosa from blood or gastroenteritis
What's hyperperistalsis?	High-pitched, tinkling sounds (also known as borborygmi) usually accompanied by crampy abdominal pain; may occur in the setting of inflammatory bowel disease and intestinal obstruction
What's tenesmus?	Crampy abdominal pain coupled with ineffective spasms of the bowel; commonly seen in inflammatory bowel disease and irritable bowel syndrome
What's Cullen's sign?	Faint hemorrhagic areas located on the skin around the umbilicus; may indicate acute pancreatitis or massive upper GI bleeding

Where is McBurney's point?

In the right lower quadrant over the appendix; one-third of the distance from the anterior superior iliac spine to the umbilicus; rebound tenderness in this area may indicate appendicitis

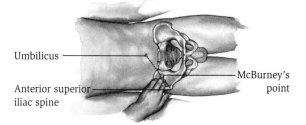

Umbilicus

Anterior superior iliac spine

McBurney's point

What are Grey Turner's spots?

Bluish discoloration at the flanks; may indicate retroperitoneal hemorrhage from pancreatitis

What's Murphy's sign and what might it indicate?

Pain causes abrupt stop midway through inspiration during palpation, which may indicate acute cholecystitis

What might involuntary rigidity of the abdomen indicate?

Peritonitis, an inflammation of the peritoneum; can occur in the setting of appendicitis

What might a concave or scaphoid abdominal contour indicate?

Malnutrition

What might tense, glistening skin and shifting dullness to percussion indicate?

Ascites, which is the abnormal accumulation of fluid within the abdominal cavity; commonly associated with cirrhosis

What might dilated, torturous superficial abdominal veins indicate?

Obstructed inferior vena cava or portal hypertension

What are cutaneous angiomas (spider angiomas) and what might they indicate?

Network of dilated capillaries that radiate out from an arteriole; may indicate liver disease, but may also be found in people on estrogen treatment or birth control pills and in children and pregnant women

What might a bluish tinge around the umbilicus indicate?

Intra-abdominal bleeding

What might strong, visible peristaltic waves indicate?	Intestinal obstruction
✎ **How do you assess for umbilical or incisional hernias?**	Observe for any bulging areas while the patient raises his head and shoulders off the examination table while remaining in a supine position
What's hepatomegaly?	Enlargement of the liver (typically greater than 12 cm), or palpation of the liver edge below the right costal margin; can result from hepatitis, a mass adjacent to the liver or from emphysematous lung disease causing displacement of the liver
What's splenomegaly?	Enlargement of the spleen, which can be associated with chronic anemia, some systemic infections (particularly mononucleosis), hyperplasia, congestion or neoplasms
What might unusual dullness to percussion indicate?	Underlying abdominal mass
✎ **What's stomatitis?**	Inflammatory process involving the oral (buccal) mucosa that can result from infections, irritants, and nutritional deficiencies as well as some medications and treatments (radiation therapy); infectious processes that cause stomatitis include herpes simplex, *Candida albicans* (thrush), and Vincent's angina or trench mouth (bleeding ulcerations related to *Borrelia vincentii*); painful erythema of the oral mucosa, a foul-taste in the mouth and halitosis (bad breath) are common manifestations, although vesicles may be present with herpes infections and white patches may be present with candidal infections
	Treatment measures include frequent alkaline mouthwashes, good oral hygiene (use of a soft toothbrush for frequent brushing), use of soft foods, and appropriate medications (antiviral agents for herpes, antifungal agents for thrush, antibiotics for Vincent's angina).
What's cheilosis?	Cracking or fissuring of the lips at the corners of the mouth; may be associated with riboflavin deficiency
What's cheilitis?	Inflammation of the lips along with fissuring, scaling, or crusting
What's leukoplakia?	Thickened, white patches that occur within the oral cavity, commonly on the tongue; typically associated with precancerous mouth lesions

What's glossitis?	A swollen and reddened tongue; commonly occurs with anemia and vitamin B deficiency
✎ **What's odyno-phagia?**	Pain with swallowing
✎ **What's dyspha-gia?**	Difficulty with swallowing
✎ **What's a mandi-bular fracture?**	A fracture of the jaw bone that typically results from trauma to the face; treatment generally consists of immobilizing the jaw with wires or rubber bands; important nursing actions include assessment for respiratory distress, prevention of nausea and vomiting, provision of routine oral hygiene, and provision of adequate nutrition (no solid foods; high-protein liquids and soft foods through a blender should be encouraged)
	⚡ *Wire cutters should be kept at the bedside at all times, and wires or rubber bands should be released if vomiting occurs to prevent aspiration.*
✎ **What's pyrosis?**	Heartburn, or an epigastric or substernal burning sensation; commonly associated with esophagitis and hiatal hernia
✎ **What's dyspep-sia?**	Indigestion or a burning sensation that may be associated with peptic ulcers or gallbladder disease
✎ **What's hemate-mesis?**	Bloody vomitus; commonly associated with erosive gastritis, bleeding ulcers (peptic ulcer disease), esophageal varices, and tears in the esophageal lining (Mallory-Weiss tear)
✎ **What's melena?**	Black, tarry, and foul-smelling stool that contains digested blood; commonly occurs as a result of *upper* GI bleeding such as from esophageal varices
✎ **What's hemato-chezia?**	Red or maroon-colored stools; commonly associated with *lower* GI bleeding that occurs with colorectal cancer
What might bright red blood per rectum indicate?	Hemorrhoids
✎ **What's jaundice?**	A yellowish discoloration of the skin, sclerae, or mucous membranes; commonly caused by diseases of the liver, but may also occur as a result of an obstruction of the bile duct

What's steator-rhea?	Frothy, fatty, foul-smelling stool that commonly occurs in association with chronic pancreatitis or malabsorption problems, including cystic fibrosis
What's irritable bowel syndrome (IBS)?	A disorder of GI motility that's manifested by alternating periods of diarrhea and constipation, abdominal pain, spasms and bloating; treatment primarily includes a high-fiber diet and elimination of or reduction in stress; an inflammatory process isn't associated with IBS
What's an anal fissure?	A split through the lining of the anal canal that's extremely tender and commonly occurs as a result of straining on defecation

keep up → at night needs to be checked

Major disease processes of the GI system

Gastroesophageal reflux disease

What's gastro-esophageal reflux disease (GERD)?	Commonly referred to as *heartburn;* a condition in which gastric acid refluxes back into the esophagus as a result of hiatal hernia, improper relaxation of the lower esophageal sphincter (LES), or decreased gastric emptying; inflammation of the esophageal lining (esophagitis) may result
mild symptom — do nothing just tums.	Pregnant women, obese people, those who do a lot of bending or straining (increases intra-abdominal pressure), habitual users of acid stimulants (caffeine, alcohol, and aspirin) and those who frequently use tobacco or ingest fatty foods, chocolate, and peppermint are at increased risk for GERD.
What's the patho-physiologic process of GERD?	Inflammatory process of the esophageal mucosa that's typically the result of improper relaxation of LES with resultant backflow of acid
What are the clinical manifestations of GERD?	Heartburn (pyrosis), discomfort behind the lower sternum or in the midepigastrium, hoarseness, sore throat, difficulty swallowing (dysphagia), and regurgitation of sour or bitter tasting material, which is worse at night and made worse by bending, stooping, or eating
What complications are associated with GERD?	*esophagitis* Esophageal stricture, GI bleeding, dysphagia, malnutrition, dehydration, hoarseness, bronchospasm, chronic pulmonary disease, and Barrett's esophagus (precancerous lesions in the lower esophagus that result from chronic irritation)

→ 5years → need to be checked

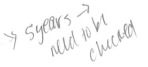

(purging)   *enamel dental erosion.*

What's the typical treatment for GERD?

1. *Behavioral modifications:* including small and frequent feedings, avoidance of irritating foods, avoidance of alcohol and tobacco, remain upright for at least 30 minutes after meals, avoidance of food within 1 hour of bedtime, weight loss, elevation of head of bed
2. *Pharmacologic agents:* proton pump inhibitors, antacids, histamine (H$_2$) antagonists, and coating agents (sucralfate)
3. *Surgery:* modified Nissen fundoplication (open or laparoscopic) in which the fundus of the stomach is wrapped around the lower portion of the esophagus, which creates a more effective valve to prevent gastric acid from refluxing into the esophagus; used for refractory GERD or GERD associated with peptic or respiratory complications

What medications should be avoided in people with GERD?

Nonsteroidal anti-inflammatory drugs (NSAIDs), calcium channel blockers, anticholinergics, and theophylline (lower LES pressure)

What are important nursing actions in the care of a patient with GERD?

1. Instruct the patient to remain upright after eating for at least 30 minutes.
2. Instruct the patient to avoid eating at least 1 hour before bedtime.
3. Instruct the patient to sleep with the head of the bed elevated 6″ (15 cm) and to avoid bending or lying in a supine position.
4. Instruct the patient to consume small, frequent meals of bland foods with high-protein and low-fat content (prevents excessive acid production).
5. Encourage smoking cessation and avoidance of alcohol.
6. Encourage the patient to lose weight if he's obese.
7. Instruct the patient to avoid constrictive clothing.
8. Instruct the patient to avoid such dietary irritants as caffeine, chocolate, peppermint, spearmint, and fat (lower LES pressure).
9. Administer medications (proton pump inhibitors, H$_2$-blockers, antacids) as ordered by the physician.

Hiatal hernia

What's a hiatal hernia?

A condition in which a portion of the stomach protrudes through an opening (hiatus) in the diaphragm into the thoracic cavity, allowing gastric acid to enter the esophagus; congenital defects, obesity, pregnancy, and age increase the risk for hiatal hernia

What's the patho-physiologic process of a hiatal hernia?

Decreased pressure or incompetence of the lower esophageal sphincter (LES) allows gastric acid to reflux into the esophagus, causing esophagitis

✎ What are the clinical manifestations of a hiatal hernia?

Heartburn (pyrosis) after eating that's worse in the recumbent position or with bending; regurgitation; sensation of a lump in the throat or sensation of food getting caught; dysphagia; and odynophagia (pain with swallowing)

What complications are associated with hiatal hernias?

Severe chronic esophagitis or GERD, ulcerations of the herniated portion of the stomach, hemorrhage from erosion, strangulation of the hernia, and regurgitation with tracheal aspiration

✎ What's the typical treatment for a hiatal hernia?

1. *Behavioral modifications:* encourage small, frequent meals of bland foods to avoid overdistention of the stomach; fatty foods, acidic foods, and foods that decrease LES pressure, such as chocolate, peppermint and coffee should be avoided; a high-protein, low-fat diet is ideal
2. *Pharmacologic agents:* proton pump inhibitors. H_2-blockers, antacids, bethanecol (to increase LES pressure)
3. *Surgery:* for failure of conservative therapy or development of complications such as stenosis, strangulation, chronic esophagitis and bleeding: fundoplication; the Nissen and the Belsey Mark IV are the two most commonly used fundoplication operations; can be performed laparoscopically

✎ What are important nursing actions in the care of a patient with a hiatal hernia?

1. Instruct the patient to remain upright after eating for at least 30 minutes.
2. Instruct the patient to avoid eating at least 1 hour before bedtime.
3. Instruct the patient to sleep with the head of the bed elevated 6″ (15 cm) and to avoid bending over or lying in a supine position.
4. Instruct the patient to consume small, frequent meals of bland foods with high-protein and low-fat content (prevents excessive acid production and overdistention of the stomach).
5. Encourage smoking cessation and avoidance of alcohol.
6. Encourage the patient to lose weight if he's obese.
7. Instruct the patient to avoid such dietary irritants as caffeine, chocolate, peppermint, spearmint, and fat (lower LES pressure).
8. Instruct the patient to avoid constrictive clothing.

Gastritis

✒ **What's gastritis?**	Inflammation of the mucosal lining of the stomach that may be either acute or chronic
What's the patho-physiologic process of gastritis?	Breakdown of the mucosal lining of the stomach occurs, which allows the entry of hydrochloric acid; histamine is released from mast cells and secretion of pepsinogen is increased, which result in edema of gastric tissues and an alteration of the capillary walls; hemorrhage from the affected areas may occur

What are the common causes of gastritis?

1. *Acute:* certain medications (NSAIDs); *Helicobacter pylori* infection; large amounts of caffeine; cigarette smoking; alcohol ingestion; severe physiologic stress (extreme illness or trauma); major surgery or organ failure; and some contaminated foods (*Staphylococcus* and *Salmonella* organisms)
2. *Chronic:* repeated alcohol abuse, certain medications (NSAIDs), chronic bile reflux, stress, presence of *H. pylori,* caustic substances, and chronic uremia

✒ **What are the clinical manifestations of gastritis?**

1. *Acute:* epigastric tenderness that's made worse by eating, a feeling of fullness, anorexia, nausea, vomiting, hiccoughs, dark stools, and hematemesis
2. *Chronic:* upper abdominal pain aggravated by eating, indigestion, anorexia, distention, nausea and vomiting after eating, and dark stools

What complications are associated with gastritis?

1. *Acute:* bleeding from the stomach lining
2. *Chronic:* GI bleeding, pernicious anemia and increased risk of gastric cancer

What's the typical treatment for gastritis?

1. *Acute:* symptomatic care; avoidance of causative factors; usually self-limited, lasting from a few hours to a few days
2. *Chronic:* administration of medications for eradication of *Helicobacter pylori* infection (two antibiotics, proton pump inhibitor, bismuth subsalicylate (Pepto Bismol), acid-neutralizing agents, and antacids

✒ **What are important nursing actions in the care of a patient with gastritis?**

1. Maintain nothing-by-mouth status during the acute phase of severe conditions until the patient can advance to a bland diet.
2. Place a nasogastric tube in severe cases for either lavage of the precipitating agent from the stomach or in conjunction with suction to keep the stomach empty and free of noxious stimuli.

3. Administer I.V. fluids and medications (antibiotics, proton pump inhibitors, antacids, H_2-blockers, antiemetics, antispasmodics, anticholinergics) as ordered by the physician.
4. Monitor for complications, including melena or hematochezia. Perform stool guaiacs to evaluate for the presence of occult blood. Monitor complete blood count periodically to assess for anemia.
5. Educate the patient about the importance of maintaining a bland diet and avoiding smoking, alcohol, and NSAIDs.
6. Administer vitamin B_{12} if pernicious anemia occurs.

Peptic ulcer disease

What's peptic ulcer disease?

A condition characterized by ulcerations in the GI mucosa and underlying tissues caused by acidic gastric secretions; primary cause of peptic ulcer disease is *Helicobacter pylori* infection, although the use of NSAIDs and Zollinger-Ellison syndrome (a condition involving gastrin-secreting tumors of the pancreas) are also possible etiologies; smoking and physical stress may increase the risk of ulcer development, and smoking also delays the healing of existing ulcers and increases the risk of recurrence; caffeine consumption may exacerbate the pain of an existing ulcer due to stimulation of gastric acid secretion, but it hasn't been proven to cause ulcer development

What's the pathophysiologic process of peptic ulcer disease?

H. pylori penetrates the mucosal lining of the stomach where it produces substances that decrease the protective actions of mucus and increase the stomach's susceptibility to hydrochloric acid pepsin. Inflammation and erosions then develop in the GI mucosa.

What's the standard treatment for *H. pylori* infection?

A combination therapy consisting of two antibiotics, including tetracycline (or amoxicillin) and metronidazole (Flagyl), bismuth subsalicylate, and a proton pump inhibitor

What are the two types of peptic ulcers?

1. *Gastric:* more commonly affects women, older adults, lower socioeconomic classes, smokers, drug and alcohol abusers, and patients with severe burns, head trauma, and major surgery; bile reflux gastritis, drug effects, autoimmune disease, and viral infections are other potential causes
2. *Duodenal:* more common among smokers, alcohol abusers, people with chronic obstructive pulmonary disease, cirrhosis, pancreatic disease, hyperparathy-

roidism, Zollinger-Ellison syndrome, chronic renal failure, and people with blood group O

How is the presence of *H. pylori* infection diagnosed?

By blood and breath tests as well as analysis of stomach tissue; breath tests are the most accurate means of testing for *H. pylori;* a drink containing urea and carbon is ingested and the amount of carbon dioxide exhaled in the breath is measured (urea is broken down if *H. pylori* bacteria are present and the carbon dioxide produced is eventually exhaled)

✎ What are the clinical manifestations of peptic ulcers?

1. *Gastric:* gnawing pain occurring 1 to 2 hours after meals (commonly occurs when the stomach is empty), radiation of pain to the back, burning or gaseous pressure high in the left epigastrium and back and upper abdomen, occasional nausea and vomiting as well as weight loss; relieved by food or antacids
2. *Duodenal:* burning, cramping, pressure-like pain across the midepigastrium and upper abdomen that typically occurs 2 to 4 hours after meals; is periodic and episodic in nature and is associated with occasional nausea and vomiting; back pain may also occur; relieved by food or antacids

What are the potential complications of peptic ulcers?

Anemia (from chronic blood loss), hemorrhage (more common with duodenal ulcers), perforation (considered the most lethal complication), penetration into neighboring organs, and obstruction (more common with duodenal ulcers)

✎ What are the clinical manifestations of an ulcer perforation?

Sudden and severe upper abdominal pain that quickly spreads throughout the abdomen, abdominal rigidity, shallow and rapid respirations, and absent bowel sounds; may experience shoulder pain if the spillage irritates the phrenic nerve

What are the potential complications of an ulcer perforation?

Bacterial peritonitis may occur within 6 to 12 hours, possibly followed by paralytic ileus and sepsis.

◤ *People with known or suspected ulcer perforations should be kept on nothing-by-mouth status during the acute phase.*

✎ What's the typical treatment for peptic ulcers?

1. *Behavioral modifications:* smoking cessation; stressor elimination; dietary changes, including several small meals per day (food acts as a buffer for gastric secretions), and avoiding substances known to irritate gastric mucosa, such as alcohol; proteins are considered the best neutralizing foods; carbohydrates and fats are the least stimulating to acid secretion; adequate rest;

calm, quiet environment, and moderation of daily activity

2. *Pharmacologic agents:* proton pump inhibitors (omeprazole, lansoprazole), antacids, H_2-blockers (cimetidine, ranitidine, famotidine), and anticholinergic agents; mucosal protective agents, including sucralfate (Carafate), misoprostol (Cytotec), and bismuth subsalicylate (Pepto-Bismol)

3. *Surgery:* for complicated cases or those refractory to conservative treatment

✎ What types of surgery may be performed in the treatment of peptic ulcer disease?

1. *Highly selective parietal cell vagotomy:* disrupts the nerves to the lower stomach, which decreases acid production and promotes ulcer healing; highest recurrence rate, but fewer complications

2. *Vagotomy or antrectomy (Billroth II):* division of both vagal nerves and removal of antrum of stomach as well as first portion of the duodenum (lowest recurrence rate but highest complication rate)

3. *Vagotomy and pyloroplasty (Billroth I):* division of both vagal nerves and cutting of pylorus to improve drainage of food from the stomach

4. *Subtotal gastrectomy:* removal of portion of the stomach

▨ *NSAIDs and high-dose steroids should be avoided in people with peptic ulcer disease.*

✎ What are common complications following a vagotomy?

Dumping syndrome (common after Billroth II), postprandial hypoglycemia, bile reflux gastritis, hemorrhage, pneumonia, and pernicious anemia

✎ What are important nursing considerations after a vagotomy?

1. Instruct the patient to consume small meals and to avoid high-carbohydrate foods to prevent gastric distention and Dumping syndrome. Encourage snacking between meals to obtain sufficient calories, if necessary.

2. Instruct the patient to drink liquids only between meals. Liquids should be consumed at least 1 hour before or after meals.

3. Maintain patency of the nasogastric tube.

4. Monitor for complications, such as hemorrhage or perforation, and notify the physician immediately if any develop.

5. Notify the physician immediately if excessive bleeding or bright red blood is noted more than 12 hours postoperatively.

✎ **What are impor-
tant nursing actions
for a patient with
peptic ulcer disease?**

1. Inform the patient that no specific diet is helpful for peptic ulcer disease but foods known to exacerbate symptoms should be avoided.
2. Monitor vital signs, especially blood pressure and temperature.
3. Monitor for complications, such as bleeding or perforation, and notify the physician immediately if any develop.
4. Educate the patient regarding the importance of compliance with medication regimen.
5. Encourage behavioral modifications, including smoking cessation and stressor elimination.
6. Instruct the patient to avoid alcohol and NSAIDs.
7. Educate the patient regarding the symptoms of ulcer complications and when to notify the physician.
8. Encourage anxiety reduction by identifying stressors as well as healthy coping mechanisms.
9. Administer medications (proton pump inhibitors, H_2-blockers, antacids, sucralfate) as ordered by the physician.

Cholelithiasis

✎ **What's choleli-
thiasis?**

A condition characterized by the presence of calculi within the gallbladder; typically composed of cholesterol, calcium, and bile pigments and result from a disturbance in their balance.

It occurs more commonly in multiparous women, people over age 40, obese people, those with a sedentary lifestyle, as well as those who are of white or Native American race and those with marked weight loss or gain.

**What's the pathophysi-
ologic process of cho-
lelithiasis?**

The precipitation of cholesterol (most common), bile salts and calcium is caused by a disturbance in their balance, resulting in the formation of stones within the gallbladder

✎ **What are the
clinical manifestations
of cholelithiasis?**

Usually produces no symptoms ("silent cholelithiasis") if immobile, but may present as indigestion; excruciating right upper quadrant pain; tachycardia; diaphoresis; bloating, nausea, and vomiting following ingestion of a heavy meal (particularly fried or fatty foods); and jaundice and fever in severe cases

⚡ *The symptoms of cholelithiasis vary greatly depending on whether the stones are stationary or mobile and whether they have produced an obstruction.*

What's biliary colic?	Severe pain in the right upper quadrant caused by spasms that occurs when a stone passes through or becomes lodged in the bile ducts; the pain typically builds to a plateau rather than waxing and waning
✎ **What's the typical timing of the pain associated with cholelithiasis?**	One or more hours after a heavy meal, and commonly at night
What are the potential complications of cholelithiasis?	Obstruction of the bile ducts, cholangitis, pancreatitis, biliary cirrhosis, and peritonitis
What are the clinical manifestations of a biliary obstruction?	Jaundice, clay-colored stools, tea-colored urine, steatorrhea, fever, and leukocytosis
What are the potential complications of obstruction?	Bleeding (prothrombin production is decreased because vitamin K isn't absorbed in the absence of bile) and infection
✎ **What's the typical treatment for cholelithiasis?**	1. *Dietary modification:* smaller, more frequent meals that are low in fat to prevent excess stimulation of the gallbladder 2. *Pharmacologic agents:* analgesics (meperidine, fentanyl); cholesterol solvents, such as ursodiol (Actigall) to dissolve stones; antispasmodics and anticholinergics to minimize gallbladder contractions; antibiotics if infection (cholecystitis) results from biliary obstruction; if chronic obstruction is present, replacement of fat-soluble vitamins and administration of bile salts (facilitates digestion and vitamin absorption) may be necessary 3. *Procedures:* laparoscopic cholecystectomy is the preferred surgical approach; extracorporeal shock-wave lithotripsy (ESWL) and endoscopic sphincterotomy are procedures commonly used in the treatment of cholelithiasis
✎ **What's extracorporeal shock-wave lithotripsy?**	Disintegration of gallstones by high-energy shock waves; the resulting stone fragments pass through the common bile duct and into the small intestine before being excreted from the body
What's endoscopic sphincterotomy (papillotomy)?	An endoscopic retrograde cholangiopancreatography procedure in which the sphincter of Oddi is widened by incision of the sphincter muscle; the stones are then removed with a basket or a balloon

✎ What are the methods of surgical intervention (cholecystectomy)?

1. *Laparoscopic cholecystectomy:* preferred surgical approach; gallbladder is removed through one of four small puncture sites in the abdomen; a fiberoptic lens is used and carbon dioxide is insufflated to create space for surgical instruments; general anesthesia is used; stable patients are discharged on the day of surgery
2. *Open cholecystectomy:* performed through a right subcostal incision; used instead of laparoscopic approach if dense adhesions from previous surgeries exist, if the gallbladder is highly inflamed (highly adherent to adjacent structures), or if the gallbladder isn't well-visualized via laparoscopy

✎ What's a T-tube?

A T-shaped biliary catheter inserted after the common bile duct has been explored; serves to decompress obstructed extrahepatic bile ducts so that bile can flow freely

▎ *Drainage from a T-tube is typically 500 to 1,000 ml for the first 24 hours, after which the amount decreases steadily.*

What are important patient teaching issues for the care of a T-tube?

The skin around the site should be cleaned daily with an antiseptic; any bile leakage at the insertion site should be reported.

✎ What are important nursing actions after a cholecystectomy?

1. Assess pain severity and administer analgesics as ordered. Evaluate patient response to therapy.
2. Place the patient in low-Fowler's position.
3. Maintain nothing-by-mouth status until bowel sounds return or passage of flatus occurs, then advance diet as ordered and as the patient tolerates.
4. Perform dressing changes as needed.
5. Provide T-tube care (if common bile duct explored) and record type and amount of drainage from T tube or any Penrose or Jackson-Pratt drains. Following T tube removal, monitor stool for normal brown color (suggests bile is entering the duodenum appropriately).

Cholecystitis

✎ What's cholecystitis?

An inflammation of the gallbladder that may result from stones obstructing the outflow of bile, adhesions, neoplasms, extensive fasting, anesthesia, and narcotics; *Escherichia coli* is the most common bacterium involved

What's the pathophysiologic process of cholecystitis?	Bile stasis results from an obstruction that produces inflammation and possibly infection
✎ **What are the clinical manifestations of acute cholecystitis?**	1. *Acute:* symptoms of indigestion; severe right upper quadrant pain (Murphy's sign), which may refer to the right shoulder and scapula, abdominal rigidity, fever, nausea, vomiting, diaphoresis, jaundice, and leukocytosis 2. *Chronic:* history of dyspepsia, heartburn, and fat intolerance
What complications are associated with cholecystitis?	Subphrenic abscess, pancreatitis, cholangitis, biliary cirrhosis, fistula formation, rupture of the gallbladder, and peritonitis (from rupture of gallbladder)
✎ **What are important nursing actions in the care of a patient with cholecystitis?**	1. Ensure nasogastric tube patency to prevent further stimulation of the gallbladder if nausea and vomiting are severe. 2. Administer medications (analgesics, antibiotics, anticholinergics) as ordered by the physician. 3. Monitor fluid and electrolyte balance. 4. Monitor for complications, including pancreatitis, cholangitis, subphrenic abscess (hiccups), and notify the physician immediately if any develop.

Pancreatitis

✎ **What's pancreatitis?**	Inflammation of the pancreas that results when chemicals produced by the pancreas attack the organ itself; acute pancreatitis can result from chronic alcoholism, cholelithiasis, some medical procedures (endoscopic retrograde cholangiopancreatography), certain infections (viral, bacterial, and parasitic), hypertriglyceridemia (triglyceride greater than 1,000), certain medications (glucocorticoids, thiazide diuretics, azathioprine, hormonal contraceptives, sulfonamides, and acetaminophen), recent blunt trauma to the pancreas, and obstruction of pancreatic duct drainage from tumors Chronic pancreatitis may occur secondary to chronic alcohol abuse, abdominal trauma, pancreatic duct obstruction, nutritional factors, genetic abnormalities (trypsinogen defect), hyperparathyroidism, peptic ulcer disease, and cystic fibrosis (many have a mutation in the same gene that causes cystic fibrosis).

What's the patho-physiologic process of pancreatitis?

Autodigestion of the pancreas occurs secondary to activation of enzymes (elastase, trypsin and phospholipase-A), which can produce inflammation, progressive destruction of the pancreatic tissue, and hemorrhagic necrosis

✎ What are the clinical manifestations of pancreatitis?

1. *Acute:* severe, sharp and stabbing epigastric or left upper quadrant pain that's typically worse after meals and may radiate to the back or left shoulder and may worsen in recumbent positions; nausea; vomiting; low-grade fever; leukocytosis; hypotension; tachycardia; rales; jaundice; ecchymosis in the flanks (Grey Turner's spots) or periumbilical area (Cullen's sign)
2. *Chronic:* repeated episodes of nausea and vomiting, abdominal pain, inability to digest fatty foods, steatorrhea, weight loss, and possible development of diabetes

✎ What complications are associated with pancreatitis?

1. *Acute:* peritonitis, ileus, fistula formation, biliary stenosis, pseudocyst and abscess (most serious) are local complications; systemic complications include pulmonary disorders, such as pleural effusions, atelectasis, pneumonia, and respiratory failure; tetany due to hypocalcemia; hypovolemia (4 to 6 L in the first 48 hours) due to fluid sequestration in the abdomen; hypotension and electrolyte imbalances (hypocalcemia, hypokalemia, hypomagnesemia) due to vasodilation; sepsis, acute renal failure, and shock from hemorrhage (from development of disseminated intravascular coagulation [DIC])
2. *Chronic:* diabetes, jaundice, malabsorption syndromes, development of strictures and obstruction of the pancreatic ducts, and the development of pseudocysts and fistulas

Why is serum lipase considered more useful than serum amylase?

More specific to the pancreas and may remain elevated for up to 2 weeks; amylase levels return to normal in 3 to 5 days

Why are serum amylase and lipase levels frequently not elevated in the patient with chronic pancreatitis?

The pancreas may be damaged to the point that it no longer produces sufficient amylase and lipase

What drugs are most likely to produce elevated amylase levels?

Opiates and thiazide diuretics

✎ What's the typical treatment for pancreatitis?

1. *Acute:* diet modification (nothing by mouth during the acute phase, but a bland, low-fat, high-carbohydrate, and high-protein diet is best when diet is resumed); and pharmacologic agents, including analgesics (fentanyl, meperidine) for pain, pancreatic enzyme replacement, and antibiotics
2. *Chronic:* diet modification (nothing by mouth during acute phases, avoidance of alcohol, use of specialized nutrition, such as jejunal tube feeding or total parenteral nutrition); administration of pharmacologic agents, including analgesics (fentanyl) for pain management, pancreatic enzyme replacements, and bile salts (facilitate absorption of fat-soluble vitamins); and nerve blocks, such as celiac plexus blocks (can be performed surgically or with endoscopic ultrasound when more conservative therapies fail)

✎ Why isn't morphine typically used for pain control in pancreatitis?

It may worsen the pain associated with pancreatitis by causing spasm of the sphincter of Oddi

What types of surgical intervention may be necessary in the setting of acute pancreatitis?

1. *Acute:* pancreatic debridement or drainage of infected, necrotic tissue
2. *Chronic:* choledochojejunostomy to divert bile around the ampulla of Vater and pancreatic drainage procedures, such as a Roux-en-Y pancreaticojejunostomy (Puestow procedure), to relieve ductal obstruction; a Whipple's operation (pancreaticoduodenectomy) may also be of benefit

✎ What are important nursing actions in the care of a patient with pancreatitis?

1. Maintain nothing-by-mouth status during acute phase to minimize pancreatic secretions.
2. Administer I.V. fluids, as ordered, to prevent dehydration from fluid loss.
3. Ensure proper nasogastric suctioning to reduce vomiting and gastric distention.
4. Anticipate the need for nutritional support with jejunal tube feeding or total parenteral nutrition (especially if nothing by mouth more than 3 days).
5. Monitor electrolytes, daily weight, and provide routine mouth care while the patient is on nothing-by-mouth status.
6. Monitor intake and output.
7. Obtain vital signs at frequent intervals.
8. Monitor for complications, including hypotension and fever, and notify the physician if any occur.
9. Assess respiratory status for pulmonary complications (crackles).
10. Assess the abdomen and back for ecchymosis (indicative of hemorrhagic pancreatitis).

11. Re-introduce food with small, frequent feedings of bland foods high in carbohydrate content (least stimulating to the pancreas) that are also low in fat and high in protein.
12. Administer medications (fentanyl, pancreatic enzyme replacements, fat-soluble vitamins for chronic pancreatitis) as ordered by the physician.
13. Instruct the patient to avoid alcohol and tobacco products.

Hepatitis

What's hepatitis?

Inflammation of the liver tissue that can result from an infection (viral, bacterial, or parasitic) and toxic chemicals, as well as alcohol and other drugs

What's the pathophysiologic process of hepatitis?

Widespread inflammation of the liver tissue leads to degeneration and necrosis of hepatic cells; cholestasis may result from obstruction of bile flow secondary to the inflammatory process

✎ What types of viral hepatitis exist?

1. *Hepatitis A:* fecal-oral route of transmission, and contact with blood or contaminated food or water
2. *Hepatitis B:* contracted through contact with contaminated blood or body fluids; primarily considered a sexually transmitted disease and one of needle-sharers, but can also result from tattoos where one needle was shared among several people, or through childbirth and breast-feeding
3. *Hepatitis C:* primarily contracted through contact with infected blood (primarily blood transfusions and needle-sharing), but can be transmitted to a lesser degree through sexual contact and childbirth; intranasal cocaine use is also a risk factor
4. *Hepatitis D:* primarily seen in people who are frequently exposed to blood and blood products, such as I.V. drug users and hemophilia patients; coexists only with hepatitis B because it needs the hepatitis B virus to replicate
5. *Hepatitis E:* primarily transmitted through the fecal oral route and in those who have recently returned from an endemic area, such as India, Africa, Asia or Central America; more common in young adults and more severe in pregnant women

What are the clinical manifestations of hepatitis?

Anorexia, nausea, vomiting, flulike symptoms, easy fatigability, jaundice, clay-colored stools, and tea-colored urine (due to impaired bilirubin excretion), pruritus (from bile salt accumulation in skin tissue), and bleeding tendencies (due to decreased prothrombin synthesis and decreased vitamin K absorption)

What complications are associated with hepatitis?

Food-borne (hepatitis A) infections are generally self-limited and don't cause long-term sequelae; blood-borne infections (hepatitis B and C) may result in a chronic infection, which can lead to cirrhosis and possibly hepatocellular carcinoma; non viral hepatitis, such as acetaminophen toxicity, can produce rapid liver failure, requiring liver transplantation

✎ What are methods of preventing contraction of viral hepatitis?

1. *Hepatitis A:* good hygiene practices, including thorough hand washing after toileting and before meal preparation; avoiding contaminated food, milk, water, and shellfish; receiving the hepatitis A vaccination series (two injections: day 0 and 6 months later)
2. *Hepatitis B:* avoid contact with contaminated blood or body fluids (don't share personal items such as a toothbrush, razor, or nail clippers with an infected person) and receive hepatitis B vaccination series (three injections: day 0, then at 1 month and 6 months after the first injection)
3. *Hepatitis C:* avoid contact with contaminated blood or body fluids (don't share personal items, such as a toothbrush, razor, or nail clippers); no vaccine for hepatitis C currently exists
4. *Hepatitis D:* avoid contact with contaminated blood or body fluids (don't share personal items, such as a toothbrush, razor, or nail clippers); no vaccine for hepatitis D currently exists
5. *Hepatitis E:* good hygiene practices, including thorough hand washing after toileting and before meal preparation, avoid activities that involve fecal-oral contact, and avoid travel to known endemic areas; when in developing countries, avoid drinking water of unknown purity (including ice), eating uncooked shellfish and uncooked fruits and vegetables that have been peeled or prepared by someone other than yourself; no vaccine for hepatitis E currently exists

What blood tests are used to screen for viral hepatitis?

1. *Hepatitis A:* a positive hepatitis A IgM indicates acute infection while a positive hepatitis A IgG indicates prior exposure and immunity
2. *Hepatitis B:* a positive hepatitis B surface antigen (HBsAg) and core antibody; positive hepatitis B surface antibody may indicate immunity due to past exposure or previous immunization
3. *Hepatitis C:* enzyme-linked immunosorbent assay detects the presence of antibodies, which denotes prior exposure to the hepatitis C virus, but it doesn't con-

firm an active infection; HCV by PCR is a more definitive test to assess for current viral activity

4. *Hepatitis D:* HbsAg, hepatitis D antibody IgM, hepatitis D antibody IgG
5. *Hepatitis E:* hepatitis E antibody IgM

What's the typical treatment for hepatitis?

1. *Hepatitis A:* primarily symptomatic care and rest
2. *Hepatitis B:* antiviral agents, such as interferon and lamivudine (Epivir) as well as liver transplantation with the administration of hepatitis B immune globulin
3. *Hepatitis C:* antiviral agents, such as interferon and rebetol (Ribavirin)
4. *Hepatitis D:* because of it's dependence on hepatitis B virus, treatment includes antiviral agents, such as interferon and lamivudine (Epivir) as well as liver transplantation with the administration of hepatitis B immune globulin
5. *Hepatitis E:* no treatment is typically recommended; usually resolves on its own over several weeks to months
6. *Nonviral hepatitis:* treatment is largely supportive; N-acetyl cysteine (Mucomyst) can be beneficial, even if acetaminophen isn't the offending agent; recovery may be rapid if the hepatotoxin is identified and removed; however, liver transplantation may be necessary if liver dysfunction progresses

✎ What are important nursing actions in the care of a patient with hepatitis?

1. Implement blood and body fluid precautions for viral hepatitis.
2. Instruct the patient to consume high-carbohydrate, high-protein, moderate-fat, high-calorie diet.
3. Educate the patient regarding importance of fat-soluble vitamin supplements.
4. Instruct the patient to avoid alcohol.
5. Administer medications as ordered by the physician.
6. Monitor liver function tests and clotting times (prothrombin time) periodically to assess for improvement or progression of condition.
7. Monitor for complications, including jaundice and excessive bleeding, and notify the physician if any occur.
8. Emphasize importance of close medical follow-up.

Cirrhosis

What's cirrhosis?

A chronic, progressive disease that involves the development of irreversible fibrosis and scarring of the liver; excessive consumption of alcohol (Laënnec's cirrhosis) is the most common cause in the United States, although it can occur as a result of many other conditions, including chronic viral hepatitis (hepatitis B and C) and chronic biliary obstruction (biliary cirrhosis or sclerosis)

What's the patho-physiologic process of cirrhosis?

Hepatic cells are permanently replaced by scar tissue, causing a nodular appearance to the liver; normal function of the liver tissue is impaired as a result of the scar tissue formation

What are the clinical manifestations of cirrhosis?

Anorexia, cachexia (muscle wasting), nausea and vomiting, dull, heavy feeling in the right upper quadrant or epigastrium, splenomegaly, jaundice, clay-colored stools, tea-colored urine, peripheral edema and ascites (accumulation of fluid within the abdominal cavity due to decreased serum albumin), gynecomastia (enlargement of breast tissue) in males and amenorrhea in females, peripheral neuropathy (more common with alcohol-associated cirrhosis), prolonged bleeding times, easy bruising, asterixis (flapping tremors of the hands when holding the arms and hands stretched out; also called "liver flap"), and fetor hepaticus (musty, sweet breath smell that results from an accumulation of the amino acid methionine)

What complications are associated with cirrhosis?

Portal hypertension (due to blood flow obstruction through a shrunken liver) with resultant esophageal varices, electrolyte abnormalities (hyponatremia, hypokalemia), ascites, hepatic encephalopathy, hepatic coma, and bacterial peritonitis (from infection of ascites) as well as renal and pulmonary complications in later stages of the disease process

What are esophageal varices?

Fragile varicosities of the esophagus that result from vascular congestion related to portal hypertension; most life-threatening complication of cirrhosis due to high risk for rupture and hemorrhage; treatments include banding, sclerotherapy, ligation of varices, and shunt therapy if the varices haven't ruptured; balloon tamponade and a Sengstaken-Blakemore tube serve to apply pressure directly onto actively bleeding varices; octreotide may also be used in the treatment of bleeding varices

What's encephalopathy?

A change in neurologic and mental responsiveness that involves irritability, memory loss, drowsiness, slow and slurred speech, emotional lability, and impaired judgment that are thought to be triggered by rising ammonia levels and other less well-understood factors; treatment may consist of protein restriction, sterilization of the intestines with antibiotics, and administration of lactulose (decreases ammonia levels)

How is cirrhosis typically treated?	1. *Pharmacologic agents:* lactulose, metronidazole (Flagyl), or neomycin to prevent or correct encephalopathy; diuretics for management of ascites and peripheral edema; beta-blockers (propranolol) to decrease risk of bleeding from varices; and fat-soluble vitamins (A, D, E, and K) 2. *Dietary modifications:* salt restriction for management of ascites and peripheral edema; protein restriction for management of encephalopathy (breakdown of protein increases ammonia levels); elimination of alcohol 3. *Invasive procedures:* paracentesis for drainage and evaluation of ascites; liver transplantation for treatment of end stage liver disease
What are important nursing actions in the care of a patient with cirrhosis?	1. Place the patient in a semi-Fowler's position to prevent ascites from causing respiratory difficulties (ascites impairs diaphragmatic movement). 2. Monitor intake and output. 3. Measure abdominal girth daily. 4. Implement measures to prevent increased intra-abdominal pressure and rupture of esophageal varices. Encourage a mechanical soft diet. Aspirin, alcohol, heavy lifting, straining with bowel movements, coughing, sneezing, and vomiting should be avoided. 5. Administer medications (lactulose, diuretics, propranolol, fat-soluble vitamins) as ordered by the physician. 6. Monitor for complications, such as excessive bleeding, hematemesis, fever and electrolyte abnormalities (hyponatremia, hypokalemia), and notify the physician immediately if any develop. Two large bore I.V. accesses should be maintained in case of need for blood transfusion or aggressive fluid replacement.

Sprue

What's sprue?	A malabsorption disorder characterized by intolerance to gluten; often classified as tropical (acquired in endemic tropical areas) or nontropical; nontropical sprue is frequently referred to as celiac sprue in children, and celiac disease and gluten enteropathy in adults
What's the pathophysiologic process of sprue?	Gluten intolerance causes flattening and blunting of the intestinal villi; the absorptive surface of the intestinal mucosa is decreased as a result
What are the clinical manifestations of sprue?	Anorexia, fatigue, abdominal pain and bloating, excessive flatulence, weight loss, chronic diarrhea, and steatorrhea

What complications are associated with sprue?	Malnutrition (vitamin deficiencies), fluid and electrolyte imbalances, tetany (from hypocalcemia), and osteoporosis (from inadequate calcium absorption)
What's the typical treatment for sprue?	Primarily consists of dietary management, but corticosteroids may be used if the disease doesn't respond to dietary measures
✎ **What types of foods should be avoided on a gluten-free diet?**	All foods that contain wheat, rye, barley, and oats; most grain, pasta, cereal, and many processed foods should be avoided
✎ **What are important nursing actions in the care of a patient with sprue?**	1. Encourage a high-protein, gluten-free diet. Stress the importance of strict compliance with dietary measures.
	2. Administer supplements of fat-soluble vitamins, folic acid and B complex vitamins, as well as iron and calcium.
	3. Encourage the use of rice, corn, and soy flours in place of wheat, rye, barley, and oats.
	4. Obtain daily weight if malnutrition is present.
	5. Monitor for complications, including malnutrition and electrolyte abnormalities.

Appendicitis

What's appendicitis?	Inflammation of the appendix that occurs secondary to circulatory compromise; causes may include obstruction of the appendix by a fecalith or foreign body
What's the pathophysiologic process of appendicitis?	Obstruction of the appendix compromises its circulation, causing necrosis and possible rupture
✎ **What are the clinical manifestations of appendicitis?**	Anorexia, nausea, vomiting, persistent and continuous periumbilical pain that eventually localizes to McBurney's point in the right lower quadrant, abdominal guarding, rebound tenderness, low-grade fever, and leukocytosis
What complications are associated with acute appendicitis?	Perforation, peritonitis, and the development of an abscess
What's the typical treatment for appendicitis?	Urgent surgical removal of the appendix (appendectomy) to prevent rupture and peritonitis

✎ What are important nursing actions in the care of a patient with acute appendicitis?	1. Maintain nothing-by-mouth status preoperatively. 2. Obtain vital signs at frequent intervals. 3. Monitor fluid and electrolyte status. 4. Administer medications (analgesics, possibly antibiotics) as ordered by the physician. 5. Monitor for complications, including perforation and infection, and notify the physician if the develop.

Diarrhea and fecal incontinence

✎ What's diarrhea?	An increase in the frequency or the looseness of stools; causes may include bacterial infections (*Clostridium difficile, Shigella, Salmonella, Escherichia coli*), viral infections (rotavirus, cytomegalovirus, adenovirus, human immunodeficiency virus), parasitic infestations (*Giardia, cryptosporidium*), fungal infections (*Candida albicans*), malabsorption conditions (lactose intolerance, sprue and cystic fibrosis), inflammatory diseases of the bowel (Crohn's and ulcerative colitis), the use of certain medications (antibiotics and chemotherapy), and certain treatments (gastrectomy, radiation therapy, and gastroenterostomy)
What's the single most common infectious cause of diarrhea in hospitalized patients?	*Clostridium difficile*
What are the clinical manifestations of diarrhea?	Loose, watery stools, abdominal cramping, and increased frequency of bowel movements
✎ What complications are associated with diarrhea?	Dehydration and electrolyte imbalances (hypokalemia, hypomagnesemia)
✎ What's the typical treatment for acute diarrhea?	1. Consumption of clear liquids to maintain adequate hydration 2. Pharmacologic agents: bismuth subsalicylate (Pepto-Bismol), loperamide (Imodium, Kaopectate), opiates (tincture of opium, paregoric, codeine), and intestinal flora modifiers (Lactinex, Bacid) 3. Avoidance of coffee, milk, and fats 4. Addition of bulk to thicken and decrease the frequency of stooling (bananas, rice, yogurt, cheese) 5. High-fiber diet (whole wheat grains and bran) 6. Use of bulk-forming agents such as psyllium products (Metamucil)

✎ **What are important nursing actions in the care of a patient with diarrhea?**	1. Encourage increased fluid intake to prevent dehydration. 2. Monitor intake and output. 3. Monitor for electrolyte abnormalities (hypokalemia, hypomagnesemia). 4. Obtain stool specimens as ordered when infectious diarrhea is suspected. 5. Isolation procedures for infections when indicated.
✎ **What's fecal incontinence?**	Inability to control expulsion of feces; may be related to neuromuscular disorders (spinal cord tumors, multiple sclerosis), anal and rectal infections, Crohn's disease, and loss of rectal sphincter control
What's the typical treatment for fecal incontinence?	Bowel training; medications, such as loperamide (Imodium) and codeine phosphate; and possible fecal incontinence pouch
✎ **What are important components of bowel training?**	1. Drink 2 to 3 qt (2 to 3 L) of fluid per day. 2. Increase fiber in diet. 3. Increase activity and perform exercises that strengthen the anal muscles. 4. Ensure privacy. 5. Administer daily mixture of cathartics. 6. Drink hot beverage before daily scheduled defecation. 7. Use cathartic suppository to stimulate defecation at the same time each day. 8. Set a time limit for defecation. 9. Apply intra-abdominal pressure during defecation.

Constipation and fecal impaction

✎ **What's constipation?**	Decreased frequency of bowel movements, retention of feces in the rectum, and difficult-to-pass stools; may be related to inadequate fluid or dietary intake, immobility, neuromuscular impairment, medication side effects, and chronic use of laxatives and enemas.
What's the pathophysiologic process of constipation?	Formation of hard, dry stool results from delayed passage of food residue through the intestines, producing difficulty with defecation
What are the clinical manifestations of constipation?	Decreased frequency of bowel movements, pain with defecation, straining with bowel movements, abdominal pain, and distention

What complications are associated with constipation?	Hemorrhoid development and elicitation of Valsalva's maneuver (can cause bradycardia and increased intra-abdominal pressure as well as increased venous, intra-thoracic, and intracranial pressures)
What's the typical treatment for constipation?	1. Cleansing enemas 2. Cathartics: bulk-forming (psyllium), lubricant (mineral oil), wetting agent (docusate sodium), stimulant (Dulcolax, Bisacodyl), or saline (magnesium citrate, Epsom Salt, Milk of Magnesia)
What are important nursing actions in the care of a patient with constipation?	1. Instruct the patient to increase dietary fiber. 2. Encourage increased physical activity. 3. Encourage increased fluid intake. 4. Administer medications (bulk-forming agents, lubricants, wetting agents) as ordered by the physician. 5. Administer enemas as ordered.
What's a fecal impaction?	Collection or mass of hardened feces, resulting in the inability to pass a normal stool and possible seepage of liquid fecal material from the anus
What's the typical treatment for an impaction?	1. Digital examination with removal (can precipitate Valsalva or vasovagal response) 2. Oil retention enemas followed by cleansing enemas 2 to 4 hours later
What complications are associated with an impaction?	Development of a fecalith (which may require surgical removal) and perforation

Inflammatory bowel disease

What's inflammatory bowel disease (IBD)?	A general term used to describe a group of chronic inflammatory disorders of the GI tract marked by characteristic periods of exacerbations and remissions; family history, immune factors, and environmental factors, such as industrialized countries with consumption of high-fat diet or refined foods; are considered contributing factors to the development of IBD *Unlike IBD, irritable bowel syndrome (IBS) isn't characterized by inflammation.*
What are the two most common forms of IBD?	1. *Ulcerative colitis:* shallow and continuous inflammation of the colonic mucosa extending from the rectum proximally, possibly involving the entire colon; bowel wall becomes thin and fragile; shallow ulcerations, bleeding, and scarring result

2. *Crohn's disease:* deep and discontinuous cobblestone ulcerations along the mucosal wall of the intestinal tract from the mouth to the anus (most often terminal ileum involved), often resulting in fibrosis and shortening of the bowel; absorption of nutrients is inhibited in diseased areas

▰ *Ulcerative colitis only affects the innermost layer of the colon and only occurs in the colon (always starts in the rectum). Crohn's disease involves "skip lesions" (patches of inflammation with normal tissue between them) that can occur anywhere in the GI tract from the mouth to the anus and can extend through every layer of affected bowel.*

✎ **What are the clinical manifestations of IBD?**

1. *Ulcerative colitis:* crampy pain in mid to lower abdomen; passage of bloody, mucoid, or watery stools; severe diarrhea; anorexia; and weight loss
2. *Crohn's disease:* severe right lower quadrant pain, malaise, weight loss, fever, and mild diarrhea generally without blood

✎ **What complications are associated with IBD?**

1. *Ulcerative colitis:* anemia, rectal hemorrhage, fever, dehydration, toxic megacolon, and increased risk of colon cancer
2. *Crohn's disease:* ulcerations may perforate the intestinal wall and form fistulas (abnormal connections between two organs); anemia; intestinal obstruction due to thickening and narrowing of the bowel; anal fissure; malnutrition due to diarrhea and inadequate nutrient absorption; and increased risk of colon cancer (but less than risk for patients with ulcerative colitis)

✎ **What's the typical treatment for ulcerative colitis?**

1. *Pharmacologic therapy:* sulfasalazine, corticosteroids, 5-aminosalicylates (Asacol, Pentasa, Rowasa, 5-ASA), balsalazide (Colazal), and immunosuppressive drugs (azathioprine, mercaptopurine, infliximab, methotrexate, cyclosporine); nicotine patches may be used for flare-ups
2. *Dietary measures:* although no specific diet is used in the treatment of ulcerative colitis, a bland diet low in fiber may cause less discomfort during exacerbations of severe diarrhea; caffeine should be avoided during exacerbations
3. *Surgery:* partial or total colectomy with a permanent ileostomy or ileoanal pouch procedure if dietary measures fail or if obstruction occurs (ulcerative colitis patients); stricturoplasty or removal of the affected portion of the intestine (ileostomy) if fistulas or intestinal obstruction occurs (Crohn's disease)

✎ What's the typical treatment for Crohn's disease?

1. *Dietary measures:* five to six small meals of low-fat, high-calorie, high-protein foods; caffeine should be avoided during flares; may avoid gas producing foods such as cabbage, beans, broccoli, and raw fruits; enteral nutrition may be necessary if absorption is severely impaired
2. *Pharmacologic therapy:* anti-inflammatory agents (aminosalicylates, steroids) antibiotics, immunosuppressants (6-MP, methotrexate), biologic therapy (infliximab), symptomatic control with anti-diarrheal agents, and vitamin B_{12} supplementation (particularly if extensive involvement of terminal ileum)
3. *Surgery:* ileostomy

◣ *Although there's no particular diet for IBD, foods that are known to exacerbate symptoms should be avoided.*

◣ *Typically, only the diseased portion of the bowel is removed in Crohn's disease, while removal of the entire colon (including the rectum) is typically performed for ulcerative colitis.*

◣ *Although removal of the large intestine typically cures ulcerative colitis, it may not be permanently curative for Crohn's disease because it can occur at other locations along the GI tract.*

What's toxic megacolon?

Life-threatening paralysis and massive dilation of the colon resulting in the inability to have a bowel movement or to pass flatus; it's the most serious acute complication of ulcerative colitis because if it's untreated the colon may rupture, resulting in peritonitis; manifestations include abdominal distention and pain, fever, or shock; treatment consists of placing an intestinal tube to decompress the bowel along with fluid replacement; a colectomy is typically performed if no improvement is noted within 24 hours

✎ What are important nursing actions in the care of a patient with IBD?

1. Emphasize the importance of strict medication compliance.
2. Inform the patient that a well-balanced diet should be consumed, but that bland and low-fiber foods as well as avoidance of caffeine may alleviate symptoms during exacerbations of diarrhea.
3. Administer medications (anti-inflammatory agents, immunosuppressants) as ordered by the physician.
4. Monitor for complications, including fluid and electrolyte imbalances as well as vitamin and mineral deficiencies (iron, calcium, zinc).

5. Provide ostomy care and teaching if colectomy is performed.
6. Encourage routine colon cancer screening.

Intestinal obstruction

What's an intestinal obstruction?	A blockage within the intestines caused by impairment of their normal peristaltic movements; surgical scar tissues (adhesions), hernias, intussusception (bowel telescopes on itself) or volvulus (twisting of the intestines), and benign or malignant tumors may be the cause
What's the pathophysiologic process of intestinal obstruction?	A neurologic or mechanical condition impairs the normal peristaltic movements of the intestines, resulting in an obstruction

What types of obstructions exist?

1. *Mechanical:* adhesions, hernias, stool impactions, intussusception (telescoping of the intestine in on itself), and neoplasms
2. *Nonmechanical:* neuromuscular or vascular disorders; most common form is a paralytic ileus
3. *Pseudo obstructions:* apparent mechanical obstruction of the intestine without demonstration of obstruction by radiographic tests

✎ **What are the clinical manifestations of an intestinal obstruction?**	Colicky abdominal pain and distention, constipation, nausea and vomiting (possibly with feculent material), inability to pass flatus, decreased or absent bowel sounds, and bowel distended with air noted on abdominal X-ray
✎ **How does the location of the obstruction affect the clinical manifestations?**	Proximal obstructions (high in the small intestine) produce bile-containing projectile vomiting; more distal obstructions result in orange-brown and foul-smelling vomitus because of bacterial overgrowth; vomitus may also be feculent in distal obstructions
What complications are associated with an intestinal obstruction?	Edema, congestion and necrosis from impaired blood supply as well as possible rupture of the bowel, resulting in peritonitis; strangulation and gangrene may also result; if the obstruction is located high (near the pylorus), metabolic alkalosis may result from the loss of hydrochloric acid in the stomach from vomiting or nasogastric intubation; if the obstruction is located in the small bowel, dehydration may occur rapidly

What's the typical treatment for an intestinal obstruction?

1. Restriction of oral intake (nothing by mouth)
2. Placement of a nasogastric or intestinal tube (Cantor or Miller-Abbott) for gastric decompression

3. Enemas, rectal tubes, sigmoidoscopy and colonoscopy
4. Pharmacologic agents: neostigmine (Prostigmin) to stimulate the passage of flatus
5. Surgery for extensive obstruction (partial or total colectomy, colostomy, or ileostomy) or correction of the underlying cause, including hernia repair and removal of adhesions

✎ Why are analgesics sometimes withheld in a patient with an intestinal obstruction?

Analgesics (particularly opioids) can mask other clinical manifestations and can result in a further decrease in intestinal motility.

✎ What are important nursing actions in the care of a patient with an intestinal obstruction?

1. Maintain nothing-by-mouth status until obstruction resolves.
2. Monitor intake and output.
3. Monitor for complications, including dehydration, electrolyte imbalances, peritonitis, and strangulation of the bowel, and notify the physician if any occur.
4. Administer medications (neostigmine, electrolytes) as ordered by the physician.
5. Provide mouth, nose, and tube care for the patient with a nasogastric tube.
6. Auscultate the abdomen for bowel sounds and inquire about passage of flatus.
7. Measure abdominal girth daily to evaluate for distention.

Diverticular disease

✎ What's diverticular disease?

A GI disorder characterized by outpouchings or saclike dilatations (diverticula) of the intestinal mucosa through the serosa; most frequently affects the sigmoid colon; a low-fiber diet may increase the risk

What's the pathophysiologic process of diverticular disease?

Out-pouchings of the intestinal wall produced by herniation of mucosa and submucosa through the serosa; believed to be a result of muscle hypertrophy with associated increased intestinal pressures that occurs secondary to constipation

What are the two forms of diverticular disease?

1. *Diverticulosis:* presence of numerous, noninflamed diverticula
2. *Diverticulitis:* inflammation of the diverticula; occurs secondary to the retention of stool and bacteria within the diverticula

What are the clinical manifestations of diverticular disease?

1. *Diverticulosis:* commonly produces no symptoms, but mild cramps, left lower quadrant (LLQ) abdominal pain that improves with bowel movement or passage of flatus, bloating, constipation, or bowel irregularity may occur
2. *Diverticulitis:* abdominal pain and cramping, rebound tenderness localized over affected portion of the colon (LLQ), bloody stools, fever, chills, leukocytosis, constipation and, possibly, a palpable mass or localized peritoneal signs with rebound tenderness

What complications are associated with diverticular disease?

1. *Diverticulosis:* brisk and painless bleeding (fairly rare, usually self-limited) and collection of intestinal contents, which may lead to infection (diverticulitis), obstruction, or perforation
2. *Diverticulitis:* development of fecalith (secondary to retention of stool and bacteria), partial or complete bowel obstructions (from scarring), colon perforations, peritonitis, formation of fistulas to the bladder and vagina, and development of a pelvic or anorectal abscess

What's the typical treatment for diverticular disease?

1. *Diverticulosis:* high-fiber diet; anticholinergic drugs, such as propantheline (Pro-Banthine) to control colonic muscle spasms; and mild analgesics
2. *Diverticulitis:* bowel rest, broad-spectrum antibiotics for treatment of infectious process, low-residue or liquid diet, as well as nasogastric suctioning and I.V. fluids if acutely ill; surgery may be necessary for the management of severe and frequent attacks, and for complications from diverticular disease

◥ *Opioids should be avoided because they may exacerbate the clinical manifestations.*

✎ **What are important nursing actions in the care of a patient with diverticular disease?**

1. Instruct the patient to increase dietary fiber (goal of 20 to 35 g/day). The consumption of whole grain breads and cereals, fruits, and vegetables should be encouraged.
2. Instruct the patient to avoid straining on defecation. Bulk-forming laxatives, such as Metamucil or Citrucel, may be recommended to prevent constipation. Adequate amounts of liquids should be consumed.
3. Administer medications (analgesics, bulk-forming laxatives, anticholinergic agents) as ordered by the physician.
4. Monitor for complications, including obstruction or peritonitis, and notify the physician immediately if any occur.

Anorectal problems

HEMORRHOIDS

What are hemorrhoids?

Internally or externally occurring varicosities of the rectum that are commonly the result of constipation, straining with defecation, prolonged sitting or standing, and pregnancy

What's the pathophysiologic process of hemorrhoids?

An increase in venous pressure causes varicosities to develop and possibly protrude from the anus

What are the clinical manifestations of hemorrhoids?

Commonly produce no symptoms, but may present with painless, bright red blood with defecation; external hemorrhoids may present with anal pain, itching, and burning

What complications are associated with hemorrhoids?

Bleeding, anemia, thrombosis, and incarceration

✎ **What's the typical treatment for hemorrhoids?**

1. Dietary modifications: high-fiber diet and adequate fluid intake; low-roughage diet during periods of exacerbation
2. Regulation of bowel regimen with high-fiber diet, especially pectin-containing fruits and vegetables
3. Consumption of at least 8 glasses of fluids per day
4. Prevention of constipation by use of psyllium bulk-forming agents as well as stool softeners and suppositories (anesthetic, steroid, and astringent)
5. Warm sitz baths for symptomatic relief
6. Rubber band ligation, injection therapy, or hemorrhoidectomy may be useful
7. Surgery for an incarcerated prolapse

✎ **What are important nursing actions in the care of a patient with hemorrhoids?**

1. Instruct the patient to increase fiber and fluid intake to soften stools. Encourage him to eat fruits, grains, and vegetables. Fiber supplements, such as Metamucil or Citrucel, may also be beneficial.
2. Instruct the patient to avoid straining on defecation and to avoid prolonged sitting to prevent worsening or recurrence of hemorrhoids.
3. Encourage the use of sitz baths, ice packs, and hemorrhoidal creams and suppositories during exacerbations.
4. Advise the patient against the long-term use of laxatives (risk of dependency).
5. Inform the patient that a small amount of bleeding immediately following hemorrhoidectomy is expected.

Other disorders of the GI tract

NAUSEA AND VOMITING

What's nausea?   A sensation of uneasiness or discomfort in the epigastrium associated with a loss of appetite and a conscious desire to vomit; causes can vary extensively, but may include infectious diseases, pregnancy, central nervous system (CNS) disorders (meningitis, CNS lesion, motion sickness, and concussion), circulatory problems (heart failure), adverse effects of medications (digoxin and antibiotics), toxic and metabolic disorders (uremia), psychological stimulation (stress and anxiety), disorders of delayed gastric emptying (diabetes), and certain GI disorders (cholecystitis, intestinal obstruction, peptic ulcer disease, gastroenteritis)

What's vomiting?   The forceful ejection of partially digested food from the stomach, through the esophagus and out the mouth that occurs secondary to overdistention, irritation, or excitation of the stomach or intestines; may also be associated with inner ear disorders (motion sickness, vertigo), brain disorders (head injuries, brain infections, or tumors), certain medications or treatments (chemotherapy) as well as pregnancy

What's the pathophysiologic process of vomiting?   The chemoreceptor trigger zone in the brain receives emetic impulses from the body and these impulses are then transmitted to the vomiting center in the medulla of the brain, stimulating the vomiting reflex

What are the clinical manifestations of nausea and vomiting?   Anorexia, desire to vomit, tachycardia, tachypnea, diaphoresis, and increased salivation

✎ What does "coffee ground" emesis indicate?   Blood has remained in the stomach and its color has changed to dark brown as a result of interaction with gastric acid

✎ What might emesis of bright red blood indicate?   Active bleeding from a Mallory-Weiss tear, bleeding gastric or duodenal ulcer or neoplasm, and bleeding esophageal varices

✎ What complications are associated with severe vomiting?   Dehydration, metabolic alkalosis (from the loss of hydrochloric acid), aspiration, and Mallory-Weiss tear (a tear in the mucous membrane at the junction between the esophagus and the stomach; commonly seen in alcoholics)

What's the typical treatment for nausea and vomiting?	Drinking small amounts of clear, sweetened liquids (flat sodas and popsicles), resting, avoiding solid food until vomiting resolves, using antiemetic or prokinetic agents, and avoiding nonessential medications

✎ What are important nursing actions for a patient with nausea and vomiting?

1. Avoid sudden changes of position and unnecessary activity.
2. Keep the patient's immediate area well ventilated and free from noxious odors.
3. Encourage nonpharmacologic interventions (guided imagery, relaxation, distraction, music, biofeedback). Promote relaxation techniques, frequent rest periods, and diversional tactics.
4. Promote oral hygiene after each episode of emesis and before each meal.
5. Instruct the patient to breathe slowly and deeply as well as change positions slowly during episodes of nausea.
6. Instruct the patient to eat small, frequent meals (low roughage foods) and to eat and drink slowly. Avoid highly seasoned foods.
7. Monitor intake and output.
8. Administer I.V. fluids to prevent dehydration or to correct electrolyte abnormalities. Encourage fluid intake.
9. Administer medications (antiemetics, promotility agents) as ordered by the physician.
10. Monitor for complications, such as dehydration and electrolyte imbalances. Assess for dehydration (skin turgor for tenting, blood pressure for hypotension). Monitor electrolytes with prolonged vomiting (hypokalemia and metabolic alkalosis can occur).

GASTROENTERITIS

✎ What's gastroenteritis?	A disorder characterized by irritation of the digestive tract that may be caused by an infection (viral, bacterial, or parasitic), medications (NSAIDs, antibiotics, corticosteroids), or excessive alcohol ingestion
What's the pathophysiologic process of gastroenteritis?	Irritants cause local inflammation of the lining of the stomach and small intestine, resulting in nausea, vomiting, and diarrhea
What are the clinical manifestations of gastroenteritis?	Nausea, vomiting, diarrhea, abdominal cramping, bloating, fever, leukocytosis and, possibly, blood or mucus in the stool

What complications are associated with gastroenteritis?	Dehydration and electrolyte imbalances (hypokalemia)
What's the typical treatment for gastroenteritis?	It's usually self-limited to approximately 3 days and treatment is therefore primarily symptomatic; antiemetics and antidiarrheals may be used for prolonged symptoms.
✎ **What are important nursing actions in the care of a patient with gastroenteritis?**	1. Monitor intake and output. 2. Follow strict medical asepsis and enteric precautions, including good hand hygiene. 3. Encourage rest and increased fluid intake. 4. Encourage clear fluids (ginger ale, broth, gelatin) for first 24 hours; a BRAT diet (foods low in fiber and residue — Bananas, Rice, Applesauce, Toast) may also be helpful. 5. Encourage the patient to consume complex carbohydrates (rice, wheat, potatoes, bread). 6. Instruct the patient to avoid fatty foods or foods with high amounts of sugar. 7. Instruct the patient to consume foods that have been cooked thoroughly and are unspoiled.

PERITONITIS

What's peritonitis?	Inflammation and possible infection involving the peritoneum within the abdominal cavity that commonly occurs after a perforation along the GI tract, or as a result of chemical stress such as occurs in pancreatitis
What's the pathophysiologic process of peritonitis?	Localized or generalized inflammation of the peritoneum occurs in response to the release of chemical irritants or bacteria into the peritoneal cavity
What are causes of bacterial peritonitis?	A traumatic injury (gunshot wound, ruptured appendix), certain procedures (large volume paracentesis), other disease processes (pancreatitis), or as a result of peritoneal dialysis
✎ **What are the common clinical manifestations of peritonitis?**	Abdominal pain, abdominal muscular rigidity, guarding, rebound tenderness, ascites, abdominal distention, nausea, vomiting, fever, leukocytosis, tachycardia, and tachypnea
What complications are associated with peritonitis?	Hypovolemic shock, septicemia, ileus, and death

What's the typical treatment for peritonitis?	Antibiotic therapy, nasogastric tube to suction, analgesics and I.V. fluids as well as bed rest in semi-Fowler's position (facilitates drainage of the affected area); surgery may be required to correct the underlying cause (appendectomy, repair of a perforation, drainage of an abscess)

What are important nursing actions in the care of a patient with peritonitis?

1. Maintain nothing-by-mouth status.
2. Maintain patency of the nasogastric tube.
3. Assess level of pain and response to treatment.
4. Obtain vital signs at frequent intervals.
5. Monitor intake and output.
6. Assess for the presence of bowel sounds and ask about passage of flatus.
7. Administer medications (analgesics, antibiotics, I.V. fluids) as ordered by the physician.
8. Monitor for complications, including hypovolemic shock or septicemia, and notify the physician if any develop.

HERNIAS

What's a hernia?

A condition in which an organ or structure protrudes through a weakened area of the abdominal wall

What's the pathophysiologic process of a hernia?

A weakening in the abdominal wall or diaphragm, which may be the result of either an acquired or a congenital defect, allows the protrusion of an underlying organ or structure

What are the primary types of hernias?

1. *Incisional:* herniation occurs through scar tissue with increased intra-abdominal pressure
2. *Umbilical:* herniation occurs through the umbilicus with increased intra-abdominal pressure due to a congenital muscular weakness or failure of the umbilicus to close at birth
3. *Inguinal:* intestinal herniation occurs through a weakened abdominal ring into the inguinal canal
4. *Femoral:* herniation occurs through the femoral canal

What are the clinical manifestations of hernias?

Appearance of a bulge or swelling upon lifting, coughing, or vigorous activity (umbilical and inguinal hernias may resolve when a recumbent position is assumed); presence of a bulge or lump along a surgical incision, or in the groin or umbilicus; pain, abdominal distention, nausea, and vomiting may occur with irritation or strangulation

🔰 **What complications are associated with hernias?**	Incarceration (not reducible), strangulation (blood supply for the structure or organ inside the hernia is interrupted), and the development of gangrenous infection (occurs secondary to strangulation)
	🔋 *Palpation of the abdomen should be avoided if a hernia is strangulated.*
What's the typical treatment for a hernia?	1. *Temporary:* manual reduction by application of gentle pressure to push the protrusion back into the abdomen, or by application of an abdominal binder to relieve symptoms 2. *Permanent:* open or laparoscopic surgical repair of the defect (herniorrhaphy) with possible placement of wire, mesh, or plastic to strengthen the abdominal wall
🔰 **What are important nursing actions after herniorrhaphy?**	1. Inform the patient that he should apply an abdominal binder before getting out of bed. 2. Instruct the patient to splint the surgical area with a pillow when coughing. 3. Instruct the patient to avoid strenuous activity and lifting until permitted by the physician. 4. Administer medications (cough suppressants, mild cathartics to prevent increasing intra-abdominal pressure with coughing or defecation) as ordered by the physician. 5. Auscultate the abdomen to assess for the presence of bowel sounds.

Cancers of the GI tract

Oral cancer

🔰 **What's oral cancer?**	Abnormal, malignant tissue growth affecting the lip and oral cavity that occurs most commonly in people who use large quantities of tobacco and alcohol products; lip cancers most commonly affect pipe smokers and fair-skinned people who have had excessive sun exposure
What's the pathophysiologic process of oral cancer?	Unregulated cellular growth and differentiation produces malignant tumors of the lip and oral cavity
🔰 **What are the clinical manifestations of oral cancer?**	A lump in the lip, mouth, or gums; a nonhealing sore of the lips or oral cavity; leukoplakia (precancerous white patches in the mouth); altered taste sensations; difficulty swallowing; and dentures that no longer fit

> ◣ *Pain is typically* not *an early manifestation of oral cancers.*

What complications are associated with oral cancer?

Disfigurement of face, head, or neck (postoperatively); dry mouth and difficulty swallowing (after radiation therapy); and metastasis to the neck or other sites

What's the typical treatment for oral cancer?

1. *Surgical resection:* removal of the tumor and any affected lymph nodes
2. *Radiation therapy:* to kill cancer cells and shrink the tumor

◣ What are important nursing actions in the care of a patient with oral cancer?

1. Advise the patient to avoid alcohol and tobacco products.
2. Provide frequent oral hygiene, including saline mouthwashes to relieve dry mouth.
3. Educate the patient preoperatively about the method of communication following surgery (writing board).
4. Administer analgesics as ordered by the physician for pain control.
5. Promote rehabilitative services, including speech therapy and learning to chew and swallow following surgery.
6. Encourage regular dental examinations (many oral cancers are found incidentally by dentists) and follow up with the physician regularly.

Esophageal cancer

◣ What's esophageal cancer?

Abnormal, malignant tissue growth within the esophagus that commonly affects people with extensive alcohol or tobacco use and chronic gastric reflux; people with hiatal hernias, Barrett's esophagus (precancerous cells of the esophagus from chronic reflux), and achalasia (a condition in which the lower esophageal sphincter can't relax adequately to allow food to pass to the stomach) are at a higher risk for the development of esophageal cancer; certain nutritional deficiencies (diets low in fruits, vegetables, vitamin A, riboflavin, and zinc) are also believed to increase the risk of esophageal cancer

What's the pathophysiologic process of esophageal cancer?

Unregulated cellular growth and differentiation produces malignant tumors within the esophageal tissues

✎ What are the clinical manifestations of esophageal cancer?	Odynophagia (painful swallowing), dysphagia (difficulty swallowing), weight loss, hoarseness and cough, pain located behind the sternum, substernal burning upon drinking hot liquids, indigestion, and pyrosis (heartburn)
What complications are associated with esophageal cancer?	Malnourishment, respiratory distress from pressure of tumor on trachea, and metastasis
What's the typical treatment for esophageal cancer?	1. *Surgical removal of the cancerous portion of the esophagus (esophagectomy):* treatment of choice; surgical removal of cancerous portion of esophagus and stomach (esophagogastrostomy) may be performed for more advanced tumors 2. *Radiation therapy and chemotherapy:* may be used prior to surgery and for palliative measures 3. *Laser therapy:* use of high-intensity light beam to kill cancer cells; photodynamic therapy is a type of laser therapy in which cancer cells absorb cancer-killing drugs when exposed to a special wavelength of light
✎ What are important nursing actions in the care of a patient with esophageal cancer?	1. Place the patient in semi-Fowler's or high Fowler's position to facilitate respirations and to prevent aspiration. 2. Monitor for respiratory distress. 3. Provide frequent oral hygiene (dysphagia can cause saliva accumulation). 4. Monitor nutritional status. Encourage the intake of high-protein liquids and administer vitamin and mineral replacements as ordered. 5. Administer analgesics as ordered by the physician for pain control.

Gastric cancer

✎ What's gastric cancer?	Abnormal, malignant tissue growth of the cells lining the stomach, which most commonly affects people with *Helicobacter pylori* infection; chronic gastritis; smoking history; a diet high in salted, pickled, or smoked (nitrates) foods and low in fruits and vegetables; advanced age; male gender; and a family history of gastric cancer
What's the pathophysiologic process of gastric cancer?	Unregulated cellular growth and differentiation causes tumor development within the gastric mucosa (inner lining); as the tumor grows, it extends outward to other layers of the stomach wall

✎ What are clinical manifestations of gastric cancer?

1. *Early:* anorexia, nausea, vague stomach discomfort, bloated sensation with meals, eructation (belching), indigestion, and pyrosis (heartburn)
2. *Late:* melena, weight loss, stomach pain, and ascites (fluid accumulation within abdomen)

▎ *Pain typically isn't an early manifestation of gastric cancer.*

What complications are associated with gastric cancer?

Weight loss, development of ascites, metastasis, and anemia, achlorhydria, and pernicious anemia (if gastrectomy is performed)

What's the typical treatment for gastric cancer?

1. Surgical removal of part of stomach and nearby lymph nodes (subtotal gastrectomy), or removal of entire stomach, nearby lymph nodes, and portions of the esophagus and small intestine (total gastrectomy)
2. Radiation therapy and chemotherapy
3. Eradication of *Helicobacter pylori*

✎ What conditions may result from a total gastrectomy?

Dumping syndrome, pernicious anemia, and osteoporosis (decreased absorption of vitamin D and calcium)

✎ What are the clinical manifestations with dumping syndrome?

Food and liquids passing too quickly into the small intestine, causing crampy abdominal pain, diarrhea (from hyperintestinal motility), early satiety (sense of fullness following a meal), nausea, tachycardia, palpitations, and diaphoresis; hyperglycemia occurs with early dumping syndrome (occurs within 30 minutes of eating); hypoglycemia occurs with late dumping syndrome (occurs within 2 hours of eating)

✎ Why does pernicious anemia develop after a total gastrectomy?

Vitamin B_{12} can't be absorbed from the digestive tract due to lack of intrinsic factor, which results in an inadequate production of red blood cells.

✎ What are important nutritional considerations after a gastrectomy?

1. Eat small, frequent meals.
2. Consume dry, low-fiber, low-carbohydrate, high-fat and high-protein foods.
3. Drink liquids between meals rather than with meals.
4. Avoid dairy products or consume low-lactose dairy products.

✎ What are important nursing actions in the care of a patient following gastrectomy?

1. Ensure patency of nasogastric tube (to decompress the remaining portion of the stomach so that the suture line can be rested). Assess gastric aspirate and report any fecal odor from the aspirate.
2. Administer tube feedings as ordered by the physician.

3. Provide care of chest tubes (if total gastrectomy is performed).
4. Assess vital signs at frequent intervals, especially blood pressure and heart rate
5. Monitor intake and output.
6. Educate the patient about anti-dumping diet (small and frequent low-carbohydrate meals).
7. Administer analgesics and vitamin and mineral supplements (vitamin B_{12}, folate, iron, calcium, vitamin D) as ordered by the physician.

> *The gastric aspirate postoperatively should be bright red at first with a gradual darkening within first 24 hours after surgery to a yellow-green color within 36 to 48 hours.*

Pancreatic cancer

What's pancreatic cancer?

Abnormal, malignant tissue growth most commonly involving the lining of the pancreatic ducts that occurs predominantly in smokers; other potential causes include advanced age, male gender, history of diabetes and chronic pancreatitis (frequently related to alcohol abuse), and a high-fat diet

What's the pathophysiologic process of pancreatic cancer?

Unregulated cellular growth and differentiation produces tumors that arise from the lining of the pancreatic ducts; tumors grow and block the ducts of the pancreas, which can cause fibrosis and obstruction of the pancreas

What are the clinical manifestations of pancreatic cancer?

Painless jaundice, weight loss, anorexia, nausea, severe abdominal pain that may radiate to the back, diarrhea, steatorrhea, clay-colored stools, or tea-colored urine (biliary obstruction); a right upper quadrant mass may be present in later stages

What complications are associated with pancreatic cancer?

Ascites, peritonitis, jaundice, hyperglycemia, hypotension (if the patient has undergone surgery), metastasis, and death

What's the typical treatment for pancreatic cancer?

1. *Surgery:* Whipple's operation (pancreaticoduodenectomy) is treatment of choice
2. *Radiation and chemotherapy*
3. *Pharmacologic agents:* analgesics, pancreatic enzymes, vitamin supplements, and anti-hyperglycemic agents (insulin) in some patients
4. *Palliative measures:* analgesics, radiation therapy to shrink tumor, nerve blocks, and sympathectomy (destruction of nerves)

🔖 **What's Whipple's operation?**

A surgical procedure that involves the removal of the head of the pancreas, the duodenum, the gallbladder, the end of the common bile duct and, possibly, part of the stomach; a connection between the end of bile duct and the remaining pancreas with small bowel is performed to allow bile and enzymes to enter the intestines

🔖 **What are nutritional considerations after Whipple's operation?**

Trial-and-error approach to foods is recommended as fatty foods may cause loose stools and abdominal cramping; a metallic taste may be experienced for the first few weeks and the patient may require insulin

🔖 **What are important nursing actions in the care of a patient with pancreatic cancer?**

1. Administer medications (anti-hyperglycemic agents if diabetes is present, analgesics for comfort measures as well as pancreatic enzymes, bile salts, and vitamin K to correct deficiencies) as ordered by the physician.
2. Encourage small, frequent, low-fat meals after surgery (fatty foods may cause diarrhea and abdominal cramping).
3. Perform soapless bathing and administer antipruritic agents to relieve itching from jaundice.

Colon cancer

🔖 **What's colon cancer?**

Abnormal, malignant tissue growth that affects the cells lining the colon; risk factors include the presence of pre-cancerous colon polyps, advanced age (over age 50), history of inflammatory disorders of the colon (Crohn's or ulcerative colitis), a low-fiber and high-fat diet low in fruits and vegetables, history of smoking and moderate consumption of alcohol, and a positive family history of colon cancer

What's the pathophysiologic process of colon cancer?

Unregulated cellular growth and differentiation in the lining of the colon produces tumors that can cause obstructions as they grow

🔖 **What are the clinical manifestations of colon cancer?**

Usually produces no symptoms initially; a change in normal bowel habits of at least 10 days' duration, rectal bleeding, bloody stools (guaiac positive or grossly bloody), persistent spasm of the bowel, weight loss, abdominal pain, and bloating may occur as the condition progresses

What are the potential complications of colon cancer?

Intestinal obstruction, anemia, metastasis, and death

What's the typical treatment for colon cancer?

Surgical resection (colectomy) of the affected portion of the colon is the preferred treatment, although radiation therapy and chemotherapy may be used in conjunction with surgery

✎ What types of colectomies may be used in the management of colon cancer?

1. *Total colectomy:* removal of entire colon and its blood supply
2. *Right hemicolectomy:* removal of last part of small bowel, the ascending colon, hepatic flexure, and small portion of transverse colon
3. *Left hemicolectomy:* removal of descending colon and adjoining portion of sigmoid colon, splenic flexure, and a portion of the transverse colon

What complications are associated with surgical procedures used in the treatment of colon cancer?

Diarrhea, irregular bowel movements, bladder dysfunction, and sexual dysfunction (in males who have undergone surgery involving the rectum)

✎ What are important nursing actions in the care of a patient with colon cancer?

1. Educate the patient about ostomy care before resection. Consult an enterostomal nurse preoperatively so that patient preparation can begin as early as possible. Inform him that colostomy drainage can be regulated through the use of dietary modifications and a regular irrigation schedule.
2. Provide an opportunity for the patient to speak with someone with an ostomy before surgery.
3. If colostomy is performed, provide colostomy care, including irrigations as ordered by the physician. Convey acceptance of ostomy to promote the patient's positive self-image.
4. Monitor vital signs and intake and output frequently in early postoperative course.
5. Monitor for complications of the disease process (obstruction, anemia) or its treatment.
6. Recommend a diet high in fruits and vegetables, and restriction of saturated fats.
7. Instruct the patient to avoid or limit use of alcohol and tobacco products.
8. Encourage folic acid and calcium supplements (unless contraindicated) to prevent complications from colon cancer.
9. Recommend colon cancer screening for the patient's family.

Pharmacology related to the GI system

Management of nausea and vomiting

PROMOTILITY AGENTS

How do promotility agents work?

Increases the threshold of the chemoreceptor trigger zone by blocking dopamine, enhances contractility of the upper GI smooth muscle, increases tone of lower esophageal sphincter, and increases gastric emptying

What's an example of a promotility agent?

Metoclopramide (Reglan)

What adverse reactions are associated with promotility agents?

Central nervous system disturbances (restlessness, drowsiness, fatigue, extrapyramidal reactions, tardive dyskinesia), dry mouth, and diarrhea; bradycardia and hypotension can result from rapid I.V. push

Diphenhydramine (Benadryl) may be used to inhibit the extrapyramidal effects of metoclopramide.

What are relative contraindications to the use of promotility agents?

Bowel obstruction or perforation, GI hemorrhage, pheochromocytoma (hypertensive crisis), history of depression, Parkinson's disease, impaired renal function, history of seizures, breast cancer, and concurrent use with other agents with extrapyramidal reactions

What are important nursing actions when administering promotility agents?

1. Inform the patient of the effects of these agents on mental alertness and coordination.
2. Keep the bedside rails up and advise the patient to call for assistance with transfers.
3. Administer promotility agents 30 minutes to 1 hour before meals for better absorption.
4. Provide mouth care at regular intervals.
5. Monitor vital signs (blood pressure during I.V. administration) and intake and output.
6. Evaluate for extrapyramidal reactions as well as GI complaints.
7. Advise the patient to avoid alcohol and other central nervous system depressants.
8. Advise the patient to report involuntary movements of the face, eyes, and extremities as well as severe depression and diarrhea.
9. Monitor complete blood count for leukopenia and neutropenia (long-term use).

Treatment of peptic ulcer disease

PROTON PUMP INHIBITORS

How do proton pump inhibitors (PPIs) work?	Block the action of the H^+,K^+–ATPase pump of parietal cells to inhibit more than 90% of hydrochloric acid production per day
What are examples of PPIs?	Lansoprazole (Prevacid), omeprazole (Prilosec), esomeprazole (Nexium), pantoprazole (Protonix), and rabeprazole (Aciphex)
✎ **What adverse reactions are associated with PPIs?**	Headache, dizziness, abdominal discomfort, nausea, vomiting, diarrhea or constipation, cough, and back pain
✎ **What are important nursing actions when administering a PPI?**	1. Administer 1 hour before meals. 2. Advise the patient not to chew or break tablets or capsules. 3. Instruct the patient to avoid alcohol and NSAIDs to facilitate healing of the ulcerations and to prevent worsening of the condition (bleeding). 4. Instruct the patient to report severe diarrhea and headache.

HISTAMINE-2 BLOCKERS

How do histamine-2 (H_2) blockers work?	Inhibit histamine action at parietal cell H_2-receptor, which in turn suppresses hydrochloric acid secretion
What are examples of H_2-blockers?	Famotidine (Pepcid), nizatidine (Axid), ranitidine hydrochloride (Zantac), and cimetidine (Tagamet)
✎ **What adverse reactions are associated with H_2-blockers?**	Diarrhea, constipation, headache, dizziness, somnolence, impotence, rash (ranitidine), and local irritation at I.M. or I.V. site (ranitidine)
✎ **What are important nursing actions when administering H_2-blockers?**	1. Administer antacids and antihistamines 1 hour apart. 2. Instruct the patient to take H_2-blockers at bedtime due to risk of somnolence. 3. Inform the patient of possible effects on mental alertness. 4. Encourage smoking cessation. (H_2-blockers are less effective in people who smoke.) 5. Monitor renal and hepatic function periodically (long-term use).

CYTOPROTECTIVE AGENTS

How do cytoprotective agents work?	Bind to ulcerated area to form a protective barrier and also absorb pepsin
What are examples of cytoprotective agents?	Sucralfate (Carafate)
✎ **What adverse reactions are associated with cytoprotective agents?**	Constipation, dry mouth, drowsiness, dizziness, and rash

✎ **What are important nursing actions when administering a cytoprotective agent?**

1. Assess for chronic renal failure before administration.
2. Advise the patient to take this medication on an empty stomach, 1 hour before or 2 hours after meals and at bedtime.
3. Administer antacids and sucralfate at least 30 minutes apart.
4. Assess mental status and intake and output.
5. Advise the patient to report severe abdominal pain, rash or decreased urination.

ANTACIDS

How do antacids work?	Neutralize hydrochloric acid and decrease rate of gastric emptying

✎ **What types of antacid formulations are available?**

1. *Aluminum hydroxide (Amphojel, AlternaGEL):* constipation and possible fecal impaction or bowel obstruction
2. *Sodium bicarbonate (Alka-Seltzer):* electrolyte imbalances and alkalosis, rebound hyperacidity and milk-alkali syndrome (contains aspirin)
3. *Calcium carbonate (Tums):* constipation, belching, flatulence, rebound hyperacidity, and milk-alkali syndrome
4. *Magnesium hydroxide (Milk of Magnesia):* diarrhea and nausea
5. *Magnesium and aluminum hydroxide (Maalox, Mylanta):* constipation or diarrhea
6. *Combination of antacid with alginic acid (Gaviscon):* constipation or diarrhea

⚡ *Aluminum- and calcium-containing antacids generally cause constipation, while magnesium-containing antacids more commonly cause diarrhea.*

What are relative contraindications for the use of antacids?	1. *Aluminum hydroxide:* gastric outlet obstruction, hypertension, heart failure, hypophosphatemia, bone pain and lactation 2. *Sodium bicarbonate:* renal impairment, heart failure, respiratory and metabolic alkalosis, hypocalcemia, and decreased serum chloride 3. *Calcium carbonate:* renal calculi and hypercalcemia 4. *Magnesium hydroxide:* renal impairment 5. *Magnesium and aluminum hydroxide:* renal impairment 6. *Combination of antacid with alginic acid:* renal impairment
✎ What are important nursing actions when administering an antacid?	1. Administer with a glass of water 1 hour before or 2 hours after other medicines. 2. Assess vital signs, intake and output, and bowel pattern. 3. Evaluate for edema, urinary output, electrolytes, urinalysis, and blood urea nitrogen and creatinine (sodium bicarbonate). 4. Monitor calcium levels periodically with long-term use of calcium products. 5. Monitor phosphorus levels with long-term use of aluminum-containing antacids (may decrease phosphate levels). 6. Monitor renal function and serum magnesium levels with chronic use of magnesium products.

Treatment of gallstones

CHOLESTEROL SOLUBILIZERS

How do cholesterol solubilizers work?	Dissolves noncalcified gallbladder stones by solubilizing cholesterol from the stones
What's an example of a cholesterol solubilizer?	Ursodiol (Actigall, URSO)
What adverse reactions are associated with ursodiol?	Diarrhea, nausea, vomiting, abdominal pain, dyspepsia, headache, dizziness, insomnia, and back pain
What are important nursing actions when administering a cholesterol solubilizer?	1. Administer aluminum antacids at least 2 hours after ursodiol. 2. Monitor hepatic function periodically throughout therapy. 3. Advise the patient that therapy may be necessary for prolonged period (9 months to 1 year).

4. Instruct the patient to report severe abdominal pain, fever, vomiting, and jaundice.

Treatment of inflammatory bowel disease

SULFA-FREE 5-AMINOSALICYLIC ACID

How does sulfa-free 5-aminosalicylic acid work?

Inhibits prostaglandin synthesis, which decreases the inflammatory reaction

What's an example of a sulfa-free 5-aminosalicylic acid?

Mesalamine (Asacol, Pentasa)

What adverse reactions are associated with mesalamine?

Abdominal cramps, nausea, diarrhea, headache, fever, dizziness, rash, pruritus, flulike symptoms, malaise, and nephrotoxicity

What are important nursing actions when administering mesalamine?

1. Assess for allergy to salicylates and for renal or hepatic impairment before administration.
2. Monitor urine output.
3. Advise the patient not to break or chew tablets.
4. Monitor renal function periodically during long-term use.
5. Instruct the patient to report bloody diarrhea, severe abdominal pain, fever, rash and chest pain.

SULFASALAZINE

How does sulfasalazine work?

Anti-inflammatory actions

What's an example of a sulfasalazine?

Azulfidine

What are the common adverse reactions to sulfasalazine?

Nausea, vomiting, diarrhea, headache, dizziness, abdominal pain, insomnia, crystalluria, hematuria, and photosensitivity

What life-threatening reactions are associated with sulfasalazine?

Anaphylaxis, seizures, hematologic disorders (thrombocytopenia, leukopenia), renal failure, and hepatotoxicity

What are important nursing actions when administering sulfasalazine?

1. Assess for allergy to sulfa, renal or hepatic impairment, and intestinal or urinary obstruction before administration.
2. Administer with food and a glass of water. Encourage fluid intake of 2 qt (2 L)/day to prevent renal crystallization.

3. Inform the patient that urine, skin, and contact lenses may become yellow-brown.
4. Monitor renal and hepatic function as well as complete blood count with long-term therapy.
5. Advise the patient to avoid prolonged sunlight or to use sunscreen with long-term therapy (photosensitivity).
6. Instruct the patient to report hematuria, rash, tinnitus, respiratory difficulties, fever, sore throat, and chills.

PANCREATIC ENZYME REPLACEMENTS

How do pancreatic enzyme replacements work?

Replace endogenous pancreatic enzymes such as protease, lipase, and amylase to promote the digestion of proteins, fats, and starches

What are examples of pancreatic enzyme replacements?

Pancreatin (Pancrezyme) and pancrelipase (Cotazym, Creon, Viokase, and Pancrease)

What adverse reactions are associated with pancreatic enzyme replacements?

Nausea, abdominal cramps, and diarrhea due to GI irritation

What are important nursing actions when administering pancreatic enzyme replacements?

1. Assess for pork allergies and pancreatitis before administration.
2. Administer with meals to minimize gastric irritation.
3. Advise the patient to avoid crushing or chewing enteric coated formulations.
4. Instruct the patient to avoid powder contact with skin or mucous membranes (irritant).

Management of diarrhea

ANTIDIARRHEAL

How do antidiarrheal agents work?

By various methods including inhibiting peristalsis, decreasing the water content of the stool and inhibiting prostaglandin synthesis

✎ What are examples of antidiarrheal agents?

1. *Antiperistaltic agents:* opium tincture (Paregoric), diphenoxylate/atropine (Lomotil), loperamide (Imodium), and codeine
2. *Adsorbents:* attapulgite (Kaopectate) and bismuth preparations (Pepto-Bismol)
3. *Intestinal flora modifiers: Lactobacillus* preparations (Lactinex)

4. *Hormonal agents:* octreotide (Sandostatin), which is reserved for treatment of profuse diarrhea associated with carcinoid tumors and certain intestinal tumors

✎ What adverse reactions are associated with antidiarrheal agents?

1. *Antiperistaltic agents:* constipation, dry mouth, central nervous system depression (drowsiness, dizziness), and physical dependency due to opium content
2. *Adsorbents:* constipation, darkened stools and tongue
3. *Intestinal flora modifiers:* constipation and flatulence
4. *Hormonal agents:* diarrhea, abdominal pain, headache, dizziness, and fatigue

✎ What life-threatening reactions are associated with antidiarrheal agents?

1. *Antiperistaltic agents:* withdrawal, respiratory depression, anaphylaxis, and paralytic ileus
2. *Adsorbents:* salicylate toxicity (bismuth subsalicylate)
3. *Hormonal agents:* bradycardia and arrhythmias

What are relative contraindications for using antidiarrheals?

Diarrhea with fever or bloody stools, poisonings, pseudomembranous enterocolitis, pregnancy, asthma, chronic obstructive pulmonary disease, renal or hepatic impairment, increased intracranial pressure, cardiovascular disease, genitourinary obstruction, and infectious conditions, such as shigella or salmonella

✎ What are important nursing actions when administering an antidiarrheal agent?

1. Assess for presence of fever, or blood- or mucous-containing stools, as well as infectious source of diarrhea (shigella or salmonella) before administration.
2. Encourage increased fluid intake.
3. Monitor intake and output, electrolyte levels, vital signs, and respiratory pattern (adsorbents).
4. Inform the patient of the effects on mental alertness (opiates).
5. Assess mental status, pupil size, urinary output, and respiratory status (opiates).
6. Advise the patient to avoid other medications that may potentiate central nervous system depression, including over-the-counter medications, such as cough and cold preparations, because they may contain alcohol (opiates).
7. Warn the patient of the habit-forming potential (opiates).
8. Advise the patient to avoid other salicylate-containing products with bismuth subsalicylate use to prevent toxicity.
9. Instruct the patient to notify the physician if fever occurs or diarrhea hasn't resolved within 48 to 72 hours.

Management of constipation

LAXATIVES

How do laxatives work?

Various methods including increasing intestinal peristalsis, increasing water retention in the stool, and reducing the surface tension of bowel contents

What are examples of laxatives?

1. *Osmotic:* glycerin suppositories, polyethylene glycol (Miralax), sorbitol, lactulose (Chronulac or Enulose), magnesium salts (magnesium citrate and Milk of Magnesia), sodium phosphate (Fleet's enema), and electrolyte solutions (GoLYTELY)
2. *Bulk-forming:* methylcellulose (Citrucel), polycarbophil (FiberCon), psyllium (Metamucil)
3. *Emollient:* docusate (Surfak and Colace)
4. *Stimulant:* bisacodyl (Dulcolax), cascara, senna (Senokot), and castor oil
5. *Lubricant:* mineral oil

What adverse reactions are associated with laxatives?

Diarrhea, abdominal cramping, and nausea

✎ What are relative contraindications to using laxatives?

Nausea, vomiting, GI obstruction or perforation, toxic colitis, megacolon, fecal impaction and rectal bleeding; certain osmotic laxatives (sodium phosphate, magnesium salts) must be used with caution in renal failure

✎ What are important nursing actions when administering laxatives?

1. Encourage nonpharmacologic interventions, such as fiber, exercise, and water.
2. Discourage chronic use and abuse of laxatives due to risk of dependence and serious electrolyte abnormalities as well as bowel atony.
3. Monitor intake and output.
4. Assess for electrolyte abnormalities (chemistry panel, muscle cramps, weakness and dizziness) with long-term therapy.
5. Administer without food for better absorption.
6. Advise the patient to avoid breaking the tablets.
7. Advise the patient to report severe abdominal pain or diarrhea.

Surgery

Bowel diversion ostomies

✎ What's an ostomy?

A surgical opening that connects an internal organ (intestine, bladder) to the skin surface; an ostomy can be temporary or permanent; the opening of the ostomy is called the *stoma*

✎ What's an enterostomy?

A surgical opening that connects the small intestine to the skin surface for the purpose of drainage (bowel diversion ostomy) or insertion of a feeding tube; enterostomies may be used in the treatment of advanced bowel cancers and inflammatory bowel disease (ulcerative colitis, Crohn's disease)

▪ *Enterostomies are named based on the portion of the intestine used to create the stoma.*

✎ How does the location of the ostomy along the intestinal tract influence the character and management of fecal drainage?

The further along the bowel, the more formed the stool

✎ What's an ileostomy?

Bowel diversion from the ileum of the small intestine to the skin surface; results in liquid fecal drainage that drains continuously and cannot be regulated; collection appliance must be emptied frequently due to large amounts of water that are excreted

✎ What's a continent ileostomy (Kock pouch)?

A type of an ileostomy involving the surgical construction of a pouch inside the abdominal cavity that allows for the storage of stool; requires irrigation on a periodic basis, but eliminates the need for an external pouch appliance and eliminates the risk of skin irritation; more common in patients with ulcerative colitis (Crohn's can recur within the pouch); the reservoir is emptied two to four times per day using a drainage catheter

✎ What are special considerations for an ileostomy?

May need increased fluid intake as the drainage contains large amounts of water and salts as well as active digestive enzymes; encourage fluids because of higher risk for dehydration, particularly in hot weather, following exercise, and during bouts of diarrhea

What's a jejunostomy?

Bowel diversion from the jejunum of the small intestine to the skin surface; performed less commonly that ileostomies and are almost always temporary

What's an ileoanal anastomosis/pull-through?

Formation of a pouch (usually called a *J* or *S pouch*) made from the small bowel that collects stool in the pelvis and permits the passage of stool through the anus; typically performed for ulcerative colitis patients after colon resection

✎ What's a colostomy?

A bowel diversion from the large intestine to the skin surface; type of fecal drainage depends on location of the ostomy but more formed stools occur with a descending colostomy as opposed to an ascending colostomy

◥ *An ostomy appliance or bag will be required if the colostomy opening is located in the* right *side of the colon.*

✎ What are normal stomal characteristics?

Shiny, wet, and dark pink skin that may bleed easily when rubbed or during cleaning due to its rich vascularity; no sensation because no nerve endings

✎ What's the expected course of a stoma?

It tends to shrink for the first few months after surgery, so it's important to remeasure it at intervals to ensure appropriate fit with the skin barrier to prevent leakage

What are the primary causes of skin problems with an ostomy?

Leakage of effluent (due to digestive enzymes), allergic reactions and improper hygiene

✎ What are important skin protection measures?

Clean, rinse, and pat dry between pouch changes; avoid oily soaps to promote a good seal; and correctly apply skin barrier to prevent leakage of effluent

When should a stoma be cleaned?

Gentle cleaning with plain soap and water should be performed when the skin barrier is changed

✎ What are nutritional considerations with an ostomy?

Few restrictions are necessary, but patients may benefit from avoiding gas-producing foods (beans, cucumbers, and carbonated drinks), avoiding the use of straws and talking or swallowing air when eating, and avoiding constipating foods with sigmoid colostomy

What foods may help control odor?

Applesauce, cranberry juice, yogurt, or buttermilk

✎ Are there any activity restrictions with an ostomy?

Contact sports should be avoided unless approval is received from the physician and heavy lifting should be avoided to prevent herniation around the stoma

✎ A patient with an ostomy may have altered absorption of which medications?

Time-released and enteric-coated medications may pass through the digestive system too quickly to be effective

✎ When should ostomy pouches be emptied?

When the pouch is one-half to one-third full or when it feels firm with gas

✎ How often should an ostomy pouch be changed?

Approximately every 3 to 5 days, depending on its durability and adhesiveness

✎ What are important considerations regarding the timing of changing an ostomy pouch?

1. Avoid times close to meals or visiting hours.
2. Avoid times immediately after the administration of any medications that may stimulate bowel evacuation.

✎ What's the proper technique for changing an ostomy appliance?

1. Explain the procedure to the patient and provide privacy, preferably a bathroom.
2. Empty the contents through the bottom of the pouch into a bedpan and remove the appliance with an adhesive remover (don't use on broken skin) or with a washcloth and warm, soapy water.
3. Assess the consistency and amount of effluent.
4. Peel the bag off slowly while holding the patient's skin taut.
5. Use warm water, mild soap, and cotton balls or a washcloth to clean and pat dry the peristomal skin and stoma.
6. Assess the stoma and peristomal skin.
7. Prepare and apply the skin barrier. Stomal opening should be $1/16''$ to $1/8''$ larger than the stoma.
8. Prepare and apply the clean appliance.

Nursing skills

Enemas

What's the purpose of an enema?

To clean the colon prior to an examination or to relieve constipation

What are the different types of enemas?

Tap water, soap suds, Harris flush or drip, high colonic irrigation and instillation

What's the proper technique for administering an enema?

1. Explain the procedure to the patient.
2. Place protective padding under the patient and have a bedpan or bedside commode readily available.
3. Lower the head of the bed to a horizontal position (if tolerated).
4. Place the patient in a left lateral position with his right leg flexed (Sims' position).
5. Lubricate the tip of the catheter with water-soluble jelly.
6. Insert the catheter 4″ to 6″ (10 to 15 cm) into the rectum directing it towards the umbilicus.
7. Allow the solution to enter slowly from a height of 12″ to 18″ (30.5 to 45.5 cm) above the rectum.
8. Instruct the patient to retain the enema as long as possible.

When should administration of an enema be temporarily stopped?

If fullness, cramping, or pain is experienced the flow should be stopped for 30 seconds and then restarted at a slower rate

When should administration of an enema be stopped entirely?

When the patient can't hold any more of the solution, if pain is experienced, or when the urge to defecate occurs

Stool samples and fecal analysis

What tests may be performed on stool samples?

1. *Guaiac:* evaluation for occult blood
2. *O & P (ova and parasites):* evaluation for ova and parasites
3. *Culture:* evaluation for abnormal bacterial growth

What are important nursing actions when obtaining stool samples?

1. Explain the procedure to the patient.
2. Place a collection "hat" in the toilet and inform the patient that urine shouldn't be mixed with a stool sample.
3. Place the sample in an appropriate container. Obtain samples from different parts of the stool if it's a formed sample.
4. Label the collection container with the patient's name and the date and time of the collection.
5. Store the sample at room temperature until it arrives in the laboratory.

18

The genitourinary system

Basic concepts of the genitourinary system

The urinary system

✎ What organs and structures comprise the urinary system?

1. *Kidneys (2):* retroperitoneal location in abdominal cavity between the 12th thoracic and 3rd lumbar vertebrae; remove wastes and excess water from blood; produce hormones that affect blood pressure and bone formation; regulate production of red blood cells
2. *Ureters (2):* ducts through which urine passes from the kidneys to the bladder; expands to for the renal pelvis as it enters the kidney
3. *Bladder:* collapsible bag of smooth muscle located behind the symphysis pubis that acts as the body's storage site for urine; 500 to 600 ml capacity in adults
4. *Urethra:* a small duct through which urine passes from the bladder and out of the body; also functions as a passageway for semen in males; external opening is called the *urinary meatus*

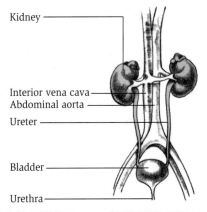

Kidney

Interior vena cava
Abdominal aorta

Ureter

Bladder

Urethra

▪ *The female urethra is much shorter than the male urethra, and this shorter length predisposes women to urinary tract infections (bacteria have a shorter distance to travel).*

✎ **What are the primary functions of the kidneys?**

Regulation of fluid balance, regulation of acid-base balance, elimination of waste products, and production of hormones that affect blood pressure (renin) and bone formation (vitamin D)

What structures comprise the kidneys?

1. *Cortex:* outer portion; contains renal corpuscles and tubules
2. *Medulla:* inner portion; consists of triangular structures (renal pyramids)
3. *Renal pelvis:* enlarged proximal portion of the ureter
4. *Calyces:* divided into major (direct extensions of renal pelvis) and minor (cuplike extensions of major calyces); channel urine into the renal pelvis; formed by collecting tubules

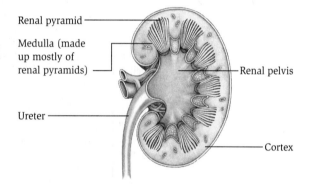

Renal pyramid

Medulla (made up mostly of renal pyramids)

Renal pelvis

Ureter

Cortex

✎ **What's the functional unit of the kidney?**

The nephron, which mechanically filters the blood of fluids, electrolytes, wastes, acids, and bases; also reabsorbs specific molecules (sodium) while secreting other specific molecules (potassium, hydrogen)

✎ **What structures make up a nephron?**

1. *Proximal convoluted tubule:* site where waste products and toxins are removed from the blood through a permeable membrane; glucose, vitamins, minerals, and amino acids are reabsorbed; osmosis (passive transport) is responsible for water reabsorption from the tubular filtrate here, while active transport methods are primarily responsible for sodium and glucose reabsorption
2. *Loop of Henle:* U-shaped extension of proximal convoluted tubule; consists of descending and ascending limbs; different sections differ in their permeability to water and other substances

3. *Distal convoluted tubule:* water permeable; another site for water and sodium reabsorption; also site for secretion of hydrogen, potassium, and ammonia into the tubular filtrate via active transport methods
4. *Collecting tubule:* receives filtrate from several distal convoluted tubule; site of final water reabsorption from urine due to effects of antidiuretic hormone
5. *Bowman's capsule:* cup-shaped; surrounds and supports the glomerulus
6. *Glomerulus:* a capillary network located within Bowman's capsule; site of filtration and removal of waste products

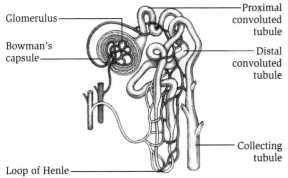

Glomerulus

Bowman's capsule

Proximal convoluted tubule

Distal convoluted tubule

Collecting tubule

Loop of Henle

▟ *Each portion of the renal tubules is responsible for a different function.*

What's urine?

A solution of inorganic salts and organic compounds produced by the kidneys as a result of glomerular filtration

✎ **What three processes are involved with the formation of urine?**

1. *Glomerular filtration:* occurs within the glomerulus; fluid and small molecules are forced through the glomerular capillary walls into Bowman's capsule as a result of high hydrostatic pressure; glomerular filtrate is the resultant fluid
2. *Tubular reabsorption:* passage of certain substances (sodium) from the glomerular filtrate into the blood
3. *Tubular secretion:* passage of certain substances (potassium, hydrogen) from the blood to the glomerular filtrate in the tubules

What's creatinine?

A waste product that results from muscle metabolism

What's urea?

A waste product produced as a result of protein and amino acid metabolism

What's glomerular filtrate?

A protein-free fluid that has been filtered by the glomerular capillaries

What hormones are produced by the kidneys?

1. *Renin:* secretion stimulated by sodium concentration in the renal tubules; ultimately increases aldosterone level via the rennin-angiotensin mechanism; regulation of blood pressure and fluid volume
2. *Erythropoietin:* produced in response to low arterial oxygen; increases erythropoiesis
3. *Vitamin D (active form):* promotes calcium absorption

What hormones influence the function of the kidneys?

1. *Aldosterone:* affects tubular reabsorption; regulates sodium retention and aids in regulating potassium secretion
2. *Antidiuretic hormone:* increases water reabsorption and urine concentration by acting in the distal tubule and collecting ducts

What's the renin-angiotensin system?

A mechanism that plays a vital role in the regulation of blood volume, arterial pressure, and cardiac and vascular function; renin is produced by the kidneys in response to decreased perfusion, decreased sodium and chloride concentrations in the kidneys, and presence of catecholamines and angiotensin II; renin converts angiotensinogen from the liver to angiotensin I, and an angiotensin-converting enzyme from the lungs converts angiotensin I to angiotensin II; angiotensin II produces a variety of effects, including stimulation of aldosterone release from the adrenal cortex and vasopressin (antidiuretic hormone) from the posterior pituitary; the end result is an increase in sodium and fluid retention, which increases the blood pressure and restores renal perfusion

What's voiding?

The elimination of waste materials from the body such as the evacuation of urine from the bladder

What's micturition?

The act of voiding or emptying the bladder; urination

Laboratory assessments of the urinary system

Serum creatinine

What does serum creatinine measure?

The amount of creatinine in the blood; it reflects the filtration ability of the kidneys

What's the acceptable range for creatinine?

Approximately 0.7 to 1.2 mg/dl for women; 0.8 to 1.4 mg/dl for men

> *Typically, a doubling of the serum creatinine level suggests a 50% reduction in the renal filtration rate.*

What bodily characteristic can influence the serum creatinine?	Muscle mass; a densely muscular person may have a slightly higher creatinine

> ⚡ *Serum creatinine can also be elevated transiently following meals with a high meat content or following the administration of some drugs, such as gentamyicin, heavy-metal chemotherapeutic agents (cisplatin), and cephalosporins.*

Creatinine clearance

What's creatinine clearance?	A test that compares the amount of serum creatinine to the amount of urine creatinine to provide information about how effectively the kidneys are functioning; typically based on assessment of a 24-hour urine specimen and a blood test (serum creatinine), which is performed at the end of the 24-hour period

> ⚡ *Creatinine clearance is an estimation of glomerular filtration rate (GFR).*

What's the GFR?	The volume of filtrate formed in both kidneys per minute; measurements of GFR are based on renal clearance of certain markers (creatinine, urea); it's the standard by which renal function is assessed; normal GFR is fairly consistent at 125 ml/minute, although normal values for women are slightly lower than those for men (88 to 120 ml/minute for women and 97 to 137 ml/minute for men)
What are some conditions that may result in an abnormally low GFR?	Dehydration, shock, acute renal failure, acute tubular necrosis, acute nephrotic syndrome, glomerulonephritis, obstructive uropathy, heart failure, and Wilms' tumor (children)
What does the blood urea nitrogen (BUN) measure?	The kidneys' ability to excrete urea waste products
What dietary factors can affect BUN?	High-protein diets and dehydration can raise BUN levels

Urinalysis

What's a urinalysis?	Examination of urine either by a dipstick technique or through a microscopic evaluation

✎ **What are normal urine characteristics?**	Light-amber or straw-colored, aromatic smell with various types of sediment, including few epithelial cells, urates, and uric acid crystals
What are examples of normal constituents of urine?	Sodium, chloride, potassium, bicarbonates, creatinine, calcium, magnesium, phosphates, ammonium ions, urea, fat-soluble vitamins (especially B and C), sulfates, uric acid, urobilinogen, some leukocytes (white blood cells) and red blood cells; the presence of a few sperm is normal for males
What's urine specific gravity?	A measurement of the concentration of particles in urine; normal range is 1.005 to 1.025, although the result can vary depending on fluid intake and amounts of solutes dissolved in the urine; abnormally low specific gravity may occur in presence of very dilute urine, as occurs in diabetes insipidus; abnormally high specific gravity may occur with diabetes mellitus because excessive quantities of glucose are dissolved in the urine

Urine cytology (culture)

When is bacterial growth considered significant on urine cytology?	When more than 100,000/ml of an organism is isolated
What's the most likely cause of mixed flora results?	Collection contamination
What's a composite urine specimen?	Collection of all urine excreted of a certain time interval (usually 12 to 24 hrs)
What tests are commonly performed through the use of composite specimens?	Creatinine clearance, total urinary protein, electrolytes (sodium, potassium, uric acid), and total glucose excretion

The female reproductive system

What structure contains the external genitalia of the female reproductive system?	Vulva, which contains the mons pubis, clitoris, labia majora, labia minora, Bartholin's glands, Skene's glands (mucous glands), and the urethral meatus

What's the perineum?

A fibromuscular area located between the vagina and anus

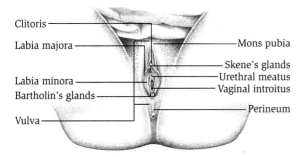

What structures comprise the internal genitalia of the female reproductive system?

1. *Vagina:* a very elastic muscular tube located between the urethra and rectum; lies in a 45-degree angle to the long axis of the body
2. *Uterus:* firm, muscular organ shaped like a pear that's located between the bladder and the rectum; lies at nearly a 90-degree angle to the vagina; divided into upper portion (fundus) and isthmus (neck), which join the fundus to the cervix
3. *Cervix:* fibrous portion of the uterus that extends into the vagina
4. *Ovaries (2):* female sex organs whose size and shape resemble large almonds; located slightly beneath the anterosuperior iliac spine near the lateral pelvic walls
5. *Fallopian tubes (2):* long and narrow tubes of muscle fibers that connect to the uterus at the fundus; contain fimbriae (fingerlike projections) at the ends closest to the ovaries

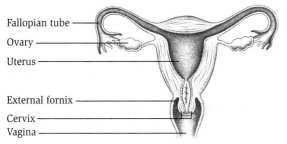

What are the two layers of the uterus?

1. *Endometrium:* mucous membrane that lines the uterus
2. *Myometrium:* muscular layer of the uterus

What's oogenesis?

Formation of a mature ovum in an ovarian follicle

What's an ovum?

Also referred to as an *egg*, it's the female reproductive cell

What hormones does the maturing ovarian follicle secrete?	Estrogen
What hormones are secreted by the corpus luteum (or "yellow body," which is the glandular structure within the ovary)?	Progesterone and estrogen
What's menarche?	The onset of the first menstrual period; typically occuring between ages 10 and 17
What's menstruation?	The cyclical shedding of the endometrium that occurs if a fertilized ovum doesn't implant itself there; lasts an average of 5 days

✎ **What are the phases of the normal menstrual cycle?**

1. *Menstrual (preovulatory) phase:* shedding of the endometrium accompanied by bleeding; first day of menstruation marks day 1 of the menstrual cycle; induced by low levels of estrogen and progesterone, which stimulate the hypothalamus to produce gonadotropin-releasing hormone (GnRH); GnRH then stimulates the anterior pituitary to release follicle-stimulating hormone (FSH) and luteinizing hormone (LH)
2. *Proliferative (follicular) phase and ovulation:* typically occurs from day 6 to 14 of the menstrual cycle; FSH and LH cause the ovarian follicle (a matured ovarian cyst that contains the ovum) to secrete estrogen; endometrium is built up as a result; later in this phase, estrogen levels peak, LH levels increase and surge around day 14, while FSH levels drop; ovulation occurs
3. *Luteal (secretory) phase:* lasts approximately 14 days; LH and FSH levels decrease; initially estrogen levels drop, but then increase in conjunction with progesterone levels; endometrium thickens in response to progesterone (which is produced by the corpus luteum) in preparation for implantation of a fertilized ovum; approximately 12 days after ovulation, drops in estrogen and progesterone levels induce menses (shedding of the endometrium) and stimulate GnRH production by the hypothalamus, which causes the cycle to begin again

◆ *The average menstrual cycle is 28 days long, although a range of 22 to 34 days is still considered normal.*

◼ *Typically, only one follicle matures and is released from the ovary during the ovulatory process of each menstrual cycle.*

What's ovulation?

The process in which an ovum is expelled from an ovarian follicle into one of the fallopian tubes; induced by high concentrations of luteinizing hormone; occurs in the middle of the menstrual cycle

What's the corpus luteum?

A glanular structure within the ovary that develops following rupture of the ovarian follicle; primarily produces progesterone

What's menopause?

The gradual cessation of menstrual periods that occurs secondary to a decrease in cyclic production of estrogen and progesterone; testosterone secretion usually increases; manifested as hot flashes or flushing sensation, atrophy of the urogenital tissues, and thinning of the vaginal walls; typically occurs between ages 45 and 60

◼ *Climacteric is a broad term used to describe the transitional period from fertility to infertility, while menopause is the term used to describe the absence of menses for 1 year.*

The male reproductive system

What structures comprise the external male reproductive system?

1. *Penis:* cylindrical shaft comprised of erectile tissue with large vascular spaces; erection occurs vascular spaces are filled with blood
2. *Scrotum:* skin covered pouch that's suspended from the perineal area; comprised of two compartments, and each compartment houses a testis, an epididymis, and a spermatic cord; site of sperm development because temperature within scrotum is maintained at 2° to 3° below body temperature
3. *Testes (2):* located within scrotum with one testis in each scrotal compartment; primary male sex glands; contain seminiferous tubules, where spermatogenesis occurs

What structures comprise the internal male reproductive system?

1. *Prostate gland:* walnut-sized gland located just beneath the bladder and surrounding the urethra; ducts open into the urethra; continuously produces the alkaline prostatic fluid, which enhances sperm motility

2. *Seminal vesicles:* convoluted pouches that are located on the posterior surface of the bladder; produce nutrient-rich fluid, which comprises semen

3. *Cowper's (bulbourethral) glands:* pea-shaped structures located just beneath the prostate gland; produce alkaline fluid that lubricates the urethra just before ejaculation occurs

4. *Seminiferous tubules:* site of spermatogenesis

5. *Epididymis:* tightly coiled tubes located at the top of each testis that serve as reservoir for sperm storage and maturation; transports seminal fluid (and mature sperm) from testes to vas deferens; secretes small portion of semen

6. *Vas deferens:* a pair of ducts that transport sperm and a small amount of fluid from each epididymis to an ejaculatory duct

7. *Ejaculatory ducts:* created by the joining of each vas with a duct from a seminal vesicle; terminate in urethra after passing through prostate gland; responsible for ejaculation of semen into urethra

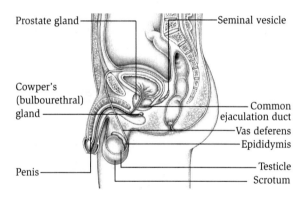

Prostate gland	Seminal vesicle
Cowper's (bulbourethral) gland	Common ejaculation duct
	Vas deferens
	Epididymis
Penis	Testicle
	Scrotum

What's spermato-genesis?

The formation of spermatozoa (sperm), the male reproductive cells

What are the three primary functions of the male reproductive system?

Sexual reproduction, secretion of male sex hormones (testosterone), and elimination of urine

What hormone do the Leydig's cells of the testes secrete?

Testosterone, the primary androgenic hormone that's responsible for the development and maintenance of male reproductive organs and secondary male sex characteristics

◥ *Male sex hormones are also called* androgens.

What are sperm?   Mature male reproductive cells that are contained in semen

What's semen?   A viscous liquid containing sperm and the fluids
                             produced by the prostate, Cowper's glands, and others

Laboratory assessment of the reproductive system

What's a Papanicolaou test?   During a gynecologic examination, the cervix is scraped
                                   or swabbed to obtain a sampling of cervical cells, which
                                   are evaluated for pathology as a screening tool for cervi-
                                   cal cancer

What screening test is used to detect prostate cancer in men?   Prostate-specific antigen (PSA) is a protein originally
                                   found in semen; certain prostate conditions, including
                                   prostate cancer, can cause high levels of PSA in the blood

How often should breast self-examination and testicular self-examination be performed?   Monthly

What are the two types of mammography?

1. *Screening mammography* is a routine procedure used
   to examine women who have no evidence of breast
   cancer; it consists of two views of each breast taken at
   an angle to each other.
2. *Diagnostic mammography* is used to examine a specific area of the breast when an abnormality, such as a
   lump, has been found. Diagnostic mammography
   includes special views and additional angles.

Physical assessment of the genitourinary system

Normal findings of the urinary system

What supplies should be available before performing a physical examination of the urinary system?   A gown and drapes to cover the patient, weight scales, a
                                   specimen cup for urine collection, a stethoscope, and a
                                   sphygmomanometer with an inflatable cuff

In what order should physical assessment techniques be performed to best evaluate the urinary system?

Inspection, auscultation, percussion, and palpation

⚡ *Palpating and percussing prior to auscultating can increase bowel motility, which can interfere with the transmission of sound during auscultation of the renal arteries.*

What are important assessment factors for inspection of the urinary system?

1. *Condition of skin and mucous membranes:* should be free of uremic frost and tenting
2. *Urethral meatus:* for males, it should be centrally located and without discharge; for females, it should be located above the vagina and appear pink and without edema or discharge

What's the purpose of auscultation in the physical examination of the kidneys?

Assessment for renal bruits (whooshing sounds)

How are the renal arteries auscultated?

By lightly placing the bell of the stethoscope over the left and right abdominal quadrants as the patient exhales deeply; auscultation should begin in the midline, work to the left, back to midline, and then to right

What organs are percussed during assessment of the urinary system?

Kidneys, to identify tenderness or pain; bladder, to determine position and contents

How is blunt percussion of the kidney performed?

1. Instruct the patient to sit upright with his back turned toward the examiner.
2. Each costovertebral angle is percussed by placing the left palm at the costovertebral over the 12th rib on the patient's right and left, and by gently striking it with the right fist.

How is percussion of the bladder performed?

1. Place the patient in a supine position.
2. Using one hand as a base placed 2″ (5 cm) above the symphysis pubis, strike the dorsal aspect of the middle third finger with two quick blows in each location to be percussed. A tympanic sound is typically produced, although a dull sound may be detected over a bladder containing urine.

⚡ *A recently emptied bladder shouldn't be percussible above the symphysis pubis.*

Why is palpation of the urinary organs performed?

To assess for the presence of any tenderness, lumps, or masses

| **How are the kidneys palpated?** | 1. Place the patient in a supine position and expose the abdominal area from the xiphoid process to the symphysis pubis. |

1. Place the patient in a supine position and expose the abdominal area from the xiphoid process to the symphysis pubis.
2. Stand at the right side of the patient and place your left hand underneath the patient's back so that it rests half way between the lower costal margin and the iliac crest.
3. Place your right hand on the patient's abdomen at a position directly above the left hand.
4. Press the right fingertips approximately 1½" (4 cm) above the right iliac crest and the left fingertips upwards into the right costovertebral angle.
5. Instruct the patient to inhale deeply; this causes the kidney to descend.
6. Assess for tenderness or masses.
7. Repeat the process on the left side to evaluate the left kidney.

◤ *The kidneys aren't usually palpable due to their deep location within the abdominal cavity; however, palpation may be possible in a thin patient.*

How is the bladder palpated?

1. Instruct the patient to void.
2. Place the patient in a supine position.
3. Using your fingertips, press deeply approximately 1" to 2" (2.5 to 5 cm) above the symphysis pubis in the midline to locate the edge of the bladder.
4. Assess for tenderness or masses.

◤ *Reassure the patient that the feeling of urinary urgency is normal during bladder palpation.*

What's the normal amount of urine produced in a 24-hour period?

1 to 1.5 L of urine in a 24-hour period

Abnormal findings of the urinary system

✎ How can the fluid status of a patient be determined on physical examination?

1. Inspect the mucous membranes of the mouth. Dryness or cracking may be suggestive of dehydration.
2. Assess skin turgor. If the skin "tents" or doesn't return to its normal position after gently pinching and releasing it, significant dehydration may be present.
3. Assess for presence of edema.
4. Monitor daily weight.
5. Record and compare intake and output daily.

6. Obtain blood pressure. Measure in both arms for comparison, and compare blood pressure results when the patient lies down and upon sitting upright.
7. Assess neck veins for distention (jugular vein distention).

◾ *A change in weight more than 2 lb (1 kg) per day suggests a change in fluid status rather than a change in body mass.*

◾ *1 ml of water is equal to 1 g. Thus, body weight should increase by approximately 2 lb (1 kg) for every 1,000 ml of excess fluid intake relative to urine output. Conversely, weight loss occurs secondary to the negative balance that occurs when urine output exceeds fluid intake.*

◾ *Weight should be obtained at the same time each day using the same scale with the patient wearing the same or similar amounts of clothing.*

◾ *Output should equal approximately two-thirds of intake in a 24-hour period.*

◾ *A drop in blood pressure more than 40 mm Hg when the patient moves from a recumbent position to a seated position may be indicative of fluid volume depletion.*

◣ What are examples of factors that should be considered when recording daily *intake*?

Volume of I.V. fluids received and oral fluids consumed

◣ What are examples of factors that should be considered when recording daily *output*?

Fluid loss from urination, vomiting, diarrhea, and wound drainage

◣ What's the normal hourly urine output range for an adult?

30 to 100 ml/hour; normal 24-hour output ranges from 720 to 2,400 ml

◣ What's edema?

The accumulation of excess water and sodium within interstitial spaces; may be pitting or nonpitting

◾ *Pitting edema is indicative of a systemic cause (commonly renal disease) and it develops most commonly in dependent portions of the body, such as the lower extremities, sacrum, and scrotum. Nonpitting edema may manifest as periorbital edema (swollen eyelids), bibasilar lung crackles, and ascites.*

How is the presence of pitting edema evaluated?

A finger is used to press against edematous skin for 5 seconds, and the finger is then quickly removed; the depth of the remaining indentation determines the degree of pitting: 1 + (barely perceptible pit) to 4 + (deep pit associated with severe foot and leg swelling)

Which renal problems are most likely to cause pitting edema in the extremities?

Hypoalbuminemic states such as nephrotic syndrome; acute nephritic syndrome such as poststreptococcal glomerulonephritis

What's anasarca?

Generalized fluid build-up throughout the body

What objective findings commonly accompany chronic renal disease?

Dry skin with a gray-yellow hue, peripheral edema, periorbital edema, ascites, and anemia

If you hear a renal bruit over the renal artery, what may be the cause?

Renal artery stenosis, an arteriovenous fistula or malformation, or a renal artery aneurysm

What's renal colic?

Severe cramplike pain usually associated with obstruction of the upper urinary tract; the obstruction is commonly due to renal calculi; radiating pain in the lower back and genital area that's unrelieved by position changes

What's hematuria?

The presence of red blood cells (RBCs) in the urine (3 to 5 RBCs per high-powered field); common causes include calculi (stones), inflammatory disorders of the kidneys and bladder (infections), tumors, enlarged prostate gland, and increased bleeding tendencies

What's glycosuria?

Excretion of glucose in the urine; occurs when the serum glucose level exceeds the renal threshold of 10 to 12 mmol/L; may be indicative of diabetes mellitus or excessive consumption of carbohydrates

What's the clinical significance of the presence of ketones in a urinalysis?

When the body can't get enough energy from sugar, fat is broken down and ketones are made; ketones in the urine may be a sign that the patient is developing diabetic ketoacidosis

What's proteinuria?

Excretion of protein in the urine; may be caused by fever and chills, exertion, and prolonged standing or running

What's leukocyturia? Elimination of white blood cells in the urine; may be caused by a urinary tract infection (UTI)

What's pyuria? Pus or cloudiness in the urine; it indicates severe inflammation of the kidneys and urinary tract

What's oliguria? Elimination of 100 to 500 ml of urine in a 24-hour period

What's anuria? Elimination of less than 100 ml of urine in a 24-hour period

What are possible causes of oliguria and anuria? Acute renal failure, obstructive uropathy, enlargement of the prostate, dehydration, or urinary catheter obstruction

Anuria is an emergency situation and requires hospitalization and immediate medical care.

What's dysuria? Pain or burning on urination; may occur secondary to a urinary tract infection or a tumor involving the bladder or urethra

What's nocturia? Increased nighttime urination; may occur secondary to high fluid intake in the evening or use of diuretics, but may also be associated with a UTI, renal disease (chronic interstitial nephritis, polycystic kidney disease), or bladder cancer

What's enuresis? Bedwetting or involuntary urination that occurs during sleep; possible causes include UTI, prostate tumor or enlargement, and relaxation of the bladder or pelvic musculature

What's polyuria? Urine output greater than 3 L in a 24-hour period; may occur with hyperglycemia associated with diabetes mellitus, as a result of diabetes insipidus, and excessive fluid intake

What's uremic frost? Formation of urate crystals on the skin that produce a pale, frostlike appearance; occurs in the presence of renal failure or uremia when metabolic waste products are unable to be excreted by the kidneys, but rather are excreted through capillaries where they accumulate on the skin

What's urinary hesitancy? Difficulty starting a urine stream; can occur as a result of an enlarged prostate gland or from obstruction by renal calculi

What's urinary urgency? The urge to urinate immediately; urine may be eliminated; commonly associated with lower UTIs and bladder dysfunction

✎ **What's vesicoureteral reflux?**	Urine reflux from the bladder back into the ureter and kidney
What's Goodpasture's syndrome?	A rare autoimmune disease in which antibodies form against basement membranes of both renal glomeruli and pulmonary alveoli; hematuria and proteinuria may result; treatment may include plasmapheresis, dialysis, and kidney transplantation, and immunosuppressive medications such as cyclophosphamide (Cytoxan)
What's Alport's syndrome?	An X-linked hereditary disease involving a genetic mutation that affects collagen formation; collagen formation is essential in forming the glomerular basement membranes, and therefore glomerular destruction occurs secondary to this disorder; may cause progressive renal failure, deafness, and vision changes
	◥ *Because Alport's is an X-linked disease, males are more likely to express a more severe form of the disease than females.*
What's nephrosclerosis?	A vascular disorder of the kidneys in which the small arteries and arterioles become sclerotic (thickened with a narrowed lumen), which results in decreased vascular blood flow; the resultant ischemia causes destruction of the glomeruli and fibrosis; chronic renal failure may occur; hypertension and atherosclerotic disease are the major contributing factors
What's renal artery stenosis?	A vascular disorder of the kidneys in which one or both renal arteries become partially occluded; an audible bruit over a renal artery may be noted on physical examination; hypertension is the primary complication

Normal findings of the female reproductive system

When should an annual pelvic examination and Papanicolaou (Pap) test begin?	1. Age 15 or younger if the patient is, or plans to become, sexually active 2. Periods are irregular or painful or if periods are delayed 3. Puberty is delayed or there's failure to begin periods 4. Unusual vaginal discharge or a possibility of sexually transmitted disease exposure 5. Suspected pregnancy, pelvic mass, or pelvic or abdominal pain

How should a patient be prepared for a pelvic examination?	1. Allow the patient time to empty her bladder before beginning the examination. 2. Provide privacy and cover the patient adequately during the examination. 3. To improve accuracy, make sure douching, intercourse, and the use of tampons have been avoided within 48 hours of the examination and that patient isn't currently menstruating.

> ◣ *A pelvic examination and Pap test should not be performed if the patient is bleeding or spotting.*

What supplies should be gathered before starting a pelvic examination?	Gloves, a speculum, lubricant, a plastic spatula or endocervical brush, glass slides and cover slides, cytologic fixative agent, culture bottles, a mirror, and a light source

What's the proper technique for performing a pelvic examination?	1. Place the patient in the lithotomy position and provide adequate draping and a mirror. 2. Carefully inspect the vulva by using a gloved hand to spread the labia majora. 3. Gently insert the speculum into the vagina for visualization of the vagina and cervix. 4. While the speculum is in place, collect samples of vaginal discharge and cervical cells with a cotton-tipped swab, brush, or plastic spatula. Remove the speculum after the samples have been collected. 5. A bimanual examination is then performed by placing one hand on the lower abdomen and one or two gloved fingers of the other hand into the vagina. Pressure is applied to the cervix, uterus, and ovaries to assess for any abnormalities, including tenderness and enlargement of any structures or organs. 6. A digital rectal examination may be performed at this time to assess for hemorrhoids, a rectal mass, blood in the stool, or to confirm condition of the uterus, fallopian tubes, or ovaries.

What's the normal appearance of the cervix?	Smooth and pink without ulcerations or other lesions

What's gravida?	The number of pregnancies irrespective of their outcomes

What's parity?	The condition of having delivered an infant (alive or dead) during the viability period (beyond 20 weeks' gestation or a birth weight more than 500 g); a multiple birth is considered a single parity

What's nulliparity?	The condition of not having delivered a viable infant

Abnormal findings of the female reproductive system

What abnormalities are screened for on visual inspection of the external female genitalia?	Discharge, foul odors, ulcerations, skin growths or nodules, excoriation, and nits or lice
What might a green or gray, frothy and malodorous discharge indicate?	Trichomonas infection
What might a green-yellow, purulent discharge from the vagina indicate?	Gonorrhea
What might a thick gray-white discharge indicate?	Chlamydia
What might a cheeselike discharge from an inflamed vulva indicate?	Candida (yeast infection)
What might a blue cervix indicate?	Pelvic congestion due to a pregnancy or tumor
What might granular, friable cervical lesions with irregular growth outward from the cervical os indicate?	Cervical cancer
When a female patient is asked to cough during the external physical examination of the genitalia what abnormality is the examiner looking for?	Rectocele, cystocele, or urinary incontinence
What's a rectocele?	A herniation of the rectum through the posterior wall of the vagina
What's a cystocele?	A herniation of the bladder through the anterior wall of the vagina

What's an enterocele?	A herniation of the intestines through the walls of the vagina
What's dyspareunia?	Pain or difficulty with sexual intercourse
What's premenstrual syndrome (PMS)?	A cyclic disorder that commonly occurs before or during menses, and typically involves fluid retention and bloating, mood swings, breast tenderness, headache, and appetite changes
What are common treatments for PMS?	Eliminating caffeine, stopping smoking, exercising regularly, eating healthily, and sleeping adequately; medications include selective serotonin reuptake inhibitors (SSRIs), such as fluoxetine and sertraline may be helpful
What's amenorrhea?	The absence of menstruation; may occur in association with menopause, pregnancy, rapid or excessive weight loss, excessive exercise, or an estrogen-secreting tumor
How does primary amenorrhea differ from secondary amenorrhea?	Primary amenorrhea is when the onset of menstruation has yet to occur at age 16; secondary amenorrhea is cessation of menstruation for at least 3 months
What's a serious complication of amenorrhea?	Lack of ovulation; results in inability to conceive
What's dysmenorrhea?	Painful menstruation; possible causes include endometriosis, pelvic inflammatory disease, uterine fibroids, benign uterine cramping, and use of intra-uterine contraceptive devices
What's menorrhagia?	Prolonged heavy menstrual flow; may be caused by complications of pregnancy, endometrial hyperplasia, hypothyroidism, and malignant tumors
What's metrorrhagia?	Spotting or intermittent bleeding between menstrual periods; may be caused by pregnancy complications, malignant tumors, and hormonal contraceptives
What's postmenopausal bleeding?	Any bleeding that occurs more than 6 months after the last normal menstrual period at menopause; may be caused by hormone replacement therapy, uterine hyperplasia, benign or malignant uterine growths (polyps, uterine cancer), and from abnormalities of the cervix or vagina
What's oligomenorrhea?	Infrequent or light menstrual flow; possible causes include severe emotional stress, chronic illness,

malnutrition, eating disorders (anorexia nervosa), excessive exercise, estrogen-secreting tumors, and illicit use of anabolic steroids

What's polymenor-rhea?
Menstruation that occurs too frequently; the menstrual cycle is consistently less than 21 days

Normal findings of the male reproductive system

What supplies should be gathered before beginning a physical examination of the male genitalia?
Gloves, a water-soluble lubricant, and a flashlight

What assessments should be made during inspection of the male genitalia?
Color and integrity of penile and scrotal skin, location of urethral meatus, size and symmetry of scrotal sac (the left testis commonly hangs lower than the right), and presence of inguinal hernias

How is a testicular examination performed?
1. Using the thumb and first two fingers, palpate the scrotal sac and compare findings on the left and right.
2. Gently roll each testis in turn between the thumb and fingers. Check for lumps or irregular swellings or changes in firmness.
3. Gently compress the testicles to elicit a dull, aching sensation that radiates to the patient's lower abdomen (normal).
4. Using a flashlight, transilluminate any abnormal findings noted in the scrotum. If light shines through the mass it's most likely cystic

How is the prostate palpated by digital rectal examination?
1. Instruct the patient to void to empty his bladder.
2. Instruct the patient to stand at the end of the examination table and rest his upper body on the table with his elbows flexed.
3. Put on a sterile glove and apply water-soluble lubricant to the gloved index finger.
4. Instruct the patient to bear down while the index finger is inserted into the rectum. Encourage the patient to breathe deeply and slowly through his mouth to promote relaxation (facilitates passage of finger through anal sphincter).
5. Palpate the prostate gland at the anterior wall of the rectum using the pad of the index finger.
6. Assess for normal characteristics, including smooth and rubbery feeling as well as a walnut-sized gland.

Abnormal findings of the male reproductive system

What abnormalities are screened for on visual inspection of the external male genitalia?	Swelling or bulges in the penis or testes, penile discharge, lesions or nodules on penis or scrotum, pain or inflammation, nits or lice
What might a palpable mass in the testicle indicate?	Spermatocele (firm or cystic mass), varicocele (soft and compressible mass), or testicular tumor (hard mass)
What might a palpable mass in the prostate indicate?	Cancer (hard nodule), advanced carcinoma (stone-hard nodule), benign prostatic hyperplasia (nontender enlargement), or acute prostatitis (tender, swollen, and firm)
What's epispadias?	A congenital condition in which the urethral opening is located on the dorsal (under) side of the penis
What's hypospadias?	A congenital condition in which the urethral opening is located on the ventral surface of the penis
What's the treatment for epispadias and hypospadias?	Surgical revision of the urethral tract and meatus; may require temporary urinary diversions
What's a hydrocele?	Benign testicular mass that's serous filled; detected as a smooth mass that encompasses the testicle; most will resolve without intervention over time, but surgical excision may be performed if significant discomfort results from the hydrocele
What's cryptorchidism?	A developmental defect in which one or both testicles fail to descend into the scrotum; infertility and an increased risk for testicular cancer may develop if the testicle fails to descend to a normal position within the scrotum by age 1 year and if isn't surgically corrected thereafter.
What's an inguinal hernia?	A condition in which a loop of the bowel protrudes through the inguinal ring of the abdominal wall into the inguinal canal; generally, the patient will have no symptoms other than a soft mass palpable in the testicle; the mass (loop of bowel) can be pushed up into the peritoneal cavity; surgical repair of the defect in the abdominal wall (herniorrhaphy) is indicated for an incarcerated inguinal hernia
How do you know if the patient's inguinal hernia is incarcerated?	The patient will experience pain, swelling and tenderness in the scrotal area; the incarcerated inguinal hernia can't be manually reduced

Major disease processes of the urinary system

Urinary incontinence

What's urinary incontinence?

A condition characterized by an involuntary loss of urine; mechanical causes include weakening of the detrusor muscles of the bladder, dysfunction of the bladder sphincter, compression of bladder, or outlet obstruction; neurologic causes include impairment of the autonomic nervous system that results in inappropriate communication to the detrusor muscle or sphincters

What's the pathophysiologic process of urinary incontinence?

The bladder sphincter can't prevent the flow of urine through it, causing leakage to occur

✎ What types of urinary incontinence exist?

1. *Urge incontinence:* sudden and intense urge to urinate; may only have a few second warning to get to a bathroom; overactive bladder because it contracts even when it isn't full; associated with urinary tract infections and neurologic disorders (stroke, multiple sclerosis)
2. *Stress incontinence:* involuntary loss of urine upon sneezing, coughing, heavy lifting, laughing, or other activity that increases abdominal pressure; most common type; commonly due to weakness of pelvic floor, and commonly occurs in women with multiple pregnancies and vaginal deliveries as well as in men following prostatectomy
3. *Overflow incontinence:* overdistension of the bladder causes involuntary loss of urine; frequent dribbling often occurs; causes include bladder outlet obstruction from tumor or prostate enlargement, underactive bladder, diabetic neuropathy, and the use of diuretics
4. *Functional incontinence:* involuntary loss of urine due to immobility, paraplegia, cognitive deficits

⬔ *Incontinence isn't normal and patients should be encouraged to discuss it with their health care provider to explore potential causes.*

What treatments are used for urinary incontinence?

1. *Pelvic floor muscle exercises (Kegel exercises):* strengthen urinary sphincter; involve squeezing the pelvic floor muscles (as if trying to stop from passing gas) and holding for a count of three; should be performed several times per day; most effective for stress incontinence

2. *Bladder training:* urination at set intervals with inhibition of urination until the scheduled time; voiding intervals initially 2 to 3 hours apart, but should be progressively increased, most effective with urge incontinence, but useful for stress incontinence as well

3. *Intermittent bladder catheterizations*

4. *Pharmacologic agents:* anticholinergic drugs, such as tolterodine (Detrol), oxybutynin (Ditropan), propantheline (Pro-Banthine), dicyclomine (Bentyl), flavoxate (Urispas), hycosamine (Levsin), or imipramine (Tofranil) to control bladder spasms; desmopressin (DDAVP) for children to slow the production of urine; and antibiotics for incontinence related to a urinary tract infection or prostatitis

5. *Medical devices:* use of urethral inserts with an air-filled balloon tip to prevent urine leakage in women; use of a stiff vaginal ring (pessary) to hold up the bladder (because of proximity of bladder and vagina) and prevent urine leakage

6. *Surgery:* prostatectomy for men with enlarged prostate glands, removal of uterine fibroids, and removal of bladder tumors, which may all cause urinary incontinence; injection of substances around the urethra may help prevent urine leakage; bladder enlargement or correction of a congenital defect may also prove beneficial; implantation of medical devices, such as an artificial urinary sphincter and a sacral nerve stimulator may also be performed

What complications are associated with urinary incontinence?

Skin problems (rashes, sores, infections) from chronic exposure to urine, psychosocial difficulties (social isolation)

What are important nursing actions in the care of a patient with urinary incontinence?

1. Assess for environmental obstacles to toileting.
2. Assess for mobility restrictions that may impede ability ambulate to bathroom.
3. Avoid the use of indwelling urinary catheters as a treatment for incontinence.
4. Obtain post-void residuals and any urine specimens as instructed by the physician.
5. Educate the patient about bladder training. Inform the patient that results may not be evident for 4 to 6 weeks.
6. Encourage voiding according to habit (morning, prior to bed).
7. Instruct the patient to avoid or minimize the use of alcohol and caffeine (both act as diuretics).
8. Instruct the patient to avoid substances that may cause bladder irritation (carbonated beverages, citrus

juices, artificial sweeteners, spicy foods), which promotes urge incontinence.

9. Prevent or treat constipation (full rectum may put pressure on bladder).

10. Encourage weight loss if the patient is obese (excess weight puts constant pressure on the bladder and weakens the muscles surrounding it).

11. Administer medications (anticholinergics) as ordered by the physician.

12. Encourage maintenance of voiding diary, if requested of patient by the physician.

13. Provide good skin care to prevent breakdown.

14. Educate the patient about the use of absorbent pads or adult diapers under regular clothing.

What's urinary retention?

Incomplete emptying of the bladder that may be an acute or chronic process; may result from autonomic nervous dysfunction (neurogenic bladder from diabetes), outlet obstruction (stones, strictures, prostate enlargement), urinary reflux, or anatomic anomalies; treatment measures may include encouraging the patient to assume a natural position when attempting to void, consuming warm drinks, running water and, possibly, catheterization

Urinary tract infections

What's a urinary tract infection (UTI)?

An infection involving the urinary system; lower urinary tract infections involve pathogen colonization in the bladder (cystitis) or urethra (urethritis), and upper urinary tract infections involve pathogen colonization in the kidney (pyelonephritis); UTIs are most commonly caused by *Escherichia coli*

What's the pathophysiologic process of a UTI?

Bacteria enter the urinary tract (most commonly through the urethra), where they begin to multiply and produce symptoms of infection

What are the clinical manifestations of UTIs?

Dysuria, urinary frequency and urgency, hematuria, suprapubic pain, bacteriuria (bacteria seen on urinalysis), and cloudy, foul-smelling urine

What complications are associated with a UTI?

Pyelonephritis (with possible permanent kidney damage) and sepsis

What's the typical treatment for a UTI?

Antibiotic therapy, commonly including co-trimoxazole (Bactrim, Septra), nitrofurantoin (Macrodantin), ciprofloxacin (Cipro), and amoxicillin (Amoxil);

phenazopyridine (Pyridium) may be prescribed for it's analgesic effects to relieve dysuria; prophylactic antibiotic therapy is considered for patients with recurrent UTIs; an increased fluid intake is also encouraged

What are important nursing actions in the care of a patient with a UTI?

1. Encourage increased fluid intake to facilitate passage of bacteria out of body.
2. Inform the patient that urine will be red-orange with Pyridium use.
3. Instruct the patient to consume large amounts of fluids when taking co-trimoxazole to prevent formation of renal crystals.
4. Encourage voiding after intercourse.
5. Instruct women to wipe from front to back.
6. Advise women to avoid douching (alters normal body flora).
7. Encourage voiding at regular and frequent intervals.
8. Instruct women to wear cotton underwear and loose-fitting clothing to prevent moisture retention; nylon underclothing and pantyhose should be avoided because they trap moisture, thereby promoting bacterial growth.
9. Encourage showers rather than tub baths.
10. Administer medications (antibiotics, Pyridium) as ordered by the physician.
11. Instruct the patient to notify the physician if symptoms persist or if they recur after completing the full course of antibiotics.

Pyelonephritis

What's pyelonephritis?

A type of urinary tract infection that affects the kidney; may be acute or chronic

What's the pathophysiologic process of pyelonephritis?

Bacterial pathogens cause inflammation of the renal parenchyma and collecting system; the inflammatory process may result in the formation of scar tissue over time, and chronic infection can result in chronic renal failure secondary to damage and atrophy of the nephrons.

What are the clinical manifestations of pyelonephritis?

Fever, chills, malaise, flank pain, nausea, vomiting, signs of a UTI, and costovertebral angle tenderness on physical exam; protein and white blood cells may be present in the urine

What complications are associated with pyelonephritis?

Acute renal failure, sepsis, and irreversible damage to the kidneys

What's the typical treatment for pyelonephritis?	1. *Antibiotics (I.V. or oral depending on severity):* cephalosporins, levofloxacin, ciprofloxacin, amoxicillin are commonly used; prophylactic antibiotics may be prescribed for chronic pyelonephritis 2. *Increased fluid intake:* 3 L/day encouraged 3. *Analgesics:* to treat severe pelvic or flank pain
What are important nursing actions in the care of a patient with pyelonephritis?	1. Emphasize the importance of seeking prompt treatment at the first signs of a UTI. 2. Stress the importance of completing antibiotic course, even if symptoms subside. 3. Administer medications (antibiotics, analgesics) as ordered by the physician. 4. Monitor for complications, including sepsis and acute renal failure, and notify the physician immediately if any develop. 5. Educate the patient about ways to prevent UTIs.

Glomerulonephritis

What's glomerulonephritis?	An antibody-mediated disorder of the kidneys characterized by inflammation of the glomeruli
What's the pathophysiologic process of glomerulonephritis?	Infection, injury, or autoantibodies stimulate an immune response within the body, and the glomeruli of the kidney become inflamed as a result of deposition of circulating immune complexes there; scar tissue forms as a result of the inflammatory reaction, and tubular atrophy and loss of renal function ultimately occur
✎ **What syndromes are associated with glomerulonephritis?**	1. *Nephrotic syndrome:* proteinuria (more than 3.5 g/24 hours), edema, hypoalbuminemia, hypercholesterolemia 2. *Acute nephritis or nephritic syndrome:* variable proteinuria, hematuria, azotemia, and hypertension 3. *Rapidly progressive glomerulonephritis:* hematuria, oliguria, and acute renal failure
What types of glomerulonephritis exist?	1. *Membranous glomerulonephritis:* deposition of immune complexes between outer aspect of basement membrane and epithelial cells; commonly associated with SLE (lupus), certain drugs (NSAIDs, gold, penicillamine), hepatitis B, leukemia, non-Hodgkin's lymphoma, melanoma; symptoms include heavy proteinuria and possibly hematuria 2. *Membranoproliferative glomerulonephritis:* a chronic, progressive form of glomerulonephritis seen in older children and adults

3. *Immunoglobulin A nephropathy:* most common form of primary glomerulonephritis; localization of immune deposits in the mesangium; symptoms include hematuria and variable proteinuria; Henoch-Schönlein purpura is a systemic form of IgA nephropathy and occurs more commonly in children

4. *Postinfectious glomerulonephritis:* onset of renal failure 2 to 3 weeks following a streptococcal infection

What are the clinical manifestations of glomerulonephritis?

Symptoms vary greatly depending on disease progression, but may include hematuria, proteinuria, oliguria or anuria, azotemia (due to impaired filtration of nitrogenous wastes), edema, hypertension, and elevated serum blood urea nitrogen and creatinine

What complications are associated with glomerulonephritis?

Renal failure, pulmonary edema, and heart failure

What are the treatment options for glomerulonephritis?

1. *Pharmacologic agents:* immunosuppressive drugs (prednisone), diuretics for moderate edema, angiotensin-converting enzyme inhibitors to reduce proteinuria and to control hypertension; acute cases of glomerulonephritis may fully recover to normal renal function with supportive therapy

2. *Renal replacement therapy:* dialysis, kidney transplantation used when disease progresses to renal failure

✎ What are important nursing actions in the care of a patient with glomerulonephritis?

1. Emphasize the importance of early detection and treatment of streptococcal infections.
2. Administer medications (immunosuppressants, angiotensin-converting enzyme inhibitors, diuretics) as ordered by the physician.
3. Educate the patient about importance of strict compliance with medication regimen.
4. Educate the patient about any recommended dietary restrictions such as sodium restriction for edema and hypertension.
5. Assess blood pressure for hypertension or to assess effectiveness of antihypertensive therapy.
6. Monitor for complications, including acute renal failure or pulmonary edema, and notify the physician immediately if any develop.

Polycystic kidney disease

What's the polycystic kidney disease (PKD)?	An inherited, progressive disorder characterized by the development of clusters of fluid-filled cysts primarily within the kidneys, but may also occur in the liver, pancreas, and other locations in the body
What's the pathophysiologic process of PKD?	The development and growth of cysts compresses healthy renal tissue and impedes renal function
✎ **What are the clinical manifestations of PKD?**	Intermittent flank pain, hypertension, palpable renal cysts, intermittent hematuria, abdominal fullness, and enlarged kidneys with multiple cysts seen on radiographic films
✎ **What complications are associated with PKD?**	Ruptured or infected cysts resulting in sepsis; renal failure; and development of aneurysms (intracranial) and organ failure (liver) from cystic involvement outside of kidneys

What are treatment options for a patient with PKD?

1. *Pharmacologic agents:* antihypertensives for high blood pressure and antibiotics for treatment of bladder or kidney infections
2. *Surgery:* drainage of cysts that cause obstructions or severe pain; removal of affected kidney (nephrectomy) may be warranted in patients with frequent ruptured cysts and infections
3. *Renal replacement therapy including dialysis or kidney transplantation:* if disease progresses to end-stage renal disease

What medications should be avoided in patients with PKD?

Estrogens should be used with caution because it's believed that estrogen may promote the growth of the cysts

✎ **What are important nursing actions in the care of a patient with PKD?**

1. Monitor blood pressure regularly.
2. Emphasize the importance of good blood pressure control, because hypertension may increase the rate of progression of renal failure and also increase the risk for rupture of aneurysms. Recommend a low-salt, low-fat diet; smoking cessation; and exercise.
3. Administer medications (antihypertensives, antibiotics) as ordered by the physician.
4. Monitor for complications, including sepsis, and notify the physician if any occur.
5. Instruct the patient to avoid hormone replacement therapy due to estrogen's ability to promote cystic growth.
6. Discuss the option of genetic counseling.

Diabetic nephropathy

What's diabetic nephropathy?	A progressive renal disorder that occurs as a result of diabetes mellitus; most common cause of renal failure in the United States
What's the pathophysiologic process of diabetic nephropathy?	Chronic hyperglycemia can cause glomerular hypertrophy, sclerosis, and loss of nephrons
What are the clinical manifestations of diabetic nephropathy?	Glucosuria, proteinuria, hypertension, and increased blood urea nitrogen and creatinine
✎ What complications are associated with diabetic nephropathy?	Progression to renal failure and need for renal replacement therapy (dialysis, kidney transplantation)

What's the typical treatment for diabetic nephropathy?

1. *Behavioral modifications:* strict blood glucose control and dietary protein restriction to 0.6 to 0.8 g/kg of body weight per day
2. *Pharmacologic agents:* angiotensin-converting enzyme inhibitors or angiotensin receptor blockers, such as losartan or valsartan, for treatment of hypertension and protection of kidneys by delaying progression of renal disease
3. *Renal replacement therapy:* dialysis or kidney transplantation; persons with type 1 diabetes mellitus may be candidates for a combined kidney and pancreas transplant (healthy pancreas cures diabetes and eliminates risk for developing diabetic nephropathy in a new kidney)

✎ What are important nursing actions in the care of a patient with diabetic nephropathy?

1. Emphasize the importance of strict blood glucose and blood pressure control to delay progression of renal dysfunction.
2. Discuss any recommended dietary protein restrictions (excessive protein may cause further damage to the kidneys).
3. Administer medications (angiotensin-converting enzyme inhibitors or angiotensin receptor blockers) as ordered by the physician.
4. Monitor renal function periodically to evaluate progression of renal dysfunction.

Urolithiasis and nephrolithiasis

✎ What's urolithiasis?

A condition characterized by the presence of calculi within the urologic system

✎ What's nephrolithiasis?

A condition characterized by the presence of kidney stones

⧉ *Kidney stones are also referred to as* renal calculi.

What's the pathophysiologic process of nephrolithiasis?

Deposits of hardened mineral crystals gradually results in the formation of stones within the bladder, ureter, or renal pelvis. Calculi form as a result of excessive levels of calcium in the urine (hypercalciuria), oxalate in the urine (hyperoxaluria), or uric acid in the urine (hyperuricosuria), or as a result of an inadequate amount of water to dissolve waste products completely in the kidneys.

What are the most common types of calculi?

Calcium oxalate stones; other types of calculi include uric acid calculi, struvite calculi (related to infections of the urinary system), and cystine calculi (cystine is an amino acid that's difficult to dissolve)

✎ What factors contribute to the formation of urinary stones?

Dehydration; high urine levels of calcium, oxalate, or uric acid; low citrate levels in the urine (citrate is believed to inhibit stone formation); reduction or obstruction of urinary flow; certain medical conditions (gout, arthritis, hyperparathyroidism, medullary sponge kidney); excessive doses of ascorbic acid (vitamin C); and a diet high in meat, fat, sodium, and sugar, and low in vegetable protein, fiber, and unrefined carbohydrates

✎ What are the clinical manifestations of urinary calculi?

Nausea and vomiting, hematuria, renal colic (pain), increased urinary frequency, dysuria, and tenderness of the abdomen or area over the kidneys; severe radiating pain from the back to the abdomen and groin may occur when a calculus is passed

✎ What complications are associated with urinary calculi?

Obstruction of urine flow (which can cause hydronephrosis, severe damage to the kidney), infection, and bleeding

✎ What's hydronephrosis?

Swelling of the kidneys due to backing up of urine secondary to an obstruction, as can occur with renal calculi, benign prostatic hyperplasia, urethral strictures, or neoplasms; treatment includes eliminating the underlying cause of the obstruction and reestablishing proper urinary drainage; stricture dilation, ureteral stents, or nephrostomy tube placement may be necessary

⬥ What are important preventative measures for the formation or recurrence of renal calculi?

1. *Calcium calculi:* use of thiazide diuretics to decrease urinary calcium levels; dietary intake of calcium should *not* be restricted unless instructed to do so by a physician
2. *Oxalate calculi:* avoid green leafy vegetables, tomatoes, nuts, berries (especially cranberries), tea, cola, and chocolate; vitamin B_6 (pyridoxine) may be prescribed to decrease oxalate excretion
3. *Uric acid calculi:* low-purine, low-protein diet; allopurinol, bicarbonate (to alkalinize the urine) or potassium citrate may be prescribed as well
4. *Cystine calculi:* bicarbonate may be used to alkalinize the urine
5. *Struvite calculi:* ammonia crystals caused by chronic urinary tract infections (causative bacteria produce an enzyme that increases ammonia in urine); have a characteristic stag horn's shape, which can result in significant damage the kidneys; prophylactic antibiotics may be used in conjunction with urease inhibitors, such as acetohydroxamic acid (AHA)

What's the typical treatment for calculi?

1. *Facilitation of calculus passage naturally:* encourage ambulation and increased fluid intake
2. *Surgery (if calculus doesn't pass on its own in 30 days):* ureteroscopy (used for calculi in the lower portion of the ureter; basket extraction of the calculi or laser fragmentation of the calculi may be performed); lithotripsy (used for calculi located in upper portion of ureter; calculi are broken up into tiny particles that can be passed out of the patient in the urine), percutaneous nephrolithotomy (calculi are removed by surgical instruments via the use of catheters through the skin), or ureteroscopic calculi removal (fiber-optic instrument is advanced into the ureter and a laser is used to break up the calculi).

⚡ *Treatment for urolithiasis depends on the size of the calculi; those smaller than 4 mm in diameter typically pass on their own, whereas those larger than 7 mm in diameter usually require some form of surgical intervention.*

What's extracorporeal shock wave lithotripsy?

A procedure that involves using highly-focused impulses to pulverize urinary calculi into sandlike granules

⬥ What are important nursing actions for caring for patients with urinary calculi?

1. Assess the patient's level of pain at frequent intervals and administer analgesics as ordered by the physician.
2. Strain the urine each time a patient voids until calculus has passed.

3. Send calculi to the laboratory for clinical analysis (helps determine how to prevent recurrence based on type of minerals present).
4. Monitor intake and output. Encourage increased fluid intake so that approximately 2 L of urine is produced each day.
5. Encourage ambulation to facilitate calculus movement through the urinary tract.

Renal failure

ACUTE RENAL FAILURE

What's acute renal failure (ARF)?

A condition characterized by an abrupt decline in renal function and the consequent build up of metabolic wastes (uremic toxins), such as creatinine and urea, in the blood; may be a reversible process that results in the return of normal renal function, but underlying cause, severity of the condition, and the timing of treatment initiation are all factors that affect the recovery rate

What's the pathophysiologic process of ARF?

Both kidneys rapidly become unable to excrete the daily accumulation of uremic (metabolic) waste, and the resultant build up of toxins damages tissues and thereby impairs the function of other organs

What are the three types of ARF?

1. *Prerenal (azotemia):* inadequate renal perfusion or hypovolemia; common causes include blood loss, atherosclerosis, heart disease, and chronic liver disease; symptoms may include decreased urine output, thirst, hypotension, dry mouth, poor skin turgor, and dizziness; usually treated with I.V. hydration to increase blood volume, although dopamine or dobutamine may be used to increase blood pressure, and hemodialysis may be necessary in severe cases
2. *Renal:* caused by damage to the glomeruli or by obstruction of the tubules; common etiologies include acute tubular necrosis from nephrotoxic agents (contrast dye, aminoglycosides), glomerulonephritis, and interstitial nephritis; symptoms include oliguria or anemia, edema, hypertension, and nocturia
3. *Postrenal:* outlet obstruction of the urinary system prevents the normal flow of urine out of the kidneys; common causes include kidney or bladder calculi, enlargement of the prostate gland, neurogenic bladder, and trauma to the kidneys; symptoms may include edema, hypertension, bladder distention (from urinary retention), difficulty with urination, hematuria, and

pain in the lower back, low abdomen, groin, or genitalia; usually treated with catheterization of the bladder and removal of calculi; placement of percutaneous nephrostomy tubes may be necessary if the calculi can't be removed

▰ *The type of ARF is determined by the location of its cause within the renal system in relation to the kidneys.*

What are some of the risk factors for the development of ARF?

Sepsis, shock, nephrotoxic agents (contrast dyes, aminoglycosides), surgery, and trauma

✎ Which diagnostic tests should be performed cautiously or avoided altogether in patients with ARF?

Those involving contrast dye (dye is nephrotoxic)

What's meant by renal-dosed medications?

Renal dosing should be considered when a patient has renal impairment, usually defined by serum creatinine greater than 2.0; medications that are excreted through the kidneys should be considered for renal-dosed calculations

✎ What's the most common manifestation of ARF?

Decreased urine output; may be oliguric (less than 500 ml of urine produced each day) or nonoliguric (more than 500 ml of urine produced each day; more favorable prognosis); other manifestations may include fluid overload, dyspnea, mental status changes, nausea, vomiting, and pruritus

✎ What complications are associated with ARF?

Severe electrolyte imbalances (metabolic acidosis, hyperkalemia), volume overload, uremic syndrome, seizures, and death

What's the typical treatment for ARF?

Renal replacement therapy, most commonly by intermittent hemodialysis or continuous hemodialysis (for critically ill patients)

✎ What are important nursing actions in the care of a patient with ARF?

1. Monitor intake and output carefully.
2. Obtain daily weight.
3. Assess respiratory status at frequent intervals for signs of volume overload or respiratory compromise.
4. Monitor serum electrolyte levels (especially potassium).
5. Administer medications as ordered by the physician.
6. Monitor for complications, including metabolic acidosis, volume overload, hyperkalemia, and seizures, and notify the physician immediately if any develop.

CHRONIC RENAL FAILURE

What's chronic renal failure (CRF)?

A chronic, progressive, and irreversible syndrome of impaired renal function that eventually leads to complete renal failure; common causes include diabetes, hypertension, glomerulonephritis, obstructive uropathy, and polycystic kidney disease

What's the pathophysiologic process of CRF?

Nephrons and glomeruli become so damaged that renal function is affected; acid-base imbalances, increases in blood urea nitrogen, and abnormalities of fluid, sodium, and potassium occur as a result of the decreased number of functioning nephrons

What are the clinical manifestations of CRF?

1. *Early:* fatigue, malaise, anorexia, nausea, vomiting, unintentional weight loss, and nocturia (frequent nighttime urination due to inability to concentrate urine; fluid is mobilized when recumbent)
2. *Late:* edema (fluid retention), dyspnea, anemia (due to erythropoietin deficiency and decreased red blood cell production), oliguria, anuria, pruritus, nocturia (frequent nighttime urination), easy bruising or bleeding (due to decreased platelets), mental status changes, uremic frost, pruritus, peripheral neuropathy, muscle twitching or cramping, hypertension, uremic fetor (characteristic breath odor), and nail abnormalities

Symptoms typically occur when the glomerular filtration rate is less than 30 ml/minute.

What diagnostic tests are frequently performed to monitor the progression of CRF?

Blood urea nitrogen and creatinine levels (progressively increase) and creatinine clearance via a 24-hour collection (progressively decreases)

What conditions can produce renal failure?

Diabetes, hypertension, glomerulonephritis, polycystic kidney disease, hemolytic uremic syndrome, certain drugs (aminoglycosides), nephrolithiasis (if obstruction occurs), and renal carcinoma

What complications are associated with CRF?

Volume overload (heart failure, pulmonary edema, anasarca), electrolyte imbalances (hypocalcemia, hyperkalemia, hyperphosphatemia, hyponatremia, decreased bicarbonate and decreased blood pH/acidosis), anemia (due to erythropoietin deficiency), renal osteodystrophy (metabolic bone disease that predisposes to fractures and bone and muscle pain; due to impaired function of vitamin D), uremic pericarditis, seizures, cardiac arrhythmias, and death

What's the typical treatment for CRF?

1. *Renal replacement therapy:* hemodialysis, peritoneal dialysis, or kidney transplantation
2. *Dietary modifications:* protein restrictions (protein may increase the rate of progression of CRF); typically restricted to 2 g/day, or 0.6 to 0.8 g/kg/day; phosphate restrictions may be useful for persons with secondary hyperparathyroidism
3. *Pharmacologic agents:* may include multivitamins, calcium supplements, phosphate binders (Renagel, calcium carbonate), vitamin D supplements (calcitriol, hexitol), sodium bicarbonate (for treatment of acidosis), iron, epoetin (Epogen or Procrit) for anemia, and diuretics; angiotensin-converting enzyme inhibitors may be used to slow the progression of CRF, particularly in patient with diabetes

What are important nursing actions in the care of a patient with CRF?

1. Educate the patient about appropriate dietary restrictions, including limiting intake of protein, phosphate and, possibly, fluids. Meats should be limited due to their high protein content, and dairy products and colas should be restricted due to their high phosphorus content.
2. Emphasize the importance of strict adherence to dialysis treatment plan and medication regimen.
3. Administer medications (vitamin and mineral supplements, iron, phosphate binders) as ordered by the physician.
4. Monitor for complications, including infection at access site and hyperkalemia, and notify the physician immediately if any occur.

Renal replacement therapy

HEMODIALYSIS

What's hemodialysis?

A process that involves removing waste products and excess fluid from the blood by passing it through a machine (dialyzer) with a semi-permeable filter, and then returning the filtered blood (without the waste products and fluid) to the patient through one of several types of access devices; may be performed at home, or through a dialysis center and it's usually performed three times per week for 3 to 4 hours per session

Ultrafiltration is the removal of excess fluid from the blood.

✎ What types of access devices may be used for hemodialysis?

1. *Temporary access:* subclavian catheter, internal jugular catheter, or femoral catheter; commonly used for urgent hemodialysis before an arteriovenous fistula or arteriovenous graft can be placed; Y-shaped with one port for carrying blood to the dialyzer and the other port for returning filtered blood to circulation
2. *Permanent access:* arteriovenous fistula (AVF), in which an artery and vein are surgically joined together; and an arteriovenous graft (AVG; commonly Gore-Tex), in which a tube is surgically placed to join an artery and a vein

⚡ *An AVF is typically allowed to mature for 3 months before it's used as an access for hemodialysis.*

⚡ *An AVG may be used once the swelling subsides, typically within 10 to 14 days of placement.*

Where are permanent access devices typically placed?

Forearms, although upper arms may also be used; the legs are typically only used after all other locations have been exhausted

Is it acceptable to draw routine laboratory work from a patient's dialysis access?

No; upper extremities with AVFs should *not* be used for needle sticks or blood pressure monitoring. If a patient has a central line access such as a Permacath, it should also *not* be used due to the line being blocked with heparin, increased risk of infections or clotting off access.

⚡ *Only during emergency situations should dialysis access devices be used for purposes other than dialysis.*

What complications are associated with dialysis access devices?

Thrombosis and infection as well as the development of a stricture or aneurysm; surgery may be required to remove a clot or to repair a stricture or aneurysm

What complications are associated with hemodialysis?

Hypotension, nausea, vomiting, leg cramps, and light-headedness are the most common complications; others may include back pain, headache, chest pain, pruritus; life-threatening complications rarely occur, but include air embolism, acute hemolysis, and anaphylaxis

✎ What are important nursing actions in the care of a hemodialysis patient?

1. Encourage exercises that facilitate the development of a newly placed AVF such as squeezing a tennis ball several times throughout each day.
2. Assess an AVF for a bruit and thrill at least once per day to evaluate its patency. Instruct the patient on how to make this same assessment. A physician should be notified if a thrill and bruit aren't detected.

3. Avoid using extremity with access device for obtaining blood pressures or for needle sticks. Inform the patient of this same information as well as the importance of avoiding tight-fitting clothing on the extremity and avoiding any direct, prolonged pressure on the site of the device (such as sleeping with head directly on the site).

4. Emphasize the importance of adhering to the dialysis treatment plan and dietary restrictions. Missed dialysis appointments should be avoided and medications should be taken exactly as prescribed.

> *The more developed and bigger an AVF is, the easier it is to access and the fewer the complications.*

> *Assessment for a bruit and thrill should be performed at least daily to evaluate the patency of an AVF.*

> *A thrill is* felt *(pulsing or buzzing flow beneath the skin) and a bruit is* heard *(swishing noise).*

What's dry weight?

Also referred to as *target weight,* it's the amount a patient would weigh after urinating if he had normal renal function; it helps to determine the amount of fluid to be removed with each dialysis session

What dietary restrictions should patients in end-stage renal failure disease follow?

A low-potassium, low-phosphorus, low-sodium and low-protein diet; some patients will need to adhere to a fluid restriction as well

PERITONEAL DIALYSIS

What's peritoneal dialysis (PD)?

A process that involves using the peritoneal lining of the abdomen as a filter; a two-way catheter (Tenckhoff) placed into the abdomen allows for fluid exchanges that removes waste products and fluids without removing the blood from the body; may be continuous ambulatory peritoneal dialysis (CAPD) or continuous cyclical peritoneal dialysis (CCPD); advantages of PD over hemodialysis include not having to travel to a dialysis center several times per week for therapy, and having fewer dietary and fluid restrictions (due to daily dialysis)

> *Dialysate must be present in the abdomen at all times with peritoneal dialysis to ensure adequate cleansing of the blood.*

What's CAPD?

A form of peritoneal dialysis in which the patient fills the peritoneum with dialysate where it remains for 3 to 6 hours; during this "dwell" time, fluid and waste products cross the peritoneal membrane, and the dialysate containing the waste products is then exchanged for fresh fluid; typically performed four times per day on a daily basis

What's CCPD?

A form of peritoneal dialysis in which a machine is used to move fluid in and out of the peritoneum; commonly performed at night while the patient sleeps because this process typically takes 8 to 12 hours to complete; because all necessary exchanges are performed during this time, the patient is free from the dialysis machine during the day

What complication is frequently associated with peritoneal dialysis?

Peritonitis; other complications include catheter infections and the development of diabetes (PD dialysate primarily contains glucose and salts)

What are important nursing actions in the care of a patient with a peritoneal dialysis catheter?

1. Instruct the patient to use clean technique to open the catheter for use (prevents infection).
2. Educate the patient about signs and symptoms of catheter infections, including fever, erythema, warmth, puslike drainage from insertion site, and bloody or cloudy drainage in dialysis fluid. Instruct the patient to notify the physician immediately if these symptoms develop.

KIDNEY TRANSPLANTATION

What's kidney transplantation?

Surgical placement of a kidney into the peritoneal cavity; kidneys for transplant may come from a cadaveric (brain dead) donor or from a living donor; typically, the two native kidneys aren't removed for a kidney transplant

What complications are associated with kidney transplantation?

Rejection, failure of the transplanted kidney (due to rejection and thrombosis of renal artery), complications associated with chronic immunosuppression (prednisone, tacrolimus, cyclosporine, azathioprine, mycophenolate mofetil, sirolimus) such as increased risk for infections and a slightly increased incidence of some cancers (skin cancer, lymphoma)

Cancers of the urinary system

Bladder cancer

What's bladder cancer?	A condition characterized by tumor formation within the bladder; most are transitional cell carcinomas that occur in the transitional cells that line the bladder wall, although tumors may also originate from the squamous cells in the bladder wall
What's the pathophysiologic process of bladder cancer?	Tumor development occurs within the bladder walls
What are the risk factors for the development of bladder cancer?	Smoking, advanced age, male gender, white, chronic bladder inflammation (repeat or chronic urinary tract infections), family history, exposure to certain chemicals used in the manufacturing industry (rubber, textiles, dyes, leather), and long-term use of certain drugs such as cyclophosphamide (Cytoxan)
✎ **What are the clinical manifestations of bladder cancer?**	Typically produces no symptoms in the early stages, but painless and intermittent hematuria, dysuria, pelvic pain, urinary frequency or urgency, and decreased urinary flow may occur as the disease progresses
What complications are associated with bladder cancer?	Anemia, urinary incontinence, hydronephrosis (due to ureteral obstruction that prevents urine from entering the bladder), and metastatic disease

✎ **What are treatment options for bladder cancer?**

1. *Surgery:* transurethral resection of the tumor via the use of a cystoscope, a small wire loop for removing the tumor and an electrical current for burning any remaining cancer cells (fulguration); removal of the bladder (cystectomy) may be segmental (removal of only the area of the bladder with cancer cells present) or radical (removal of entire bladder, part of the urethra and some lymph nodes as well as possibly the ovaries, fallopian tubes and a portion of the vagina in women and the prostate gland, seminal vesicles, and part of the vas deferens in men); bladder reconstruction is performed with radical cystectomy

2. *Radiation therapy:* may involve an internal or external source; commonly used following surgery to destroy remaining cancer cells

3. *Chemotherapy:* may be intravesical (instillation of chemotherapeutic drugs into the bladder through a catheter) or systemic; used before or after surgery to

shrink tumor and possibly spare the bladder, or to destroy any remaining cancer cells
4. *Biological therapy:* use of immune stimulant Bacillus Calmette-Guerin to inhibit development and growth of new bladder tumors

What complications are associated with the surgical treatments used for bladder cancer?

1. *Transurethral resection:* temporary hematuria or dysuria for first few postoperative days
2. *Segmental cystectomy:* increased urinary frequency
3. *Radical cystectomy:* induction of menopause for women; infertility and possibility of impotence in men; men may want to bank their sperm prior to surgery

✎ What are common types of urinary diversions?

1. *Nephrostomy tubes:* tube is placed percutaneously (through the skin) into the renal pelvis to allow for an unobstructed urinary drainage system; may be temporary or permanent
2. *Ileal conduit:* segment of small intestine is removed and used to attach a ureter to a stoma in the lower abdomen to allow urine drainage into a small collection bag (urostomy); urine is then collected in an ostomy pouch
3. *Kock or Indiana pouch:* urine reservoir is created internally by using a portion of the ileum or a combination of the terminal ileum and ascending colon; need for an external ostomy pouch is eliminated; requires regular catheterization of the stoma

What's a neobladder?

A surgical technique in which a portion of the bowel is used to create a completely new bladder, which is directly attached to the urethra for normal outflow of urine

Aside from bladder cancer, what other conditions may necessitate urinary diversion?

Urethral strictures, congenital anomalies, chronic pyelonephritis, neurogenic bladder, and ureteral or bladder trauma

✎ What are important nursing actions in the care of a patient with bladder cancer?

1. Educate the patient preoperatively about need for bladder reconstruction after a radical cystectomy. Patients will need assistance in coping with body image changes as well as care of the new urinary outlet device.
2. Promote smoking cessation.
3. Emphasize the importance of close medical follow-up and regular screening with cystoscopies every 3 to 6 months (90% of superficial bladder tumors recur).

Renal cancer

What's renal cancer?

A condition in which cancerous cells develop within the kidney; most common type in adults is renal call carcinoma, which begins within the renal tubules; transitional cell carcinoma involves the development of a tumor in the renal pelvis; Wilms' tumor is the most common form of renal cancer in children

What's the pathophysiologic process of renal cancer?

Unregulated cell growth and proliferation occurs (commonly in the lining of the renal tubules), forming a tumor; begins most commonly within the renal tubules in renal cell carcinoma, but may also occur at the site where the kidney joins with the ureter (renal pelvis), as occurs in transitional cell carcinoma

What risk factors are associated with development of renal cancer?

Advanced age (ages 50 to 70), black race, male gender, history of smoking (cigarettes, cigars, pipes), hypertension, chronic dialysis, exposure to certain chemicals (asbestos, cadmium) increase the risk of renal cancer; a genetic predisposition is also suspected, because people with a positive family history of renal cancer appear to be at increased risk; a high-fat diet and obesity may also increase the risk

✎ What are the clinical manifestations of renal cancer?

Usually produces no symptoms in the early stages, but intermittent hematuria, flank pain, unintentional weight loss, fever, and a palpable mass of the kidney may be present as the condition progresses

What complications are associated with renal cancer?

Hypercalcemia, polycythemia (excessive red blood cell production due to release of erythropoietin), and metastatic disease

What's the typical treatment for renal cancer?

1. *Surgery:* removal of the entire kidney (nephrectomy; partial or radical) and possibly its associated adrenal gland; may be performed laparoscopically; nephron-sparing surgery involves removing only the tumor as opposed to the entire kidney
2. *Arterial embolization:* substance is injected into the renal artery in order to deprive the tumor cells of oxygen and other nutrients; may be performed prior to surgery or to relieve pain and bleeding in a nonsurgical candidate
3. *Radiation therapy:* typically used to relieve pain related to metastatic bone disease
4. *Chemotherapy:* usually used for treatment of metastatic disease
5. *Immunotherapy:* biological response modifiers (interferon, interleukin-2) may be used in some instances

✎ What are important nursing actions in the care of a patient with renal cancer?

1. Encourage smoking cessation.
2. Encourage weight loss and maintenance of healthy weight.
3. Encourage exercise to decrease blood pressure.
4. Emphasize the importance of close medical follow-up.
5. Monitor the patient for complications, including hypercalcemia and polycythemia and notify the physician if any occur.

Major disorders of the female reproductive system

Vaginitis

What's vaginitis?

Inflammation of the vagina; may be caused by an infectious process (bacterial, viral, fungal), a disturbance in the normal bacterial flora of the vagina, or by chemical irritants; douching, poor hygiene, antibiotic therapy, pregnancy, diabetes, and multiple sex partners can increase the risk of vaginitis

What's the pathophysiologic process of vaginitis?

Inflammation of the vaginal tissue occurs in response to an infection, an irritant, or a disturbance in the normal vaginal flora

What are the clinical manifestations of vaginitis?

Malodorous discharge, vaginal itching, and lower abdominal pain

What complications are associated with vaginitis?

Painful intercourse (dyspareunia)

What's the typical treatment for vaginitis?

Treatment is specific to the organism identified: antibiotics such as metronidazole (Flagyl) for bacterial infections; antifungals such as miconazole (Monistat, Lotrimin) for fungal infections.

What are important nursing actions in the care of a patient with vaginitis?

1. Encourage the patient to reduce her risk factors by encouraging safer sex and proper hygiene.
2. Instruct the patient to refrain from intercourse during treatment and until symptoms subside.
3. Inform the patient that lying recumbent for 15 to 30 minutes after vaginal suppository or cream insertion increases its effectiveness.
4. Advise women taking metronidazole to avoid alcohol during therapy and warn that the urine may become dark or reddish brown.

Endometriosis

What's endometriosis?

A painful gynecologic disorder in which uterine tissue (endometrium) becomes implanted outside of the uterus, typically the fallopian tubes, ovaries or throughout the pelvis; most common cause of pelvic pain in women

What's the pathophysiologic process of endometriosis?

Unknown exact cause; a common theory is that menstrual blood flow containing endometrial cells occasionally backs up into the fallopian tubes and becomes implanted in the surrounding pelvic wall tissue, which results in new endometrial cell growth outside the uterus

What are the clinical manifestations of endometriosis?

Menstrual pain (dysmenorrhea); abdominal pain; heavy menstrual periods (metrorrhagia); pain with intercourse (dyspareunia), bowel movements, urination, and ovulation; and an irregular menstrual cycle

Displaced endometrial tissue functions just as the endometrial tissue within the uterus does: it breaks down and bleeds each month according to the rise and fall of hormone levels.

What complications are associated with endometriosis?

Formation of cysts from trapped blood may cause adhesions and scarring; infertility can result

What are treatment options for endometriosis?

1. *Analgesics*
2. *Hormone therapy:* oral contraceptives containing low-dose estrogen and high progestin; medroxyprogesterone (Depo-Provera) to inhibit menstruation, which relieves symptoms associated with endometriosis
3. *Surgery:* removal of adhesions for infertility problems; total hysterectomy (uterus and cervix removal), oophorectomy (ovary removal), or salpingectomy (fallopian tube removal) for severe, painful cases

Pregnancy and menopause may halt or slow disease progression due to amenorrhea.

What are important nursing actions in the care of a patient with endometriosis?

1. Emphasize the importance of compliance with medication regimen.
2. Inform the patient of the potential for infertility related to endometriosis.

Cancers of the female reproductive system

Cervical cancer

What's cervical cancer?

A malignant condition of the cervix that typically occurs in women ages 30 to 55; cervical cancer is strongly associated with the human papilloma virus, but other risk factors include early onset of intercourse, multiple sexual partners, history of sexually transmitted diseases, and pregnancy at a young age

What's the pathophysiologic process of cervical cancer?

Neoplastic changes occur within the epidermis of the cervix

What are the clinical manifestations of cervical cancer?

Commonly produces no symptoms and only detected on routine Papanicolaou (Pap) tests; symptoms may include vaginal bleeding after intercourse, between menstrual periods, or after menopause; watery, bloody or malodorous vaginal discharge; and pelvic pain (late)

What complications are associated with cervical cancer?

Metastatic disease if untreated or detected late in disease progression

What are treatment options for cervical cancer?

1. *Conization of cervix:* cone-shaped piece of diseased cervix is removed with a scalpel
2. *Laser surgery:* narrow beam of intense light is used to destroy cancerous and precancerous lesions
3. *Loop electrosurgical excision procedure:* a wire loop is used to pass an electrical current and remove cancerous cells
4. *Cryosurgery:* uses freezing to destroy cancerous and precancerous cells
5. *Hysterectomy:* removal of cervix and uterus; radiation, and chemotherapy may be used in advanced cases

▲ *A Pap test is the single most important screening tool in the evaluation for cervical cancer.*

What are important nursing actions in the care of a patient with cervical cancer?

1. Encourage regular Pap tests.
2. Educate the patient regarding preventative measures. Advise the patient to practice safer sex by using condoms and limiting the number of sex partners.
3. Encourage routine medical follow-up and compliance with any treatment regimen.

Ovarian cancer

What's ovarian cancer?	A malignant condition affecting the ovaries; common risk factors include a positive family history, advanced age (age 60 and older), and nulliparity or late age of first pregnancy
What's the patho-physiologic process of ovarian cancer?	Uncontrolled cellular growth and proliferation of the cells within the ovaries result in tumor formation; as the tumor grows, it may exert pressure on nearby organs and interfere with their function
What are the clinical manifestations of ovarian cancer?	Most women remain asymptomatic until the disease is advanced, but symptoms may include abdominal pain and swelling (ascites), pressure sensation in pelvis, urinary frequency, constipation or diarrhea, abnormal vaginal bleeding, weight loss, pelvic and back pain, and pain with intercourse (dyspareunia)
What clinical sign in postmenopausal women warrants a malignancy work up?	Palpable ovaries
The elevation of what tumor marker may be associated with ovarian cancer?	CA-125; elevations of CA-125 may also be associated with endometriosis and breast cancer
What complications are associated with ovarian cancer?	Impairment of normal function of nearby organs, and metastatic disease
What are the treatment options for ovarian cancer?	Typically a combination of surgery and chemotherapy; surgery may include total hysterectomy, oophorectomy, or salpingectomy
What are important nursing actions in the care of a patient with ovarian cancer?	1. Promote good nutritional intake of protein-rich foods. 2. Emphasize the importance of close medical follow-up. 3. Discuss the option of attending support groups.

Major disorders of the male reproductive system

Epididymitis

What's epididymitis?	An acute inflammation of the epididymis and possibly the scrotal sac; possible causes include infections caused by surgical or diagnostic procedures or sexually transmitted diseases; urinary reflux may also cause inflammation
What's the pathophysiologic process of epididymitis?	An infection begins in the urethra and ascends to the epididymis, where it causes inflammation.
What are the clinical manifestations of epididymitis?	Testicular pain or tenderness (usually affects only one testes), scrotal edema and erythema, Prehn's sign (testicular pain relieved by elevation), low-grade fever, and chills
What complications are associated with epididymitis?	Painful ejaculation, scrotal abscess, chronic epididymitis, and infertility
What's the typical treatment for epididymitis?	Antibiotic therapy for bacterial infections in conjunction with supportive measurements, such as the use of nonsteroidal anti-inflammatory drugs, application of ice packs to the area, and elevation of the scrotum to relieve discomfort
What are important nursing actions in the care of a patient with epididymitis?	1. Emphasize the importance of completing the full course of antibiotics. 2. Instruct the patient to elevate the scrotum and apply ice packs to relieve discomfort. 3. Instruct the patient to take analgesics, such as nonsteroidal anti-inflammatory drugs for pain relief.

Prostatitis

What's prostatitis?	Inflammation of the prostate gland, which is classified as bacterial or nonbacterial (most common form)
What's the pathophysiologic process of prostatitis?	An infection typically spreads from the bladder or urethra and causes inflammation of the prostate gland.

What are the clinical manifestations of prostatitis?	Dysuria, urinary frequency or urgency, hematuria, low-grade fever, chills, urethral discharge
What complications are associated with prostatitis?	Painful ejaculation, chronic infection, possible infertility, and increased risk of prostate cancer
What's the typical treatment for prostatitis?	Broad-spectrum antibiotics, such as co-trimoxazole (Bactrim) and ciprofloxacin (Cipro) as well as anti-inflammatory drugs; sitz baths may also offer some pain relief

What are important nursing actions in the care of a patient with prostatitis?

1. Emphasize the importance of completing the full course of antibiotics.
2. Advise the patient about the use of analgesics (nonsteroidal anti-inflammatory drugs) for relief of discomfort.
3. Instruct the patient on the use of a sitz bath for symptom relief.
4. Encourage the patient to increase his fluid intake.
5. Advise the patient to restrict the intake of alcohol, caffeine, and spicy foods.

Benign prostatic hyperplasia

What's benign prostatic hyperplasia (BPH)?	Noncancerous hyperplasia (enlargement) of the prostate gland due to the abnormal growth of benign prostate cells; the enlarged prostate may compress the urethra and bladder, impeding the normal flow of urine
What's the pathophysiologic process of BPH?	Although the underlying cause isn't well understood, enlargement of the prostate gland may result in obstruction of the urethra, and subsequently, the flow of urine
What are the clinical manifestations of BPH?	Difficulty starting urinary stream, smaller and weaker urinary stream, urinary frequency, nocturia, and leakage or dribbling of urine
What are complications associated with BPH?	Urinary difficulties, including urine retention and incontinence, urinary tract infections, and renal damage

What are treatment options for BPH?

1. *Pharmacologic agents:* finasteride (Proscar) to inhibit production of hormone dihydrotestosterone; alpha blockers, such as tamsulosin (Flomax), terazosin (Hytrin), and doxazosin (Cardura), may be used to relax the smooth muscle of the prostate and improve urine flow

2. *Nonsurgical procedures:* TransUrethral Microwave Therapy (TUMT) or thermotherapy uses microwaves to heat and destroy excess prostate tissue; transurethral needle ablation uses low-level radiofrequency energy delivered through two needles to destroy excess prostate tissue

3. *Surgery:* transurethral resection of the prostate involves the insertion of an instrument through the urethra to remove the prostate tissue that's obstructing the flow of urine

What are important nursing actions in the care of a patient with BPH?

1. Instruct the patient to urinate upon earliest urge to do so.
2. Instruct the patient to avoid alcohol or excessive fluid consumption, particularly in the evening.
3. Encourage a low-fat diet and encourage the consumption of fruits and vegetables.
4. Instruct the patient to avoid over-the-counter cough and cold medications that contain decongestants (may worsen symptoms of BPH).

Erectile dysfunction

What's erectile dysfunction (impotence)?

The inability to maintain an erection sufficient for intercourse; may occur secondary to some disease processes (diabetes, hypertension, hypercholesterolemia), injury, or medication adverse effects (antihypertensives)

What's the pathophysiologic process of erectile dysfunction?

An interruption in the sequence of events that produces an erection occurs, inhibiting the achievement of an erection firm enough for sexual intercourse

What are the clinical manifestations of erectile dysfunction?

Inability to achieve an erection and difficulty with ejaculation

What complications are associated with erectile dysfunction?

Psychological concerns, including depression, low self-esteem, stress, and anxiety; infertility

What are treatment options for erectile dysfunction?

1. *Pharmacologic:* addition of drugs, such as sildenafil (Viagra), or intracavernosal injections and testosterone therapy; deletion of contributory medications such as antidepressants and beta-adrenergic blockers may also be useful
2. *Psychologic:* psychotherapy and stress reduction techniques

3. *Mechanical:* vacuum erection devices, external penile prosthetics
4. *Surgical:* inflatable penile prosthetic implant, arterial revascularization and penile venous ligation

What are important nursing actions in the care of a patient with erectile dysfunction?

1. Promote stress reduction.
2. Explain the need for evaluating levels of testosterone in the blood.
3. Educate the patient about various treatment options and encourage open discussion with partners.

Cancers of the male reproductive system

Prostate cancer

What's prostate cancer?

A slowly progressive, malignant condition affecting the prostate gland; the most common type of cancer in males in the United States each year

What's the pathophysiologic process of prostate cancer?

A malignant tumor develops in the tissues of the prostate gland, typically in the outer portion; as the tumor enlarges it may cause obstruction of the urinary flow

Who is most at risk for prostate cancer?

Blacks, men age 55 and older, men with a family history of prostate cancer and possibly, a high-fat diet (may increase production of testosterone)

What are the clinical manifestations of prostate cancer?

Although commonly produces no symptoms, elevated serum prostate-specific antigen levels, symptoms of BPH (urinary frequency, difficulty starting a stream, weak urine flow, dysuria, dribbling), blood in urine or semen, painful ejaculation, difficulty having an erection, and an abnormal prostate mass noted on digital rectal exam may occur; bone pain, fatigue, and myalgias can occur late in the disease and may be indicative of metastatic disease

What complications are associated with prostate cancer?

Erectile dysfunction (impotence), urinary incontinence, recurrence, and metastasis

What are treatment options for prostate cancer?

1. *Pharmacologic agents:* tamsulosin (Flomax), terazosin (Hytrin), and doxazosin (Cardura) to minimize symptoms of prostate enlargement
2. *Surgery:* transurethral resection of the prostate is the most common surgery and involves the insertion of an instrument through the urethra to remove the

prostate tissue that's obstructing the flow of urine; radical prostatectomy, involving the complete removal of the prostate gland and seminal vesicles, may be performed

3. *Radiation therapy:* via external beam or by implanted radioactive seeds (brachytherapy)

4. *Hormonal therapy:* luteinizing-hormone-releasing hormone agonists, such as leuprolide (Lupron Depot); anti-androgens, such as flutamide and bicalutamide; orchiectomy (surgical removal of testicles) may be performed to eliminate the primary source of male hormones

What complications are associated with surgeries performed for prostate cancer?

Urinary incontinence, rectal injury, impotence, and infertility (due to potential inability to produce semen)

What are nursing considerations for the postsurgical prostatectomy patient?

1. Assess the urinary catheter for patency due to its tendency to clot with blood. Irrigation may be necessary.

2. Monitor intake and output as well as urine characteristics. Urine will be pinkish red in the immediately postoperative period but should clear 3 to 4 days after surgery.

3. Administer analgesics and antispasmodic agents for bladder spasms.

4. Promote bowel regimen to minimize straining and damage to surgical site due to close proximity of prostate to bowel.

5. Instruct the patient to avoid sexual activity and heavy lifting for 3 weeks, to use stool softeners, to get adequate hydration, and to notify the physician if blood in urine reoccurs.

6. Implement chemotherapy precautions when handling patient waste if radioactive seed implants have been placed.

Testicular cancer

What's testicular cancer?

A malignant condition that affects the cells within a testis; most commonly affects white males ages 15 to 35

What's the pathophysiologic process of testicular cancer?

A malignant tumor forms from the uncontrolled growth and differentiation of cells within the testicles

What are the clinical manifestations of testicular cancer?	A scrotal mass or nodule in a testicle, a heavy sensation in the scrotum, pain or discomfort in the affected testis or in the scrotum, a dull aching sensation in the abdomen or groin, and an abrupt accumulation of fluid within the scrotum
What complications are associated with testicular cancer?	Infertility (only if both testicles are removed as a means of treatment) and metastatic disease
What are screening guidelines for testicular cancer?	Performance of monthly self-testicular examinations beginning at age 15, with clinical testicular examinations by a health care provider performed annually

How should a patient be instructed to perform a testicular self-examination?

1. Instruct the patient to perform an examination following a warm bath or shower (relaxes the scrotum).
2. Instruct the patient to use his thumb and fingers to palpate each testicle thoroughly for lumps.
3. Tell the patient to visually inspect the scrotum for any color changes or asymmetry.
4. Instruct the patient to report any suspicious nodules to the physician promptly.

What are treatment options for testicular cancer?

1. Surgery — radical inguinal orchiectomy, in which one or both testes are removed through an incision made in the groin
2. External beam radiation therapy
3. Chemotherapy

What are important nursing actions in the care of a patient with testicular cancer?

1. Emphasize the importance of close medical follow-up and performance of monthly testicular examinations.
2. Promote good nutritional habits, including consumption of protein-rich foods, fruits, and vegetables.

Pharmacology related to the genitourinary system

Diuretics

How do diuretics work?	Increase the rate of urine flow, typically by increasing the rate of sodium excretion in the urine

▶ *Water follows sodium and because sodium is the primary determinant of extracellular fluid (ECF) volume, a diuretic that induces sodium excretion in the urine will decrease ECF volume.*

◥ *The primary classes of diuretics act on different sections of the nephron, which gives the drugs within these classes their unique characteristics.*

What are examples of diuretics?

1. *Loop diuretics:* furosemide (Lasix), bumetanide (Bumex), torsemide (Demadex)
2. *Thiazide diuretics:* hydrochlorothiazide, chlorothiazide (Diuril)
3. *Potassium sparing diuretics:* spironolactone (Aldactone), triamterene (Dyrenium), amiloride (Midamor)
4. *Osmotic diuretics:* mannitol (Osmitrol)
5. *Combination agents:* hydrochlorothiazide with triamterene (Dyazide, Maxzide)

What adverse reactions are associated with diuretics?

1. *Loop diuretics:* polyuria, nocturia, dehydration, hypotension, hypokalemia, ototoxicity, muscle cramps, paresthesias, hyperglycemia, hypercholesterolemia, hypertriglyceridemia
2. *Thiazide diuretics:* polyuria, nocturia, dehydration, hypotension, hyperkalemia, hyperglycemia, precipitation of gouty attack (due to decreased renal excretion of uric acid), photosensitivity
3. *Potassium-sparing diuretics:* polyuria, nocturia, hyperkalemia, gynecomastia (breast enlargement), breast tenderness, decreased libido, menstrual irregularities
4. *Osmotic diuretics:* hypotension, urine retention, edema, dehydration

What life-threatening reactions are associated with diuretics?

1. *Loop diuretics:* allergic reactions (most loop diuretics are sulfonamides), arrhythmias (secondary to hypokalemia and hypocalcemia)
2. *Thiazide diuretics:* sulfa allergies, arrhythmias (secondary to hyperkalemia and hypercalcemia)
3. *Potassium-sparing diuretics:* arrhythmias (secondary to hyperkalemia)
4. *Osmotic diuretics:* precipitation of heart failure and pulmonary edema

What are important nursing actions when administering a diuretic?

1. Monitor intake and output and blood pressure.
2. Obtain daily weight.
3. Monitor for complications, including electrolyte abnormalities. Serum sodium, potassium, calcium, magnesium, phosphate and bicarbonate levels should be evaluated periodically throughout diuretic therapy, including following dosage adjustments.
4. Recommend that the patient take diuretics in the morning to minimize nocturia.
5. Instruct the patient to avoid taking nonsteroidal anti-inflammatory drugs (NSAIDs) simultaneously with loop or thiazide diuretics, because NSAIDs may reduce the effectiveness of these diuretics.

6. Instruct the patient to change positions slowly to prevent or minimize orthostatic hypotension.
7. Instruct the patient to avoid alcohol, excessive exercising, and prolonged exposure to heat to prevent dehydration.
8. Instruct the patient to limit dietary intake of potassium and avoid potassium supplements (including salt substitutes) while taking potassium-sparing diuretics.
9. Encourage the use of sunscreen, particularly with thiazide diuretics.

Contraception

What's contraception?

Commonly referred to as *birth control,* it's the act of preventing pregnancy

What methods of contraception exist?

1. *Hormonal agents:* oral contraceptive pills (estrogen and progestin), hormonal injections (Depo Provera), transdermal hormonal patches (Ortho Evra), vaginal contraceptive rings (Nuva Ring), and emergency contraceptive pills; hormonal agents prevent ovulation (the release of an egg from an ovary); emergency contraceptive pills use hormones to prevent contraception, but don't induce miscarriage (not an abortion pill); 98% to 99% effective if used consistently
2. *Barrier methods:* male and female condoms, diaphragms, cervical caps, intrauterine devices (IUD); prevent sperm from entering the uterus; IUDs may contain copper or progesterone that alter the lining of the uterus, making implantation of a fertilized egg difficult; condoms are 75% to 85% effective if used alone, but are 97% effective when used correctly in combination with spermicides; diaphragms and cervical caps are 82% to 94% effective; IUDs are 99% effective
3. *Chemical agents:* spermicidal foams, jellies, tablets, or suppositories; chemically destroy sperm and may offer some protection against sexually transmitted diseases; 79% effective if used alone and 97% effective if used in combination with condoms
4. *Surgical sterilization:* tubal ligation for women (fallopian tubes are sealed shut through laparoscopic surgery), or the placement of a springlike device into the fallopian tubes through the vagina, which produces scarring and blockage of the fallopian tubes (Essure); vasectomy for men (vas deferens is cut and sealed to prevent the passage of sperm out of the testes); all are approximately 99% effective at preventing pregnancy,

and are considered permanent because these procedures are difficult to reverse

5. *Withdrawal:* involves removing the penis completely from the vagina prior to ejaculation; unreliable because it's impossible to make sure that no semen has been released into the vagina before withdrawal of the penis; offers no protection from sexually transmitted diseases; approximately 75% effective at preventing pregnancy, but this varies greatly

6. *Rhythm method:* a woman's body temperature and consistency of vaginal discharge are tracked to determine when she's ovulating; the man and woman abstain from sexual intercourse for several days during this time; offers no protection from sexually transmitted diseases; approximately 75% effective at preventing pregnancy, but this varies greatly (may be as low as 50%) depending on the tracking method used and the regularity of the woman's menstrual cycles

⚑ *Contraceptive methods are effective at preventing pregnancy, but they aren't necessarily as effective at protecting against sexually transmitted diseases.*

ORAL CONTRACEPTIVES

What is an emergency contraceptive pill?

Commonly referred to as the *morning after pill,* the emergency contraceptive pill, such as mifepristone (Mifeprex, formerly known as *RU486*), is a high dose of an oral contraceptive pill that should be administered within 72 hours of unprotected sex to be effective at preventing pregnancy; nausea and vomiting are the most common adverse reactions

How do oral contraceptives work?

Oral contraceptives prevent pregnancy by using estrogen and progesterone to inhibit ovulation

What are examples of oral contraceptive pills?

1. *Combined hormonal therapy:* Ortho-Cyclen, Ortho Tri-Cyclen, Nordette, Yasmin, Levlen, Lo/Ovral, Ortho-Novum
2. *Progestin-only therapy:* Minipill, Ovrette, and Micronor; adverse reactions include weight gain and breast tenderness

What adverse reactions are associated with oral contraceptive pills?

Combined hormonal therapy may produce nausea, breast tenderness, weight gain, headache, acne, spotting, hypertension, and thromboembolic events; adverse reactions to progestin-only pills may include weight gain and breast tenderness

What life-threatening adverse reactions are associated with oral contraceptive pills?	Thromboembolism, pulmonary embolism, stroke, pancreatitis, and liver tumors

What are important teaching points for a patient taking an oral contraceptive pill?

1. Start taking the first pill on day 1 after the start of menses.
2. Use a second form of contraception during first 3 months of oral contraceptive pill use.
3. Take the oral contraceptive pill at the same time each day.
4. Take any missed pills as soon as possible, and take the next dose at its regularly scheduled time. When two pills are missed, two pills should be taken for the next 2 days in order to catch up.
5. If prescribed an antibiotic, ask about interference with oral contraceptive pill effectiveness. A second form of contraception should be used during this therapy.
6. Inform the patient that oral contraceptive pills don't offer protection from contracting a sexually transmitted disease. A latex male or female condom should be used to reduce the risk.

Nursing skills

Urine specimens

What are important nursing considerations in the collection of urine samples?

1. Assess the patient's ability to perform collection independently.
2. Instruct the patient on proper technique to minimize contamination.

How is a urinalysis collected in a non-catheterized patient?

1. The first morning void is desirable because it's most likely to show formed elements.
2. Urine is collected by midstream or clean catch technique.
3. Male patients are instructed to clean the glans penis with cotton balls moistened with sterile saline. Female patient are instructed to separate the labia and wash the urethral orifice with several single downward strokes using sterile moistened cotton balls and then collect the urine with the labia still separated.

How is a midstream urine collection obtained?

The patient should begin passing urine into the toilet and, without interrupting the flow, 30 ml of urine should be collected in a sterile container

How would you instruct a patient to collect a 24-hour urine specimen?	1. Obtain the appropriate collection container from the laboratory or physician's office. 2. On waking, empty your bladder and discard the urine. 3. Collect all of the urine passed after the first morning voiding until the same time the following morning. 4. Write the start and stop date and time of the collection on the container and follow the directions for storage because many specimens need to be kept chilled before analysis. 5. The collection container should be gently shaken each time a new urine sample is added.

◤ *The first morning void at the start of the 24-hour collection should be discarded.*

What should you tell the patient to do if they forget to save one urine sample during the 24-hour collection period?	Throw away all of the urine collected and start again the following morning
What patient position is used to catheterize a female patient?	Dorsal recumbent, the patient lies on her back with her knees flexed and her soles flat on the bed
What types of indwelling urinary catheters exist?	1. *Coudé catheter:* tapered tip catheter commonly used to facilitate insertion when an enlarged prostate is known or suspected 2. *Foley catheter:* balloon-tipped catheter that's inflated after it's inserted, which prevents accidental removal 3. *Simple catheter:* straight catheter designed for use in in-and-out catheterizations 4. *Three-way catheter:* balloon-tipped catheter that's inflated after insertion to maintain it's position in the bladder; another lumen is present for use in continuous bladder irrigations 5. *Suprapubic catheter:* surgically inserted catheter that enters the bladder through the abdominal wall above the symphysis; diverts urine from the urethra
How is a urinary catheter inserted in a female patient?	1. Inspect the perineum and wash the area if needed. 2. Spread the labia and locate the urinary meatus. 3. Remove the paper wrapped urinary catheter tray and place it on the bed between the patient's legs, near the perineum. 4. Prepare the sterile field by opening the inner wrap of the catheter tray. 5. Pick up the sterile absorbent under pad by one corner and slip it under the patient's buttock.

6. Put on the sterile gloves.
7. Place the sterile drape over the genital area exposing the labia.
8. Open the antiseptic solution pack and apply the solution evenly over the cotton balls.
9. Open the package of lubricant and squirt it on to the tray.
10. Attach the sterile water filled syringe to the balloon port on the catheter and instill the water to test for patency of the balloon.
11. Remove the water from the balloon to deflate it but leave the syringe attached to the catheter balloon port.
12. Separate the labia minora exposing the meatus. Hold this position until the catheter is inserted.
13. Using the forceps, pick up on antiseptic saturated cotton ball and clean one side of the labia majora then the other. Repeat for the labia minora. Work from the top to the bottom.
14. Clean the urinary meatus last.
15. Pick up the catheter about 3″ (7.5 cm) from the tip and lubricate it.
16. Insert the catheter into the urinary meatus 2″ to 3″ (5 to 7.5 cm) until the urine is seen in the catheter.
17. Instill water into the balloon port of the catheter.
18. Attach the catheter to the thigh of the female patient with tape.
19. Coil the excess catheter tubing on the bed.

What should you do if there's no urine flow from the catheter?

Rotate the catheter and advance it slightly

◤ *Never force a urinary catheter.*

What should you do if the catheter is inadvertently inserted into the vagina?

Leave the catheter in place to mark the vaginal opening, and obtain a new sterile urinary catheter kit and start the process again.

How is a urinary catheter inserted in a male patient?

1. Hold the shaft of the penis with your nondominant hand throughout cleaning.
2. Using forceps to hold cotton balls soaked in an antiseptic solution, stroke from the front to the back.
3. Lubricate and insert the catheter with your dominant hand while continuing to hold the penis with your nondominant hand.
4. Drain urine from the bladder and remove catheter, or inflate catheter balloon if an indwelling urinary catheter is inserted.
5. Attach the drainage bag if an indwelling urinary catheter is inserted.

What condition might cause resistance upon insertion of a catheter into a male?

Prostatitis

How is a male condom catheter applied?

1. Prepare the urinary drainage system.
2. Wash and dry the penis and surrounding skin.
3. Roll the wider tip of the condom sheath toward the narrower end.
4. Apply the skin preparation to the penis and allow it to dry.
5. Grasp the penis along the shaft and smoothly roll the sheath on to the penis.
6. Leave 1″ to 2″ (2.5 to 5 cm) of space between the tip of the penis and the drainage tube of the condom catheter.

⚡ *Don't apply the condom sheath too tightly because it may restrict blood flow to the penis.*

How should the urinary catheter collection bag be secured?

Attach the drainage collection bag to a part of the bed frame that doesn't move

In what position should the urine collection bag be placed in relation to the patient?

The collection bag should be lower than the level of the patient's urinary bladder to facilitate drainage

What should the nurse do if a component of the sterile catheter kit falls outside the sterile field and becomes contaminated?

Obtain a new sterile urinary catheter kit and start the procedure again

What type of urinary catheter care should patients routinely receive?

Gentle cleaning of the perineum or penis with soap and water; remove any debris with minimal manipulate to the catheter

Why are urinary catheters irrigated?

To maintain the patency because debris can cause obstructions

What are the different types of bladder irrigation?

Intermittent bladder irrigation and continuous bladder irrigation

How is intermittent bladder irrigation performed?

1. Position the patient and drape him appropriately.
2. Open the irrigation tray while maintaining sterile technique.
3. Pour the sterile irrigating solution into sterile graduated container and recap the solution bottle.
4. Put on sterile gloves.
5. Place a sterile basin between the patient's legs.
6. Disconnect the drainage system from the catheter, and insert a sterile plug.
7. Clean the end of the catheter with an antiseptic swab.
8. Draw up 30 ml of sterile solution into the syringe, and slowly inject it into the catheter.
9. Withdraw the syringe, and allow the catheter to drain into the sterile basin.
10. Repeat the procedure until the amount of fluid ordered is injected and returned.
11. Reconnect the catheter to the drainage system.
12. Measure the solution to determine the amount of sterile solution and the amount of urine returned.

How is continuous bladder irrigation performed?

1. Insert a three-way urinary catheter.
2. Verify the patency of all the ports on the catheter.
3. Using sterile technique, clamp the tubing and connect the irrigation solution to the tubing. The irrigation bag should be hanging on an I.V. pole so that it flows by gravity.
4. Prime the tubing with the irrigation solution and connect it to the urinary catheter.
5. Attach the drainage bag to the frame of the bed.
6. Manually open the clamp on the irrigation solution and regulate the flow.
7. Clean the spigot of the continuous bladder irrigation collection bag with alcohol before and after draining it.

What assessments should the nurse perform on a patient with continuous bladder irrigation?

1. Proper rate of flow of the irrigation solution
2. Uninhibited flow of urine into the collection bag
3. Presence of bladder distention, pain, color and clarity of urine, and blood clots in the urine

When the bladder irrigation is stopped, does the urinary catheter need to be changed to a standard catheter?

No; the three-way catheter may remain in place with a cap on the irrigation port

▧ *Continuous bladder irrigation tubing should be changed every 24 hours.*

How is a urine specimen obtained from a urinary catheter?	1. Clamp the urinary drainage tubing below the port for approximately 15 minutes. 2. Put on gloves and clean the port with an alcohol swab. 3. Insert the needle into the port and aspirate the appropriate amount of urine required for the laboratory test. 4. Drain the urine from the syringe into the labeled specimen bottle. 5. Unclamp the urinary catheter.
✎ What potential complication may occur after obtaining a urine specimen from a urinary catheter?	The patient is at risk for developing a urinary tract infection if any part of the catheter is contaminated during the specimen collection.
✎ How is a postvoid residual obtained?	1. The patient is asked to void completely. 2. Immediately following voiding, the nurse should have the patient lie in a supine position and perform an intake and output catheterization. 3. The urine is collected and measured to obtain the residual urine volume. 4. In some instances, a postvoid ultrasound is used and urine volume is estimated.
How much urine normally remains in the bladder after voiding?	Less than 50 ml
What are the indications for long-term indwelling urinary catheter?	1. Neurogenic bladders experiencing complication from urinary retention such as frequent urinary tract infection 2. Bladder outlet obstructions 3. Severe complications of incontinence such as skin breakdown 4. Use in palliative care
What nursing actions can be taken to ensure free flow of urine from the bladder?	1. Kinking of the catheter and collecting tube should avoided. 2. Collecting bag should be emptied regularly. 3. Poorly functioning or obstructed catheters should be replaced, if necessary. 4. Urine collection bags should always be kept below the level of the bladder.
For what conditions would a suprapubic urinary catheter be recommended?	For patients who require long-term urinary catheterization, those who have undergone certain types of gynecologic or urologic surgeries, and those who have urethral injury or obstruction

What observations should the nurse include in the assessment of a patient with a suprapubic catheter?

Leakage of urine around the skin insertion site of the suprapubic catheter, skin erosion, and problems with catheter reinsertion

What's appropriate care for a suprapubic catheter?

1. Remove the old dressing covering the catheter.
2. Assess the catheter insertion site for swelling, foul odor, bleeding, and skin irritation.
3. Wash around the shield with soap and water.
4. Clean under the shield and around the exit site of the catheter with hydrogen peroxide. Start at the exit site and clean outward. Let the area dry.
5. Apply a thin coat of antibiotic ointment around the insertion site of the catheter.
6. Place a split 4″ × 4″ dressing around the catheter.
7. Tape the dressing in place.

How often should the dressing on a suprapubic catheter be changed?

Daily (or if the dressing becomes soiled)

What should the patient do to retrain his bladder after suprapubic urinary catheterization?

1. Attempt to empty his bladder at least every 3 hours.
2. Collect the urine in a container in order to measure and record the amount voided.
3. Unclamp the suprapubic catheter, drain the urine into a collection container, and record the amount of urine.
4. Clamp the catheter.

When is it safe to remove the suprapubic catheter?

Typically, when less than 50 ml of urine is drained from the suprapubic catheter

NCLEX practice questions

1. A nurse conducts a chart review in order to gather information on a new client. Which component of the nursing process does this action fulfill?

☐ **1.** Assessment
☐ **2.** Diagnosis
☐ **3.** Planning
☐ **4.** Evaluation

2. A nurse is checking on clients during the night shift and finds a client on the floor next to his bed. He informs her he had gotten up to go to the bathroom, but slipped on the way back and couldn't get back into bed on his own. The nurse suggests calling the physician and having the client examined, but he insists that he isn't injured and asks that the physician not be bothered. The most appropriate nursing action would be to:

☐ **1.** assist the client back to bed and document the fall in the chart.
☐ **2.** notify the physician and the charge nurse of the fall.
☐ **3.** notify the physician and complete an incident report.
☐ **4.** notify the physician so that he may complete an incident report.

3. A client admitted for diabetic ketoacidosis becomes stuporous and develops bradycardia and deep, rapid respirations. Laboratory studies reveal a pH of 7.55, a Pco_2 of 27 mmHg, and a HCO_3^- of 16 mEq/L. Treatment for this client's condition would likely include:

☐ **1.** sodium bicarbonate.
☐ **2.** potassium chloride.
☐ **3.** magnesium oxide.
☐ **4.** calcium chloride.

4. Which finding might indicate a fluid volume deficit?

☐ **1.** Blood pressure of 162/94 mm Hg
☐ **2.** Pulse of 112 beats/minute
☐ **3.** Urine output of 85 ml/hour
☐ **4.** Respiratory rate of 22 breaths/minute

5. A client develops acidosis due to inadequate ventilation and, as a result, experiences fatigue and altered consciousness. Because of the client's compensatory rapid and deep respirations, the nurse expects:

☐ **1.** Pco_2 of 36 mmHg.
☐ **2.** pH < 7.32.
☐ **3.** Pco_2 of 18 mm Hg.
☐ **4.** Po_2 72 mm Hg.

6. A client is diagnosed with iron deficiency anemia and has been instructed to take ferrous sulfate 325 mg three times a day with meals. A nutritionist has educated the client about iron-rich foods. Which food would likely be recommended to enhance the absorption of iron?

☐ **1.** Legumes
☐ **2.** Raisins
☐ **3.** Oranges
☐ **4.** Apple

7. A 53-year-old male client has been diagnosed with hypertension and is placed on a 2 g per day sodium diet. Which item should be eliminated from his diet?

☐ **1.** Whole wheat bread
☐ **2.** Canned green beans
☐ **3.** Bananas
☐ **4.** Baked chicken

8. A client has been diagnosed with moderately impaired kidney function and has been placed on a renal diet. Which food would be allowed on this diet?

☐ **1.** Lean chicken
☐ **2.** Orange juice
☐ **3.** Potatoes
☐ **4.** Milk

9. A 16-year-old client diagnosed with anorexia nervosa has been started on total parenteral nutrition (TPN). Which statement regarding TPN therapy is true?

☐ **1.** Insulin may be necessary temporarily during TPN therapy.
☐ **2.** Hyperglycemia may result if TPN is stopped abruptly.
☐ **3.** A TPN catheter may be used to administer medications, but may not be used to draw blood.
☐ **4.** The nurse may inject electrolyte solutions into the TPN solution using aseptic technique.

10. A client is diagnosed with mild hypercholesterolemia and a low-cholesterol diet is recommended before cholesterol-lowering medications are begun. Which statement made by the client would demonstrate understanding of nutritional counseling to the nurse?
- ❑ 1. "I'll avoid food items that contain egg whites."
- ❑ 2. "I'll avoid meats and milk products."
- ❑ 3. "I'll avoid canned vegetables."
- ❑ 4. "I'll avoid foods high in fiber."

11. A head computed tomography (CT) scan has been ordered for a client with suspected stroke. What would be a contraindication to giving a client a CT scan with contrast medium?
- ❑ 1. The client had a previous reaction to barium.
- ❑ 2. The client is allergic to shellfish.
- ❑ 3. The client has a creatinine level of 1.0 mg/dl.
- ❑ 4. The client has been diagnosed as claustrophobic.

12. A 58-year-old male is about to undergo cardiac catheterization to evaluate chest pain. Which statement by the client displays to the nurse that he understands the educational preparation for the test?
- ❑ 1. "I took my warfarin last night at the scheduled time."
- ❑ 2. "I ate a light breakfast about 1 hour ago, but I didn't take my morning medications."
- ❑ 3. "I'll have a small incision made in the left side of my neck through which the catheter will be threaded to my heart."
- ❑ 4. "I'll have to lie flat in bed for at least 4 hours after the test."

13. A 34-year-old female is admitted after a 2-day history of severe headache, photophobia, and temperature of 103° F (39.4° C). Meningitis is suspected and a lumbar puncture is planned to confirm the diagnosis. The nurse explains to the client that she'll be placed in which position for this procedure?
- ❑ 1. Supine position with the head of the bed slightly elevated
- ❑ 2. Prone position with the knees tucked underneath
- ❑ 3. Side-lying position with knees bent to chest and head flexed
- ❑ 4. Side-lying position with the bottom leg straight and the top leg flexed at the knee

14. Two hours after a bronchoscopy, a client returned to the nursing unit. He's now developing severe respiratory distress. The nurse is aware that this is a life-threatening reaction most likely related to which complication of a bronchoscopy?
- ❑ 1. Inspiratory stridor
- ❑ 2. Laryngeal edema

- ❑ 3. Pharyngitis
- ❑ 4. Absent gag reflex

15. A client with an empyema has undergone a right thoracentesis to aspirate fluid for a cytologic examination. After the procedure the client should be placed:
- ❑ 1. on his left side for at least 1 hour.
- ❑ 2. on his right side for at least 1 hour.
- ❑ 3. in a semi-Fowler's position for at least 1 hour.
- ❑ 4. in a Sims' position for at least 1 hour.

16. A liver biopsy is planned for a 54-year-old male client with suspected hepatitis C. Which statement made by the client regarding a liver biopsy is true?
- ❑ 1. "The procedure will be performed in my hospital room."
- ❑ 2. "I'll be placed in a supine position with my arms at my sides."
- ❑ 3. "I'll be placed on my right side for the biopsy."
- ❑ 4. "I should avoid lifting heavy objects for 24 hours after the biopsy."

17. A 25-year-old client is scheduled for a lumbar puncture to rule out meningitis. What's an appropriate nursing action for a client after a lumbar puncture?
- ❑ 1. Make sure the client remains flat in bed for at least 1 hour after the procedure.
- ❑ 2. Make sure the head of the bed is slightly raised to prevent a spinal headache.
- ❑ 3. Encourage oral fluid intake.
- ❑ 4. Turn the client from side-to-side every hour.

18. Which assessment finding in a client who had a colonoscopy would require the nurse to notify the physician immediately?
- ❑ 1. Respiratory rate of 20 breaths/minute
- ❑ 2. Blood pressure of 96 mm Hg/65 mm Hg
- ❑ 3. Temperature of 102.5° F (39.2° C)
- ❑ 4. Pulse of 58 beats/minute

19. A 26-year-old female client diagnosed with asthma is receiving steroid therapy to decrease her immune response. Which adverse reaction is associated with steroid use?
- ❑ 1. Diabetes mellitus
- ❑ 2. Diabetes insipidus
- ❑ 3. Alopecia
- ❑ 4. Goiter

20. A 13-year-old male is diagnosed with an endocrine disorder involving an overproduction of growth hormone. Which clinical manifestation would the nurse expect to find?
- ❑ 1. Dwarfism
- ❑ 2. Acromegaly
- ❑ 3. Cretinism
- ❑ 4. Giantism

21. A client is diagnosed with adrenal hyperplasia affecting the adrenal cortex. The production of which of the following would most likely be affected by this condition?
❐ 1. Epinephrine
❐ 2. Dopamine
❐ 3. Cortisol
❐ 4. Norepinephrine

22. A client with hyponatremia, blurred vision, abdominal pain, and muscle weakness is diagnosed with syndrome of inappropriate antidiuretic hormone (SIADH). The diagnosis was based on a urine sodium of 24 mEq/L and a urine osmolality of 108 mOsm/kg. The nurse should question which order for this client?
❐ 1. Encourage oral fluids.
❐ 2. Administer demeclocycline.
❐ 3. Administer sodium chloride replacement I.V.
❐ 4. Administer furosemide I.V. push

23. A 36-year-old female client with type 2 diabetes has a fasting blood glucose of 145 mg/dl, an Hb A_{1c} of 9.2%, and a weight gain of 13 lb (5.9 kg) since her last appointment 3 months ago. What's the most appropriate statement the nurse can make to this client?
❐ 1. "Your blood sugar control over the past 3 months has been excellent, although you need to try to lose some of the weight you have gained to prevent needing more insulin in the future."
❐ 2. "Your blood sugar has been too high over the past 3 months and we need to add an oral hypoglycemic agent to help lower it."
❐ 3. "Your blood sugar has been too high over the past 3 months and you are at risk for developing a severe metabolic disorder called diabetic ketoacidosis."
❐ 4. "Your blood sugar hasn't been well-controlled over the past 3 months and we need to discuss your diet and insulin use."

24. A 54-year-old female with hypothyroidism is admitted to the hospital for management of left lower lobe pneumonia. The nurse is aware that the client is at risk for:
❐ 1. thyroid storm.
❐ 2. thyrotoxicosis.
❐ 3. myxedema coma.
❐ 4. adrenal crisis.

25. The nurse observes facial twitching in a post-thyroidectomy client. After laboratory analysis of his blood chemistry, it's determined that he has developed hyperparathyroidism secondary to the surgical procedure. Which laboratory finding would be expected in this client?

❐ 1. Parathyroid hormone (PTH) level of 15 pcg/ml
❐ 2. Calcium level of 7.1 mg/dl
❐ 3. Phosphorus level of 3.5 mg/dl
❐ 4. Sodium level of 135 mEq/L

26. A 40-year-old female client with systemic lupus erythematosus has been diagnosed with Cushing's syndrome. What would be appropriate care for this client?
❐ 1. Corticosteroid therapy
❐ 2. Volume resuscitation
❐ 3. Seizure precautions
❐ 4. Low-sodium diet

27. A client with diabetes reports feeling shaky and weak and he's noted to be diaphoretic. The nurse checks his blood glucose level, which is determined to be 47 mg/dl. What's the most appropriate nursing action for this client?
❐ 1. Administer metformin at the regularly scheduled time.
❐ 2. Provide the client with a glass of orange juice.
❐ 3. Administer 4 units of regular insulin according to a sliding scale.
❐ 4. Administer 25 g of 50% dextrose (D_{50}).

28. The nurse is assigned to care for a client with hyperthyroidism. Which order for this client should the nurse question?
❐ 1. Levothyroxine 50 mcg by mouth daily
❐ 2. Propylthiouracil 300 mg by mouth daily in three divided doses
❐ 3. Propranolol 40 mg by mouth daily
❐ 4. Lugol's solution 0.2 ml by mouth three times a day

29. Two days after a craniotomy for a brain tumor, a 42-year-old male is receiving dexamethasone, phenytoin, and famotidine. The nurse explains to the client's family that insulin injections are required because of the client's persistently elevated blood glucose levels. When the family questions why insulin is necessary, the best response from the nurse would be:
❐ 1. "The physical stress of the surgery has temporarily caused diabetes."
❐ 2. "He obviously had borderline diabetes before the surgery, but the condition only became apparent because of the stress of the surgery."
❐ 3. "People with a family history of diabetes can develop the condition if they're overweight."
❐ 4. "His blood glucose elevations are the result of the steroid he's receiving, but the insulin won't likely be necessary when the steroid therapy is stopped."

30. A 38-year-old client has been prescribed prednisone to control his immune response after a kidney transplant 3 months ago. Because of his steroid therapy, he has developed Cushing's syndrome. The nurse is aware that a client with Cushing's syndrome is at risk for:

❑ 1. addisonian crisis.
❑ 2. compression fractures of the spine.
☑ 3. hypertensive crisis.
❑ 4. rheumatoid arthritis.

31. A client presents with hypertension, tachycardia, palpitations, and café au lait spots. Pheochromocytoma is suspected, but the physician wants to perform a test that will confirm the diagnosis of pheochromocytoma? Which test would help confirm the diagnosis of pheochromocytoma?

☑ 1. 24-hour urine for metanephrine and vanillylmandelic acid (VMA)
❑ 2. 24-hour urine for cortisol
❑ 3. Dexamethasone suppression test
❑ 4. Water deprivation test

32. A client with hyperthyroidism undergoes a subtotal thyroidectomy to remove a thyroid adenoma. Which statement is true regarding this client's postoperative course?

❑ 1. The client will require a tracheal stoma.
❑ 2. The client will require permanent steroid therapy.
❑ 3. The client will need to have an alternative means of communicating temporarily.
☑ 4. The client will require permanent thyroid replacement therapy.

33. The nurse is preparing a teaching session for a client with diabetes mellitus. Which instruction would be appropriate to include in this teaching session?

☑ 1. Take regular insulin 30 minutes before meals.
❑ 2. Eat meals of simple carbohydrates.
❑ 3. Exercise at peak insulin times.
❑ 4. Administer insulin injections at the same site for the most consistent absorption.

34. The nurse is assigned to care for a client with pheochromocytoma. The client complains of persistent nasal congestion and asks the nurse to call the physician for an order of a decongestant. The nurse is aware that decongestants may predispose a client with pheochromocytoma to which complication?

❑ 1. Infection
❑ 2. Bronchospasm
❑ 3. Stroke
☑ 4. Hypoglycemia

35. A 64-year-old male client has been prescribed ibuprofen 800 mg twice per day for long-term management of his rheumatoid arthritis. Which statement is true for this medication?

Select all that apply:
☑ 1. The client should report a sustained decrease in urine output during ibuprofen therapy.
☑ 2. The client should avoid alcohol during ibuprofen therapy.
☑ 3. The client should inform his rheumatologist that he has peptic ulcer disease before taking the medication.
☑ 4. The client should notify his rheumatologist that he currently takes phenytoin (Dilantin) before taking the ibuprofen.
❑ 5. The client should take this medication with food or milk.

36. A client is found to have a blood pressure of 105/65 mm Hg, a pulse of 68 beats/minute, a respiratory rate of 9 breaths/minute, and a temperature of 101.2° (38.4°C). The client is due for his scheduled doses of 1 g vancomycin I.V., 2 mg morphine I.V., and 50 mg atenolol (Tenormin) by mouth. Based on the client's status, what's the most appropriate nursing action?

❑ 1. Administer the medications as ordered and document the time they were given.
❑ 2. Withhold the I.V. vancomycin and notify the physician.
☑ 3. Withhold the morphine and notify the physician.
❑ 4. Withhold the atenolol and notify the physician.

37. A client who had a splenectomy 2 days ago after a motor vehicle accident is noted to have altered level of consciousness, pinpoint pupils, and a respiratory rate of 8 breaths/minute. The nurse notifies the physician immediately and anticipates that which drug will be administered?

❑ 1. Naltrexone (ReVia)
☑ 2. Naloxone (Narcan)
❑ 3. N-acetylcysteine (Mucomyst)
❑ 4. Clonidine (Catapres)

38. An unconscious client arrives in the post-anesthesia care unit. In what position should this client be placed?

❑ 1. Supine position with head slightly elevated
❑ 2. Supine position without a pillow beneath the head
❑ 3. Side-lying position with head slightly elevated
☑ 4. Side-lying position with the face in a slightly downward position

39. One day after an open cholecystectomy, a client is instructed by her physician to ambulate at least twice today. When the nurse attempts to get the client out of bed, the client complains of pain and asks why it's necessary for her to walk so soon after surgery. What's the most appropriate nursing response?

❏ 1. "Walking helps stimulate your appetite and prevents nausea and vomiting."

❏ 2. "Walking is necessary because it prevents many types of surgical complications, including pneumonia and constipation."

❏ 3. "Walking is necessary because it helps to dislodge blood clots that may have formed in your legs during the operation."

❏ 4. "Walking is necessary because it minimizes postoperative pain"

40. A client is placed in Buck's traction for a femur fracture and develops constipation 3 days after surgery. Which factors may be responsible for his decreased peristalsis?
Select all that apply:

❏ 1. Administration of I.V. famotidine to prevent gastrointestinal irritation.

❏ 2. Use of Percocet tablets for pain management.

❏ 3. Nothing-by-mouth status before the surgery.

❏ 4. Anesthesia administered used during the surgery.

❏ 5. Immobility related to prescribed bedrest.

41. A 46-year-old female is 6 hours postoperative from an abdominal appendectomy. Which finding would require immediate notification of the surgeon?

❏ 1. Temperature of 99.2° F (37.3° C)

❏ 2. Pulse of 90 beats/minute

❏ 3. Blood pressure of 90/56 mm Hg

❏ 4. Urine output of 25 ml over the past hour

42. A nurse is caring for a client 2 days after the client's liver resection surgery. When the nurse empties the two Jackson-Pratt drains, she notes that the drainage from drain #1 is 10 ml, and drain #2 contains 70 ml for an 8-hour period. She compares these findings to the previous shift calculations and notes that drain #1 had drained 56 ml and drain #2 had drained 68 ml. The nurse is aware that the most likely explanation for these findings is that:

❏ 1. drain #1 has effectively drained the affected area and it's ready to be pulled.

❏ 2. drain #1 has become clogged with tissue debris or clot formation.

❏ 3. drain #2 is draining a larger fluid collection within the abdomen.

❏ 4. an infection has occurred in the area of drain #2.

43. A client is being discharged to home 2 days after a complicated umbilical herniorrhaphy. Which statement made by the client during discharge teaching would indicate the need for additional teaching?

❏ 1. "I can bathe in a tub right away, but I shouldn't get in the shower for 2 weeks."

❏ 2. "I shouldn't drive a car until my surgeon tells me I may do so."

❏ 3. "I should avoid picking up my 3-year-old son until my incision has healed adequately."

❏ 4. "I should expect to see clear or light red drainage from the incision for the first few days."

44. A nurse is caring for a client who had abdominal surgery 2 days ago. The client calls for the nurse, stating he just felt a popping sensation and pain at the incision site. Upon inspection of the area, the nurse notes that the wound has separated and a small portion of bowel is visible. The nurse's first priority should be to:

❏ 1. notify the surgeon.

❏ 2. soak towels with normal saline and cover the exposed portion of bowel.

❏ 3. obtain the client's vital signs, particularly his temperature.

❏ 4. gently attempt to reinsert the exposed portion of bowel to prevent ischemic damage.

45. A client develops severe pain and pallor of the affected extremity 24 hours after a surgical repair of a fractured tibia. A 2 mg I.V. morphine (Duramorph) was administered 1 hour ago. An as-needed order for 1 mg of I.V. morphine is written for breakthrough pain every 2 hours. The most appropriate nursing action for this client would include:

❏ 1. administering the additional dose of morphine as ordered.

❏ 2. applying warm compresses to the affected area.

❏ 3. positioning the affected extremity at the level of the heart.

❏ 4. applying cold packs to the affected extremity.

46. A client in reverse isolation has leukemia and is found to have cold and clammy skin, hypotension, and a weak, but rapid pulse. The nurse suspects that the client has developed septic shock. In which position should this client be placed?

❏ 1. Trendelenburg

❏ 2. Reverse Trendelenburg

❏ 3. Semi-Fowler's

❏ 4. Left lateral

47. A 58-year-old male in the emergency department complains of indigestion associated with nausea, diaphoresis, dyspnea, and left arm numbness. An acute myocardial infarction (MI) is suspected. Which action should receive the highest priority?

❏ 1. Order a stat electrocardiogram (ECG).

❏ 2. Administer 2 mg I.V. morphine (Duramorph).

❏ 3. Administer 81 mg of aspirin orally.

❏ 4. Administer oxygen at 4 L via nasal cannula and place the client in an upright position.

48. A client who was recently admitted to the hospital after a syncopal episode has had a series of blood studies. Which laboratory value would require immediate intervention?
- ❑ **1.** Sodium level 137 mEq/L
- ❑ **2.** Potassium level 6.2 mEq/L
- ❑ **3.** Calcium level 8.5 mg/dl
- ❑ **4.** Hematocrit 44%

49. A client is noted to have these laboratory results: sodium 135 mEq/L, potassium 3.7 mEq/L, calcium 7.2 mg/dl, and a magnesium level 1.9 mEq/L. Which symptoms is this client most likely to exhibit?
- ❑ **1.** Muscle cramps and paresthesia
- ❑ **2.** Hypertension and bounding pulse
- ❑ **3.** Lethargy and dry, sticky mucous membranes
- ❑ **4.** Analgesia and seizures

50. A client with end stage renal disease is admitted to the hospital for management of electrolyte abnormalities. Laboratory tests reveal: sodium 139 mEq/L, potassium 6.9 mEq/L, chloride 100 mEq/L, HCO_3^- 25 mEq/L, calcium level 8.6 mg/dl, phosphorous 2.8 mg/dl, and magnesium 2.1 mEq/L. The nurse would anticipate which treatment to be ordered?
- ❑ **1.** Sevelamer (Renagel)
- ❑ **2.** Magnesium sulfate
- ☑ **3.** Sodium polystyrene sulfonate (Kayexalate)
- ❑ **4.** Sodium bicarbonate

51. A 19-year-old female has a severe headache associated with photophobia and a fever of 103.2° F (39.6° C). She's diagnosed with bacterial meningitis based on the results of a lumbar puncture. An appropriate neurologic status assessment for this client would include:
- ❑ **1.** level of consciousness.
- ❑ **2.** Babinski reflex.
- ❑ **3.** tonic neck reflex.
- ❑ **4.** paresthesia.

52. A client with a severe brain injury displays extension of the arms and legs with internal rotation, hyperextension and plantar flexion of the feet, and a backward arching of the head. What best describes the condition the client has developed?
- ❑ **1.** Decorticate posturing
- ☑ **2.** Decerebrate posturing
- ❑ **3.** Nuchal rigidity
- ❑ **4.** Dysesthesia

53. A 58-year-old female who suffered a subarachnoid hemorrhage 3 days ago is found to have an intracranial pressure (ICP) of 22 mm Hg. What's an appropriate intervention for this client?
- ❑ **1.** Position the client flat in bed.
- ☑ **2.** Assess the client's vital signs and neurologic status every 4 hours.

- ❑ **3.** Minimize the client's movement.
- ❑ **4.** Suction the client every 2 hours prophylactically.

54. A client with bacterial meningitis experiences a seizure. During the postictal state, what primary assessment should the nurse make?
- ❑ **1.** Level of consciousness (LOC)
- ❑ **2.** Vital signs, especially temperature
- ❑ **3.** Pupillary responses
- ☑ **4.** Respiratory status

55. A client experiences a stroke related to a ruptured cerebral aneurysm. What would be appropriate nursing care for this client?
- ❑ **1.** Administer I.V. urokinase (Abbokinase) within 3 hours of the stroke.
- ❑ **2.** Position the client in Trendelenburg's position to increase blood flow to the brain.
- ❑ **3.** Monitor intake and output carefully to avoid overhydration.
- ☑ **4.** Implement bleeding precautions.

56. A 26-year-old male suffers a diving accident and a spinal cord injury is suspected. What's the immediate neurologic assessment that should be made?
- ❑ **1.** Palpating the spine to detect abnormalities
- ❑ **2.** Instructing the client to turn his head slowly from side to side
- ❑ **3.** Instructing the client to roll onto his left side
- ☑ **4.** Instructing the client to wiggle his toes and move his hands

57. A 62-year-old male undergoes cataract removal with placement of an intraocular lens implant. In what position should this client be placed postoperatively?
- ❑ **1.** On the operative side
- ☑ **2.** On the inoperative side
- ❑ **3.** In Sims' position
- ❑ **4.** In the prone position

58. Stimulation of the sympathetic nervous system causes a release of epinephrine. What effects do epinephrine and norepinephrine have on the body?
Select all that apply:
- ☑ **1.** Dilation of pupils
- ❑ **2.** Excitation of the bladder
- ☑ **3.** Increased diaphoresis
- ☑ **4.** Slowing of digestion
- ❑ **5.** Decreased heart rate

59. The nurse is caring for a client who has just undergone a craniotomy. The nurse is aware that increasing intracranial pressure (ICP) is a potential complication after this procedure. Which manifestation would be an early sign of increasing ICP?

☐ **1.** Headache with projectile vomiting

☑ **2.** Pupillary changes

☐ **3.** Slurring of speech

☐ **4.** Fluctuations in vital signs

60. A Tensilon test using edrophonium chloride determines that a client is experiencing a myasthenic crisis rather than a cholinergic crisis. What's the primary concern for this client?

☐ **1.** Decreased gag reflex

☑ **2.** Respiratory failure

☐ **3.** Severe psychosis

☐ **4.** Syndrome of inappropriate antidiuretic hormone (SIADH)

61. A client with a detached retina undergoes scleral buckling to correct the condition. In what position should this client be placed postoperatively?

☐ **1.** With the operative side down

☐ **2.** With the operative side up

☐ **3.** In a lateral position

☑ **4.** In a semi-Fowler position

62. A client suffers a closed head injury from a motor vehicle accident. He's admitted to the neurologic intensive care unit and scores a 5 on the Glasgow Coma Scale based on his neurologic assessment. Based on this information, what clinical manifestations would most likely be present?

☐ **1.** The client can open his eyes and follow commands, but is confused.

☐ **2.** The client can open his eyes when instructed to do so and withdraws from pain, but uses inappropriate words.

☑ **3.** The client can open his eyes, follow commands, or make verbalizations.

☐ **4.** The client can open his eyes and follow commands.

63. What neurologic condition is characterized by bradykinesia, jerking movements, pill-rolling, and a shuffling gait?

☐ **1.** Muscular dystrophy

☐ **2.** Alzheimer's disease

☐ **3.** Huntington's disease

☑ **4.** Parkinson's disease

64. A 40-year-old client with spinal cord injury at level T8 has bladder distention. What's the primary concern in a paralyzed client with bladder distension?

☐ **1.** Spinal shock

☑ **2.** Autonomic dysreflexia

☐ **3.** Dystonia

☐ **4.** Tardive dyskinesia

65. A 61-year-old male is diagnosed with mitral valve prolapse. When the patient asks where the mitral valve is located, the nurse should point at what area of the heart, using the diagram at the top of the next column?

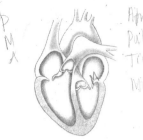

66. A client who suffered a myocardial infarction (MI) 4 years ago is admitted for chest pain. Which assessment finding should be of most concern?

☐ **1.** Heart rate of 96 beats/minute

☐ **2.** Heart rate of 60 beats/minute

☑ **3.** Blood pressure of 84/52 mm Hg

☐ **4.** Pulse oximetry of 93% on room air

67. A client undergoes a pulmonary lobectomy for lung cancer. Three days after the surgery, she complains of swelling, redness, warmth, and tenderness over her left calf. What primary nursing intervention should be performed?

☐ **1.** Apply heat to the affected extremity and encourage more frequent ambulation.

☐ **2.** Apply a cool pack alternating with sequential compression devices to the affected extremity.

☐ **3.** Elevate the affected extremity and encourage leg flexion.

☑ **4.** Elevate the affected extremity and maintain bed rest.

68. A client undergoes three-vessel coronary artery bypass grafting and is taken to the coronary care unit immediately after surgery. When the client's wife inquires about the purpose of the catheter that's placed in the right side of his neck, the nurse's best response would be:

☑ **1.** "It's used to monitor pressures within his heart."

☐ **2.** "It's used to administer I.V. fluids."

☐ **3.** "It's used to administer I.V. medications."

☐ **4.** "It's used to provide nutritional support until he can eat on his own again."

69. The nurse prepares to auscultate the aortic area as part of the cardiovascular assessment. Where should the stethoscope be placed to make this assessment?

☑ **1.** Second intercostal space along the right sternal border

☐ **2.** Second intercostal space along the left internal border

☐ **3.** Fourth intercostal space at the left sternal border

☐ **4.** Fifth intercostal space near the midclavicular line

70. A 65-year-old male client has been diagnosed with right-sided heart failure. When performing a physical assessment on this client, what physical finding would be associated with this diagnosis?

☐ 1. Bilateral crackles in all lung fields
☑ 2. Bilateral neck vein distention in a semi-Fowler position
☐ 3. Paroxysmal nocturnal dyspnea (PND)
☐ 4. Unilateral neck vein distention in a supine position

71. What should the nurse ask a client to most accurately assess for the presence of intermittent claudication?

☐ 1. "How does the position of the extremity affect the pain?"
☑ 2. "How does activity involving the extremity affect the pain?"
☐ 3. "How does the environmental temperature affect the pain in the extremity"
☐ 4. "How does the time of the day affect the pain in the extremity?"

72. A client on telemetry in the cardiac care unit is suspected of having a re-infarction. The nurse immediately notes that the monitor shows his blood pressure is 148/95 mm Hg, his pulse is 102 beats/minute, and his oxygen saturation is 97% on room air. What primary action should be taken for this client?

☑ 1. Administer supplemental oxygen at 4 L/minute via nasal cannula.
☐ 2. Administer oral propranolol.
☐ 3. Administer sublingual nitroglycerin.
☐ 4. Administer I.V. morphine.

73. The nurse is caring for a client who had a hip replacement 2 days ago. Assessment findings reveal a positive Homans' sign in the right leg. What's the appropriate nursing intervention for this client?

☐ 1. Ambulate the client and assist with performance of leg exercises.
☐ 2. Apply warm compresses to the right lower extremity.
☐ 3. Apply sequential compression devices to both lower extremities.
☑ 4. Maintain bedrest and elevate the right lower extremity.

74. A client is admitted to the coronary care unit after an acute myocardial infarction. A series of seven premature ventricular contractions (PVCs) is noted on the client's telemetry monitor 3 hours after his admission. The immediate response of the nurse is to:

☐ 1. prepare the client for cardioversion.
☐ 2. administer I.V. calcium chloride, according to physician's orders.

☐ 3. administer I.V. lidocaine, according to physician's orders.
☑ 4. place the client in semi-Fowler's position.

75. A client suffers an acute myocardial infarction (MI) and tissue plasminogen activator (tPA) is ordered. The nurse is aware that the purpose of this drug is to:

☐ 1. prevent blood clot formation.
☑ 2. dissolve existing blood clots.
☐ 3. decrease the mean arterial pressure (MAP).
☐ 4. induce coronary vasodilation.

76. A client with long-standing emphysema is now diagnosed with hypertension. Which group of antihypertensive agents should be avoided in this client?

☐ 1. Angiotensin-converting enzyme (ACE) inhibitors
☐ 2. Calcium channel blockers
☐ 3. Vasodilators
☑ 4. Beta-adrenergic blockers

77. When would performance of Valsalva's maneuver be appropriate?

☐ 1. In the treatment of bradycardia
☐ 2. In the training of a client after a myocardial infarction (MI) to fully empty his bladder
☑ 3. During the insertion of a central venous catheter
☐ 4. During treatment of cardiogenic shock

78. A client has just returned from a cardiac catheterization with a pressure bandage on his right groin. He reports to his nurse that the bandage is too tight. What primary nursing action should be taken for this client?

☐ 1. Loosen the dressing slightly, but monitor for bleeding or hematoma formation.
☐ 2. Notify the physician immediately of the client's complaint.
☑ 3. Assess pulses below the dressing.
☐ 4. Ask the client to flex his right foot.

79. Which laboratory value is the best indicator of myocardial damage?

☑ 1. Troponin
☐ 2. Lactate dehydrogenase (LD)
☐ 3. Aspartate aminotransferase (AST)
☐ 4. Creatine kinase (CK)

80. Myocardial ischemia would most likely appear on an electrocardiogram as:

☐ 1. wide and irregular ventricular complexes.
☐ 2. erratic, wavy baseline between ventricular complexes with no definable P waves.
☐ 3. ST-segment depression.
☑ 4. ST-segment elevation.

81. A client has persistent blood pressure readings in the 145 to 155 mm Hg/92 to 99 mm Hg range despite implementing appropriate dietary restrictions, exercising, and losing 12 lb (5.4 kg) over the past 3 months. Which classification of medications should be started first for this client?

☑ **1.** Beta-adrenergic blocker

☐ **2.** Angiotensin-converting enzyme (ACE) inhibitor

☐ **3.** Calcium channel blocker

☐ **4.** Thiazide diuretic

82. A client is found to have total cholesterol level of 260 mg/dl at the time of his annual physical examination. What nutritional information would be appropriate for the nurse to provide this client during educational sessions? Select all that apply:

☐ **1.** Encourage stanol esters.

☐ **2.** Encourage trans fatty acids.

☐ **3.** Encourage omega-3 fatty acids.

☑ **4.** Encourage fat intake of less than 30% of calories.

☐ **5.** Encourage more polyunsaturated fats than saturated fats.

83. A client is diagnosed with atrial fibrillation; he isn't a candidate for cardioversion. Which medication would likely be prescribed for this client's long-term management?

☐ **1.** Captopril (Capoten)

☑ **2.** Warfarin (Coumadin)

☐ **3.** Hydrochlorothiazide (HydroDIURIL)

☐ **4.** Metoprolol (Lopressor)

84. A client with stable angina is prescribed nitroglycerin. Which statement made by the client would indicate the need for additional teaching?

☐ **1.** "If I have chest pain, I'll take one nitroglycerin and wait 5 minutes before taking another."

☐ **2.** "If I still have chest pain after three doses of nitroglycerin I should call an ambulance."

☑ **3.** "If the nitroglycerin feels tingly on my tongue, I should throw it away and get another tablet."

☐ **4.** "I should sit down when I take nitroglycerin."

85. A client is admitted to the hospital for treatment of bacteremia. On the second hospital day, the client reports a sharp chest pain that worsens when she takes a deep breath. On physical examination, a harsh creaking sound is detected over the left third intercostal space. Which condition has this client most likely developed?

☐ **1.** Pneumonia

☐ **2.** Pulmonary embolus

☐ **3.** Endocarditis

☑ **4.** Pericarditis

86. A client with hypercholesterolemia is started on pravastatin (Pravachol). Which action would be appropriate for a client on this medication?

☐ **1.** Monitor troponin, lactate dehydrogenase (LD), and myoglobin.

☑ **2.** Monitor blood urea nitrogen (BUN) and creatinine.

☐ **3.** Monitor aspartate aminotransferase, alanine aminotransferase, alkaline phosphatase, and total bilirubin.

☐ **4.** Monitor partial thromboplastin time (PTT).

87. A client who has recently recovered from rheumatic heart disease is noted to have a heart murmur that's heard best in the aortic area that radiates to the neck. After an echocardiogram is performed, the physician explains to the client that an abnormal stiffening of one of his heart valves has developed, which impairs the flow of blood through it. The nurse recognizes that this client most likely has what valvular disorder?

☑ **1.** Aortic stenosis

☐ **2.** Aortic insufficiency

☐ **3.** Mitral stenosis

☐ **4.** Mitral insufficiency

88. A client receiving digoxin for atrial fibrillation is noted to have a digoxin level of 3.4 ng/ml. What clinical finding would be expected in this client?

☐ **1.** Tachycardia, confusion, and seeing a yellow haze

☐ **2.** Tachycardia, anorexia, and seeing a green haze

☑ **3.** Bradycardia, confusion, and seeing a yellow haze

☐ **4.** Bradycardia, increased appetite, and seeing a green haze

89. A client with a known abdominal aortic aneurysm (AAA) suddenly develops a severe, stabbing sensation in his abdomen that radiates to his neck. The nurse is aware that the client needs urgent medical attention because he has likely developed what complication of an AAA?

☐ **1.** Pulsus paradoxus

☐ **2.** Arteriospastic disease

☑ **3.** Aortic dissection

☐ **4.** Thromboangiitis obliterans

90. A 62-year-old male with a history of angina is admitted to the coronary care unit for evaluation of chest pain refractory to nitroglycerin. Which statement is true regarding angina?

☑ **1.** Stable angina is a symptom of underlying coronary artery disease (CAD).

☐ **2.** Unstable angina is typically more responsive to medications than stable angina.

☐ **3.** Angina is diagnostic of a myocardial infarction (MI).

☐ **4.** Stable angina is caused by coronary artery spasms.

91. A 26-year-old male client undergoes tuberculosis (TB) skin testing for a new job. An occupational health nurse reads the test 2 days later and notices the area of injection has a 10-mm induration and associated erythema. The most accurate statement that the nurse can make to this client at this time would be:

❏ 1. "Your TB skin test is negative."
❏ 2. "Your TB skin test is positive, which means that you'll require at least 9 months of treatment with isoniazid (INH) and possibly other medications."
❏ 3. "Your TB skin test is indeterminate, so you'll need to have a chest X-ray to determine whether you have active TB."
❏ 4. "Your TB skin test is positive, which indicates that you have been exposed to TB in the past, but it's uncertain whether you have active disease. You'll need to have a chest X-ray to determine whether you have active TB."

92. A 56-year-old male is admitted for an acute exacerbation of his emphysema. What's a characteristic of chronic obstructive pulmonary disease (COPD)?

❏ 1. Decreased anteroposterior diameter
❏ 2. Increased tactile fremitus
❏ 3. Prolonged inspiratory phase
❏ 4. Prolonged expiratory phase

93. A 32-year-old female with diabetes mellitus is admitted for treatment of metabolic acidosis related to diabetic ketoacidosis (DKA). What type of respirations is a client with metabolic acidosis most likely to exhibit?

❏ 1. Cheyne-Stokes
❏ 2. Kussmaul
❏ 3. Bradypnea
❏ 4. Bronchophony

94. A client with laryngeal cancer and lymph node involvement undergoes a total laryngectomy with radical neck dissection. Which nursing interventions would be appropriate in the postoperative care of this client?

❏ 1. Place the client in a supine position.
❏ 2. Instruct the client to avoid Valsalva maneuver.
❏ 3. Provide tracheostomy care.
❏ 4. Provide chest tube care.

95. Thirty hours after abdominal surgery, a client develops a cough, dyspnea, and a temperature of 101.2° F (38.4° C). The nurse is aware that this client has most likely developed what postoperative complication?

❏ 1. Pleuritis
❏ 2. Pleural effusion
❏ 3. Bronchiectasis
❏ 4. Atelectasis

96. A 58-year-old male with a long-term history of smoking is diagnosed with emphysema. Which statement is true regarding this condition?

❏ 1. Persons with emphysema use pursed-lip breathing because of the prolonged inspiratory phase.
❏ 2. Emphysema is a reversible process if the client quits smoking.
❏ 3. Persons with emphysema are known as "blue bloaters."
❏ 4. Hyperventilation is a characteristic feature of emphysema.

97. A client with a new diagnosis of tuberculosis has been prescribed rifampin (Rifadin), isoniazid (Laniazid), ethambutol (Myambutol), and pyrazinamide. What would be an appropriate teaching point for this client?

❏ 1. "The ethambutol will turn your urine and tears a reddish-orange color."
❏ 2. "The rifampin will turn your urine and tears to a reddish-orange color."
❏ 3. "The ethambutol will turn your skin and sclerae a yellow-orange color."
❏ 4. "The rifampin will turn your skin and sclerae a yellow-orange color."

98. What would be an inappropriate nursing action for a client with a 5-year history of chronic bronchitis who's found to have an oxygen saturation level of 92% on room air and a heart rate of 92 beats/minute?

❏ 1. Place the client in an upright position to facilitate the respiratory effort.
❏ 2. Administer 3 L/minute of oxygen via nasal cannula to decrease the client's oxygen demands.
❏ 3. Encourage the client's fluid intake of 2 L/day by mouth to thin secretions.
❏ 4. Administer (fluticasone) Flovent, as ordered by the physician, to dilate the bronchioles

99. The nurse is preparing a client for chest tube removal. Which instruction would be appropriate for this client?

❏ 1. "Exhale slowly as the tube is being pulled out."
❏ 2. "Cough as the tube is being pulled out."
❏ 3. "Lean forward as much as possible as the tube is being pulled out."
❏ 4. "Take a deep breath and hold it as the tube is being pulled out."

100. A client is diagnosed with asthma and the nurse is providing education about the medications that have been prescribed. Which statement made by the client would indicate the need for additional teaching?

❏ 1. "I'll use my albuterol for asthma attacks."
❏ 2. "I'll wait at least 2 minutes between inhalations from my two asthma inhalers."

3. "Overuse of my albuterol may actually worsen my asthma."

4. "I'll use my theophylline for asthmatic attacks."

101. A client with a persistent cough has been prescribed an expectorant. Which medication is an expectorant?
- **1.** Dextromethorphan (Robitussin DM)
- **2.** Codeine elixir
- **3.** Guaifenesin (Robitussin)
- **4.** Benzonatate (Tessalon Perles)

102. A client is experiencing an acute exacerbation of chronic bronchitis. In what position should this client be placed to increase his ventilatory efforts?
- **1.** Low Fowler's
- **2.** High Fowler's
- **3.** Sitting upright and slightly leaning over a bedside table
- **4.** Reverse Trendelenburg

103. A client with emphysema has been ordered to receive 3 L/minute of oxygen through a nasal cannula. This client should be monitored closely for which symptom?
- **1.** Cyanosis
- **2.** Anxiety and tachypnea
- **3.** Lethargy and bradypnea
- **4.** Hemoptysis

104. A physician informs a client that the client's pulmonary function tests revealed an increased residual volume. When the client asks the nurse what residual volume means, she explains that it's the amount of air:
- **1.** trapped in the alveoli that can't be exhaled.
- **2.** exhaled normally after a normal inspiration.
- **3.** exhaled forcibly after a normal expiration.
- **4.** exhaled during the first second of a forced expiration from a position of full inspiration.

105. A 16-year-old female with cystic fibrosis is scheduled for postural drainage four times per day. After this procedure, which nursing intervention would be appropriate to maximize the client's respiratory efforts?
- **1.** Administer a bronchodilator.
- **2.** Instruct the client to cough deeply.
- **3.** Place the client is a seated position.
- **4.** Encourage oral intake or fluids.

106. An accident victim is found to have a deep puncture wound on the left side of his chest. The client is alert, but dyspneic and tachypneic; a pneumothorax is suspected. What primary action should the nurse take for this client?
- **1.** Begin rescue breathing until help arrives.
- **2.** Apply an occlusive dressing over the wound site.

3. Position the client in an upright position to facilitate breathing.
- **4.** Place an I.V. line and administer fluids to prevent hypovolemic shock.

107. When a client with a tracheostomy is being suctioned, the nurse should remember to do which intervention?
- **1.** Remove the inner cannula before introducing the suction catheter.
- **2.** Begin suctioning as the catheter is being withdrawn.
- **3.** Insert the suction catheter until the gag reflex is stimulated.
- **4.** Change the suction catheter with each insertion.

108. A client with a spontaneous pneumothorax has a chest tube inserted. Within which chambers of the drainage system would bubbling be considered normal?
- **1.** First and second drainage collection chambers
- **2.** First drainage collection and suction control chambers
- **3.** Second drainage collection and water seal chambers
- **4.** Water seal and suction control chambers

109. The nurse is caring for a client with heart failure. The presence of which symptom may indicate that the client is developing pulmonary edema?
- **1.** Diminished or absent breath sounds
- **2.** Bradycardia
- **3.** Lethargy
- **4.** Pink and frothy sputum

110. A client with emphysema is diagnosed with hypertension. Which group of medications should be avoided in this client?
- **1.** Beta-adrenergic blockers
- **2.** Beta agonists
- **3.** Angiotensin-converting enzyme (ACE) inhibitors
- **4.** Angiotensin receptor blockers

111. The nurse is caring for a client with cystic fibrosis. She's aware that the least appropriate time for postural drainage is:
- **1.** in the morning.
- **2.** at bedtime.
- **3.** before a meal.
- **4.** after a meal.

112. A client is receiving cyclophosphamide, vincristine, Adriamycin, and prednisone (CHOP) therapy for non-Hodgkin's lymphoma. Which laboratory result is most likely to be due to the adverse effects of the client's chemotherapy?
- **1.** Potassium of 4.5 mEq/L
- **2.** Creatinine of 1.8 mg/dl
- **3.** Prothrombin time of 15.7 seconds
- **4.** Platelet count of 43,000/μl

113. A male client undergoing chemotherapy has these laboratory results: white blood cell (WBC) count of 1.3/µl, hemoglobin of 14.6 g/dl, hematocrit of 44%, and a platelet count of 95,000/µl. Based on these findings, the nurse is aware that the physician will likely order which therapy?

☐ 1. A six pack of platelets
☐ 2. Two units of packed red blood cells
☐ 3. Filgrastim (Neupogen)
☐ 4. Erythropoietin (Epogen, Procrit)

114. A client is undergoing radiation therapy of the pelvis and develops radiation enteritis as a result. Which finding would be expected in this client?

☐ 1. Diarrhea
☐ 2. Constipation
☐ 3. Dysgeusia
☐ 4. Xerostomia

115. A client with cancer is found to have an absolute neutrophil count of 440 and is placed on appropriate isolation precautions. What would be permitted for this client?

☐ 1. Fresh cut flowers
☐ 2. Consumption of peeled apples
☐ 3. Vaccination against measles, mumps, and rubella
☐ 4. Visit from his brother who received the chicken pox vaccination 3 days ago

116. A client with advanced lung cancer develops severe pain upon leg raising, paresthesia of the lower extremities, and urinary incontinence. The nurse is aware that this client has likely developed which condition?

☐ 1. Superior vena cava syndrome
☐ 2. Tumor lysis syndrome
☐ 3. Paraneoplastic syndrome
☐ 4. Spinal cord compression

117. Which vaccination would be safe to administer to a severely immunocompromised person?

☐ 1. Tetanus toxoid
☐ 2. Oral polio virus (OPV)
☐ 3. Measles
☐ 4. Mumps

118. A client has chronic allergies. Which immunoglobulin (Ig) is most likely responsible for this type of reaction?

☐ 1. IgA
☐ 2. IgD
☐ 3. IgE
☐ 4. IgG
☐ 5. IgM

119. A client receiving gentamicin (Garamycin) would most likely develop which adverse reaction?

☐ 1. Ototoxicity
☐ 2. Red man syndrome
☐ 3. Disulfiram (Antabuse)-like reaction
☐ 4. Permanent discoloration of teeth

120. The most recent CD4+ count for a client with human immunodeficiency virus (HIV) was 225/µl and her physician recommended initiation of HAART therapy. Which statement would provide accurate information to this client?

☐ 1. HAART therapy is the combination of two types of HIV drugs.
☐ 2. HAART therapy will produce an immediate increase in CD4+ counts.
☐ 3. Treatment with antiviral drugs that results in a decreased or nondetectable viral load doesn't mean that the virus can't be passed on to other people.
☐ 4. HAART therapy is effective at lowering the viral load of HIV in the blood, but it doesn't decrease the risk of developing an opportunistic infection.

121. A child develops pruritic skin lesions and is diagnosed with chickenpox. Which statement regarding chickenpox is correct?

☐ 1. It's spread only through direct contact with open lesions.
☐ 2. It's spread through coughing or sneezing as well as by direct contact with open lesions.
☐ 3. It's contagious until all the scabbed areas have disappeared.
☐ 4. It's contagious for several days after the scabbed areas have disappeared.

122. A client has been prescribed a 1-week course of co-trimoxazole (Bactrim) for a urinary tract infection. Which condition would be a contraindication to the use of this medication?

☐ 1. Photosensitivity
☐ 2. Chronic asthma
☐ 3. Warfarin therapy
☐ 4. Allergy to sulfa

123. Two units of packed red blood cells have been ordered for a client with a hematocrit of 22%. The nurse is aware that adverse reactions associated with blood transfusions include which of the following?
Select all that apply:

☐ 1. Hemolytic reaction
☐ 2. Hypertensive crisis
☐ 3. Hypothermia
☐ 4. Hypocalcemia
☐ 5. Malignant hyperthermia

124. A nurse is educating a 17-year-old male with sickle cell anemia about the prevention of sickling crises. Which teaching topic would be the most appropriate for the nurse to include?

1. Encourage the client to participate in aerobic exercises, such as swimming or walking.

2. Instruct the client to maintain adequate hydration and adequate oxygenation.

3. Encourage the use of iron and folate supplements.

4. Encourage the client to consider living at high-altitude locations.

125. Two units of packed red blood cells (RBCs) are to be transfused for a client with lower GI bleeding who's O negative. The blood arrives from the blood bank and on inspection, the nurse notes that it was collected 36 days ago and that it's O positive. What's the most appropriate nursing action?

1. Hang the O positive blood that was delivered because O is the universal recipient.

2. Throw out the blood that arrived because it's too old. Request that the blood bank deliver new blood products.

3. Throw out the O positive blood because it's incompatible with the client's blood type. Request O negative blood from the blood bank.

4. Administer the first unit of O positive blood to prevent treatment delay. However, request that the second unit of blood be changed to O negative to better match the recipient's blood type.

126. A client with hemophilia suffers a puncture wound to his left foot. Once the bleeding is controlled it's discovered that the client's last tetanus immunization was 8 years ago. How should a tetanus booster be administered?

1. Injections shouldn't be given to a client with hemophilia due to the increased risk of hemorrhage.

2. The injection should be administered subcutaneously rather than intramuscularly (I.M.).

3. The injection should be administered using the standard I.M. technique followed by application of cold packs to the area.

4. The injection should be administered using the Z-track method for I.M. injections and cold packs should be applied to the area afterwards.

127. A client with leukemia is scheduled for a bone marrow biopsy to evaluate treatment response. Which intervention is an appropriate nursing action for this client?

1. Maintain nothing-by-mouth status for 12 hours before the biopsy.

2. Notify the physician of the need to cancel the biopsy when the client's prothrombin time (PT) is 11.2 seconds.

3. Apply pressure at the biopsy site for at least 10 minutes after the procedure.

4. Administer analgesics after the biopsy and encourage ambulation to minimize discomfort and prevent complications of immobility.

128. A client had a partial gastric resection 4 months ago for gastric cancer. Laboratory studies reveal a decreased hemoglobin and hematocrit. The nurse is aware that this client has most likely developed which type of anemia?

1. Pernicious anemia

2. Aplastic anemia

3. Iron deficiency anemia

4. Acquired hemolytic anemia

129. Which intervention would be contraindicated for a client with polycythemia vera?

1. Intermittent phlebotomy

2. Administration of epoetin (Epogen, Procrit)

3. Administration of anagrelide (Agrylin)

4. Administration of hydroxyurea (Droxia)

130. A nurse is caring for a client who has severe burns covering 25% of his body surface area (BSA). The physician has ordered premedications to be administered before debridement. The nurse is aware that the most appropriate medication and route for this client is:

1. oral codeine.

2. subcutaneous morphine (Duramorph).

3. I.V. morphine.

4. I.M. meperidine (Demerol).

131. A client is admitted for management of arterial ulcers of the toes. Which nursing intervention would be appropriate for this client?

1. Apply compression stockings to reduce edema and minimize pain.

2. Elevate the affected extremity.

3. Maintain bedrest with the affected extremity in a slightly dependent position.

4. Change the Unna boot once per week.

132. A 72-year-old thin woman is admitted for a pressure ulcer that developed 2 weeks after right internal hip fixation. The physician has ordered a bed with circulating air. The nurse's main priority when it comes to caring for this client should be:

1. skin assessments twice per day.

2. hydration and intake and output assessment every shift.

3. range-of-motion (ROM) exercises twice per day.

4. vital signs assessment every shift.

133. A client has clusters of small fluid-filled blisters located on the right side of his abdomen that he describes as mildly painful. Crusting of some of the lesions is present. What medication will likely be prescribed for this client?

❏ **1.** Mupirocin (Bactroban)

❏ **2.** Silver sulfadiazine (Silvadene)

❏ **3.** Tazarotene (Tazorac)

❏ **4.** Acyclovir (Zovirax)

134. A 52-year-old male with diabetes is admitted for management of several painful ulcerations on his left lateral malleolus. Upon examination, the wound bed is found to be deep, but pale and dry, and the dorsalis pedis pulse is noted to be weaker on the left. The most likely cause of this client's ulcerations is:

❏ **1.** arterial ulcers.

❏ **2.** venous insufficiency ulcers.

❏ **3.** pressure ulcers.

❏ **4.** decubitus ulcers.

135. An escharotomy is planned for a client who suffered deep partial-thickness (second-degree) burns over 15% of his body. The client's family asks why this procedure is necessary. The nurse's best response would be:

❏ **1.** "Removal of eschar minimizes the risk of infections."

❏ **2.** "Removal of eschar prevents the development of compartment syndrome."

❏ **3.** "Removal of eschar prevents the dramatic fluid shifts that occur commonly in a client with burns."

❏ **4.** "Removal of eschar minimizes the need for skin grafting later."

136. A client who has had a purified protein derivative (PPD) skin test placed 48 hours ago is noted to have localized edema beneath the skin at the injection site. This clinical manifestation is best described as:

❏ **1.** undermining.

❏ **2.** tunneling.

❏ **3.** induration.

❏ **4.** nodule.

137. A 66-year-old female underwent surgery to repair a hip fracture with an internal fixation device. In what position should the affected extremity be placed the next day in order to facilitate restoration of normal anatomical function?

❏ **1.** Normal body alignment

❏ **2.** Slight external rotation using a trochanter role

❏ **3.** Moderate adduction using a trochanter role

❏ **4.** Moderate abduction using a trochanter role

138. A client with a comminuted fracture is placed in skeletal traction. The nurse explains that pin care is required because the pin sites provide a direct avenue for the entry of microorganisms into the bone, which can cause osteomyelitis. What's the most appropriate manner in which pin care should be provided?

❏ **1.** Hydrogen peroxide or normal saline solution and sterile applicators will be used to gently remove crusting at the pin sites.

❏ **2.** An antibiotic ointment will be applied to the pin sites twice a day to prevent infections.

❏ **3.** A Betadine solution will be used to remove crusting at the pin sites.

❏ **4.** A solution of half-peroxide and half-Betadine will be used to remove crusting at the pin sites.

139. A client with rheumatoid arthritis develops an acute exacerbation. What's the most important nursing action for this client during the acute episode?

❏ **1.** Encourage the use of the affected extremity to prevent immobility.

❏ **2.** Maintain flexion of the affected extremity by placing a pillow beneath it.

❏ **3.** Encourage rest of the affected extremity and maintain its functional alignment.

❏ **4.** Elevate the extremity on a pillow to minimize edema.

140. A soft tissue injury involving the excessive stretching of a muscle is best described as:

❏ **1.** a sprain.

❏ **2.** a strain.

❏ **3.** a subluxation.

❏ **4.** tendonitis.

141. A 20-year-old male suffers a right shoulder injury while playing football. A dislocation is suspected because movement of the right extremity is painful and restricted, and because the right extremity appears to be slightly shorter than the left. The nurse explains to the client that re-alignment of the shoulder joint should be performed as soon as possible because:

❏ **1.** pain medications won't be as effective the longer the dislocation exists.

❏ **2.** surgery may be required the longer the dislocation exists.

❏ **3.** the risk for carpal tunnel syndrome increases the longer the dislocation exists.

❏ **4.** the risk for avascular necrosis of the joint increases the longer the dislocation exists.

142. A 72-year-old male sustains a fall in his home and is later diagnosed with a left hip fracture. Which finding would typically be associated with this type of injury?

❏ **1.** The left leg is slightly shorter than the right leg.

❏ **2.** The left leg is slightly longer than the right leg.

❏ **3.** The left leg is slightly internally rotated.

❏ **4.** The left hip area is ecchymotic.

143. A 58-year-old female is diagnosed with osteoporosis and is prescribed alendronate (Fosamax). What are the most common adverse reactions associated with this group of medications?
- ☐ **1.** Neurologic disturbances
- ☐ **2.** Hematologic disturbances
- ☐ **3.** Cardiovascular disturbances
- ☑ **4.** GI disturbances

144. A nurse is preparing a client for a total hip replacement that's scheduled the following week. Which option would be an appropriate teaching point for this client regarding the postoperative routine?
- ☐ **1.** Flat bed rest will be required for 1 week after surgery.
- ☑ **2.** Crossing of the legs or ankles should be avoided.
- ☐ **3.** Ambulation will be encouraged on postoperative day 3.
- ☐ **4.** Turning to the unaffected side without assistance will be permitted after the first 48 hours.

145. A client describes a 2-day history of severe lower back pain that shoots down her left leg. She also mentions that she has experienced some mild urinary incontinence since the pain began. A herniated disc is suspected, and the nurse recognizes that the most likely cause of this condition is the client's:
- ☐ **1.** family history of back problems.
- ☐ **2.** history of osteoporosis.
- ☐ **3.** history of arthritis.
- ☑ **4.** job that involves heavy lifting and frequent bending at the waist.

146. A client suddenly develops pain, swelling, and stiffness of his left ankle; he's diagnosed with gout. Which medication should be prescribed first?
- ☐ **1.** Probenecid (Benemid)
- ☑ **2.** Colchicine (Colgout)
- ☐ **3.** Allopurinol (Zyloprim)
- ☐ **4.** Sulfinpyrazone (Anturane)

147. A 63-year-old female is diagnosed with compression fractures related to osteoporosis. Her physician prescribes risdronate (Actonel) and instructs her to increase her dietary intake of calcium and to stop smoking. Other treatment measures that would be appropriate include:
- ☐ **1.** non–weight-bearing exercises.
- ☐ **2.** decreased consumption of vitamin D.
- ☐ **3.** increased consumption of phosphates.
- ☑ **4.** decreased consumption of soda.

148. A client with diabetes undergoes a below-the-knee amputation (BKA) on his left leg related to ischemia from his peripheral vascular disease. Which nursing step would be considered appropriate stump care for this client?
- ☐ **1.** Instruct the client to dangle the left leg over the side of the bed a few times each day beginning postoperative day 1 to prevent contractures.
- ☑ **2.** Instruct the client to lie on his abdomen for 30 minutes each day to prevent contractures.
- ☐ **3.** Instruct the client to apply baby powder to the stump once per day to absorb moisture.
- ☐ **4.** Encourage the client to sit in a chair for at least 1 hour several times per day to prevent contractures.

149. A 67-year-old male is diagnosed with osteogenic sarcoma. The nurse is aware that this client is at risk for developing what complication?
- ☐ **1.** Bursitis
- ☐ **2.** Crepitation
- ☑ **3.** Pathologic fracture
- ☐ **4.** Pathologic contracture

150. A client who has mild residual neurologic deficit after a recent stroke is instructed to ambulate at least twice per day. On which side of the client should the nurse stand when assisting him with ambulation when no assistive device is used?
- ☐ **1.** On his right side
- ☐ **2.** On his left side
- ☑ **3.** On his stronger side
- ☐ **4.** On his weaker side

151. A client with a newly placed cast on his left forearm complains of increasing pain and states that the cast is too tight. The primary nursing action should be to:
- ☐ **1.** notify the surgeon immediately.
- ☐ **2.** check capillary refill of the left digits.
- ☐ **3.** apply a cold pack above the casted portion of the forearm to minimize edema.
- ☐ **4.** attempt to insert two fingers into the proximal and distal ends of the cast.

152. A 56-year-old male with a recent history of rectal bleeding has just returned from a colonoscopy. Which finding should the nurse report immediately to the physician?
- ☐ **1.** Mild abdominal pain and cramping
- ☐ **2.** Sudden temperature of 103.4° F (39.7° C)
- ☐ **3.** Thirst and hoarseness
- ☐ **4.** Complaint of light-headedness and dizziness

153. A nurse is teaching a client with chronic pancreatitis about appropriate dietary interventions. Which statement by this client would indicate the need for additional teaching?
- ☐ **1.** "I should avoid alcoholic beverages."
- ☐ **2.** "I'll eat a high-calorie diet."
- ☐ **3.** "I'll eat a high-fat diet."
- ☐ **4.** "I'll eat more often, but in smaller portions."

154. A nurse is preparing a client for a colectomy. Which statement by the client would indicate an appropriate understanding of the procedure?
- ❏ **1.** "The colostomy should begin to function 2 to 3 hours after the surgery."
- ❏ **2.** "The colostomy should begin to function 2 to 3 days after the surgery."
- ❏ **3.** "I won't be allowed to eat greasy foods after my surgery."
- ❏ **4.** "I should eat a bland, low-residue diet after my surgery."

155. A 20-year-old female is diagnosed with sprue. Which food selection should the nurse instruct this client to avoid?
- ❏ **1.** Broiled fish
- ❏ **2.** Grapefruit juice
- ❏ **3.** Baked potato
- ❏ **4.** Spaghetti

156. A 21-year-old male is admitted with right lower quadrant pain with rebound tenderness, nausea, vomiting, and a fever of 101.4° F (38.6° C). A ruptured appendix is suspected. In which position should this client be placed?
- ❏ **1.** Trendelenburg
- ❏ **2.** Semi-Fowler's
- ❏ **3.** Sims'
- ❏ **4.** Reverse Trendelenburg

157. A 22-year-old female is admitted for an exacerbation of her ulcerative colitis. The nurse recognizes that the most likely reason for development of this flare is:
- ❏ **1.** severe psychologic distress.
- ❏ **2.** increased exercise frequency in the past 2 weeks.
- ❏ **3.** increased dietary fiber.
- ❏ **4.** increased protein intake.

158. A 56-year-old male has liver failure secondary to chronic hepatitis C infection. He's admitted for management of worsening encephalopathy as evidenced by increasing confusion and somnolence. Which substance should be restricted in the treatment of this client's encephalopathy?
- ❏ **1.** Sodium
- ❏ **2.** Fluid
- ❏ **3.** Protein
- ❏ **4.** Potassium

159. A 42-year-old male with a history of peptic ulcer disease is suspected of having peritonitis from a ruptured ulcer. What's the most common finding with peritonitis?
- ❏ **1.** Diarrhea
- ❏ **2.** Constipation
- ❏ **3.** Jaundice
- ❏ **4.** Abdominal muscular rigidity

160. Pernicious anemia would be expected after which type of surgery?
- ❏ **1.** Nissen fundoplication
- ❏ **2.** Colectomy
- ❏ **3.** Gastrectomy
- ❏ **4.** Cholecystectomy

161. A nurse is caring for a client with liver disease who has developed ascites. Which laboratory finding would best correlate with this client's condition?
- ❏ **1.** Serum sodium of 150 mEq/L
- ❏ **2.** Serum total bilirubin of 2.2 mg/dl
- ❏ **3.** Serum sodium of 118 mEq/L
- ❏ **4.** Serum albumin of 2.6 g/dl

162. A female client has intractable vomiting. The nurse's primary concern would be:
- ❏ **1.** metabolic alkalosis.
- ❏ **2.** metabolic acidosis.
- ❏ **3.** hyperglycemia.
- ❏ **4.** hyperkalemia.

163. A 43-year-old male with advanced liver disease undergoes esophagogastroduodenoscopy and is found to have esophageal varices. Which group of medications would you expect to use in the management of esophageal varices?
- ❏ **1.** Loop diuretics
- ❏ **2.** Beta-adrenergic blockers
- ❏ **3.** Angiotensin-converting enzyme (ACE) inhibitors
- ❏ **4.** Calcium channel blockers

164. A nurse is assigned to care for a 36-year-old male who's jaw has been immobilized to treat a mandibular fracture incurred in a motor vehicle accident. The nurse should be aware of what possible life-threatening complication?
- ❏ **1.** Malignant hyperthermia
- ❏ **2.** Hypertension
- ❏ **3.** Stomatitis
- ❏ **4.** Vomiting

165. A 65-year-old client has been diagnosed with chronic esophagitis. Which treatment instruction is appropriate for this client?
Select all that apply:
- ❏ **1.** Eat a bland diet to minimize mucosal irritation.
- ❏ **2.** Eat just before bedtime to ensure food on the stomach to buffer hydrochloric acid.
- ❏ **3.** Sleep with the head of the bed on blocks to prevent reflux of gastric contents.
- ❏ **4.** Avoid smoking and alcohol consumption to preserve the lower esophageal sphincter (LES) pressure.

166. Which symptom is an early sign of gastric cancer?
- ❏ **1.** Dysphagia
- ❏ **2.** Dysphonia

☐ **3.** Dyspepsia

☐ **4.** Dysuria

167. In addition to pernicious anemia, which outcome is expected after a gastrectomy?

☐ **1.** Hiatal hernia

☐ **2.** Pancreatitis

☐ **3.** Dumping syndrome

☐ **4.** Vasovagal syndrome

168. A patient with persistent dyspepsia and vague abdominal pain is diagnosed with peptic ulcer disease. Which medication should be avoided in this client?

☐ **1.** Ranitidine (Zantac)

☐ **2.** Metoclopramide (Reglan)

☐ **3.** Sucralfate (Carafate)

☐ **4.** Indomethacin (Indocin)

169. A 43-year-old female with cholelithiasis develops right upper quadrant pain that's aggravated by greasy foods, a temperature of 102.4° F (39.1° C), and clay-colored stools. The nurse is aware that the client most likely has developed:

☐ **1.** intestinal obstruction.

☐ **2.** cholecystitis.

☐ **3.** peritonitis.

☐ **4.** hepatitis.

170. A client has been diagnosed with cholelithiasis. Which dietary recommendation would *not* be appropriate for this client?

☐ **1.** Consume smaller portions at more frequent intervals.

☐ **2.** Consume low-fat meals.

☐ **3.** Avoid fried, greasy foods.

☐ **4.** Increase intake of dairy products.

171. What's the primary nutritional concern for a client with chronic pancreatitis?

☐ **1.** Malabsorption of water-soluble vitamins

☐ **2.** Malabsorption of fat-soluble vitamins

☐ **3.** Malabsorption of minerals

☐ **4.** Malabsorption of essential proteins

172. A 40-year-old woman is diagnosed with cholelithiasis. Which medication is typically used to treat gallstones?

☐ **1.** Probenecid (Benemid)

☐ **2.** Ursodiol (Actigall)

☐ **3.** Cholestyramine (Questran)

☐ **4.** Colchicine (Novocholcine)

173. A client with obstructive jaundice has just returned from an endoscopic retrograde cholangiopancreatography (ERCP). What's the most common complication of this procedure?

☐ **1.** Pancreatitis

☐ **2.** Cholelithiasis

☐ **3.** Pancreatic abscess

☐ **4.** Bowel perforation

174. An 28-year-old male with severe Crohn's disease has been receiving total parenteral nutrition (TPN). What's the primary concern with abrupt discontinuation of TPN?

☐ **1.** Hypoglycemia

☐ **2.** Hyperglycemia

☐ **3.** Hypernatremia

☐ **4.** Hypokalemia

175. A 58-year-old female comes to the hospital with upper GI bleeding. She's later found to have elevated liver function tests and a positive hepatitis C screening test. The nurse is aware that the client's exposure to hepatitis C most likely resulted from:

☐ **1.** sharing eating utensils with an infected person 2 weeks ago.

☐ **2.** having unprotected sex with a high-risk person 1 month ago.

☐ **3.** eating raw oysters 3 days ago.

☐ **4.** sharing needles while using I.V. drugs 20 years ago.

176. A 42-year-old male admitted with nausea, vomiting, and abdominal pain is diagnosed with an intestinal obstruction. Which nursing action is appropriate for this client?

☐ **1.** Administer morphine to reduce the client's discomfort.

☐ **2.** Administer metoclopramide to facilitate bowel movements.

☐ **3.** Encourage the client to increase his dietary fiber over the next several days until the obstruction has resolved.

☐ **4.** Auscultate for bowel sounds at least once per shift.

177. A client who just returned from an endoscopic procedure is complaining of a dry mouth; his family members offer him a glass of water. The nurse explains to the family that before fluids or food are permitted, she must assess for the presence of:

☐ **1.** bowel sounds.

☐ **2.** a gag reflex.

☐ **3.** a distended bladder.

☐ **4.** a distended abdomen.

178. A 38-year-old female has had a total colectomy for severe ulcerative colitis. Which instruction is an appropriate nutritional consideration for a client with an ostomy?

☐ **1.** Avoid spicy foods.

☐ **2.** Increase fluid intake.

☐ **3.** Increase dietary fiber.

☐ **4.** Avoid gas-producing foods.

179. Which order should the nurse question, when it comes to a client with active diverticulosis?

❑ 1. "Please provide a high-fiber diet."

❑ 2. "Acetaminophen 1,000 mg every 8 hours as necessary for pain."

❑ 3. "Chlordiazepoxide and clindinium (Librax) 1 tab orally every 12 hours."

❑ 4. "Morphine sulfate 2 mg I.V. every 8 hours prn pain."

180. A client is receiving intermittent tube feedings every 8 hours. When the nurse checks for residual stomach contents before the next tube feeding is administered, she obtains 210 ml of gastric fluid. Which action by the nurse would be the *most* appropriate in this setting?

❑ 1. Administer the tube feeding as scheduled because this volume is acceptable.

❑ 2. Continue the tube feeding, but at a slower rate.

❑ 3. Hold the tube feeding and recheck the residual stomach contents in 1 hour.

❑ 4. Hold the tube feeding and recheck the residual stomach contents in 4 hours.

181. Enteral tube feedings have been ordered for a client who recently had a stroke. Which option states the most appropriate manner to initiate this type of feeding?

❑ 1. Half-strength formula at 20 ml/hour, increasing by 20 ml/hour every 8 hours as tolerated, until target rate is achieved

❑ 2. Full-strength formula at 20 ml/hour, increasing by 20 ml/hour every 8 hours as tolerated, until target rate is achieved

❑ 3. Half-strength formula at 30 ml/hour, increasing by 10 ml/hour every 2 hours as tolerated, until target rate is achieved

❑ 4. Full-strength formula at 30 ml/hour, increasing by 10 ml/hour every 2 hours as tolerated, until target rate is achieved

182. A client with a colitis exacerbation is admitted to the hospital and placed on a low-residue diet to minimize colonic irritation. Which food selection would be permitted on this diet?

❑ 1. Whole wheat toast

❑ 2. White rice

❑ 3. Apple

❑ 4. Cooked carrots

183. A client is diagnosed with a hiatal hernia. Which instruction is an appropriate teaching point?

Select all that apply:

❑ 1. Avoid caffeine-containing products to preserve sphincter pressure.

❑ 2. Elevate the head of the bed to prevent reflux of gastric contents.

❑ 3. Increase dairy products to neutralize hydrochloric acid.

❑ 4. Eat smaller portions more frequently to prevent overdistention of the stomach.

184. A client underwent a large volume paracentesis for severe ascites that caused moderate respiratory distress. Which physiologic response should the nurse anticipate in this client immediately after the procedure?

❑ 1. Tachycardia

❑ 2. Bradycardia

❑ 3. Orthopnea

❑ 4. Platypnea

185. Which type of surgery would be indicated in the management of intractable pain from severe peptic ulcer disease?

❑ 1. Nissen fundoplication

❑ 2. Billroth I

❑ 3. Vagotomy

❑ 4. Whipple procedure

186. A client with pulmonary edema has been ordered to receive 40 mg furosemide via I.V. push. What nursing action is a priority before this drug is administered?

❑ 1. Insert an indwelling urinary catheter.

❑ 2. Obtain the client's weight.

❑ 3. Check the results of that morning's electrolytes.

❑ 4. Obtain an order to decrease the client's I.V. fluids.

187. A client with renal calculi would be experiencing which symptoms if he were developing renal colic?

❑ 1. Urinary urgency and frequency

❑ 2. Tea-colored urine and dull pain

❑ 3. Hematuria and sharp pain

❑ 4. Malodorous urine with gross hematuria

188. A client is admitted for treatment of acute renal failure. The physician writes an order for the client to receive 6 units of regular insulin followed by 50% dextrose. When the client inquires about the need for these medications, the nurse's best response would be:

❑ 1. "You have developed diabetes related to your kidney failure."

❑ 2. "The dextrose and insulin will prevent you from developing diabetes related to your kidney failure."

❑ 3. "The dextrose and insulin is needed to correct your low blood sugar."

❑ 4. "The insulin will help lower excessive levels of potassium in your blood."

189. A client is diagnosed with advanced bladder cancer and undergoes an ileal conduit after a total cystectomy. Which statement is true regarding this client's postoperative care?

❑ 1. "The urinary diversion is only temporary."

❑ 2. "Urine should flow constantly from the stoma."

❑ 3. "The stoma will require daily irrigation."

❏ **4.** "Bladder retraining should be initiated as soon as the client is psychologically ready."

190. A client with end stage renal disease has an arteriovenous fistula (AVF) placed in the left forearm in preparation for hemodialysis. Which instruction would be an appropriate teaching point for this client?
❏ **1.** Advise health care personnel to use the right arm for blood pressure measurements.
❏ **2.** Advise health care personnel to use the left arm for drawing blood.
❏ **3.** Clean the Tenckhoff catheter insertion site daily.
❏ **4.** Assess for the presence of a thrill and bruit once a week.

191. A 28-year-old female is concerned about vague abdominal pain and a persistent vaginal discharge that have been present for the past week. On physical examination, it's noted that she has a purulent yellowish green discharge from her vagina, and samples are obtained for cultures. Based on these preliminary physical findings, the nurse is aware that this client most likely has:
❏ **1.** candidiasis.
❏ **2.** chlamydia.
❏ **3.** gonorrhea.
❏ **4.** trichomoniasis.

192. Which phase of the menstrual cycle is characterized by endometrial thickening secondary to progesterone secretion from the corpus luteum, in preparation for a fertilized ovum?
❏ **1.** Menstrual (preovulatory) phase
❏ **2.** Ovulatory phase
❏ **3.** Luteal (secretory) phase
❏ **4.** Degenerative phase

193. A male neonate is noted to have a urethral opening on the underside of the penis. Which condition best describes this situation?
❏ **1.** Cystocele
❏ **2.** Hydrocele
❏ **3.** Hypospadias
❏ **4.** Epispadias

194. A client with a recent history of a bladder infection has developed a temperature of 102.6° F (39.2° C), chills, severe flank pain, vomiting, and costovertebral angle tenderness. White blood cells and protein are present on urinalysis. The nurse is aware that the most likely cause of this client's symptoms is:
❏ **1.** nephrolithiasis.
❏ **2.** pyelonephritis.
❏ **3.** glomerulonephritis.
❏ **4.** urethritis.

195. A client is diagnosed with benign prostatic hyperplasia (BPH). The client requires additional teaching if he makes which statement?
❏ **1.** "I should avoid over-the-counter cough and cold medications with decongestants."
❏ **2.** "I'll likely need to undergo radiation treatments."
❏ **3.** "I may experience some dribbling of urine periodically."
❏ **4.** "I may have difficulty starting a urine stream or notice that the stream is weaker than usual."

196. A client with glomerulonephritis is found to have a serum albumin of 2.8 g/dl, a total cholesterol of 260 mg/dl, and 4 g of protein in a 24-hour urine collection. Which syndrome associated with glomerulonephritis is this client most likely to have developed?
❏ **1.** Nephrotic syndrome
❏ **2.** Nephritic syndrome
❏ **3.** Rapidly progressive glomerulonephritis
❏ **4.** Diabetic nephropathy

197. A client with prostate cancer undergoes a prostatectomy. Which topic would be appropriate for the nurse to teach the client?
❏ **1.** Fluids should be restricted to 1.5 L/day after surgery.
❏ **2.** Heavy lifting should be avoided for 1 week after surgery.
❏ **3.** Pink-red discoloration of the urine will be normal for the first several days after surgery .
❏ **4.** Stool softeners should be avoided for the first 2 weeks after surgery.

198. A client presents with severe abdominal pain that radiates to the lower back and genital area and is unrelieved by changing positions. A kidney-ureter-bladder X-ray is performed and he's diagnosed with nephrolithiasis. Further testing reveals that the calculi are composed of oxalate crystals. What intervention would be appropriate to prevent the formation of additional oxalate calculi in this client?
❏ **1.** Administer thiazide diuretics
❏ **2.** Follow a low purine diet
❏ **3.** Encourage green, leafy vegetables
❏ **4.** Avoid teas and colas

199. A client with prostate cancer undergoes a transurethral resection of the prostate. Continuous bladder irrigation (CBI) is instituted after the procedure to flush the bladder. What appearance of the urine would indicate that the CBI flow rate is appropriate?
❏ **1.** Clear, but contains some small clots
❏ **2.** Colorless to light pink with no clots
❏ **3.** Amber-colored urine with small clots
❏ **4.** Amber colored urine with no clots

200. A client is diagnosed with urinary incontinence and is being educated about therapeutic interventions for the condition. Which statement made by the client would alert the nurse that he needs additional teaching?

☐ **1.** "I'll need a Foley catheter placed to prevent leaking urine."

☐ **2.** "I should limit my caffeine intake."

☐ **3.** "I should use stool softeners to prevent constipation."

☐ **4.** "I should try to urinate according to a schedule."

Answers and rationales

1. Correct answer: 1
The assessment phase of the nursing process consists of collecting objective and subjective data about a client through a history and physical, interview, or chart review. The diagnosis phase consists of analyzing the data collected and identifying actual or potential health problems. Planning involves setting goals and priorities as well as determining what interventions should be used to accomplish the goals. Evaluation consists of analyzing the effectiveness of the previous steps by determining the extent to which the goals were met.

2. Correct answer: 3
The physician should be notified so that the client can be examined after any fall. An incident report should be completed after any accident or unusual occurrence that either results in or has the potential to cause injury to a client, employee, or visitor. While the fall should be documented in the chart and the charge nurse should be notified, additional action is required on the part of the nurse.

3. Correct answer: 2
This client has developed metabolic acidosis secondary to DKA; sodium bicarbonate would help to neutralize the acid concentration of the blood and help to restore the normal pH. Potassium, magnesium, and calcium would help to correct deficiencies of these electrolytes but wouldn't correct the acidosis.

4. Correct answer: 2
Tachycardia would be indicative of hypovolemia because the heart must work harder and pump faster to provide adequate oxygen and to maintain adequate perfusion throughout the body. Hypertension, an increase in urine output, and tachypnea would be suggestive of hypervolemia, not a fluid volume deficit.

5. Correct answer: 1
Hyperventilation helps to eliminate CO_2 and corrects acidosis; consequently, the PCO_2 is reduced to normal or slightly low levels (normal range is 35 to 40 mm Hg). Option 2 is incorrect because the compensatory mechanism of hyperventilation would correct these values to normal (normal pH greater than or equal to 7.35 to 7.45; normal HCO_3^- 22 to 26 mEq/L; and normal PO_2 80 to 95 mm Hg.

6. Correct answer: 3
Oranges contains large amounts of vitamin C, which enhances the absorption of iron. Legumes and raisins contain large quantities of iron, but aren't rich in vitamin C. Apples contain only minimal amounts of both iron and vitamin C.

7. Correct answer: 2
Canned, cured, and processed foods contain large quantities of salt, which is used as a preservative. Bananas are high in potassium content, but not sodium. Whole wheat bread and baked chicken aren't considered high sodium foods, and would therefore be permitted on a 2-gram sodium diet.

8. Correct answer: 2
Sodium, potassium, and phosphorus are restricted on a renal diet, and lean chicken contains low quantities of each of these. Orange juice and potatoes should be restricted because they're high in potassium, and milk products are high in phosphorus content.

9. Correct answer: 1
TPN solutions typically have high glucose concentrations, and temporary insulin injections may be necessary during TPN therapy. Because of their high glucose content, hypoglycemia (not hyperglycemia) can develop if TPN solutions are stopped abruptly; rather, gradual tapering over 4 to 6 hours should be performed. TPN catheters should only be used for administration of TPN solutions; no medications should be given and no blood should be drawn through this line. Nothing should be added to the TPN solution; it must be prepared by a pharmacist or trained technician using aseptic technique under hooded laminar airflow.

10. Correct answer: 2
Meats and milk products, including cheese, are high in cholesterol and should be avoided on a low-cholesterol diet. Although egg yolks contain large quantities of cholesterol, egg whites don't contain cholesterol and would be permitted on a low-cholesterol diet. Canned vegetables have a high-sodium content, which should be restricted for persons on a low-sodium diet and those with hypertension. Foods high in fiber should be encouraged.

11. Correct answer: 2

Allergies to iodine-containing foods, such as shellfish, iodized salt, and kale, and previous reactions to iodine-containing contrast agents are contraindications to CT scans. Barium isn't used in CT scans. Clients with renal impairment (creatinine more than 1.4 mg/dl) are at increased risk for renal failure associated with contrast agents but a creatinine level of 1.0 mg/dl is with a normal range. In clients diagnosed with claustrophobia, magnetic resonance imaging would be contraindicated but typically not a CT scan, because it's performed in a more open donut-shaped machine.

12. Correct answer: 4

Clients who have undergone a cardiac catheterization must lie flat in bed for 4 to 6 hours without flexion of the affected extremity after the procedure in order to prevent bleeding at the puncture site. Blood thinners, such as aspirin, platelet inhibitors, and warfarin should be discontinued several days before an angiographic procedure due to the increased risk of hemorrhage. A client should be on nothing-by-mouth status at least 2 hours before an angiographic procedure, and the femoral artery in the groin is the most commonly used access site for cardiac catheterization.

13. Correct answer: 3

A side-lying position with the knees and head tucked toward the chest increases the space between the vertebrae and allows easier access to the spinal canal. Non-side-lying positions don't increase the intervertebral space and shouldn't be used because they would increase the risk of complications.

14. Correct answer: 2

Laryngeal edema is a complication of bronchoscopy, and is marked by moderate to severe dyspnea, inspiratory stridor, and decreased oxygenation. Inspiratory stridor is more accurately described as a symptom of laryngeal edema, rather than a complication of bronchoscopy. Pharyngitis is a sore throat that may occur after a bronchoscopy, but it isn't life-threatening. The presence of the gag reflex should be assessed after any endoscopic procedure before food or beverages are offered, but its absence alone doesn't cause severe respiratory distress.

15. Correct answer: 1

The client should be placed on the unaffected side with the affected side up for at least 1 hour after a thoracentesis in the event that air was introduced during the procedure. This position will enable the air to escape. The other positions won't facilitate the escape of air.

16. Correct answer: 2

Liver biopsies are commonly performed at the bedside, with the client in a supine or left lateral position with his right arm raised over his head so that it doesn't obstruct the physician's access to the biopsy site. He should assume a right side-lying position after the biopsy is performed in order to splint the puncture site; this position should be maintained for at least 2 hours after the procedure. Heavy lifting and strenuous activities should be avoided for 1 week after a liver biopsy.

17. Correct answer: 3

Fluid intake should be encouraged to prevent or minimize a spinal headache that can occur after a lumbar puncture. The client should remain flat in bed for at least 4 hours after this procedure to prevent or minimize a spinal headache.

18. Correct answer: 3

A fever or sudden temperature spike after an endoscopic procedure are suggestive of a perforation and the physician should be notified immediately. Hypotension and bradycardia can occur secondary to sedatives administered for the procedure, but a blood pressure of 96 mm Hg/ 65 mm Hg and a pulse of 58 beats/minute don't warrant immediate notification of a physician. The respiratory rate is normal in this client.

19. Correct answer: 1

Diabetes mellitus is a syndrome of disordered metabolism characterized by inappropriate hyperglycemia due to the development of insulin resistance, which can be induced by long-term steroid use. Diabetes insipidus is a disorder of water metabolism caused by decreased or ineffective secretion of antidiuretic hormone and is characterized by marked polyuria. Hirsutism (excessive hair growth)—not alopecia—is associated with steroid use. A goiter is an enlargement of the thyroid gland that results from its constant stimulation to release more hormones, such as occurs in Hashimoto's thyroiditis, Graves' disease, or thyroid cancer.

20. Correct answer: 4

Giantism is a disorder associated with hyperpituitarism that results from the overproduction of growth hormone (GH) resulting in the overgrowth of the long bones and a very tall stature. Dwarfism is incorrect because it's found in hypopituitary disorders and involves a short stature related to a deficiency in GH in children. Acromegaly is a disorder of hyperpituitarism involving an excessive production of GH in adults. Exophthalmos (protruding eyeballs) is a common manifestation of hyperthyroid conditions, such as Grave's disease, whereas prognathism (protrusion of the jaw) is more commonly associated with acromegaly. Cretinism is a disorder associated with insufficient thyroid hormone secretion in infants, which results in impaired physical and mental development.

21. Correct answer: 3

Glucocorticoids (cortisol), mineralocorticoids (aldosterone), and sex hormones (androgens, such as testosterone) are produced by the adrenal cortex. Epinephrine, norepinephrine, and dopamine are produced by the adrenal medulla.

22. Correct answer: 1

SIADH is an endocrine disorder characterized by water retention, volume expansion, and hyponatremia that result from the body's inability to suppress the secretion of vasopressin (ADH). Volume overload, including hypertension, heart failure, pulmonary edema, and anasarca, can occur. Fluid restriction is therefore the foundation of treatment for SIADH. Demeclocycline (Declomycin) is an ADH antagonist that may be used to help treat people with chronic SIADH. Persons with central nervous system manifestations of hyponatremia associated with SIADH may be treated with loop diuretics, such as furosemide, to promote diuresis or with hypertonic sodium chloride solutions.

23. Correct answer: 4

An Hb A_{1c} level reflects blood glucose control over a 3-month period, and an Hb A_{1c} greater than 8% indicates that better glucose control is warranted, despite the current fasting level. While weight loss would be somewhat effective, it isn't the only blood glucose-controlling measure indicated for this client. This client is already taking insulin, so the addition of an oral hypoglycemic agent to help control blood sugar isn't indicated; rather, an adjustment of insulin dose and type may be necessary. Persons with type 2 diabetes typically don't develop diabetic ketoacidosis because they generally produce some amount of exogenous insulin; rather, people with type 2 diabetes are at risk for developing hyperosmolar hyperglycemic nonketotic syndrome either from the inhibition of insulin's action or as a result of noncompliance with hypoglycemic agents.

24. Correct answer: 3

Myxedema coma is an advanced and life-threatening form of hypothyroidism that results from the undertreatment of hypothyroidism or its non-diagnosed state, and it's often preceded by stress, infections, exposure to cold, and sedative use. Thyroid storm is a life-threatening endocrine disorder that's characterized by a marked increase in the symptoms associated with hyperthyroidism (high fever, altered mental status) that's commonly precipitated by infections, trauma, diabetic ketoacidosis, or thyroiditis. Thyrotoxicosis is an endocrine disorder of slow onset

hyperthyroidism that results from exposure of tissues to excessive amounts of unbound thyroid hormone. An adrenal crisis, or addisonian crisis, is an acute and potentially fatal condition involving extreme manifestations of adrenal insufficiency, including vomiting, high fever, confusion, and shock from cardiovascular collapse.

25. Correct answer: 2

Loss of active parathyroid tissue can result after surgery that involves either the thyroid or parathyroid glands. This loss of active parathyroid tissue can result in hypoparathyroidism. The inadequate amounts of PTH produced ultimately result in hypercalcemia. Other diagnostic features of hypoparathyroidism include a decreased serum PTH level and hyperphosphatemia.

26. Correct answer: 4

Adverse effects of steroid therapy include alterations in glucose metabolism, fluids, and electrolytes. A client with Cushing's syndrome would benefit from a sodium-restricted diet in order to prevent fluid retention and hypertension. Steroid therapy should be slowly discontinued because it can induce the disorder. Volume resuscitation would be inappropriate due to the propensity for fluid retention.

27. Correct answer: 2

Standard treatment for an alert client with hypoglycemia is to replace glucose by administering 15 g of carbohydrates, such as a $1/2$ cup of fruit juice or regular soda (not diet), 1 cup of milk, or several pieces of hard candy. If the blood glucose level remains below 70 mg/dl 15 minutes later, another 15 g of carbohydrates should be provided. Administration of D_{50} is typically reserved for unconscious clients or those who don't respond to more conservative therapy. Insulin and oral hypoglycemic agents, such as metformin or rosiglitazone, would be contraindicated in this situation because they lower blood glucose.

28. Correct answer: 1

Levothyroxine is used in thyroid hormone replacement therapy and would be contraindicated in a client with hyperthyroidism. Propylthiouracil and Lugol's solution are thyroid hormone antagonists and would be appropriate for this client. Beta-adrenergic blockers, such as propranolol, may be used to alleviate the symptoms of hyperthyroidism, particularly palpitations, tremor, and heat intolerance.

29. Correct answer: 4

A common adverse reaction to the use of glucocorticosteroid is temporary diabetes mellitus, and insulin injections may be necessary for its treatment. While the physical stress of surgery may be contributing somewhat to the rise in glucose, the steroid administration is the most prominent cause. Although obesity and borderline diabetes increase the risk of developing diabetes mellitus, there's no indication that this patient is overweight or had borderline diabetes before surgery.

30. Correct answer: 2
People with Cushing's syndrome are at risk for fractures due to their predisposition for osteoporosis. Addisonian crises (or adrenal crises) occur in those with adrenal insufficiency; Cushing's syndrome is a disorder of hyperadrenal function. While hypertension may be a complication of Cushing's syndrome, a hypertensive crisis isn't common to this disorder, but is more commonly associated with pheochromocytoma. The treatment of rheumatoid arthritis with long-term steroid use may actually cause Cushing's syndrome, but it isn't a complication of it.

31. Correct answer: 1
Pheochromocytomas are catecholamine-secreting tumors, and metanephrine and VMA are the metabolites of catecholamines. Thus, elevated levels of these substances in 24-hour urine collections are indicative of pheochromocytoma. 24-hour urinary cortisol levels and dexamethasone suppression tests can be useful in the diagnosis of Cushing's syndrome, but not pheochromocytoma. A water deprivation test is used in the differentiation of central versus nephrogenic causes of diabetes insipidus. It involves the collection of hourly samples for measurement of plasma and urine osmolality after the administration of antidiuretic hormone.

32. Correct answer: 4
Lifelong thyroid replacement therapy will be necessary for a client who has undergone a subtotal thyroidectomy. A tracheal stoma and an alternative means of communicating would be associated with a total laryngectomy rather than a subtotal thyroidectomy. Permanent steroid therapy isn't indicated in this client.

33. Correct answer: 1
Regular (short-acting) insulin, such as Humulin-R or Novolin-R, should be taken 30 minutes before meals because the onset of action in these medications is 30 to 60 minutes. Immediate acting insulin, such as lispro (Humalog) or aspart (Novolog), should be taken immediately before meals because the onset of action in these medications is approximately 15 minutes. Complex carbohydrates, rather than simple carbohydrates, should be consumed, and exercise should ideally be timed to correspond to avoid peak insulin times so that hypoglycemic episodes are prevented or minimized. Insulin injections should be administered using a rotation of injection sites to avoid lipodystrophy.

34. Correct answer: 3
A client with pheochromocytoma is at increased risk for stroke related to hypertension or a hypertensive crisis, and cold medications containing pseudoephedrine may precipitate a hypertensive crisis. Decongestants containing pseudoephedrine aren't associated with the development of infections, bronchospasm, or hypoglycemia.

35. Correct answer: 1, 2, 3, 5
Nonsteroidal anti-inflammatory drugs (NSAIDs) can cause nephrotoxicity and GI bleeding from peptic ulcerations, particularly in the presence of alcohol and steroid therapy. Food and milk will help to minimize the gastric irritation that may occur with NSAID ingestion. The use of phenytoin isn't a contraindication to NSAID use.

36. Correct answer: 3
Opioid analgesics cause respiratory depression, and should be withheld if the respiratory rate is less than 10 breaths per minute. Vancomycin should be withheld if a client develops "red man" syndrome (pruritic rash and hypotension), tinnitus, or renal dysfunction during therapy. Beta-adrenergic blockers such as atenolol should be withheld if the pulse is less than 60 beats per minute or if the systolic blood pressure is less than 100 mm Hg.

37. Correct answer: 2
Naloxone is an opioid antagonist and is used in the treatment of opioid overdose. Naltrexone is used in the treatment of opioid addiction and clonidine may be used in the management of withdrawal symptoms. N-acetylcysteine is used in the treatment of acetaminophen overdose and pulmonary conditions that produce thick and viscous mucous secretions, such as septic fibrosis and tuberculosis.

38. Correct answer: 4
A side-lying position in which the face is slightly downward is preferred for unconscious clients because it allows drainage of mucus or vomitus out of the mouth, thereby preventing aspiration. A supine position could be assumed once the client is responsive enough to protect his own airway. The other options are incorrect because these positions would increase the risk of aspiration.

39. Correct answer: 2
Early ambulation after surgery is necessary in the prevention of respiratory, circulatory, GI, and urinary complications. The administration of analgesics before ambulation will minimize the discomfort. Ambulation would be contraindicated in a client with known or suspected blood clots because dislodgment may result in a pulmonary embolus and death. Although walking can stimulate the appetite and may help minimize the pa-

tient's perception of pain, option 2 is the most appropriate response.

40. Correct answer: 2, 3, 4, 5
Opioids, anesthetic agents, immobility, and alterations in fluid and food ingestion may all cause decreased peristalsis and constipation. I.V. famotidine doesn't contribute to constipation.

41. Correct answer: 4
Urine output less than 30 ml/hour requires immediate notification of the surgeon. A low-grade temperature can be a normal occurrence as a result of the inflammatory process after surgery, and mild hypotension may occur secondary to sedatives and analgesics administered in the perioperative period. Although these findings should continue to be monitored, this client's temperature, pulse, or blood pressure wouldn't require immediate notification of the physician.

42. Correct answer: 4
A sudden cessation of drainage from a surgical drain is most likely due to obstruction from clot formation or tissue debris. If the area has been effectively drained to the point that the drain was ready to be pulled, drainage would be expected to have slowly decreased over time, rather than to have slowed abruptly. Option 3 is incorrect because larger fluid collections don't necessarily drain at a faster rate than smaller collections. An infection would most likely be associated with cloudy, discolored, and foul-smelling drainage.

43. Correct answer: 1
Tub bathing isn't permitted for approximately 2 weeks after an open surgical procedure, although sponge bathing is permitted right away and showering may be performed if the water is allowed to gently run over the incision. The other options are appropriate discharge instructions for a surgical client.

44. Correct answer: 2
Any exposed organ or body structure should be covered with warm gauze or towels soaked in normal saline in order to keep them moist. Another nurse should be instructed to notify the physician that an evisceration has occurred so that the client's primary nurse can remain with him and obtain vital signs at frequent intervals until the surgeon arrives. The client should also be covered with blankets to prevent hypothermia; taking the client's temperature isn't a priority nursing action. No attempt should be made to reinsert exposed organs because this action may actually cause ischemic damage.

45. Correct answer: 3
Severe pain, pallor, pulselessness, paresthesia, and paresis of an extremity after an orthopedic procedure or crushing injuries is indicative of compartment syndrome. The affected extremities should be positioned at the level of the heart, not above it, because this may worsen the ischemia. Application of heat to the affected area may worsen the underlying edema, and application of cold packs may worsen the ischemia. Although analgesics are indicated for the severe pain, the finding of pallor is suggestive of ischemic damage, which requires immediate intervention and notification of the surgeon.

46. Correct answer: 1
The Trendelenburg position is the most appropriate position for a client in shock because it improves blood flow to the brain. The reverse Trendelenburg and semi-Fowler's positions would further impair cerebral blood flow, and are therefore contraindicated in this situation. A side-lying position wouldn't facilitate blood flow as effectively as would the Trendelenburg position.

47. Correct answer: 4
Oxygen should be administered immediately for a client suspected of having an acute MI. While a stat ECG and morphine and aspirin administration are important interventions, the primary treatment goal for this client is to minimize the oxygen demands.

48. Correct answer: 2
The normal range for potassium is 3.5 to 5.0 mEq/L (although this varies according to laboratory technique) and hyperkalemia predisposes a client to cardiac arrhythmias or cardiac arrest. A sodium level of 137 mEq/L, calcium level of 8.5 mg/dl, and a hematocrit of 44% are all within normal ranges and wouldn't require intervention.

49. Correct answer: 1
Hypocalcemia may be manifested as muscle cramps, twitching, hyperactive reflexes, tetany, and paresthesia. Hypotension rather than hypertension would be expected with hypocalcemia. Lethargy and dry, sticky mucous membranes would be more commonly associated with hyponatremia, and analgesia and seizures is more characteristic of hyperphosphatemia.

50. Correct answer: 3
Treatment for hyperkalemia would likely include Kayexalate and possibly insulin because these agents lower the serum potassium level. Sevelamer (Renagel), a phosphate-binding agent, would be indicated for the treatment of hyperphosphatemia. Sodium bicarbonate is an alkalinizing agent and would be used in the management of metabolic acidosis. Magnesium sulfate is indicated for hypomagnesemia but this client's serum magnesium level was within normal limits.

51. Correct answer: 1
Altered mental status, including a decreased level of consciousness, may signify increasing intracra-

nial pressure (ICP), a complication of meningitis. Babinski reflex is a test of the corticospinal tract that involves dorsiflexion of the great toe and fanning of the other toes when a stimulus is applied from the heel and runs to the great toe; it's normal in children up to age 2 and abnormal in adults but isn't associated with meningitis. A tonic neck reflex is a normal finding in neonates, but typically disappears by age 3 to 4 months. Paresthesia is a tingling, numbness, or prickly sensation that can occur in association with nerve disorders but isn't associated with meningitis.

52. Correct answer: 2

Decerebrate posturing results from the disruption of motor nerve fibers in the midbrain and brain stem, and is manifested as downward pointing toes, backward arching of the head, and extension of the arms and legs with internal rotation. Decorticate posturing is manifested as flexion of the arms, hyperextension of the legs, and clenching of the fists. Nuchal rigidity, or "stiff neck" is a symptom of meningitis and isn't related to head trauma. Dysesthesia is an abnormal painful sensation that results from a stimulus that isn't typically painful.

53. Correct answer: 3

Unnecessary movement, straining, and suctioning of the client should be avoided because these activities can cause temporary, but sharp increases in ICP and should be performed only when necessary. Vital signs and neurological status of clients with increased ICP should be assessed at least once per hour. A client with increased ICP should be positioned with the head of the bed elevated 15 to 30 degrees with his head in a neutral position.

54. Correct answer: 4

Respiratory status is always the priority assessment. LOC, pupillary responses, and vital signs are also important assessment factors, but aren't the primary assessments the nurse should make.

55. Correct answer: 3

Overhydration would raise the blood pressure, which may cause further neurologic damage. Avoid giving thrombolytic agents to clients who suffer a hemorrhagic stroke, such as those involving a ruptured aneurysm or that result from uncontrolled chronic hypertension or anticoagulant use. Stroke victims should be positioned with the head slightly elevated to prevent increased intracranial pressure. Bleeding precautions aren't specifically indicated for this client.

56. Correct answer: 4

Asking the client to wiggle his toes, move his hands, and bend his elbows helps determine the level of cord injury without causing further injury. Palpating the spine wouldn't necessarily detect a spinal cord injury. Asking the client to turn his head from side to side may cause additional cord injury and possibly cord severance; similarly, instructing the patient to roll on his left side is incorrect because the spinal cord shouldn't be moved if a cord injury is known or suspected.

57. Correct answer: 2

A client should be placed on the inoperative side or in a semi-Fowler's position after cataract surgery to avoid increasing pressure on the suture line. The other choices are incorrect because they would cause unnecessary pressure on the operative site.

58. Correct answer: 1, 3, 4

The sympathetic nervous system's release of epinephrine and norepinephrine produces the characteristic "flight or fight" responses of pupillary dilation, increased diaphoresis, increased heart rate, stimulation of glucose release from the liver, relaxation of the bladder smooth muscle, and decreased blood flow to the abdominal organs, which delays digestion and gastric emptying. The other choices are incorrect because epinephrine would produce relaxation of the smooth muscles of the bladder and an increased heart rate.

59. Correct answer: 3

Slurring of speech, delayed responses, lethargy, and a decreased level of consciousness are all early manifestations of rising ICP. In contrast, a headache with projectile vomiting, pupillary changes, and fluctuations in vital signs are late manifestations of increasing ICP.

60. Correct answer: 2

Myasthenia gravis is a progressive neurologic disorder characterized by generalized muscle weakness that improves with rest, and a myasthenic crisis involves the rapid development of respiratory muscle weakness. A decreased gag and cough reflex is a manifestation rather than a complication of myasthenia gravis. SIADH can occur after a head injury but isn't related to myasthenic crisis.

61. Correct answer: 1

The detachment area should be positioned lowermost both preoperatively and postoperatively in order to prevent further detachment and to facilitate approximation of the two retinal layers, respectively. The other choices are incorrect because they wouldn't prevent further detachment or facilitate approximation of the retinal layers.

62. Correct answer: 3

A Glasgow Coma Score of 8 or less indicates a severe head injury in which the client's motor, verbal, and eye responses are severely impaired.

63. Correct answer: 4
The three cardinal symptoms of Parkinson's disease include slow movements (bradykinesia), cogwheel rigidity (stiff, jerking movements), and a resting tremor (pill-rolling), although a stooped posture, a shuffling gait, masked facies, and dementia may also be present. Muscular dystrophy is a genetic neurologic disorder involving symmetrical muscle weakness and atrophy. Alzheimer's disease is characterized by cognitive dysfunction, including forgetfulness, disorientation, repetition of ideas, and behavioral changes, including irritability and combativeness. Huntington's disease is manifested as choreiform movements (abnormal and excessive involuntary movements), a shuffling gait, and a deterioration of mental function.

64. Correct answer: 2
Autonomic dysreflexia is an exaggerated autonomic nervous system response to a noxious stimulus, such as a distended bladder or a full bowel, which involves vasoconstriction secondary to catecholamine release. Vasodilation occurs above the level of the injury, goose bumps occur below, and hypertension and bradycardia may result. Spinal shock occurs shortly after the initial spinal cord injury, and often produces vasodilation, hypotension, and bradycardia. Dystonia is a hyperkinetic disorder characterized by sustained or repetitive involuntary movements. Tardive dyskinesia is a drug-induced dystonia.

65. Correct answer:
The mitral valve is located between the left atrium and the left ventricle.

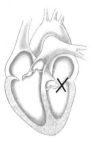

66. Correct answer: 3
A decreased blood pressure reflects a decreased cardiac output and should be the most concerning finding in this client. A heart rate of 96 beats/minute is at the high end of the acceptable range. A heart rate of 60 beats/minute in this patient would be in the desirable range, because a slower heart rate decreases the afterload and the myocardial workload, which can prevent further tissue damage. A pulse oximetry of 93% on room air isn't necessarily diagnostic of hypox-

ia (levels <90% on room air are diagnostic of hypoxia). In addition, oxygen should be administered to a patient experiencing an MI despite pulse oximetry readings in order to meet myocardial oxygen demands.

67. Correct answer: 4
Thrombophlebitis occurs when a blood clot forms in one or more veins and causes irritation or injury to the vein. Immobilization of the affected extremity would prevent the clot from becoming dislodged, whereas ambulation or flexion of the leg or use of sequential compression devices would promote its dislodgment and could result in a pulmonary embolism.

68. Correct answer: 1
A Swan-Ganz catheter is commonly used in the intensive care setting. It's inserted into the subclavian vein and is advanced into the pulmonary artery so that pressures within the heart may be monitored. Swan-Ganz catheters aren't used for I.V. fluid administration or medication or to administer nutritional support. Nutritional support is usually administered through a catheter for total parenteral nutrition.

69. Correct answer: 1
The aortic area is located in the second intercostal space along the right sternal border. The pulmonic area is located at the second intercostal space at the left sternal border. The tricuspid area is located at the fourth intercostal space along the left sternal border, and the mitral area is located at the fifth intercostal space near the midclavicular line.

70. Correct answer: 2
Bilateral neck vein distention when the client is in a semi-Fowler's position is called *jugular vein distention,* which is associated with advanced cardiopulmonary disease related to right-sided heart failure. Crackles may be associated with pulmonary edema (which can result from left-sided heart failure), pneumonia, and pulmonary fibrosis. PND is a condition in which a person is awakened with shortness of breath from being in a supine position, which is associated with left-sided heart failure. Unilateral neck distension would more likely be related to trauma involving the neck or chest.

71. Correct answer: 2
Intermittent claudication is pain or cramping in the legs that occurs with activity and is relieved by rest. The condition is caused by poor circulation and may be indicative of atherosclerosis. While the other questions can be helpful in the assessment of various vascular diseases, inquiring about how activity affects the pain in the ex-

tremity is the most accurate manner in which to assess for intermittent claudication.

72. Correct answer: 1
Oxygen administration decreases the workload of the heart, even when the blood oxygen levels are normal. While the administration of nitroglycerin, propranolol, and morphine would be appropriate for this client, they aren't the primary intervention.

73. Correct answer: 4
A positive Homans' sign is suggestive of a deep vein thrombosis. Immobilization and elevation of the extremity should be performed to prevent dislodging the clot and to minimize pain and edema, respectively. Ambulation and the use of sequential compression devices would risk dislodging the clot, resulting in a possible pulmonary embolism. Application of warm compresses may minimize some of the discomfort, but it isn't the first intervention that should be taken; it's also an action that usually requires a physician's order.

74. Correct answer: 3
Lidocaine decreases ventricular irritability. Cardioversion is typically used in the treatment of atrial fibrillation or flutter by suppressing ventricular depolarization and would be an appropriate intervention for this client's PVCs. I.V dopamine is primarily used to treat hypotension unrelated to hypovolemia and wouldn't be used to treat this client. While placing the client in a semi-Fowler's position may facilitate his respiratory efforts, it wouldn't affect the underlying ventricular irritability that caused the PVCs.

75. Correct answer: 2
If administered within 6 hours of an acute MI, tPA may dissolve existing blood clots, thereby preventing irreversible tissue damage caused by ischemia. Heparin would prevent the formation of blood clots, but this isn't the action of tPA. Coronary vasodilation can be caused by nitrates, calcium channel blockers, adenosine, and dipyridamole.

76. Correct answer: 4
Beta-adrenergic blockers can cause bronchospasm and should therefore be avoided in persons with asthma or emphysema. ACE inhibitors may cause hyperkalemia in persons with renal insufficiency, but aren't contraindicated in clients with emphysema. Calcium channel blockers can induce arrhythmias and heart failure, and should be avoided in persons with histories of these disorders but aren't contraindicated in clients with emphysema. Vasodilators, such as clonidine, may cause rebound hypertension if they're stopped abruptly, but they aren't contraindicated in emphysema.

77. Correct answer: 3
Valsalva's maneuver prevents air emboli during insertion of central venous catheters or during tube changes. Valsalva's maneuver actually causes bradycardia and should be avoided in a person with a recent MI, a significant reduction in blood volume, and a history of severe coronary artery disease. It may be used to help persons with multiple sclerosis to fully empty their bladders. Cardiogenic shock is a complication of an MI that's characterized by a reduced pumping action of the heart, which results in inadequate tissue perfusion.

78. Correct answer: 3
By assessing pulses below the dressing, the nurse can determine if the circulatory status of the affected extremity has been compromised. Notification of the physician is warranted if circulatory compromise occurs. Pressure dressings should be loosened after an arterial puncture unless circulatory compromise has been demonstrated. The client shouldn't flex his foot; he should keep his right leg straight.

79. Correct answer: 1
Troponin is more specific to heart damage than LD, AST, or CK because these enzymes may also reflect muscle damage from sources other than the heart.

80. Correct answer: 3
ST-segment depression is more characteristic of myocardial ischemia, while ST-segment elevation, new Q waves, and T-wave inversions are more characteristic of myocardial infarction. Option 1 is more characteristic of premature ventricular beats or other arrhythmias that originate in the ventricles. Option 2 is characteristic of atrial fibrillation.

81. Correct answer: 4
Thiazide diuretics are generally the first antihypertensive agents started for persons with stage 1 hypertension that's been refractory to lifestyle modifications. Consideration of other antihypertensive agents, such as ACE inhibitors, beta-adrenergic blockers and calcium channel blockers, is made if high blood pressure persists despite diuretic therapy.

82. Correct answer: 1, 3, 4, 5
Stanol esters, including margarine substitutes such as Benechol, and omega-3 fatty acids, such are found in fish, would be appropriate teaching points for this client. Polyunsaturated fats are preferred over saturated fats for persons who are trying to lower cholesterol levels. Trans fatty acids should be minimized, and total fat intake should comprise less than 30% of total caloric intake.

83. Correct answer: 2

Anticoagulation is necessary for atrial fibrillation because of the potential for thrombus formation secondary to the inability of the atria to contract properly. Captopril would be appropriate for the preliminary treatment of a client experiencing a myocardial infarction. Hydrochlorothiazide is a diuretic and would be appropriate as a first-line treatment for hypertension. Metoprolol is a beta-adrenergic blocker that may be used in the treatment of hypertension.

84. Correct answer: 3

A tingling sensation on the tongue when nitroglycerin is taken is indicative that the tablet hasn't expired. If no tingling sensation is noted when nitroglycerin is taken, another bottle of nitroglycerin should be opened and another tablet taken. Nitroglycerin tablets should be replaced every 6 months if not used to ensure their effectiveness when needed. The other options are incorrect statements regarding nitroglycerin.

85. Correct answer: 4

Pericarditis is an inflammatory condition of the pericardial sac, and can result from viral or bacterial infections, open-heart surgery, myocardial infarction, or trauma. Manifestations include a pericardial friction rub and sharp substernal chest pain that worsens with deep inhalation. While pneumonia can be associated with sharp or stabbing chest pain that worsens with deep breathing or coughing, this patient's symptom of a harsh creaking sound over the left third intercostal space is more consistent with pericarditis. Symptoms of pulmonary embolus include shortness of breath sometimes accompanied by chest pain. Endocarditis is an inflammatory condition of the lining of the heart chambers and valves and is manifested by fever, shortness of breath with activity, fatigue, myalgias, and edema of the lower extremities.

86. Correct answer: 3

Clients on statin drugs or HMG-coA reductase inhibitors, such as pravastatin (Pravachol), atorvastatin (Lipitor), and simvastatin (Zocor), should have baseline hepatic function tests performed before initiation of therapy and periodically during therapy to monitor for adverse effects. Troponin, LD, and myoglobin are enzymes useful in diagnosing ischemic damage to the heart related to a myocardial infarction. BUN and creatinine are markers for renal function, which isn't affected by statin drugs. PTT isn't affected by statin drugs, but should be monitored in persons receiving heparin therapy.

87. Correct answer: 1

Valvular stenosis as in mitral stenosis is a stiffening of a valve, the resultant narrowing of its opening that impedes the flow of blood through it. Valvular insufficiency results in the backward flow of blood through a closed valve. Rheumatic fever is associated with various types of valvular disorders, but the physical examination is more descriptive of aortic stenosis.

88. Correct answer: 3

This patient's digoxin level exceeds the drug's therapeutic levels of 0.5 to 2 ng/ml. Symptoms associated with digoxin toxicity include bradycardia, confusion, and seeing either green or yellow hazes or halos around objects.

89. Correct answer: 3

AAA is a ballooning of a portion of the aorta that extends into the abdominal area. Aortic dissection is a potential complication of AAA that involves a tearing of the arterial lining secondary to leakage of blood into the arterial wall. Manifestations include a sharp, stabbing, or tearing pain that develops suddenly and may radiate to the shoulder, neck, jaw, arm, abdomen, or hips. Pulsus paradoxus is an exaggerated inspiratory decrease in systolic blood pressure that's associated with cardiac tamponade. Arteriospastic disease, also known as *Raynaud's phenomenon,* is a vascular disorder that involves arterial spasms and transient ischemia of the fingers and toes. Thromboangiitis obliterans, also known as *Buerger's disease,* is an inflammatory vascular disorder characterized by discoloration of the fingers or toes upon exposure to cold and the resultant intermittent claudication.

90. Correct answer: 1

Angina is chest pain or discomfort that occurs secondary to decreased oxygen delivery to the myocardium, typically due to a blockage within the coronary arteries, and can therefore be a symptom of underlying CAD. Unstable angina is typically less responsive to medications than stable angina, occurs without a precipitating event, and is generally of longer duration than stable angina. Angina is a symptom of myocardial ischemia, but isn't necessarily diagnostic of MI. Prinzmetal's angina is a rare form of unstable angina that's caused by spasms of the coronary arteries.

91. Correct answer: 4

A positive TB skin test is read as a 10-mm or larger induration in persons with low risk factors, and is only indicative of previous exposure to someone with TB. A chest X-ray will need to be performed in order to determine whether active disease is present and whether medical therapy is necessary.

92. Correct answer: 4

COPD is characterized by air trapping, a prolonged expiratory phase, decreased tactile fremitus, and an increased anteroposterior diameter. The other options aren't characteristic of COPD.

93. Correct answer: 2

Kussmaul respirations are very deep respirations (similar to gasping) that can occur with metabolic acidosis, such as DKA and coma. Cheyne-Stokes respirations consist of apneic periods followed by respirations of increasing depth and frequency. They are more commonly associated with drug-induced respiratory depression or with the final stages of life. Bradypnea is a general term used to describe a respiratory rate that's less than normal for the age. Bronchophony is a type of voice sound that can be detected on physical examination of the respiratory system.

94. Correct answer: 3

A permanent tracheostomy is performed after a total laryngectomy, and tracheostomy care should be performed routinely in this client. Option 1 is incorrect because positioning the client in a supine position would predispose him to edema at the surgical site; a semi-Fowler's position in the postoperative period is preferred because it minimizes edema and tension placed on the suture line. Option 2 is incorrect because the Valsalva maneuver may need to be performed after a laryngectomy in order to swallow (it compensates for the loss of the epiglottis). Option 4 is incorrect because chest tubes aren't inserted for this type of surgery.

95. Correct answer: 4

Atelectasis is a respiratory condition characterized by collapsed, airless alveoli that occurs most frequently within the first 48 hours after surgery and is manifested as dyspnea, cough, and fever. Bronchiectasis is a condition marked by chronic abnormal dilation of bronchial walls. It's often associated with bacterial infections and obstructive processes, including lung or thoracic tumors. A pleural effusion is a fluid accumulation that occurs in the pleural space secondary to blocked lymphatic drainage or a change in colloid osmotic pressure. Pleuritis, or pleurisy, is an inflammation of the pleura that causes pain with breathing and, possibly, a pericardial friction rub.

96. Correct answer: 4

Emphysema is an irreversible destruction of the airways distal to the terminal bronchioles, and hyperventilation prevents the development of cyanosis. In fact, persons with emphysema are known as "pink puffers" because hyperventilation prevents the development of cyanosis. Prolonged expiration (rather than inspiration) is a characteristic of emphysema. While emphysema is irreversible, smoking cessation should be encouraged to prevent further damage to the lung tissue.

97. Correct answer: 2

Rifampin will cause a reddish-orange discoloration to body fluids, including urine, tears, and sweat. If a yellow-orange discoloration of the skin or sclerae occurs, the medication should be discontinued and the physician should be notified immediately, because this may represent jaundice secondary to hepatic toxicity. Ethambutol's adverse effects commonly include fever, malaise, headaches, nausea and vomiting, rash, and optic neuritis.

98. Correct answer: 2

Oxygen should be used with caution in persons with chronic obstructive pulmonary disease (COPD) because its overuse may take away the client's respiratory drive. For this reason, it isn't typically administered for oxygen saturation levels greater than 90% on room air in clients with COPD. Placing the client in an upright position, encouraging increased fluid intake (unless otherwise contraindicated), and administering inhaled bronchodilators are all appropriate therapeutic interventions for a client with chronic bronchitis.

99. Correct answer: 4

Taking a deep breath and holding it would minimize the risk of developing a new pneumothorax. Option 1 is incorrect because it would lower the intrathoracic pressure and increase the risk of developing a new pneumothorax. The other options aren't as effective at preventing the development of another pneumothorax as is taking and deep breath and holding it.

100. Correct answer: 4

Theophylline shouldn't be used for rescue therapy during an asthma attack because its actions aren't immediate. Typically, a beta$_2$-agonist, such as albuterol, is used for rescue therapy for acute asthmatic attacks. The other options are all true statements regarding asthma medications.

101. Correct answer: 3

Guaifenesin (Robitussin, Humabid L.A.) is an expectorant, while dextromethorphan, codeine, and benzonatate are all antitussive agents used for cough suppression.

102. Correct answer: 3

Sitting up and slightly leaning forward allows for maximal lung expansion. While a low or high Fowler's position does allow for some lung expansion, it doesn't facilitate lung expansion to the degree that option 3 does. Reverse Trendelenburg is incorrect because it impedes lung expansion.

103. Correct answer: 3

Administration of oxygen to persons with chronic obstructive pulmonary disease can eliminate the stimulus to breathe, which results in drowsiness and decreased respirations. Cyanosis would likely be reduced with the administration of oxygen. Rising carbon dioxide levels would result in drowsiness rather than anxiety. Hemoptysis isn't associated with oxygen therapy in clients with emphysema.

104. Correct answer: 1
Residual volume is the amount of air trapped in the alveoli that can't be exhaled. Option 2 describes tidal volume, option 3 describes expiratory reserve volume, and option 4 defines forced expiratory volume in 1 second (FEV_1).

105. Correct answer: 2
Deep coughing facilitates the expectoration of secretions and would therefore provide optimal results after postural drainage. Bronchodilators are more effective if used before postural drainage, rather than afterwards. A seated position would inhibit the expectoration of secretions. Encouraging oral intake of fluids wouldn't be appropriate until the secretions have been expectorated.

106. Correct answer: 2
Application of an occlusive dressing prevents air from entering the area. Rescue breathing isn't appropriate because the client is still breathing on his own. Although the other options would be appropriate for this client, they aren't the primary actions that should be taken.

107. Correct answer: 2
In order to prevent depleting excessive oxygen, suctioning should be performed only as the catheter is being withdrawn. Removal of the inner cannula is performed for routine tracheostomy care, but isn't necessary for suctioning. Gag and cough reflexes may be absent or diminished in some clients, so these reflexes aren't a reliable means of assessing how far to insert the catheter. Instead, suction catheters should be inserted approximately $4^{1}/_{2}''$ (12 cm). Changing the suction catheter with each insertion isn't necessary, although a new sterile catheter should be used with each suctioning session.

108. Correct answer: 4
Bubbling would be expected in the water seal and suction control chambers due to the removal of air from the pleural space. Bubbling in other areas within the drainage system would be abnormal.

109. Correct answer: 4
Pink and frothy sputum, a rapid and thready pulse, anxiety or restlessness, and wheezes or crackles are suggestive of pulmonary edema. Diminished or absent breath sounds are more commonly associated with pleural effusions or pleural thickening as well as decreased air movements, such as occurs with pneumothorax, severe asthma, or emphysema. Tachycardia rather than bradycardia is more commonly associated with

heart failure and pulmonary edema. Lethargy may be indicative of impaired oxygenation but isn't specific for pulmonary edema.

110. Correct answer: 1
Non-selective beta-adrenergic blockers, such as metoprolol or propranolol, should be avoided in persons with chronic obstructive pulmonary disease (COPD) due to the risk of bronchospasm. Calcium channel blockers, ACE inhibitors, and angiotensin receptor blockers aren't contraindicated in persons with COPD because bronchospasm isn't a common adverse reaction associated with their use.

111. Correct answer: 4
Coughing induced by postural drainage can precipitate nausea and vomiting; therefore, it should be avoided after meals. Performance of postural drainage upon awakening and approximately 1 hour before meals is the most beneficial because mucus secretions are abundant and are thicker and tenacious in the morning and dietary intake is least likely to be affected at this time.

112. Correct answer: 4
Chemotherapeutic agents cause pancytopenia, including neutropenia, anemia, and thrombocytopenia. Although chemotherapeutics may also cause hyperkalemia secondary to cellular rupture, this client's potassium is within normal limits. Potassium and creatinine elevations more typically occur in persons with impaired renal function or end-stage renal disease, or they may occur as an adverse effect of certain medications, such as aminoglycosides. A prolonged prothrombin time is more commonly associated with the use of warfarin or hepatic dysfunction.

113. Correct answer: 3
The client's WBC count is extremely low, which places him at high risk for infection. Filgrastim (Neupogen) accelerates neutrophil recovery in the bone marrow, thereby raising the overall WBC count. Epoetin (Epogen, Procrit) is used in the treatment of anemia, and isn't indicated for this client. Although this client's platelet count is slightly low, it isn't the primary laboratory value in this instance.

114. Correct answer: 1
Diarrhea is a manifestation of radiation enteritis caused by inflammation and damage to the GI mucosa. Constipation may occur in cancer clients secondary to obstruction of the bowel by tumor compression, from impairment of peristalsis by some chemotherapeutic agents, or as a result of immobility. Dysgeusia is more commonly associated with chemotherapeutic agents, and although xerostomia (dry mouth) is associated with radiation therapy, it isn't a manifestation of radiation enteritis.

115. Correct answer: 2
Peeled fruits and vegetables are typically permitted for clients on isolation precautions. Unpeeled fruits and vegetables and fresh cut flowers are contraindicated due to the large number of microorganisms they can carry. Live attenuated vaccinations, including the measles vaccine, and persons who have recently received vaccinations should be avoided by a client on isolation precautions due to the theory that they may contract the illness.

116. Correct answer: 4
Spinal cord compression in a cancer client occurs secondary to extension of an adjacent bony or soft tissue lesion. This direct pressure on the spinal cord typically produces severe pain that worsens with movement, straining, or leg raising. Other symptoms, such as lower extremity weakness and paresthesia, paralysis, and loss of bowel or bladder control may occur, but are dependent on the level of the spinal cord compression (cervical, thoracic, or sacral). Superior vena cava syndrome is a condition that occurs secondary to obstruction of blood flow from the superior vena cava to the right atrium and is manifested as facial edema, jugular vein distention, edema of the upper extremities, a nonproductive cough, and hoarseness. Tumor lysis syndrome is a complication of cancer therapy that results from the rapid release of cellular components into the bloodstream, producing metabolic disturbances, such as hyperkalemia, hyperphosphatemia, hyperuricemia, and hypocalcemia. Paraneoplastic syndrome occurs secondary to the release of hormones by cancer cells, and may be manifested as hypercalcemia, syndrome of inappropriate antidiuretic hormone, and inappropriate secretion of corticotropin and insulin.

117. Correct answer: 1
Tetanus toxoid doesn't contain a live virus and would therefore be considered safe for administration to those with severely impaired immune systems. Antitoxins and killed viruses are generally considered safe for these individuals. In contrast, OPV, measles, and mumps vaccines contain live attenuated viruses, which could result in the development of infection in immunocompromised persons. They should be avoided. However, inactivated polio vaccine contains a killed virus and would be safe to administer in those who are immunocompromised.

118. Correct answer: 3
IgE is most closely associated with allergic responses. IgA is found in body secretions, such as saliva and breast milk, and it lines the mucous membranes. IgD participates in the differentiation of B-lymphocytes and acts as an antigen receptor for them. IgM is the first antibody produced after exposure to an antigen and is responsible for antibody production to ABO antigens. IgG is responsible for the antibody response that occurs after subsequent exposure to the same antigen, and it crosses the placenta to provide neonates with passive acquired immunity for approximately 3 months.

119. Correct answer: 1
Aminoglycosides, such as gentamicin (Garamycin) and tobramycin, are associated with ototoxicity. Red man syndrome is most commonly associated with vancomycin, and disulfiram-like reactions are more likely to occur in people who drink alcohol during metronidazole therapy. Permanent discoloration of the teeth may occur in a child born to a mother who took tetracycline during the last half of pregnancy.

120. Correct answer: 3
While HAART therapy has been shown to decrease viral shedding and viremia in semen and vaginal secretions, it may still be possible to infect other persons with HIV. Option 1 is incorrect because HAART therapy is the combination of three drugs: typically, two nucleoside analogues and a protease inhibitor. Option 2 is incorrect because it may take several weeks to months to see the effects of HAART therapy on CD4+ counts. Option 4 is incorrect because HAART therapy has been proven to improve clinical outcomes, including reducing the incidence of opportunistic infections and HIV-associated neoplasms such as Kaposi's sarcoma.

121. Correct answer: 2
Chickenpox is spread via respiratory droplets and direct contact with open lesions caused by chickenpox. A person is considered noncontagious once all the lesions have scabbed over.

122. Correct answer: 4
Co-trimoxazole should be avoided in people with known or suspected sulfa allergies. Photosensitivity is incorrect because it's a potential adverse effect associated with the use of sulfonamides, but it isn't a contraindication. Bactrim doesn't cause bronchospasms, which would be a contraindication in clients with chronic asthma. Although sulfonamides may enhance the affects of oral anticoagulants such as warfarin, their use isn't a contraindication. Rather, dosage adjustments of the oral anticoagulant should be anticipated, and prothrombin time and International Normalized Ratio results should be followed closely.

123. Correct answer: 1, 3, 4
Adverse reactions associated with the administration of blood products include transfusion reactions (hemolytic reactions), hypothermia (from administration of blood products that haven't

been warmed), and hypocalcemia (due to citrate additive in blood products). Hypertensive crises are more commonly associated with pheochromocytomas, but hypotension is more commonly experienced with adverse reactions to blood transfusions. Malignant hyperthermia is a life-threatening hypermetabolic state affecting the skeletal muscles and is associated with the use of general anesthesia.

124. Correct answer: 2
Adequate hydration and oxygenation will minimize or prevent lung infections, which may precipitate a sickling crisis. Aerobic activities may result in tissue hypoxia, and high altitudes have low oxygen concentrations, both of which would induce sickling. Iron and folate supplements won't prevent sickling.

125. Correct answer: 3
Incompatible blood types (including Rh mismatches) would precipitate an acute hemolytic reaction (type II hypersensitivity reaction). The shelf life of whole blood is 42 days, so the blood delivered by the blood bank isn't too old to administer.

126. Correct answer: 4
The Z-track method of I.M. injections followed by cold packs to the affected area is the safest approach for this client because these actions are most effective at preventing or minimizing bleeding and hematoma formation. Although injections should be avoided whenever possible for hemophiliacs, option 1 is incorrect because this client has suffered a dirty puncture wound and his last tetanus booster was more than 5 years ago.

127. Correct answer: 3
Direct pressure should be applied to the biopsy site for at least 10 minutes after the procedure to prevent bleeding and hematoma formation. This client's PT is normal, which wouldn't necessitate cancellation of the biopsy. Analgesics should be administered before the biopsy (not afterwards), and ambulation immediately after the procedure is contraindicated due to the risk of bleeding.

128. Correct answer: 1
Pernicious anemia is due to a deficiency of intrinsic factor secondary to the removal of its site of production or absorption, as occurs with gastric or intestinal resections. Aplastic anemia is characterized by pancytopenia that results from bone marrow hypoplasia or anaplasia. Acquired hemolytic anemia occurs secondary to the premature destruction of red blood cells (RBCs), as can occur with certain medications, infections, autoimmune processes, and some inherited disorders. Iron deficiency anemia is most commonly caused by inadequate nutritional intake of iron, poor absorption of iron by the body, and blood loss.

129. Correct answer: 2
Polycythemia vera is primarily characterized by the overproduction of RBCs; epoetin stimulates the production of RBCs. Phlebotomy sessions, which are used to maintain a hematocrit of 45% or less, are the first line of treatment for a client with polycythemia vera. Although RBCs are the predominant blood cells overproduced in polycythemia vera, white blood cells and platelets are overproduced as well; myelosuppressive agents, such as anagrelide and hydroxyurea, may be used in the treatment of these conditions.

130. Correct answer: 3
Morphine administered I.V. would provide this client with immediate relief due to its more reliable absorption. Oral medications are absorbed slowly, and with much variability. Because of the tissue damage associated with extensive burn injuries, injectable medications are poorly and unpredictably absorbed in these clients.

131. Correct answer: 3
Bedrest with placement of the affected extremity in a slightly dependent position increases circulation to the ischemic area. The other options would be useful in the treatment of venous insufficiency ulcers, but are contraindicated for arterial ulcers because they would further impair circulation.

132. Correct answer: 2
Insensible fluid loss can occur secondary to the high airflow associated with special circulating air beds. Therefore, the client's hydration status should be monitored carefully. Option 1 is incorrect because skin assessments for this client should be performed at least every 8 hours. Range-of-motion exercises for this client's right extremity would require a surgeon's orders. Option 4 is incorrect because even though this action is indicated for many types of clients, it isn't specific for this situation.

133. Correct answer: 4
This client likely has herpes zoster (shingles), which is caused by the varicella zoster virus and is characterized by clusters of small vesicles that occur in a dermatome (area of skin innervated by a single peripheral sensory nerve). Acyclovir would most likely be prescribed for this client because of its antiviral effects. Mupirocin is an antibacterial cream commonly used for bacterial skin infections. Silver sulfadiazine is a cream that's commonly used in the treatment of burns. Tazarotene is an agent commonly used in the treatment of psoriasis.

134. Correct answer: 1

Arterial ulcers are caused by ischemia from arterial occlusions and are characterized by deep, painless lesions with minimal edema, and pale, dry, and necrotic eschar. Pulses in the affected extremity may be diminished or absent, and loss of hair may be present. Venous insufficiency ulcers are caused by blood stasis and are characterized by painless, shallow ulcerations with moderate serous exudates and palpable pulses. Pressure ulcers and decubitus ulcers are the same process and are characterized by distinct stages of development, ranging from hyperemia to crater formation that's usually painless.

135. Correct answer: 2

Eschar (dead skin) can function as a tourniquet, reducing blood flow to distal sites and compressing nerves. Compartment syndrome can occur as a result. Cutting into the eschar (escharotomy) is primarily performed to treat compartment syndrome by relieving pressure from the underlying swelling and inflammation, but it doesn't minimize the risk of infection or prevent fluid shifts. Eschar must be completely removed by debridement (which does minimize the risk of infection) before skin grafting can occur. An escharotomy doesn't minimize the need for skin grafting.

136. Correct answer: 3

Induration is localized edema and thickening that occurs beneath the skin and can result from an inflammatory response such as occurs after the administration of a PPD test in people previously exposed to the disease. Undermining is a cavity formation beneath the periwound (area surrounding the wound opening) that occurs secondary to shearing forces. Tunneling is an extension of a sinus or tract beneath the skin under a wound that's accompanied by inflammation and infection. A nodule is a firm, circumscribed lesion that extends deeper into the dermis than a papule.

137. Correct answer: 4

Proper positioning of the affected extremity after a hip repair should be moderate abduction using a trochanter role, which maintains the head of the femur in the acetabulum and prevents external rotation. The other options may cause dislocation of the femur head and would be contraindicated in this client.

138. Correct answer: 1

Gentle removal of crusting at the pin sites is best performed through use of sterile applicators dampened with hydrogen peroxide or normal saline solution. Ointments could block drainage from the pin sites, which may facilitate the development of an infection. Betadine or other iodine substances would cause corrosion of the metal pins.

139. Correct answer: 3

Maintenance of the extremity's functional alignment using resting splints prevents the development of contractures and deformities. Use of the affected extremity should be minimized or prevented because it may exacerbate the inflammatory process. A flexed position should be avoided because it may result in the development of contractures.

140. Correct answer: 2

Strains are soft tissue injuries caused by abnormal stretching or tearing of a tendon or muscle, whereas sprains are soft tissue injuries involving ligaments. A subluxation is a partial dislocation and tendonitis is more accurately defined as an inflammatory process affecting a tendon.

141. Correct answer: 4

A complication of dislocations is the development of avascular necrosis, and the risk increases the longer the joint remains maligned. While the risk for surgical intervention (open reduction) may increase the longer the dislocation exists, it may also be required regardless of the length of the dislocation. Carpal tunnel syndrome is pain and weakness in the hands that results from median nerve compression at the wrist, commonly related to repetitive movements of the wrist. The length of time the dislocation exists doesn't affect the pain medication's effectiveness.

142. Correct answer: 1

Because of overriding of bones, the affected extremity is slightly shorter after a hip fracture. External rotation of the affected extremity would be associated with a hip fracture, rather than internal rotation. Ecchymosis results from soft tissue injuries and the associated blood vessel trauma, but isn't unique to hip fractures.

143. Correct answer: 4

GI disturbances, including diarrhea, abdominal cramps, acid reflux, esophagitis, dyspepsia, and gastritis are the most common adverse reactions to bisphosphonates. Neurologic, hematologic, and cardiovascular disturbances aren't associated with these medications.

144. Correct answer: 2

Crossing the legs or ankles after a total hip replacement may cause a dislocation, so it should be avoided. Clients who have undergone a total hip replacement are typically out of bed on postoperative day 1 and not day 3. Side-lying may not be permitted at all.

145. Correct answer: 4

Disc herniation is commonly related to frequent bending and twisting movements, particularly those that involve a combination of lifting objects using a lateral bending or twisting motion. A family history of back problems and a history of osteoporosis are associated with degenerative disk disease and can predispose a client to a herniated disk but herniation is more commonly associated with bending, twisting, and lifting things.

146. Correct answer: 2
Colchicine minimizes or prevents the inflammation associated with uric acid crystal deposition in joints, and is therefore used to treat acute episodes of gout. Probenecid, allopurinol, and sulfinpyrazone lower the uric acid levels in the blood by various methods, and therefore would be used more effectively for the chronic management of gout.

147. Correct answer: 4
Soda contains high amounts of phosphates and many contain large quantities of caffeine as well, both of which promote bone loss. A client with osteoporosis should be encouraged to participate in weight-bearing exercises (prevents bone loss), to increase consumption of vitamin D (enhances absorption of calcium), and to decrease consumption of phosphates (promotes calcium loss from bones).

148. Correct answer: 2
Lying on the abdomen for at least 30 minutes each day helps to prevent hip contractures. Dangling the affected extremity over the side of the bed should be avoided in the immediate postoperative period to prevent edema and pressure on the surgical incision. Powders, oils, and lotions should be avoided in the stump area, unless otherwise prescribed by a physician. Sitting for prolonged periods of time promotes the development of hip contractures.

149. Correct answer: 3
Osteogenic sarcoma is a malignant condition of the bone, which predisposes an individual to pathologic fractures. Bursitis is an inflammatory process affecting the synovial fluid sacs that typically occurs in areas subject to friction. Crepitation is a palpable or audible grating sensation that occurs when irregular bone edges rub together. Pathologic contractures are the permanent tightening of muscles, tendons, ligaments, or skin that often occurs secondary to lack of use, scarring or nerve damage.

150. Correct answer: 3
The nurse should stand on the client's stronger side when assisting with ambulation without an assistive device; however, the nurse should stand on the client's weaker side if an assistive device, such as a cane or walker, is being used.

151. Correct answer: 2
Assessment of the neurovascular status of the left forearm and fingers, including checking the capillary refill and making sure that the skin is warm and that the client can move the fingers, would provide the most accurate information. The surgeon should be notified if the skin is dusky or cool or if the capillary refill is delayed. Although option 4 is an appropriate action for this client, it isn't the primary action because it doesn't provide direct information about the neurovascular status of the affected extremity.

152. Correct answer: 2
A sudden temperature spike within the first several hours after an endoscopic procedure could indicate a perforation and would require notification of the physician. Mild abdominal cramping, thirst, hoarseness, and dizziness are potential complications that can occur temporarily after an endoscopic procedure, but they don't necessitate immediate physician notification.

153. Correct answer: 3
Clients with chronic pancreatitis should follow a low-fat diet to avoid over-stimulation of the pancreas. Overstimulation increases the pressure within the pancreatic duct and results in worsening pain. Eating smaller, more frequent meals with high-caloric content and avoidance of alcohol are appropriate interventions for a client with chronic pancreatitis.

154. Correct answer: 2
A colostomy should begin functioning properly 2 to 3 days postoperatively because peristalsis returns after abdominal surgery at this time. Clients with colostomies should be allowed to resume a regular diet as soon as possible for psychologic support, and they won't necessarily have dietary restrictions. These clients should be allowed to determine for themselves which types of foods they can tolerate; it's usually varies greatly among clients.

155. Correct answer: 4
Clients with sprue should avoid gluten-containing grains, such as wheat, rye, barley, and oats. Rice, corn, and soy flours should be substituted in place of gluten-containing grains. The other foods don't need to be avoided.

156. Correct answer: 2
Semi-Fowler's position facilitates localization of the drainage to the pelvic area and minimizes the spread of infection throughout the abdomen. The Trendelenburg position is useful for some postural drainage. Sims' position is appropriate for unconscious clients because it facilitates drainage from the mouth; it's also frequently used to administer an enema. The reverse Trendelenburg position is used for clients with arterial circulatory difficulties of the lower extremities.

157. Correct answer: 1
While it isn't a specific cause for the development of ulcerative colitis, psychologic stress is a

common cause of an acute exacerbation of this condition. Causes of ulcerative colitis include heredity, environment, and immunologic factors. The other options aren't causes of ulcerative colitis.

158. Correct answer: 3
Protein should be restricted in clients with liver dysfunction who experience worsening encephalopathy. Normal protein metabolism is hindered in a client with liver disease, and blood ammonia levels will rise as a result of the liver's inability to convert it to urea. Sodium and fluids would be restricted in a client with ascites. Potassium would be restricted in a client with renal insufficiency.

159. Correct answer: 4
Abdominal muscular rigidity with moderately severe abdominal pain is the classic sign of peritonitis, and it results from intraperitoneal inflammation. Patients often attempt to pull their knees to their abdomen to minimize the strain on the tender peritoneum. Diarrhea and constipation aren't common findings associated with peritonitis. Jaundice would occur in the setting of advanced liver disease or obstructed bile ducts but it isn't a common manifestation of peritonitis.

160. Correct answer: 3
Pernicious anemia can occur after a gastrectomy. The parietal cells of the gastric mucosa are responsible for secreting intrinsic factor, which is necessary for the absorption of vitamin B_{12}. A Nissen fundoplication involves the wrapping of a portion of the stomach (fundus) around the lower portion of the esophagus to create a new valve that relieves chronic heartburn in persons with gastroesophageal reflux disease, but it isn't associated with pernicious anemia. A colectomy is the removal of a diseased portion of the bowel, such as may occur in people with ulcerative colitis, diverticulitis, or colon cancer, but it isn't associated with the development of pernicious anemia. A cholecystotomy isn't associated with pernicious anemia.

161. Correct answer: 4
Hypoalbuminemia results from the impaired synthesis of albumin by the diseased liver. This deficiency causes oncotic edema. Normal ranges for albumin are 3.5 to 5.0 g/dl. A serum sodium level of 150 mEq/L, which indicates hypernatremia, can cause edema and hypertension. Hyponatremia as evidenced by a serum sodium level of 118 mEq/L may result in dehydration, hypotension, muscle cramps, and seizures. Hyperbilirubinemia (total bilirubin of 2.2 mg/dl) is manifested as jaundice and pruritus.

162. Correct answer: 1
Metabolic alkalosis results from the excessive loss of hydrochloric acid from the stomach contents. Hydrochloric acid acts to neutralize sodium bicarbonate secreted into the duodenum by the pancreas. Other potential complications of intractable vomiting include hypokalemia, hypochloremia, pulmonary aspiration, and the development of a Mallory-Weiss tear. Metabolic acidosis occurs most often in association with diabetic ketoacidosis, renal failure, hepatic failure, poisonings or overdoses (aspirin), shock, and severe diarrhea. Transient hypoglycemia (until gluconeogenesis occurs within the liver) and hypokalemia (from GI losses) would be associated with intractable vomiting.

163. Correct answer: 2
Beta-adrenergic blockers reduce portal hypertension in clients with mild liver disease thereby decreasing the risk of esophageal rupture and hemorrhage. Loop diuretics decrease vascular volume by increasing excretion of water and potassium. ACE inhibitors block the conversion of angiotensin I to angiotensin II. Calcium channel blockers block the influx of calcium to the cell and act as a smooth muscle relaxer. All of the options will decrease peripheral blood pressure but only option 2 will have more than a minimal effect on portal hypertension.

164. Correct answer: 4
Vomiting can result in aspiration when the jaw is immobilized. Wire cutters should be kept at the bedside and the wires should be cut immediately if the client develops vomiting. Malignant hyperthermia is a complication from anesthesia. Hypertension could have a number of causes but none are related to immobilization of the jaw. Stomatitis commonly occurs in association with chemotherapy and radiation therapy of the head and neck but it isn't a life-threatening complication related to immobilization of the jaw.

165. Correct answer: 1, 3, 4
In addition to pharmacologic therapy with proton pump inhibitors, antacids, histamine-2 antagonists, and coating agents, other appropriate treatment measures for chronic esophagitis include consuming a bland diet, sleeping with the head of the bed elevated, cessation of smoking and alcohol consumption, and losing weight if obese. Option 2 is incorrect because preferably, food should be avoided 3 hours before bedtime.

166. Correct answer: 3
Dyspepsia or indigestion is an early symptom of gastric cancer. Dysphagia is a symptom of esophageal cancer. Dysphonia is a symptom of a stroke, and dysuria is a symptom for urinary, not GI, problems.

167. Correct answer: 3
Dumping syndrome results from the rapid emptying of hypertonic food products into the upper small intestine, causing movement of plasma water into the gut lumen, which results in hypovolemia. The other disorders aren't associated with gastrectomy.

168. Correct answer: 4
Nonsteroidal anti-inflammatory agents, such as ibuprofen (Advil, Motrin, Nuprin), naproxen sodium (Aleve), and indomethacin (Indocin), irritate the mucosa and may cause bleeding. The other medications aren't contraindicated for use in clients with peptic ulcer disease.

169. Correct answer: 2
Cholecystitis can result from cholelithiasis if the stone obstructs the common bile duct (choledocholithiasis) and is manifested as right upper quadrant pain that may relate to the right shoulder, nausea, vomiting, and fever. An intestinal obstruction is characterized by abdominal pain and distention and the inability to pass stools, and isn't a common complication of cholelithiasis. Peritonitis is manifested as abdominal muscular rigidity, pain, and fever.

170. Correct answer: 4
Foods that are high in fat or cholesterol should be avoided in clients with gallstones. Therefore, dairy products should be avoided. Appropriate interventions for a client with cholelithiasis would include eating smaller portions more frequently, consuming low-fat foods, and avoiding fried or greasy foods.

171. Correct answer: 2
Such fat-soluble vitamins as A, D, E, and K aren't well absorbed by clients with chronic pancreatitis. Bile salts may be required to enhance their absorption. The absorption of water-soluble vitamins, minerals, and essential proteins aren't directly affected by chronic pancreatitis.

172. Correct answer: 2
Ursodiol dissolves cholesterol gallstones by decreasing biliary cholesterol secretion and desaturating bile. Probenecid is used for the treatment of chronic gout. Cholestyramine is useful as a cholesterol-lowering agent and for the relief of pruritus from bile stasis. Colchicine is used in recurrent gout or in acute gouty flares.

173. Correct answer: 1
Pancreatitis is the most common complication of an ERCP. It's characterized by severe abdominal pain, nausea, vomiting, and fever. Mild jaundice and fatty stools may also be present. Cholelithiasis is the formation of gallstones and may be an indication for ERCP but it isn't a complication. Although infections and bowel perforations are potential complications of an ERCP, they are rare.

174. Correct answer: 1
Hypoglycemia can occur if TPN is discontinued abruptly because of its high glucose content; the pancreas has been excreting increased insulin to cover the hyperglycemic solutions. Hypokalemia and hypernatremia shouldn't occur because potassium and sodium levels should remain unchanged and aren't affected by discontinuation of the solution.

175. Correct answer: 4
Hepatitis C is transmitted by blood and body fluids. Previous blood transfusions and I.V. drug use involving needle-sharing are major risk factors for the development of hepatitis C. Options 1 and 3 are risk factors for hepatitis A. Option 2 would make the client at risk for human immunodeficiency virus infection. The client's hepatitis C tests probably wouldn't be positive only one month after exposure.

176. Correct answer: 4
The presence of bowel sounds would indicate resolution of the bowel obstruction. Narcotics should be avoided because they may mask other symptoms as well as worsen the obstruction. Promotility agents such as metoclopramide should be avoided as well. Clients with an intestinal obstruction will remain in a nothing-by-mouth status until the obstruction has resolved.

177. Correct answer: 2
Because the throat is anesthetized with a spray before the endoscope is inserted, the presence of a gag reflex must be assessed before food and fluids are provided to prevent aspiration. The presence of bowel sounds should be assessed before food is reintroduced after abdominal surgery to prevent a distended abdomen from lack of peristalsis. A distended bladder isn't a complication of an endoscopic procedure.

178. Correct answer: 4
Gas-producing foods should be minimized. Avoiding spicy foods and increasing fluid intake aren't typical recommendations for persons with ostomies, and increasing dietary fiber is contraindicated.

179. Correct answer: 4
Narcotics should be avoided in clients with diverticulosis because they may exacerbate the clinical findings. High-fiber diets, mild analgesics, and anticholinergic agents are useful treatment options.

180. Correct answer: 4
An intermittent tube feeding should be held if the residual stomach contents volume is greater than 150 ml. The residual should be checked again in 3 to 4 hours. If the volume is less than 150 ml at that time, the tube feeding can be reinitiated.

181. Correct answer: 2
Enteral tube feedings should be initiated at full-strength at 10 to 30 ml/hour, increasing by 20 to 30 ml/hour every 6 to 8 hours as tolerated until the target rate is achieved. Half-strength formulas won't deliver the caloric needs of the client. Tube feedings should begin slowly to decrease the chance of dumping syndrome from increased osmolality of tube feeding. Increased osmolality pulls water into the intestinal tract leading to diarrhea.

182. Correct answer: 2
White rice, white bread, and lean meats are permitted on a low-residue diet. Whole grain foods, fruits, and vegetables should be avoided during a colitis exacerbation because they aren't low residue and have the potential to harm the intestinal lining.

183. Correct answer: 1, 2, 4
Caffeine decreases the lower esophageal sphincter pressure, which can result in an increased incidence of reflux. Elevating the head of the bed prevents reflux of gastric contents into the esophagus, and overdistention of the stomach increases the likelihood of reflux. Option 3 is incorrect because dairy products increase gastric acid secretion.

184. Correct answer: 1
A large volume paracentesis may cause a fluid shift from the intravascular space to the abdomen, resulting in hypovolemia, hypotension, and tachycardia. Bradycardia isn't a consequence of fluid shifts related to paracentesis. Orthopnea and platypnea are both forms of dyspnea but aren't complications of fluid shifts.

185. Correct answer: 3
A vagotomy is useful in managing peptic ulcer disease because the vagus nerve stimulates hydrochloric acid secretion by the stomach. A Nissen fundoplication is useful in the treatment of gastroesophageal reflux disease. A Billroth I is used in the management of gastric cancer. The Whipple procedure is used in the management of pancreatic cancer.

186. Correct answer: 3
Because furosemide is a potassium-wasting diuretic, it shouldn't be administered to a client who's already hypokalemic. Checking the results of the most recent serum electrolytes would ensure that the client wasn't already hypokalemic, which would predispose the client to life-threatening arrhythmias. Although options 1 and 2 may be appropriate interventions, they aren't the priority nursing action in this setting. In addition, option 1 would require a physician's order in most institutions.

187. Correct answer: 3
Symptoms of renal colic include slight hematuria (pink-tinged urine), sharp pain, and urinary frequency (due to the inability to completely empty the bladder). While urinary frequency is a symptom of renal colic, urinary urgency typically isn't; the combination of urinary frequency and urgency would be more characteristic of bladder infections or an enlarged prostate. Tea-colored urine and dull pain can occur in some liver diseases and with bile obstructions but they aren't associated with renal colic.

188. Correct answer: 4
Hyperkalemia is a frequent complication of renal failure due to inefficient glomerulofiltration; administration of insulin is one method that can be used to decrease the serum potassium concentration. Insulin causes potassium to move inside cells, thereby lowering the serum potassium level. Glucose is typically administered after insulin in this situation to prevent hypoglycemia. Diabetes is often a contributing factor to the development of chronic renal failure, but it isn't a complication of it. Dextrose and insulin wouldn't be administered together to correct a low blood sugar.

189. Correct answer: 2
Urine is formed continuously and should therefore flow from the stoma continuously. The absence of urine should be reported immediately because it may indicate an obstruction or other complication. Because the bladder has been removed in this client, the urinary diversion is permanent and bladder retaining won't be possible. An ileal conduit doesn't require irrigation.

190. Correct answer: 1
Health care personnel should be informed of the AVF in the left forearm; blood pressure measurements, needlesticks for blood draws, and placement of an I.V. line in this arm should be avoided due to the risk of damaging the fistula. Option 3 is incorrect because a Tenckhoff catheter is one that's placed in the peritoneum for peritoneal dialysis. Option 4 is incorrect because clients should be taught to assess for the presence of a thrill and bruit in the AVF at least once per day.

191. Correct answer: 3
Although it may be asymptomatic, gonorrhea can present as a green or yellow purulent discharge from the vagina or male urethra. Vaginal candidiasis typically presents with a cheeselike appearance associated with an inflamed vulva. Chlamydia more commonly presents with a thick gray-white discharge, and trichomonas is more often associated with a frothy, malodorous, greenish grey discharge.

192. Correct answer: 3

The luteal phase typically occurs during the last 14 days of the menstrual cycle and is characterized by thickening of the endometrium in preparation for implantation of a fertilized ovum. The menstrual phase is characterized by shedding of the endometrium if pregnancy doesn't occur, and the ovulatory phase involves the release of an ovum by an ovary. There's no degenerative phase in the menstrual cycle.

193. Correct answer: 4

Epispadias is a condition in which the urethral opening is located on the dorsal (underneath) side of the penis, which typically requires surgical correction. When the urethral opening is located on the ventral side of the penis, the condition is known as *hypospadias.* A cystocele isn't a condition that occurs in males because it's a herniation of the bladder through the anterior wall of the vagina. A hydrocele is a benign testicular mass of serous fluid.

194. Correct answer: 2

Pyelonephritis is an infection involving the kidneys and can result from an incompletely treated (or untreated) urinary tract infection. Nephrolithiasis is a condition related to kidney stones. Glomerulonephritis is an antibody-mediated disorder of the glomeruli that causes inflammation. Urethritis is an inflammatory condition of the urethra that can lead to pyelonephritis.

195. Correct answer: 2

BPH is a noncancerous enlargement of the prostate gland, so radiation treatments wouldn't be necessary. Over-the-counter cough and cold medications with decongestants should be avoided because they may exacerbate symptoms of BPH. Because the enlarged prostate often compresses the urethra or bladder, urinary symptoms, including urinary frequency, dysuria, difficulty starting a urine stream, experiencing a smaller or weaker stream, and post void dribbling may all be noted.

196. Correct answer: 1

Nephrotic syndrome is characterized by proteinuria (> 3.5 g/24 hours), hypercholesterolemia, and edema related to hypoalbuminemia. Nephritic syndrome involves hematuria, azotemia, and hypertension with variable degrees of proteinuria. Rapidly progressive glomerulonephritis is characterized by hematuria, oliguria, and acute renal failure. Diabetic nephropathy is a progressive renal disease associated with diabetes mellitus that involves glucosuria, proteinuria, and hypertension.

197. Correct answer: 3

A pink-red discoloration of the urine is expected for the first 3 days after a prostatectomy. Option 1 is incorrect because fluids should be encouraged rather than restricted after a prostatectomy. Heavy lifting should be avoided for at least 3 weeks after this type of surgery to prevent damage to the surgical site. Straining with bowel movements should also be avoided for this reason and, therefore, stool softeners are typically recommended after a prostatectomy.

198. Correct answer: 4

Teas, colas, tomatoes, berries, chocolate, and green, leafy vegetables should be avoided in persons at risk for developing oxalate calculi. Thiazide diuretics would be useful in the management of calcium calculi because they decrease urinary excretion of calcium, but they wouldn't be effective in the management of oxalate calculi. A low purine diet is used in the management of uric acid calculi. Green, leafy vegetables should be avoided in clients with oxalate calculi.

199. Correct answer: 2

Urine that's colorless to light pink with no clots would indicate that the flow rate of the CBI was appropriate. The other options aren't indicative of adequate flow rates.

200. Correct answer: 1

The use of indwelling catheters should be avoided as a treatment option for persons with urinary incontinence due to the risk for urinary tract infections. Intermittent urinary catheterizations, on the other hand, may be used to facilitate emptying of the bladder for persons with incontinence. Caffeine and alcohol should be avoided as they act as diuretics, and citrus juices, carbonated beverages, and artificial sweeteners may cause bladder irritation. Bladder training, or urinating according to a schedule, is often used in the management of incontinence. Constipation should be avoided because a full rectum can exert pressure on the bladder, worsening urinary incontinence.

Index

i refers to an illustration.